Atlas of Full Breast Ultrasonography

Aristida Colan-Georges

Atlas of Full Breast Ultrasonography

Springer

Aristida Colan-Georges
Department of Radiology and Imaging Diagnosis
County Emergency Clinical Hospital
Craiova, Dolj
Romania

ISBN 978-3-319-31417-4 ISBN 978-3-319-31418-1 (eBook)
DOI 10.1007/978-3-319-31418-1

Library of Congress Control Number: 2016945363

Printed on acid-free paper

This Springer imprint is published by Springer Nature
The registered company is Springer International Publishing AG Switzerland

"The missing link in classical breast imaging: the systematic correspondence with anatomy," as says Teboul, who renewed the breast US since 1995. Moreover, "It is not possible to assess that a breast has been adequately investigated if its ductal-lobular structures have not been observed."

Michel Teboul

"No classic method in routine allows the differentiation of a ductal lesion and a lobular one. Only DUCTAL echography is a technique which offers us, with its remarkable accuracy, the possibility of analysis and comprehension of the ANATOMY and thus of a better approach of the pathological alterations at an early stage. Already used successfully by some European teams, Ductal Echography is a method not operator dependant, it is only anatomical-dependant."

Dominique Amy

To my family who believed in my dreams,
to my teachers who helped me accomplish them,
and to my patients who believed in Life.

Contents

Abbreviations

ABVS	Automated breast volume scanner
ACR	American College of Radiology
BI-RADS	Breast Imaging Reporting and Data System
BRCA1 and BRCA2	Breast cancer gene 1 and breast cancer gene 2
CAD	Computed-aided diagnosis
CAFs	Cancer-associated fibroblasts
CEUS	Contrast-enhanced US
CIN	Cervical intraepithelial neoplasia
CR	Computed radiography
CT	Computed Tomography
DCIS	Ductal carcinoma in situ
DE	Ductal Echography
DOI	Digital object identifier
DR	Digital radiography
E2	Estradiol
ER	Estrogen receptor
FBU	Full Breast Ultrasonography
FDG-PET	(Fluorine-18) fluorodeoxyglucose positron emission tomography
FFDM	Full-field digital Mammography
FLR	Fat-to-lesion ratio
FNAB	Fine-needle aspiration biopsy
FOV	Field of view
FSH	Follicle-stimulating hormone
IBC	Inflammatory breast cancer
IDC	Invasive ductal carcinoma
ILC	Invasive lobular carcinoma
LCIS	Lobular carcinoma in situ
LDP	Largest diameter plane
LS	Large format section in pathology
MPR	Multiplanar reconstruction
MQSA	Mammography Quality Standards Act
MRI	Magnetic Resonance Imaging
NPV	Negative predictive value
PET	Positron Emission Tomography
PPV	Positive predictive value
PR	Progesterone receptor
RIS	Radiology Information System
ROI	Region of interest
RTSE	Real-Time Sonoelastography
SE	Sonoelastography
TBG	Thyroxin-binding globulin

TDLUs	Terminal ductal-lobular specific units
THI	Tissue Harmonic Intensifier
TNM staging system	Classification of the solid malignant neoplasia based on the tumor, lymph nodes, and metastases
UICC	Union for International Cancer Control
US	Ultrasound

Introduction: Actual Possibilities and Limits of Modern Imaging Diagnosis in Breast Cancer

Diversity of Modern Imaging Diagnosis in Breast Cancer

There are many possibilities of imaging diagnosis of the breast, in continuous faster evolution than ever known in the medical imaging, because of the continuous improvement of technology based on computer sciences, on one hand, and because of the unsatisfactory results of each method in use, on the other hand. When we will be able to use a performing technique, feasible for all patients, opened to all practitioners, with high accuracy and low costs, then the other techniques will be no more useful, such as the "forgotten" breast thermography. This would be ideal for breast diagnosis, but there are already in use new performing imaging and interpreting techniques, which are only based on the technological progress and which are trying to reach a significant irrational goal, to discover as early as possible almost all cancers developing in the breast. This goal is not enough, because the incidence of breast cancer is the same after 40 years of screening mammography in the developed countries, and it will remain the same in the future projected with digital mammography and computer-aided diagnosis (CAD), breast CAD magnetic resonance imaging (MRI), computed tomography with positron emission tomography (CT/PET), ultrasonography (US) with Doppler techniques, contrast-enhanced imaging, automatic 3D acquisitions, and sonoelastography (SE). The incidence of the breast cancer will be the same because these methods could not accurately illustrate neither normal parenchyma of the breast nor the earliest premalignant lesions, which must be treated to prevent breast cancer and thus to decrease its incidence.

Another reason of limited results of these expansive techniques of imaging diagnosis is the wrong anatomical assessment of the breast.

The normal breast has a particular structure, with radial lobes of different shapes and dimensions; thus, a good diagnosis must firstly characterize the normal lobar architecture and then has to precisely identify abnormalities the earliest. Prevention by early diagnosis and treatment of the premalignant breast lesions will really reduce the breast cancer incidence; this will be possible with a cheap, performing, and available for all technique, represented by the full ductal breast ultrasonography (FBU), consisting of ductal/radial US mapping of the whole breast, completed with Doppler, and SE for the characterization of the lesions.

We will briefly present the new developments of the most important imaging diagnostic techniques of breast cancer, to realize their possibilities and their limits, as a basis for comparison for the yet less known concept of the ductal FBU.

Mammography

Mammography is one of the most formerly and actually used diagnostic methods and practically the unique method for large screening of breast cancer. It is not our intention to describe the benefits of this method, because it has a lot of supporters and it is still recommended by the most scientific societies in the Europe and especially in the United States as the first examination method in the screening of breast cancer.

We will discuss the limits of the mammography, more or less recognized by the published researches, in order to demonstrate the necessity to develop new techniques and methods of examination. While great strides have been made in recent years in reducing the mortality rate of breast cancer, this disease is still a leading cause of cancer deaths in women, second only to lung cancer.

One of the most important limits is that mammography is not for all, because of anatomical characteristics or because of irradiation risk: children, young women, men, and pregnant women are formerly not recommended. *In conclusion, we need another method of breast diagnostic for all.*

Other limits of the risk of exposure on X-rays are some restrictions of the frequency of examinations. It is admitted that for any 8 lives saved using screening mammography, we are losing 1 life because of cancer induced by X-rays used in mammography. A large trial directed by the American College of Radiology enrolled 49,528 women to compare the radiation dose in the full-field digital mammography (FFDM) and in the screen-film mammography for screening [1]. The results demonstrated a mean glandular dose per view averaging 2.37 mGy for screen-film mammography and 1.86 mGy for FFDM, with a reduction of 21 % for the last. The dose seems not very high, but the exposure risk is increased by the number and the interval of examinations during the screening. *In conclusion, we need another method that is not dangerous but is available anytime, without side effects.*

Another very important limit of mammography is the restriction in the diagnosis of dense breasts. Studies show that mammography can miss up to 15 % of cancers in certain women. In some models, the number of cancers not visible is even higher for high-risk women with dense breasts, up to 25 %. It is often younger women who have dense breast tissue, and younger individuals tend to have more aggressive breast cancer. The "lifetime risk" is the estimated probability to achieve a cancer during the reminder of the life; so, the risk depends on the age when a person is exposed to radiation. It is estimated that the risk at age 70 is less than half the risk exposure at age 50 but for younger person is much more and difficult to calculate.

Older women can present congenital dense breast or increasing breast density following hormonal substitutive therapy. It is assumed the sensibility of the mammography in dense breasts is less performing. Moreover, studies confirmed dense breasts have an elevated risk to develop cancer, as compared with fatty breasts. One of the largest studies about dense breast risk, published in 2007, suggests that high breast density is the number 1 risk for breast cancer [2]. There were used data from 3 Canadian nested case-control studies carried out in populations screened with modern mammography. Subjects were 1112 women with histological verified invasive breast cancer, included in 6 categories of breast density: 0%, <10 %, 10% to <25 %, 25% to <50 %, 50% to <75%, and ≥75 %. The authors found that women with a high breast density (≥75 %) had a nearly fivefold increased risk for breast cancer compared with women having a low density (<10 %); moreover, the risk for breast cancer in women with high breast density is markedly increased (by 17-fold) in the 12 months after a negative mammogram finding. It is then logical that annual mammographic screening will not increase the rate of detection of cancers, even with the most performing digital mammography. It seems that the association between the extensive mammographic density and an increased risk of breast cancer is due not only to a masking effect but also to a biologic connection between breast density and breast cancer. Dense breast may include normal ductal-lobular structures or abnormal premalignant lesions (which should be evaluated with another imaging method), and the conclusion of this study was a recommendation to perform an alternative method of diagnosis such as digital mammography, US, and MRI, in order to increase the detection rate of breast cancer.

We think early detection is not enough but represents the goal for all methods which cannot visualize normal breast parenchyma. *In conclusion, we need another method that is sensitive both for dense and for fatty breasts.*

It is well known after screening mammography the incidence of breast cancer is the same, or higher, as compared with the cervical or prostate cancer that have lower incidence because of efficient screening and treatment of the premalignant lesions [3]. The most breast cancers are ductal or lobular adenocarcinomas. In fact, mammography can visualize neither the normal breast parenchyma nor 4 of the most important benign premalignant lesions: ductal ectasia, papillomatosis without microcalcifications, adenosclerosis, and especially ductal or lobular hyperplasia, which are considered as histological earliest abnormalities which may develop to fibroadenoma, cysts, or breast cancer [4]. Since mammography could not diagnose the most important premalignant lesions, consequently these lesions were not treated systematically, as is the use for cervical intraepithelial neoplasia (CIN) or for endometrial hyperplasia. *In conclusion, we need another imaging method that could visualize both normal breast parenchyma and benign lesions, to select premalignant from nonmalignant ones and to improve the prevention of the breast cancer.*

It is assumed that mammography is a standardized method, which is a necessary condition for screening, and European guidelines stipulate that each examination must be read/interpreted independently by two radiologists and, in the case of disagreement, by a third. It was usual to have double reading diagnosis, in the classical practice with 2 independent experts or, in the last years, with a computer-aided detection (CAD) added to a human diagnosis expert. Mammography CAD system scans, digitizes, and analyzes conventional analog films. CAD seems to improve cancer detection in screening and diagnostic mammograms. In the move to digital, mammography providers will be choosing computed radiography (CR) imaging solutions, between plain-film radiography and digital radiography (DR) technologies, which are represented by FFDM systems. For that reason, we must be sure our facility has enough digital storage capacity, since the average file size of one mammogram on a CR system may be as high as 200 megabytes. For example, a facility with 20 screenings a day needs to plan to manage up to 20 gigabytes of new images a week. Viewing mammography images has special requirements, including 5-megapixel monitors, and some specialized functionality. Therefore, standard PACS workstations cannot be used for mammography reading. Multimodality breast imaging workstations streamline workflow by enabling the reading of all breast imaging modalities, including CR, DR, ultrasound, and MRI. These workstations can also be used for general radiology exams, which creates an ideal platform for many healthcare providers.

There are some advantages in digital diagnosis such as the high-resolution image quality and especially the availability in flexible point-of-care CR imaging devices or as a central system with multiple workstation software options, which allows us to access a central patient database from multiple sites. The software can easily be configured to enable the extraction of statistical data for workflow analysis, evaluation, and improved administration, e.g., participation rates, number of detected carcinomas, tumor size, type of tumor, false positives, and false negatives. The capability for real-time web conferencing also facilitates case discussions and is of particular benefit in achieving multiple radiologist consensuses. The new double-blind reading functionality of the Radiology Information System (RIS) Mammography module streamlines this process improving workflow and productivity.

Despite all huge developments of technology, mammography seems to attain some limits even in the detection and the characterization of the most important radiological findings for depicting breast cancer. One of the most important advantages of the digital mammography was presented as the possibility to zoom the images, to avoid supplementary X-ray exposure. However, the results were not satisfactory, because some studies revealed that images zoomed from digital contact mammography cannot become an alternative to direct magnification digital mammography [5].

A majority of U.S. mammography screening sites are considering implementing digital technology for mammography screening within the next years. A report of 2008 affirmed that RIS is improving mammography screening administration in three of Denmark's five regions. There are arguments that improved algorithm produces more efficient detection with improved workflow, more breast cancers screened months sooner, and fewer false-positives markers. But CAD for breast imaging has generated controversy of late, with dueling studies producing different results regarding its accuracy. CAD diagnosis is still a controversial method, and it seems logically better programs will not improve too much the diagnosis, because of the limits of mammography itself. *In conclusion, we need another standardized method aside from mammography, allowing follow-up exams and double-reading diagnosis, eventually CAD.*

Classical Breast Ultrasonography

Instead of becoming the most useful imaging method of diagnosis in breast pathology, US is disappointing because of the lower sensibility, despite its good specificity, so it is still recommended as the second method of choice in case of unclear aspects on mammography or MRI. This undervalue is due to the classical approach of US, with less standardized acquisitions scans of the breast, usually in the axial and the sagittal planes, or randomly, without standardized reporting of the precise location of the abnormalities and without correlation with the radial anatomical architecture of the breast; thus, the imagist "watches" for the lesion without "seeing" the breast itself. Even those ultrasonographers who apply the radial and antiradial technique of US examination recommend these scans after the axial and sagittal approach; they are using radial scans only around the nipple (because they are using ordinary short linear transducers) or targeted for the lesion, without visualization of the entire mammary lobe, so they do not realize the assembly; we compare them with "someone missing the forest because he is looking just for the special trees."

Classical US is generally acknowledged to be a highly operator-dependent modality that requires a skilled practitioner, high-quality examinations, and state-of-the-art equipment. These limits are easily vanquished by the standardized ductal US technique, with the actual available equipment that will always be inevitably more performing and cheaper than any MRI equipment. Moreover, there is a considerable variability in the description and assessment of lesions demonstrated on sonograms. More uniform and clearly understandable examination reports are needed to improve patient care and to facilitate research in the use of breast US [6]. In 2003, the American College of Radiology (ACR) published the Breast Imaging Reporting and Data System (BI-RADS) Atlas [7]. This document is an extended version of the Third Edition of the BI-RADS lexicon used in mammography. The BI-RADS Atlas includes new sections on US (ACR BI-RADS – US) and MRI (ACR BI-RADS – MRI). ACR BI-RADS – US may help standardize the terms used for characterizing and reporting lesions, thereby facilitating patient care, the characterization of lesions, and the development of possible screening applications. This lexicon is very useful, especially in the screening US, but this achievement is not enough for classical US considered, because of lack of precision in the location of the lesion regarding the nipple, the ducts/lobules, and the breast lobe by one hand, and of uncertainty of whole breast exploring by the other hand. These limits are imposed by the short transducers and by the inevitable uncontrolled slipping of them during the axial and sagittal scanning of the convex breast surface, with possible blind/missed regions of the breast, which are the reasons of the low sensibility of US.

Originally, US was primarily used as a relatively inexpensive and effective method of differentiating cystic from solid breast masses seen on mammography or suspected on clinical examination. However, even in classical US, it is now well established that we can diagnose the nature and the extension of solid masses and of other breast lesions [8].

One of the most important advantages of using US is the avoidance to expose a patient to X-rays, a factor that is particularly important for pregnant or young patients, whom breast is more sensitive to ionizing radiation; this would mean that in comparison with US, mammography would be associated with a slight increase in the risk of acquiring radiation-induced neoplasm [9]. Furthermore, young women's breasts tend to appear dense on mammograms and that reduces the diagnostic sensitivity of mammography. In addition, breast US is superior to mammography in the evaluation of breast abscess, breast with implants, and male breast. In women less than 50 years old with a family history of breast cancer, mammographic sensitivity is appreciated to only 68.8% after Kerlikowske et al. [10]. Otherwise, Buchberger et al. found that, when performed carefully, (classical) US may be useful in detecting occult breast cancer in dense breasts [11]. When used regularly along with the mammogram, for the appropriate indications and with proper technique, breast ultrasound proved to lower breast cancer mortality and decreased the benign biopsy rate.

US is used to guide procedures such as cyst aspiration, percutaneous biopsy, harpoon localization of masses for surgical excision, abscess drainage in selected cases, and therapeutic intratumoral radiofrequency or cryoablation. US provides effective guidance for percutaneous breast biopsy without ionizing radiation. The guidance was firstly performed with special mammographic pads, but the technique is more laborious and painful, with less precision than in US due to the breast distortion by compression during the image acquisition and to the whole volumic projection in complementary plans, while US is a sectional technique of imaging. US also offers the advantages of real-time visualization of the needle and target lesion, multidirectional imaging, faster procedure with less pain and patient discomfort, and also low cost. With US, the patient does not need to undergo mammographic compression, and the examination may usually be performed with the patient in the recumbent position rather than sitting, as is often the case with procedures involving mammographic guidance.

Some authors showed the possible benefit of combining preoperative whole-breast US with mammography for breast-conservation surgery [12]. Classical US demonstrated some additional sites of multicentric carcinoma, and this allowed facilitating preoperative planning, but this technique is operator dependent and the lesion mapping has a more risk to be incomplete as compared with ductal US.

Several investigators have studied the role of US in the assessment of axillary lymph nodes for tumor staging. Normal lymph nodes usually have a prominent echogenic fatty hilum and a hypoechoic cortex. Lymph nodes that lack a fatty echogenic hilum or are heterogeneous are considered suspicious. The US-guided fine-needle aspiration biopsy (FNAB) of suspicious lymph nodes has been advocated. Krishnamurthy et al. found that in approximately 12 % of cases, false-negative results occur with guided axillary lymph node FNAB [13]. Contrarily, the new SE added to Doppler US performs more in the characterization of malignant lymph nodes, and a reduction of the number of node biopsies is expected.

Classical US can provide additional information about implants, and it may also help in evaluating breast masses that are unrelated to the implant. US may demonstrate the *stepladder sign*, consisting of multiple echogenic parallel lines within the implant lumen, which is highly suggestive of a broken and collapsed implant shell; when an intracapsular or an extracapsular rupture occur, they are producing the snowstorm increased echogenicity within the breast tissue [9]. Other authors consider MRI more accurate than ultrasound for the evaluation of silicone gel implant integrity and recommend US as initial evaluation. Sometimes we can find areas of moderate-to-marked homogeneous low-level echogenicity within the implant, but this sign is not highly specific for rupture.

In some clinical cases, we can find abnormalities related to postsurgical changes or other breast pathologies that are difficult to describe in classical US; the panoramic views (type SieScape) or better the ductal US with long water-bag probe is advantageous.

The use of quantitative Doppler, with arterial systolic and diastolic velocimetry, or even the use of velocity indices was abandoned because of low specificity, with benign and malignant lesions presenting both high- and low-flow values. This aspect is determined by many factors, such as tumoral size and various grades of stromal reaction, and by different pathological tumoral cellularity. Otherwise, the qualitative Doppler ultrasound vasculature probing, consisting in the number and the orientation of the vascular branches displayed as 2D or 3D images, contributes considerably to the diagnostic evaluation of suspicious breast lesions [14]. The limit of Doppler is still related to the low sensibility of the classical breast US technique of examination itself, which is operator dependent and thus nonreproducible; there are possible missing areas of scanning and lack of precise relationship with the surrounding structures especially the ductal-lobular parenchyma. That results frequent misinterpreting of the small lesions. The overdiagnosis by Doppler criteria is rare, usually in cases with breast focal or diffuse infections, and the SE is recommended as noninvasive method for the differential diagnosis.

SE is the last acquisition in US and MRI techniques, with good results in the differential diagnosis of the benign from the malignant lesions, especially with the quantitative analysis using the fat-to-lesion ratio (FLR). SE is improving accuracy of US, because the Stavros criteria are not valid in all cases, for example, benign appearance of cancers without desmoplastic reaction or some malign sonographic aspects of fibrocystic dysplasia are better characterized by measuring/quantification of their elasticity.

Breast ultrasound computer-aided detection (US CAD) appears to help doctors more consistently find lesions smaller than 1 cm, according to a study conducted by Chinese researchers. Using a single reader completed with CAD seems to produce comparable results as using two readers to interpret breast ultrasound. The group affirmed CAD was able to increase diagnostic accuracy in identifying lesions less than 1 cm. Accuracy increased by 44 % when single readers using CAD and single readers not using the technology were compared [15]. For lesions greater than 1 cm, there was no difference in diagnostic accuracy between the three reading techniques: a single physician without the use of CAD, a single physician using CAD, and two physicians performing double reading without CAD.

However, there are many discordant reports about US CAD systems, because of the perpetuated confusion between mammography and US techniques. For example, a study presented differences of breast ultrasound CAD performance in ethnic populations [16]: one incriminated factor is the higher breast density of Asian women that may have an effect on sonographic feature extraction. Previous studies have shown that Asian women tend to have increased breast density, and this higher average density may change the average value of a feature in the CAD software that is linked to or dependent upon density. It is assumed that the measurement for shadowing isn't working as well: in North America, shadowing is an important factor, but in Asia, it may not be as important. By consequence, if the software will not give as much importance to shadowing with the Asian database, the results may be more comparable after Gruszauskas.

A study made by Lehman and colleagues, which prospectively determined cancer yield, callback and biopsy rates, and positive predictive value (PPV) of mammography, MRI, and US in women at high risk for breast cancer, concluded that screening MRI had a higher biopsy rate but helped detect more cancers than either mammography or US. (Classical) US had the highest false-negative rate compared with mammography and MR, enabling detection of only one in six cancers in high-risk women. Those results were predictable, because the authors performed classical breast US, which may produce void areas on breast mapping examination. Some authors presented screening sonography being especially beneficial in women less than 50 years old with dense breasts, for example, whereas mammography depicted only 21 (50 %) of 42 cancers, and sonography diagnosed 33 (79 %) of 42 cancers [17]. Younger age seems to be predictive of increased prevalence of cancers seen only on sonography, independent of breast density.

3D targeting should be a reduction of needle passes without an increase of miss rate due to objective three-dimensional demonstration of correct or incorrect core- or fine-needle position.

Newly developed software allows real-time 4D US needle guidance during breast biopsy. The three-dimensional permanent analysis of lesion position as well as needle position in all three planes allows one to navigate the core needle in an optimal preferred position [18, 19]. We can use the precise positioning to perform some treatment interventional US techniques, such as cryoablation, needle aspiration, or intratumoral chemotherapy.

3D US and 4D US are very useful in optimal resection of tumors with the minimal and cancer-negative surgical margins in breast-conserving surgery [20] or to detect the spiculation. It is proven that spiculations are more easily seen in the coronal view than other two views. Moreover, 16% of benign cases and 90% of malignant cases are detected with spiculations [21].

3D was proposed in Paget disease, in patients with nipple discharge [22]. It is proven that the availability of high-frequency high-resolution linear transducers enables us nowadays to visualize the mammary duct in detail. The three-dimensional volume images can be reviewed immediately in the bedside ultrasound machine or in the computer retrospectively, so that the relationships among the nipple, the duct, and the tumor can be clearly identified. It is logical that 3D US directs us towards ductal US. Moreover, 3D was combined with CAD. All parameters: accuracy, sensitivity, specificity, positive predictive value, and negative predictive value for CAD are improved using 3D US instead of 2D US with statistical significance. The proposed system is expected to be a useful CAD tool for classifying benign and malignant tumors in sonograms and can provide a second reading to help reduce misdiagnosis [23].

The general expectations in breast US is the development of the technologies and engineering and computational soft programs [24], but future trends should be oriented towards the perfectionning of the physicians themselves, by restarting the learning of breast US from the anatomical bases. In fact, not only is US less performing, but the operators and the lexicon are worse functioning.

A study of Wendie and col. [25], published in 2006, about the operator dependence of physician-performed whole-breast US lesion detection and characterization, concluded that larger lesions (>11 mm) are most consistently detected, with fewer than half of lesions 5 mm or smaller in mean diameter identified; substantial agreement was found for the description of lesion size, location, and key features, and moderate agreement was found for lesion management but comparable with those at mammography and breast MR imaging. We understand the limits in the detection of the smaller lesions in classical US, because their relationship with the ducts and lobules is not demonstrated; thus, the examination is researching only the detectable masses and could not visualize the intraductal dissemination.

The practical use of breast US needs guidelines more than other applications of US examination, but there are no consensus. The limits of breast US in the classical technique are thought to be absolute, so US is generally limited as an additional method of diagnosis, and it is recommended only in some circumstances, such as palpable breast mass or abnormal screening mammogram that requires further diagnostic evaluation [26]. The less sensitivity of the classical breast US leads to recommendation to not perform adjunct US in the follow-up of probably benign lesions or for symptomatic complaints, such as pain, skin or nipple abnormalities, or patients referred for positive family history of breast cancer. Contrarily, these cases are well diagnosed by ductal ultrasonography, because its sensitivity is almost 99% if trained operator, and the specificity is improved by the use of Doppler and SE, the actual results confirming specificity over 95%.

According to other studies [27], in nonfatty breasts, US and MRI were more sensitive than mammography for invasive cancer, but both MRI and US involved the risk of overestimation of tumor extent. Combined mammography, clinical examination, and MRI were more sensitive than any other individual test or a combination of tests. Classical US showed higher sensitivity than did mammography for IDC, depicting 104 of 110 (94%) cases, and for ILC, depicting 25 of 29 (86%) cases ($P<.01$ for each). US showed higher sensitivity for invasive cancer than DCIS (18 of 38 [47%], $P<.001$). This study does not present US technique but is presumed to be the classical US, possible with Doppler characterization of the lesions and surely without SE. We think better scanning using ductal/radial US technique, completed with Doppler US and SE, briefly named the full breast US (FBU), will improve the characterization both of the first 5mm diameter lesion and of the malignancy risk and will be the future first method of breast screening [27, 28].

In conclusion, we need a better ultrasound technique, which could be standardized, with better sensibility, applicable as screening, with the possibility of CAD in small lesions and the advantages of computing storage and web transmission of data; these aims are realizable if we will change the classical US scanning technique with Doppler ductal US, using the radial and antiradial whole breast scanning with a same equipment! Upgrading SE, the diagnosis accuracy becomes the best of all noninvasive imaging techniques, FBU being more precise and cheaper than contrast enhancement US, tomosynthesis, or breast MRI.

Breast Tomosynthesis

Digital mammography offers a cancer detection benefit for specific subgroups of patients: women under 50 years of age, pre- and perimenopausal women, or women with dense or heterogeneously dense breast tissue. Using annual mammography, the mortality rate from breast cancer is reduced in a population by almost 20 % in the USA between 1990 and 2000 and by 25 % in 2005 [29], but as many as 20 % of breast cancers will be missed by it [30]. The true value of digital mammography lies not in its conventional use but rather in its ability to serve for the development of other mammography-based breast imaging applications, such as tomosynthesis.

Tomosynthesis is the best X-ray exposing technique in breast diagnosis, which uses the digital platform to capture a series of images of the breast that are then reconstructed into a three-dimensional image. Indeed, the conventional analog or digital mammograms, which use two-dimensional imaging, have the same inconvenience: areas of concern are sometimes difficult to visualize because of tissue overlap. Though tomosynthesis consists of multiple exposures, each acquisition requires only 5–10 % of the normal dose on a single-view mammogram. Using a selenium detector, tomosynthesis performs a three-dimensional examination with a total radiation dose similar to the conventional mammography.

Digital tomosynthesis is expected to help detect cancers earlier than mammography, because its images can be taken apart and examined without additional acquisitions and thus additional irradiation. However, tomosynthesis is a promising method; perhaps new technologies will improve cancer detection, but it is unbelievable that this exam will be able to detect normal ducts or lobules, as well as premalignant lesions, because of low X-ray absorption of the breast parenchyma.

In addition to diagnosis improvement, tomosynthesis requires less compression than the mammography; thus it is less painful and the architectural deformation parallel with the detector is less important.

Moreover, even with lower dose, the irradiation will not allow using tomosynthesis for all, children, young patients, or pregnant women; as well it will be not possible to use it anytime and anywhere, because its availability could not increase significantly. Another limitation is presumably the less sensitivity in detecting the relationship of the simultaneous cancers, for the differential diagnosis of the multifocal cancers from the multicentric cancers, such as demonstrated by FBU. Another limit is related to the detection of an in situ cancer, which can lack microcalcifications and usually presents a branching development.

Despite the large agreement about the advantages of this method of diagnosis, there are some limitations or potential disadvantages that restrain the availability and the overall accuracy as compared with other methods:

- Special training of technologists.
- Prolonged time of radiological interpretation and additional training for radiologists.
- Motion artifacts more likely to occur due to the less tissue compression and to an increased exposure time.
- Despite no substantial artifacts for small calcifications, there are significant artifacts for large calcifications, considered usually benign [31].
- No significant additional information for the lesions will be visible in 2D mammography.
- Follow-up examination after tomosynthesis is recommended to be performed with the same method, the images being difficult to compare with 2D acquisition in mammography [31]; therefore, it could be impossible to obtain sections identically, at the same level, to compare small lesions or small clusters of microcalcifications in consecutive tomosynthesis, eventually performed with different equipments.
- Problems of optimizing of the angular range of tube motion, of optimal number of exposures, or of the optimal thickness of reconstructed sections.

- Limitations of the reconstruction planes: currently the reconstructions available are parallel to the detector, neglecting the radial breast anatomy; even if the ducts are better illustrated than in mammography, they are visualized only segmental, without interconnections and without demonstration of their relationship with the benign or malignant lesions.
- The use of contrast agents for tomogalactography or of contrast-enhanced 3D imaging is promising and may be cheaper than breast MRI, but they are more expansive and less accurate than 2D or 3D Doppler acquisitions.

Breast Magnetic Resonance Imaging

During the last two decades, important advances have been made in the performance and interpretation of breast magnetic resonance imaging (MRI). Recently, there has been an increase in the use of MRI in screening for breast cancer and taking biopsies. An initial study presented at the American Society of Clinical Oncology meeting in June 2006 reported that following lumpectomy for cancer, a woman can expect an average recurrence rate of 10–15 %, and only 8 % after preoperative MRI. Indeed, in patients with invasive lobular carcinoma (ILC), who represent 7–15 % of breast carcinomas, breast MRI has proven to be a better tool for preoperative assessment than mammography and/or classical US.

Top 10 recommendations for breast MRI generally accepted are:

1. *All newly diagnosed breast cancer patients: to define the extent of disease multifocality and/or presence of contralateral abnormalities and to assist with planning or surgical treatment.* However, multifocality can easily be demonstrated on breast ductal ultrasonography, with precise location and high intraobserver and interobserver agreeability.
2. *Adjunct to Mammography and US in women with clinically difficult exam and dense breasts on these examinations (women younger than 40).* Nevertheless, dense breast is a limit only in the mammographic examination, while in US and especially in ductal US exam, a dense breast is really easier to examine than a fatty breast.
3. *Preoperative assessment in patients with mammographic abnormalities or dense breast tissue (i.e., preoperative breast reduction or revision reconstruction).* But the best anatomical technique of examination, which can visualize normal and abnormal ducts and lobules and the connection of the lesions with the ductal tree is ductal US, which could be completed with 3D or 4D acquisitions, to realize the reproducible mapping of the breast.
4. *Yearly follow-up for breast cancer patients.* There are many benign lesions associated with breast cancer; practically, there is a continuous pathology between benign-no-risk lesions, benign premalignant lesions, and malignant breast lesions, which could not be well differentiated by MRI and needle biopsy; otherwise, ductal US can be repeated on short intervals, and when completed with Doppler techniques and SE (the concept of FBU), it allows making the differential diagnosis between multiple associated lesions easier.
5. *Screening patients at high risk for breast cancer, especially those with suspected or proven mutations of BRCA1 and BRCA2.* The high cost and low availability of MRI screening are prohibitive for large areas of populations, while full-breast US is available and cheaper.
6. *Further evaluation of suspicious clinical findings or imaging results, those remain indeterminate after mammographic and (classical) US evaluation.* This seems a rational indication, in limited number of cases, as a complementary non-invasive exam.
7. *Evaluation of silicone gel implants integrity, after recent U.S. Food and Drug Administration recommendations.* We think this evaluation can be as easier performed by ductal US with Doppler technique, with and without water-bag probe, which allows better evaluation of the contours, shape and internal echoes of the implants, of the surrounding small parts including the pectoral muscles and fat and of the breast itself, with its ductal trees and eventually associated pathology.

8. *Breast cancer screening in women with breast implants as adjunct to mammography.* Mammography is less performing in breast implants (due to the difference in the penetration of the X-rays between the implant and the tissue) and MRI has low specificity, so this recommendation means double screening, while water-bag ductal US is safe and cheaper and do not requires additional imaging.
9. *Monitor response to new adjuvant hormonal therapy and/or chemotherapy.* The best short interval monitor could be performed by the ductal US.
10. *To determine primary site in patients with axillary nodal disease and unknown primary disease.* This is a really good indication for breast MRI as first examination, especially for large breasts, and in some types of diffuse breast cancer.

Breast MRI is proved to be a very useful diagnostic tool, especially for women who have dense breasts and/or those that may be at high risk for developing breast cancer; it is proved that MRI can detect numerous incidental lesions, unapparent on mammography or misdiagnosed on the classical US [32].

The *American Cancer Society March 2007 recommendations for annual breast MRI screening as an adjunct to their annual mammography screening* refer especially for women who have the following:

- A BRCA1 or BRCA2 mutation
- A first-degree relative who has a BRCA1 or BRCA2 mutation
- A lifetime risk of 20–25 % or greater, as defined by BRCAPRO or other models that are largely dependent on family history
- A history of chest radiation between ages 10 and 30

The ACR BI-RADS (Breast Imaging Reporting and Data System) lexicon for breast MRI has brought uniformity to the interpretation of breast MRI examinations. With these advances in imaging technique, interpretation guidelines, and increasing availability of MR-compatible breast biopsy systems, MRI of the breast is rapidly gaining popularity in clinical practice in both the diagnostic setting and, more recently, in the screening setting. There is some inconvenience for screening breast MRI, relating to the technical issues that vary significantly across practices: magnet field strength, breast coil specifications, pulse sequences, and other parameters such as contrast agent mode of administration and dose or dynamic scan parameters. Other elements of the BI-RADS MRI lexicon are better defined: standardized terminology (morphology of lesions: focus/foci <5 mm, mass, non-mass-like enhancement, associate findings and kinetic curve assessment) and standardized reporting (assessments and recommendations) [33].

We will reproduce below the report on BI-RADS MRI because it is a proof of unification in the attitude towards the patient following mammography, MRI, and US, as we will present in the following chapters:

The BI-RADS MRI categories

	Assessment	Recommendation
0	Incomplete	US, mammography
1.	Negative	Routine follow-up
2.	Benign	Routine follow-up
3.	Probably benign	Short interval follow-up
4.	Suspicious	Biopsy
5.	Highly suggestive of malignancy	Biopsy
6.	Known biopsy/proven malignancy	Treatment

The clinical indications for breast MRI, however, remain to be defined [34]. There are clinical indications that have emerged where MRI, as an adjunct to mammography, seems to be the imaging study of choice. All those recommendations represent in fact a confirmation of low accuracy of mammography and a less confidence in breast MRI, which is not recommended as the only method for screening. In fact, there are multiplied disadvantages: X-ray exposure risk of mammography added to MRI high costs, which estimates to 1,000–1,500$. *In conclusion, we need a method with higher accuracy and lower costs for screening.*

Breast MRI could be used as a second method of breast diagnosis in:

- Further evaluation of suspicious clinical findings or imaging results, those remained indeterminate after mammographic and ultrasound evaluation
- The determination of the primary site in patients with axillary nodal pathology and unknown primary disease's location
- Particular cases

One of the most important disadvantages of breast MRI is the less specificity of the lesions. Many studies report increasing biopsies after breast MRI. Technically, MRI-guided biopsies are more challenging. Discordance was found at higher rates with MRI, which may in part be attributed to a lack of experience by examiners in performing MRI-guided biopsies, and because when using MRI-guided imaging, once one is in there, it's very hard to see the lesion. It is confirmed by most of the authors that despite contrast enhancement curves and MRI-elastography, the number of biopsies in MRI of the breast still increased. High recall rates and a high level of false positives are considered the Achilles' heels of breast MRI [35], but we have to take truly the prevalence of both can be reduced when studies are read by more experienced radiologists.

Some authors consider this application is not appreciated feasible for lower risk women, and we agree with their reasons: there are not enough qualified radiologists to interpret breast MRI nor the facilities to perform them anywhere; the procedure averages at least $1,000, and the examination must be performed annually, mainly without reimbursement of the costs; positive predictive value will be lower, with higher risk of unnecessary biopsies. There is an exception for reimbursement in developed countries, where MRI exams for patients who have tested positive for the BRCA1 and BRCA2 gene mutations – which have a 60–80 % risk of developing breast cancer in their lifetime – receive unquestioned reimbursement. The problem for those patients is whether that individual can pay the approximately $2.800 cost for the genetic testing if it's not covered by their current health insurance provider, as is the reality for most countries.

Moreover, the breast examination with MRI is not possible without paramagnetic contrast agents' administration, which has some contraindications, adverse reactions, and significant limits. The only approved contrast agent for breast MRI is Gadavist® (gadobutrol), which has the following limits:

- Administration contraindicated in patients with history of severe hypersensitivity reactions to Gadavist®, other contrast agents, or history of bronchial asthma and allergic disorders; risk of mild to severe reactions, including death (rarely)
- Acute kidney injury in patient with chronic renal impairment
- Extravasation and injection site reactions: moderate irritation
- Adverse reactions, according to the producers: headache (1.5 %), nausea (1.2 %), and dizziness (0.5 %)
- Overestimation of the extent of the malignant disease in breast MRI in up to 50 % of the patients according to the contrast agent manufacturer, resulting to a recognized low accuracy, which determine an increase of the unnecessary biopsies, with raising of the overall diagnostic costs
- No specific information about the benign breast pathology, which may be associated with breast cancer or may be symptomatic and could be treated; no information about the premalignant breast lesions, such as ductal-lobular hyperplasia

Another problem is this expansive MRI could not replace the other methods of diagnostic. It is recommended to not skip mammography because mammography does contribute information and acts as a reference point. If some isolate a suspicious finding on MRI, then return for a mammogram (or perform a "second-look" ultrasound) and search the best way to biopsy the suspected lesion by mammographic or ultrasonographic guidance. We think it is not reasonable to do so many expansive exams (MRI, mammography, classical US, biopsy), instead of using a cheaper, accessible, and safer method, which reduces the complementary exams such as MRI and biopsies. This new method proposed as the anatomical ductal echography, imagined by Teboul and col., will be illustrated in the next chapters as FBU; in the last years, more practitioners were trained to perform it.

Nowadays, there are available dedicated spiral units for breast MRI, faster and generating better images, all obtained at 1mm thickness sections being more accurate than general MRI vendors with more than 2.5 mm thickness. Because image acquisition is so fast in the dedicated machines, there are no significant issues with patient motion artifact that plagues others. The ability to acquire 1 mm thick scans means that it is possible to not omit many lesions and to see subtle areas of abnormality such as ductal carcinoma in situ (DCIS), which is a noninvasive (low-grade) cancer, while other machines often have detecting problems. However, the interval between scans is larger for all manufacturers. The dedicated workstations provide for meaningful subtracted images and the ability to evaluate lesions in different projections simultaneously. In fact, these equipments are so efficient and comprehensive that usually experts read a study relatively quickly and then review the results of the scan with the patient at the time of her visit. Seeing all lesions, rapidly, almost nonoperator dependent and without irradiation is the greatest advantages of breast MRI; but the low availability is the most important limit of this method.

MRI was proposed in the differential diagnosis of the inflammatory breast carcinomas (IBC) from acute mastitis. There are clinical different histories but sometimes clinical similar findings: breast enlargement, diffuse skin thickening, tenderness, abnormal nipple configuration, prominent vessels, and also cutaneous/subcutaneous, perimamillar, and diffuse edema. Mammography or classical US is less specific, but MRI can better differentiate these entities: in IBC, more masses with a greater average size are detected, with T2 hypointensity (rarely in acute mastitis), the presence of the blooming sign, infiltration of pectoralis major muscle (interruption of fat plane usually is malignant), pathological enhancement (when present is suggestive), and edema present perifocal and in the great pectoral muscle. While the main localization of the acute mastitis is subareolar, related to infected ducts, in IBC, the localization is predominantly central or dorsal. However, MRI is not reassuring, and the discrimination between acute mastitis and IBC remains a diagnostic challenge because of overlapping imaging features.

There are many other technical developments engaged in the fight against breast cancer, such as F-18 FDG-PET (fluorine-18 fluorodeoxyglucose positron emission tomography) combined with CT to improve the modality's sensitivity, specificity, and overall accuracy for detecting breast cancer [36, 37]; for lesions smaller than 10 mm, best results were obtained with dual-time-point PET/CT, whose overall accuracy, sensitivity, and specificity were 89, 88, and 100 %, while MRI proved 95 % accurate, 98 % sensitive, and 80 % specific. These efforts oriented for better diagnosis may be combined with CAD in MRI, but it was claimed that breast MRI CAD doesn't improve accuracy, due to poor DCIS detection [38]. For example, sensitivities and NPV were better for invasive cancers only (100 % and 100 %, respectively), compared to DCIS only (54 % and 76 %, respectively). Other authors confirm that the presence of threshold enhancement at computer-aided evaluation is sensitive for malignancy, while the absence of threshold enhancement at computer-aided evaluation improves the discrimination between benign and malignant lesions when compared with those at initial interpretation by the radiologists.

In fact, we can observe the efforts of the engineers and computer scientists to develop new and more accurate techniques of exploring and interpreting imaging data of the breast, but every new technique is the proof that all the others are not so good to be used as replacements of the unsatisfactory mammography. Indeed, if only one of them would be good enough, the other ones will be eliminated, as inefficient. The efforts of engineers could help, but they are not able to solve the problem without medical experts, and up till now all of them have forgotten the essence of the diagnostic: the object of the examination, we mean the breast particular radial branching structure, with particular physiological and pathological changes.

Up to this day, the goal of the breast examination was "to see the lesion." We are on the side of those which recommend as a goal "to see the breast" with its anatomical structures and after that to identify and characterize the eventual lesions of any type [39]. "Anatomy, the anatomy firstly" is the key, as recommended by the promoters of breast ductal US.

Conclusions

We summarized some of the advantages and the disadvantages of the most used present diagnostic methods of breast cancer. The breast pathology is increasing due to long lifetime survive, to hormonal replacement treatments and to more polluted ambient in the modern society, impose the use of a method more efficient than the screening mammography and more available than the breast MRI. No method will be very soon as performing and as confident to replace all the others, but we have to chose the best cost/performing method for the huge number of examination, to offer to each woman an earlier and no dangerous screening, and to preserve the most sophisticated techniques for the selected cases.

These arguments are the most important reasons for the new approach, the complete and anatomical breast US, because we are living "The 'Coming of Age' of Nonmammographic Screening for Breast Cancer" [40]. The establishing of standardized diagnostic criteria and the widespread use of the BI-RADS lexicon should help to demystify the practice and application of breast US. Taking all clinical and imaging information into consideration, most masses meeting benign criteria can be followed clinically or by short-term interval ultrasound follow-up in the evaluation of the response to the conservatory therapy. Lesions meeting criteria for complex cysts or solid masses with malignant characteristics should be aspirated or biopsied, most readily by ultrasound-guided core biopsy. Increasing the rate of diagnosis of DCIS or LCIS and of small multicentric lesions will decrease the mortality rate. Making possible the diagnosis of the breast cancer by noninvasive techniques, such as SE, we will reduce the unnecessary biopsies.

The benign lesions were largely neglected to treatment, and the premalignant breast lesions are still incidental pathological findings. Only by detecting the premalignant lesions, we will reduce the incidence of the breast cancer, and till now this was not systematically possible.

References

1. Hendrick RE, Pisano DE, Averbukh A et al (2010) Comparison of acquisition parameters and breast dose in digital mammography and screen-film mammography in The American College of Radiology Imaging Network Digital Mammographic Imaging Screening Trial. AJR 194(2):362–369. doi:10.2214/AJR.08.2114
2. Boyd N (2007) High breast density is a major risk factor for breast cancer. N Engl J Med 356:227–236, 297–299
3. Tot T (2007) Clinical relevance of the distribution of the lesions in 500 consecutive breast cancer cases documented in large–format histologic sections. Cancer 110:2551–2560
4. Teboul M (2010) Advantages of Ductal Echography (DE) over Conventional Breast Investigation in the diagnosis of breast malignancies. Med Ultrason 12(1):32–42
5. Kim MJ, Kim E-K, Kwak JY et al (2009) Characterization of microcalcification: can digital monitor zooming replace magnification Mammography in full-field digital Mammography? Eur Radiol 19:310–317
6. Mendelson EB, Berg WA, Merritt CR (2001) Toward a standardized breast ultrasound lexicon, BI-RADS: ultrasound. Semin Roentgenol 36(3):217–225
7. Mendelson EB, Baum JK, Berg WA et al (2003) Breast imaging reporting and data system BI-RADS: ultrasound, 1st edn. American College of Radiology, Reston
8. Bassett LW, Ysrael M, Gold RH, Ysrael C (1991) Usefulness of mammography and sonography in women less than 35 years of age. Radiology 180(3):831–835
9. Perlmutter S (2008) Breast cancer, ultrasonography. Article Last Updated: Jul 31. www.emedicine.com/radio/TOPIC795. HTM 10/5/2008
10. Berg WA (2003) Rationale for a trial of screening breast Ultrasound: American College of Radiology Imaging Network (ACRIN) 6666. AJR 180:1225–1228. © American Roentgen Ray Society
11. Buchberger W, Niehoff A, Obrist P et al (2000) Clinically and mammo-graphically occult breast lesions: detection and classification with high-resolution sonography. Semin Ultrasound CT MR 21(4):325–336
12. Berg WA, Campassi CI, Ioffe OB (2003) Cystic lesions of the breast: sonographic- pathologic correlation. Radiology 227(1):183–191, http://radiology.rsnajnls.org/cgi/content/full/227/1/183

13. Krishnamurthy S, Sneige N, Bedi DG et al (2002) Role of ultrasound-guided fine-needle aspiration of indeterminate and suspicious axillary lymph nodes in the initial staging of breast carcinoma. Cancer 95(5):982–988 [Medline]
14. Le Carpentier G (2008) 3D Doppler evaluation helps identify malignant breast lesions. Reuters Health November 6, Radiology, p 249
15. Madden Yee K (2008) Breast ultrasound CAD helps doctors find smaller lesions. AuntMinnie.com staff writer, October 10
16. Keen C (2008) Breast ultrasound CAD performance varies in ethnic populations. AuntMinnie.com staff writer, September 5
17. Kolb TM, Lichy J, Newhouse JH (2002) Comparison of the performance of screening mammography, physical examination, and breast US and evaluation of the factors that influence them: an analysis of 27,825 patient evaluations. Radiology 225:165–175
18. Rotten D, Levaillant J-M, Zerat L (1998) Use of three-dimensional ultrasound Mammography to analyze normal breast tissue and solid breast masses. In: Merz E (ed) 3-D ultrasonography in obstetrics and gynecology. Lippincott Willams&Wilkins, Philadelphia, Chap. 11, pp 73–78
19. Rotten D, Levaillant J-M, Zerat L (1999) Analysis of normal breast tissue and of solid breast masses using three-dimensional ultrasound mammography. Ultrasound Obstet Gynecol 14:114–124
20. Tamaki Y, Inoue T, Tanji Y, Noguchi S (2003) 3D Ultrasound navigation for breast cancer surgery. 13th international congress on the ultrasonic examination of the breast. International Breast Ultrasound School. The 10th Meeting of Japan Association of Breast and Thyroid Sonology
21. Chang R-F, Huang SF, Chen D-R, Moon WK (2003) Detection of spiculation in three-dimensional breast Ultrasound. 13th international congress on the ultrasonic examination of the breast. International Breast Ultrasound School. The 10th Meeting of Japan Association of Breast and Thyroid Sonology
22. Lee CC, Chen D-R, Chang R-F, Lee J-H, Jeng L-B (2003) Three-dimensional breast Ultrasound imaging in patient with nipple discharge: a pictorial review of 36 patients. 13th international congress on the ultrasonic examination of the breast. International Breast Ultrasound School. The 10th Meeting of Japan Association of Breast and Thyroid Sonology
23. Chang R-F, Chen W-M, Chen D-R, Moon W-K (2003) Three-dimensional breast Ultrasound Computer Aided Diagnosis. 13th international congress on the ultrasonic examination of the breast. International Breast Ultrasound School. The 10th Meeting of Japan Association of Breast and Thyroid Sonology
24. Rizzatto G (2007) US-advanced technical aspects and future trends. ECR A-123
25. Berg WA, Blume JD, Cormack JB, Mendelson EB (2006) Operator dependence of physician-performed whole-breast US: lesion detection and characterization © RSNA, 2007. Radiology 241:355–365. © RSNA, 2006
26. Vercauteren LDB, Kessels AGH, van der Weijden T et al (2008) Clinical impact of the use of additional ultrasonography in diagnostic breast imaging. Eur Radiol 18(10):2076–2084
27. Georgescu AC, Enachescu V, Bondari S (2010) The full breast ultrasonography: an anatomical standardized imaging approach of the benign and malignant breast lesions. doi:10.1594/ecr2010/C-0434
28. Georgescu AC, Enachescu V, Bondari A, Bondari S, Manda A, Simionescu C (2011) A new concept: the Full Breast Ultrasound in avoiding false negative and false-positive sonographic errors. doi:10.1594/ecr2011/C-0449
29. Kopans DB (2006) Breast imaging, 3rd edn. Lippincott Williams &Wilkins, p 121
30. Tabár L, Vitak B, TonyChen H-H et al (2001) Beyond randomized controlled trials. Organized mammographic screening substantially reduces breast carcinoma mortality. Cancer 91(9):1724–1731
31. Park JM, Franken AE, Garg M et al (2007) Breast tomosynthesis: present considerations and future applications. RadioGraphics 27(suppl 1):S231–S240. doi:10.1148/rg.27si075511
32. Cilotti A, Iacconi C, Marini C et al (2007) Incidental MR findings: which role for ultrasonography? ECR B-280
33. Lehman CD, Isaacs C, Schnall MD, Pisano ED (2007) Cancer yield of mammography, MR, and US in high-risk women: prospective multi-institution breast cancer screening study. Radiology 244:381–388, © RSNA, 2007
34. Orel S (2008) Who should have breast magnetic resonance imaging evaluation? J Clin Oncol 26(5):703–711. © 2008 American Society of Clinical Oncology. doi:10.1200/JCO.2007.14.3594
35. Pal S (2007) MR-guided breast biopsy results need careful correlation with histology for on-time diagnosis. AuntMinnie.com staff writer, September 24
36. Madden Yee K (2008) Dual-time-point FDG-PET/CT improves breast imaging accuracy. AuntMinnie.com staff writer, November 18
37. Madden Yee K (2008) PET/CT and breast MRI. AuntMinnie.com staff writer, November 18
38. Madden Yee K (2008) Breast MRI CAD doesn't improve accuracy due to poor DCIS detection. AuntMinnie.com staff writer, February 18
39. Teboul M, Halliwell M (1995) Ductal echography: the correct ultrasonic approach to the breast. In: Teboul M, Halliwell M (eds) Atlas of ultrasound and ductal echography of the breast. Blackwell Scientific, Oxford, p 83
40. Kuhl CK (2008) The "coming of age" of nonmammographic screening for breast cancer. JAMA 299(18):2203–2205

Breast Doppler Ductal Ultrasonography: Definition, History, and Advantages

1

1.1 Definition and History: Galactography and Ductal Echography

The only method of diagnosis of the breast ductal pathology used in the past and still recommended is galactography/ductography of the breast, considered as an underused procedure that often helps define the cause of unilateral, single-pore, spontaneous nipple discharge [1]. It is recommended to search papilloma or carcinomas that can be responsible for nipple discharge and to help guide accurate surgical intervention. Galactography is useful because it refers to ducts, but it has some inconvenient facts:

- It increases the effects of the X-ray exposure, as follow-up a mammography.
- It is an interventional procedure, with risk of complications and with possible artifacts such as air bubbles or extravasations of the contrast iodinate agents.
- It cannot measure the thickness of the duct's wall nor the ductal tree distal from a stenosis.
- Most importantly, this procedure cannot visualize the surrounding tissues, the lobules, nor the lymph nodes or the pathological nearby vasculature.
- The optimal quantity of iodinated contrast agent and the best degree of breast compression could not be calculated: too much or too less?
- The lobar ductal branching is distorted by the compression of the tissues; indeed, the lobar projection appears too large in all views, with the false perception of the lobar volume and a wrong conservative therapy planning.
- The ductal enlargement is overestimated, because the initial content is increased by the iodinated contrast agent added by instillation; moreover, there are ductal ectasias misdiagnosed in cases without salient nipple surge; thus, not all ectasias are evaluated.

With regards to performance, galactography/ductography is as limited for the breast diagnosis as the urography for the urinary system, or barium meal for the upper digestive tube.

The breast pathology was redefined by T. Tot and L. Tabar, which developed *the theory of the* "sick lobe" [2–4]: the breast carcinoma is a lobar disease, with simultaneously or asynchronously appearance (either in situ or infiltrative type) of multiple tumor foci originated in a single lobe of the breast. This theory affirms that the malignant process is initiated when the *sick lobe* is differentiated, in early embryonic life, as an explanation for the almost simultaneous transformation of the whole lobe. *The sick lobe theory* is proved by the frequent *multifocality* of the lesions in the same lobe, while the *multicentricity* with two or more lobes simultaneously involved is rarely found. The branching ducts inside the lobe were reproduced by Ichihara and Ohitake [5] and demonstrated by numerous pathologists. The explanation of the origin of the *sick lobe* in the embryonic life is nevertheless unbelievable, because there is not any small embryonic or fetal model of the breast with little lobes, similar to the embryonic cartilaginous model of the bones, for example, or an embryonic branching tracheal-bronchial tree; indeed, the newborn has a not divided mammary bud, and the branching process during thelarche is progressive: initially the homogeneous bud becomes heterogeneous, and then the main ducts appear at the periphery and are surrounded by the simultaneously growing glandular stroma; in the next stage, the secondary segmental ducts develop and finally appear in the lobules, with the terminal ductules and the acini. If the moment of the origin of the *sick lobe* seems to be thelarche, it is possible to be determined by the amount of hormonal and neural receptors or by a mutation of the responsible genes during the cellular multiplication. The *sick lobe* could be determined even later, related to pregnancy, dishormonal pathology, substitution hormonal therapy, or other unknown factors. We find this explanation concordant with the statistically risk factors for breast malignancies such as precocious thelarche, late pregnancy, birth control pills, or postmenopausal substitution therapy.

The greatest value of the "sick lobe theory" consists in removing the concept of "breast cancer as a lump;" thus, the radical excision of the whole "sick lobe" should theoretically

A. Colan-Georges, *Atlas of Full Breast Ultrasonography*, DOI 10.1007/978-3-319-31418-1_1

represent the best conservative curative intervention. This is sustained by the fact the mammary lobes may overlap, but there are not directly communications between their ductal-lobular trees, so the cancer is spreading initially via the lobar tree inside the same lobe before to extend to the surrounding lobes or other tissues. For achieving this target, we need a technique of imaging able to visualize the anatomy of the breast lobe, and the only technique that is noninvasive, in real time, operator independent, and accessible for all is the ductal echography (DE) imagined by M. Teboul and his collaborators and further developed by promoters such as D. Amy.

In 1995, the first *Atlas of Ultrasound and Ductal Echography of the Breast,* by Michel Teboul and Michael Halliwell, was published [6, 7]. The new technique was presented as a *newer, more effective diagnostic tool in breast disease*. Despite the argued challenges in the technique of examination and diagnosis of breast pathology related to the normal anatomical lobes of the breast, with the description of the ductal US features, of the lobules, and their relationship with the surroundings tissues, this method of diagnosis rested almost unknown until the publication in 2003, in Spain, of the *Practical Ductal Echography (D.E.): Guide to Intelligent and Intelligible Ultrasonic Imaging of the Breast,* by Michel Teboul and F. Javier Amorós Oliveros [8]. This was a best seller, the ductal approach became more familiar, and many specialists from Europe, Japan, and the USA became adepts of this method.

M. Teboul sustained his method in Congresses and Conferences such as *The 13th International Congress on the Ultrasonic Examination of the Breast, April 6–8, 2003* [9]. He revealed the progress of the technique, especially after 2000, when the release of high-quality fully digitized equipment has still further increased DE performance. *New digital equipment has highlighted the superior aspects of DE over conventional investigation and reinforced the sense of reliability in the relationship between the DE display and the macroscopic pathological situation.* With better resolution, the visual evaluation of lesions was improved to such a point that the use of needle aspiration was often bypassed, and surgical biopsies were directly performed with a high rate of reliability. This method is opposed to breast MRI, for instance, which increased biopsies and needs a complementary method such as mammography or US to complete diagnosis. DE added confidence to surgeons in the US technique, so that the *American College of Breast Surgeons* has recommended adopting, teaching, diffusing, and utilizing ultrasound and DE for the management of breast diseases [9]. It seems the *American College of Radiologists* was more conservator, because it is easier to learn a new technique than to change an old, well-known technique with another newer, even better one. This is an observation of one of the most active promoters of DE, Dominique Amy, who worked formerly in DE at the Francophone Center of Formation in the USA, of Aix-en-Provence, coordinated by the University of Nimes, France.

However, we can read many publications about breast US that are referring of the radial and antiradial scans in classical breast US, but used as complementary targeted scans, after the "classical" longitudinal and transversal scans; this approach has as goal to *find the lesion*, while DE intends to analyze *the breast anatomy*, because only searching the whole "forest," we are able to localize, recognize and characterize all its "trees" as normal elements, and thus we become able to detect all the abnormal changes. By using DE, it proves a feasible diagnostic procedure of the subcentimeter breast carcinoma, as presented by Amy at the *13th International Congress on the Ultrasonic Examination of the Breast: Thanks to its systematic anatomical analysis it's a perfectly reproducible technique and moreover it became interpretable by everyone*.

In the studies of Amy, 2003 [10, 11], with 1400 files analyzed, focused on the lesions of 4–5 mm to 10 mm, DE was evaluated in comparison with mammography. There were classified three categories of cases:

- Positive mammography: the US was used to confirm a carcinoma and to search additional lesions.
- Doubtful mammography: US allowed the identification of suspect zones and a wide lesion assessment.
- Negative mammography: US made it possible to detect lesion clinically and radiological dumb.

Contrary to certain publications, this author never met a mammographically visible lesion which was not detected by US. Moreover, the analysis of the multicentric cancers confirmed and raised the literature data that affirms more than 43 % of multiple lesions, this percentage increasing with the new equipment to be above 55 %. The very significant number of multifocal cancer (more than 1 out 2), of infracentimetric dimensions, certainly will involve surgical and chemotherapeutic treatment adaptations.

The DE is not a different technique of examination, but an US with another method of acquisition and interpreting the images, based on the anatomy and sustained by the most recent theories of breast pathology. There are some models of the primary site and the spreading ways of ductal and lobular cancers [12], which offered a three-dimensional network showing the ductal-lobular system, where the papilloma develops in the main ducts, while the cancers arise in the periphery, in *the terminal ductal-lobular specific units (TDLUs)*. This model explains the branching ductal-lobular system, where several duct systems overlap one another in the same radius of the breast, and may mimic a multilobar simultaneous pathology.

We must remember, in 1842, Doppler presented his paper to the Royal Bohemian Society with his most famous idea entitled: "On the Coloured Light of the Double Stars and Certain Other Stars of the Heavens." This paper presented for the first time the Doppler principle which relates the frequency of a source to its velocity relative to an observer. Nowadays, it is not conceivable to perform US without Doppler, and for the breast, this technique is very useful in the differential diagnosis of the benign and malignant changes. Doppler will be part of the full ductal Doppler US or simply the full breast ultrasonography (FBU), represented by breast US in radial scanning and interpreting (DE), completed with Doppler and sonoelastography. The last was developed from the beginning of the 1990s in Japan and almost simultaneously in the USA. There is almost a consensus about the value of the qualitative Doppler, eventually associated with 3D acquisitions, in the differential diagnosis of the malignant breast lesions; despite the differences of opinions at the beginnings, sonoelastography both qualitatively and quantitatively demonstrated its contribution in increasing the overall accuracy of US.

1.2 The Advantages of the Breast Doppler Ductal Echography

Breast Doppler DE represents a useful diagnostic tool, both for the diagnosis of the infracentimetric breast cancer and fibroadenoma and for the group of four benign lesions that are generally omitted/underdiagnosed by the mammography and the classical US, *ductal ectasias*, *papillomatosis*, *adenosis*, and especially *ductal hyperplasia*, which are considered forerunner for fibroadenomas, cysts, and breast cancer [8]. The noninvasive diagnosis of these benign but not mammographically visible lesions allows the treatment of the symptomatic patients, usually referred for painful breast mostly related to the endocrine disorders [13]. The most important progress is the opportunity to develop differential diagnosis criteria between infracentimetric benign and malignant lesions, with these small lesions generally having less specific features upon the Stavros criteria, and thus to reduce unnecessary biopsies and to prevent the advanced breast cancer.

We present the most important risk factors for breast cancer upon the analysis of OMS published in 2005 [14]; these factors increase 4–5-folds the risk of breast cancer by determining the premalignant changes of breast parenchyma:

- Oral birth control pills
- Hormonal substitution treatment
- Food with animal fat (steroids depot), contaminants (xeno-estrogens and some pesticides, these factors being controversial)
- Beast irradiation (especially the therapeutically irradiation associated with the epithelial proliferative lesions, the most important being atypical hyperplasia)

Doppler DE is able to diagnose small parenchymal lesions with better characterization of the premalignant ones and of the less 10 mm diameter cancers; contrary, following the mammographic screening any 2 years in patients after 50-year old, in the advanced countries, the breast cancer incidence is constant and the mortality was reduced with only 30 % [15].

The most important argument for using Doppler DE is the fact that 90 % of the human cancers are carcinomas, epithelial or glandular tumors, which in the breast are related to the ductal-lobular system; from these, 80 % are ductal carcinomas, 15 % are lobular, and the rest of 5 % are tubular, medullar, or other types. "In situ" carcinomas without microcalcifications are difficult to detect by mammography, but they are visible on Doppler DE, supposing that the findings are not yet proved to be malignant. There are either the ductal-type (ductal carcinoma "in situ"—DCIS), whom 30 % develop to invasive ductal carcinomas, or the lobular-type (lobular carcinoma "in situ"—LCIS), usually multifocal/multicentric, uni-/bilateral, with estrogens receptors in young woman, considered on high risk of raising invasive cancer, in despite of discordant opinions of different authors [14]. In the future, it is presumed Doppler DE could represent an alternative to IRM in the diagnosis of the multicentric breast cancer.

Doppler DE visualizes less 5 mm diameter lesions, either dysplastic, without visible vasculature, or tumoral, with salient suspect new vasculature, offering an anatomical precise localization and characterization (shape, volume, structure, ductal connection).

Doppler DE is superior to 3D/4D US in the diagnosis of the following:

- Nipple discharge
- Symptomatic ductal ectasia
- Diffuse or segmental ductal hyperplasia
- Breast-feeding pathology
- "True" gynecomastia, generally difficult to diagnose on mammography or MRI
- Breast pathology in children and teenagers
- Multifocal cancer, the disease spreading by the ductal way in a centripetal or centrifugal direction toward the intraluminal lowest pressure

3D/4D US is useful in the diagnosis of solid tumors, adenosis, sclerosing adenosis, and fibro-micro-cystic dysplasia, with less than3 mm cysts, which may not be mammographically recognized, especially in the nodular form. Doppler DE better visualizes the complex cysts, with differentiation between the intracystic papilloma, septae, pseudo-septae, debris, and peripheral inflammation.

Ductal and lobular hyperplasia, associated or not with ductal ectasia, despite the presence of the estrogen receptors is not related to the menstrual cycle; otherwise, diffuse/localized increasing breast vasculature associated with ductal-lobular hyperplasia is suspected for atypical hyperplasia, and the short-interval Doppler DE follow-up associated with the dynamic research of the tumoral serum markers such as CA 15-3 may be useful, because the biopsy cannot be used as screening of the premalignant lesions.

Diffuse increasing vasculature associated with ductal ectasia with/without significant hyperplasia is usually related to the physiological or pathological hyperprolactinemia, while ectasia without hyperemia is found in chronic infections either with saprophyte bacteria, which become resistant to antibiotics (opportunistic infections), such as *Staphylococcus epidermidis* and *Staphylococcus albus*; or with pathogen bacteria such as *Staphylococcus aureus*, *Streptococcus haemolyticus*, and *Escherichia coli*; or even with fungus such as *Candida albicans*.

In the painful breast with ductal ectasia on Doppler DE and without spontaneous nipple discharge, it is useful to actively squeeze out the nipple for the cytological and bacteriological tests; in galactorrhea, the hyperprolactinemia may direct to a pituitary prolactinoma.

The malignant microcalcifications are less than 0.1 mm and are better visualized on mammography; high-resolution Doppler DE could detect small intraductal or intratumoral calcifications, which appear as hyperechoic spots. For the actual probes, it is possible to detect microcalcifications over 0.4 mm, and when present, the benign lesion is defined. There were not proved US microcalcification features highly corresponding to the radiological findings; most cases of so-called microcalcifications on US represent in fact artifacts of the fibro-micro-cystic dysplasia, explained by the posterior tiny enhancement effect with marginal small shadowing of the millimetric cysts and proved on sonoelastography, which demonstrates a summation-BGR scoring upon Ueno.

The presence on Doppler DE of a multiple subcentimeter nodules attached to the same duct, with salient vasculature, with a centripetal or centrifugal descending scale of rank development, is highly suspicious for ductal carcinoma with intraductal dissemination, even without the classical signs of probable malignant breast lesion (acoustic shadowing, marginal spicules, taller-than-wide, etc.). The connection of a lesion with the ductal tree is essential in the diagnosis, and this aspect was introduced by ED, while the classical US and the 3D US, including the automated breast volume scanner (ABVS) with the plane "C," cannot visualize simultaneously all the foci related to the same ductal tree.

The proven connection of the most lesions with the ductal-lobular tree allows a better definition of the isoechoic lesions, such as fibroadenoma or atypical cancers, with differentiation from the lipomatous tissues especially in fatty breasts, while these lesions are usually misdiagnosed in the classical US; once the isoechoic lesion is found on DE, we can improve the contrast by using the tissue harmonic intensifier (THI), and when available, the sonoelastography demonstrates this particular strain.

Doppler DE is the sectional imagery with the best resolution, with continuous scans less than 1 mm thick and measurements less than 0.5 mm, as compared with MRI that usually, without dedicated machines, has a resolution of several millimeters and does not allow the scanning in the axis of the main ducts.

Doppler DE is useful in the monitoring, guided biopsies, and conservatory surgical treatment [16], being proved that large surgical mastectomies did not significantly improve the lifetime of the patients.

For illustration, we will present some images related to the technique, the results of ductal echography compared with the MRI aspect in the same case, and the influence of the imaging diagnostic approach to the surgical therapy (Figs. 1.1, 1.2, 1.3, 1.4, and 1.5).

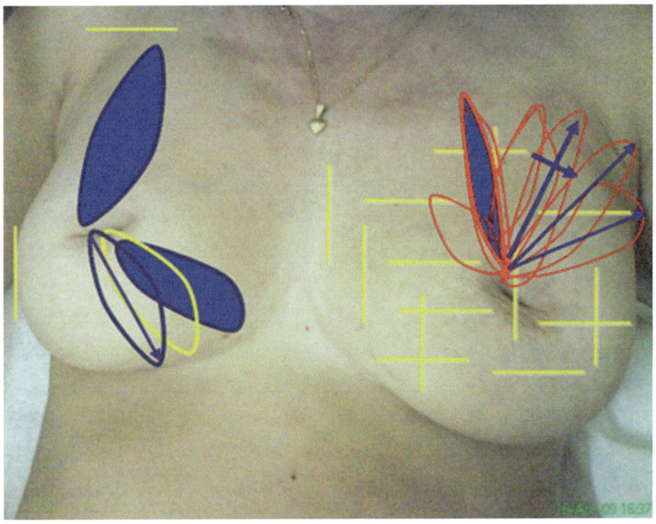

Fig. 1.1 Radial and antiradial scan planes used in DE (examples colored in *blue*) are logical, repeatable, and easy to locate; we visualize on the first intention the normal anatomy, and consequently, we are able to identify eventually a lesion; the transversal and sagittal planes which are still used by the large majority of ultrasonographers (examples colored in *yellow*) are nonanatomical, are difficult to analyze, and are looking just for a lesion in an unknown surrounding "breast tissue"

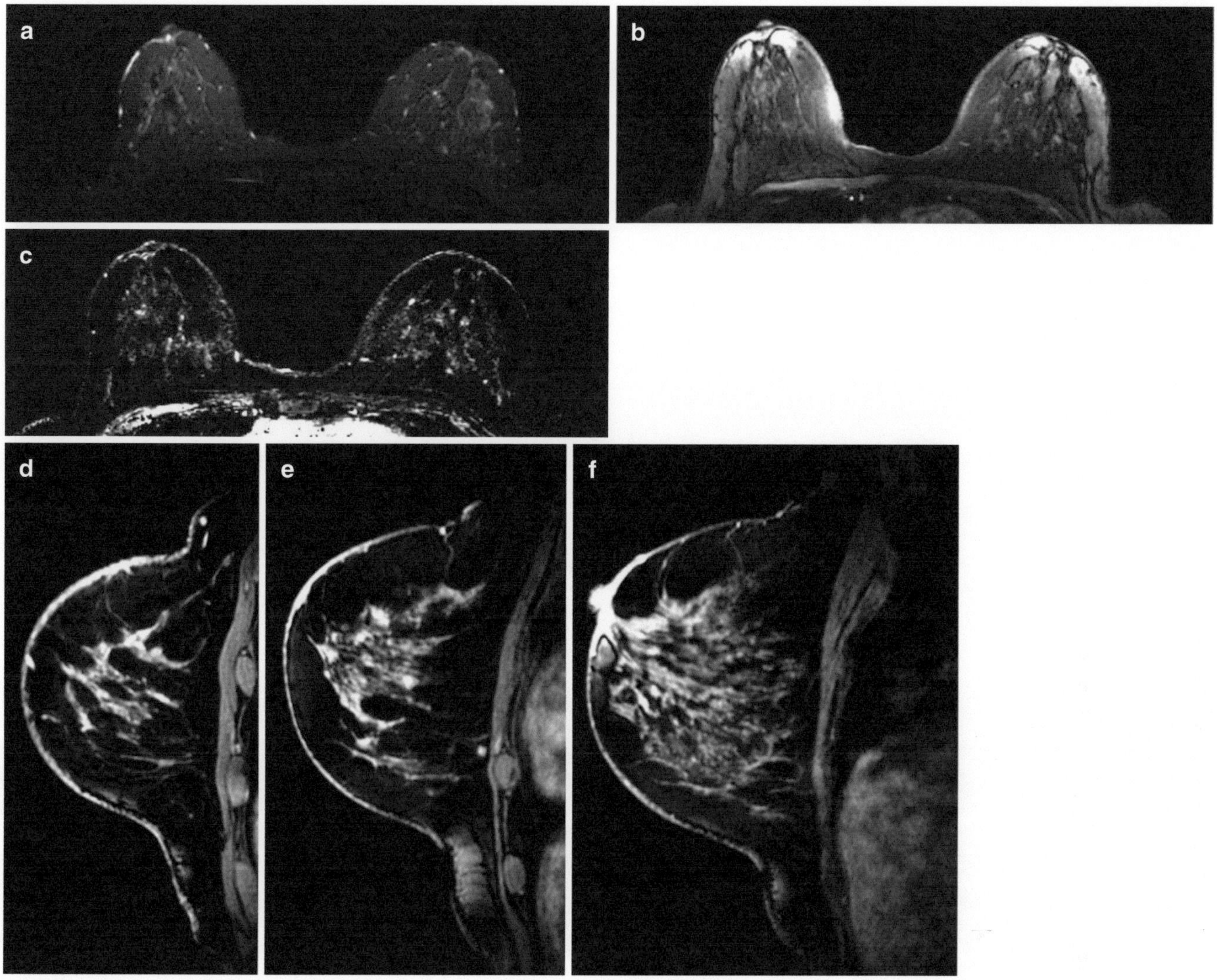

Fig. 1.2 Breast MRI in a 40-year-old patient: upper acquisitions in the axial plane on T2-fat sat, T1 with contrast and T1 with contrast agent and subtraction weighted sequences (**a–c**); lower sequences in the sagittal plane T1 with contrast and fat suppression (**d–f**). MRI exam is suggesting bilateral multiple small lesions, with unspecific character, but no section is able to present the anatomy inside a mammary lobe, despite the resolution enough for visualization of the normal Cooper ligaments. The enhancement curves were more specific for benignity, but they must be performed for each lesion before the final diagnosis, with higher costs due to the contrast agent and being time consuming than a ductal echography with Doppler and sonoelastography (FBU)

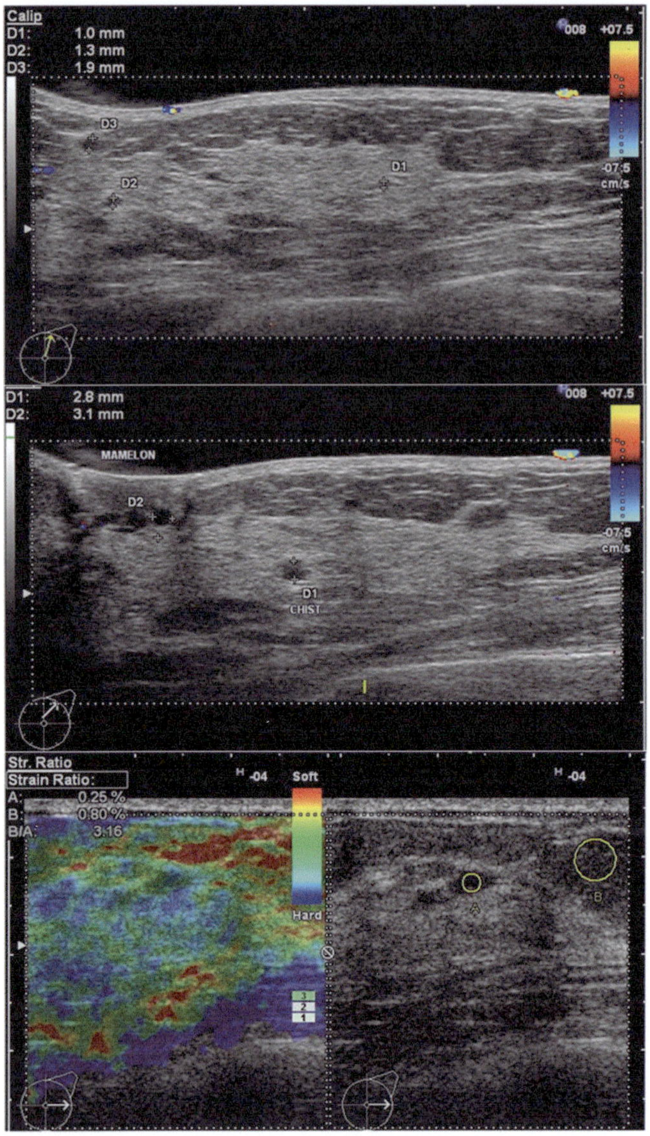

Fig. 1.3 The same case: Doppler DE and sonoelastography present the lobar anatomy with tiny ducts connected to the abnormal findings of 1–3 mm corresponding to microcystic fibrous dysplasia, scored 2 Ueno with "benign" FLR of less 4.70

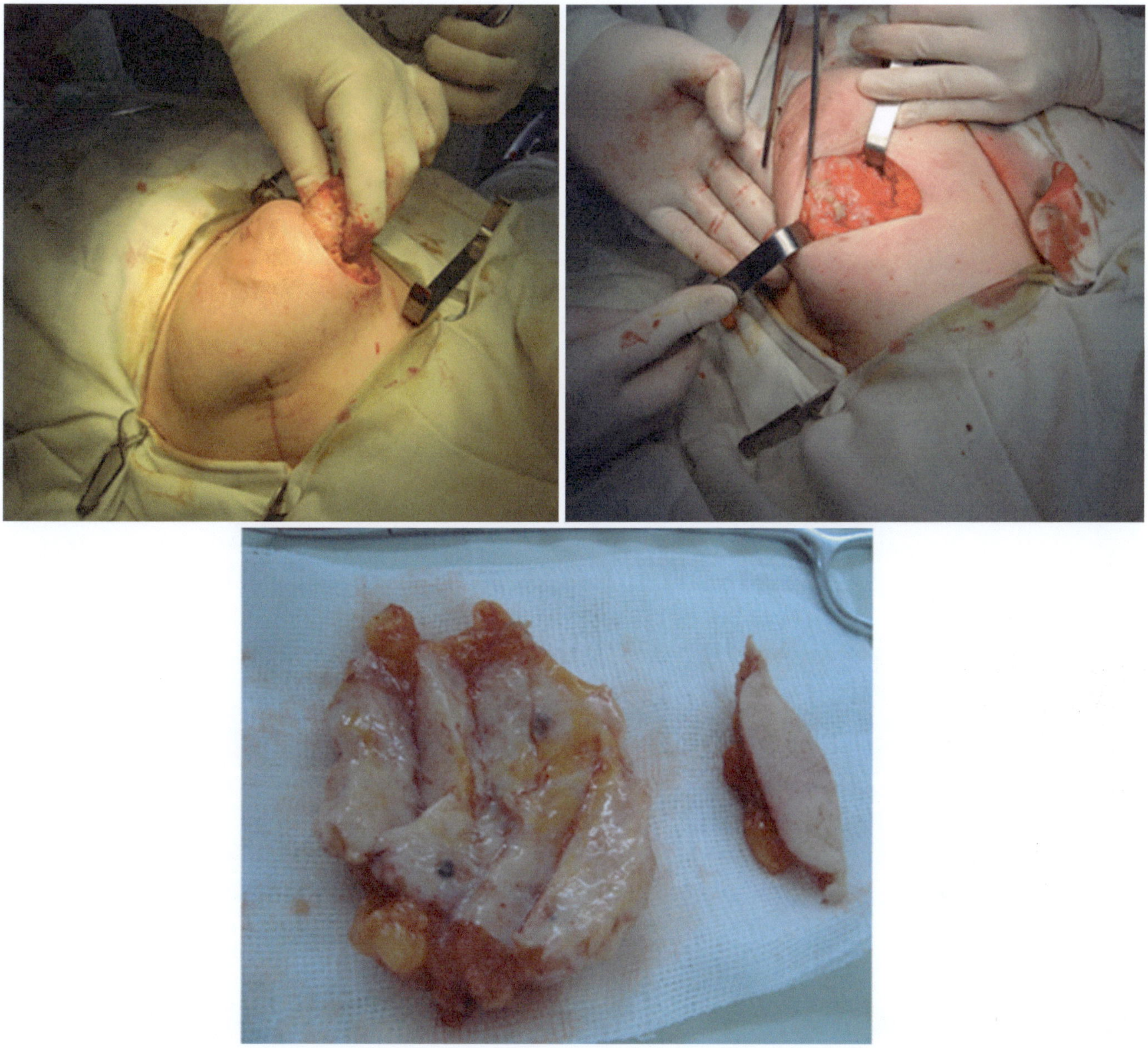

Fig. 1.4 A wrong imaging approach, referred only to the lesion, leads to a wrong therapeutic approach, such as lumpectomy, or segmentectomy. Misinterpreting the anatomy and ignoring the "sick lobe" are proved by the incomplete, repeated lumpectomy with random axes and by illogical random section of the specimen

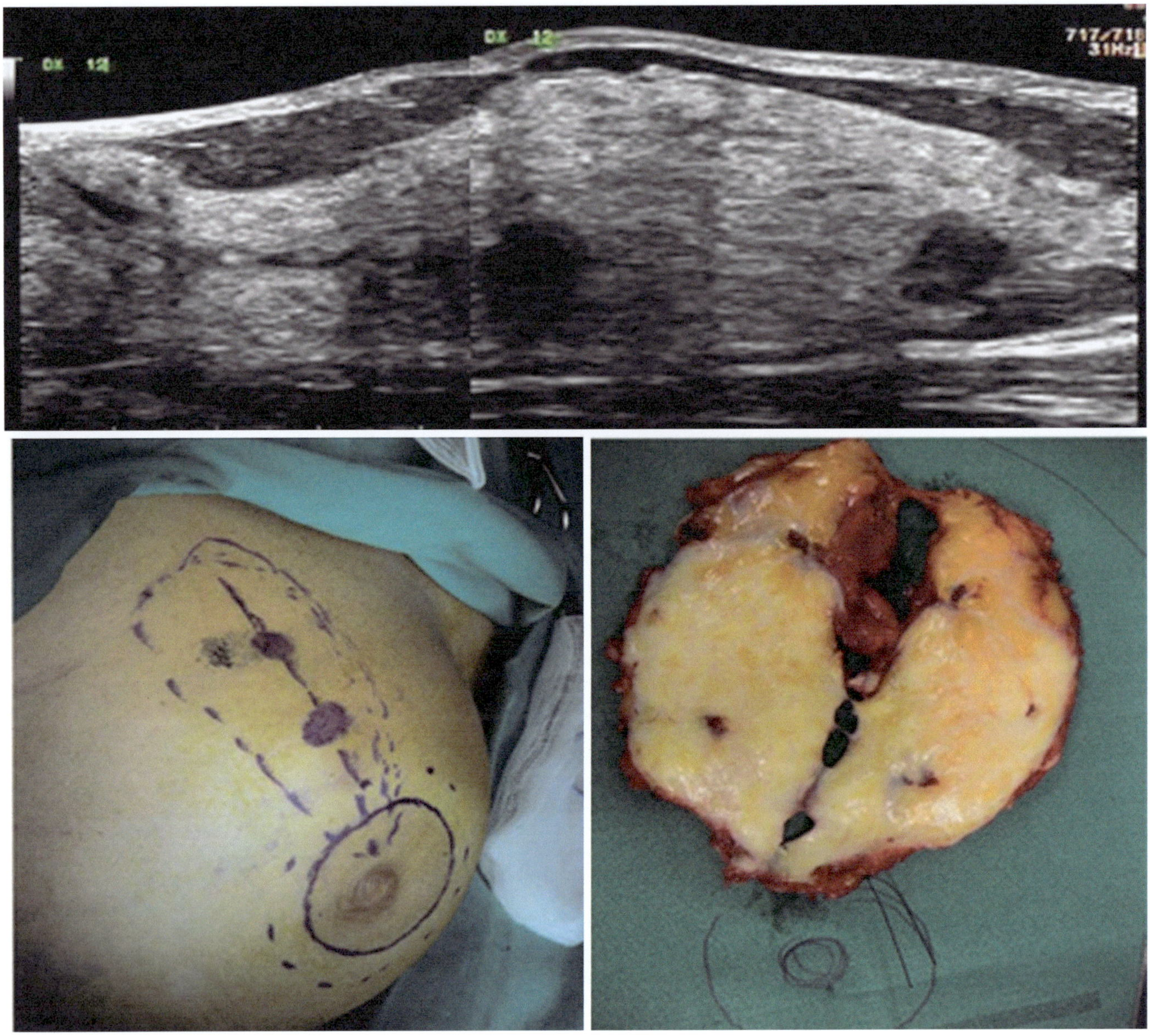

Fig. 1.5 The "intelligent and intelligible" DE of Teboul offers the best therapeutic approach, lobectomy being the ideal treatment for multicentric carcinoma. Conservatory surgery involves not only the lesions but also the whole sick lobe, confirmed by the radial section of the specimen (Courtesy of M. Teboul)

References

1. Slawson SH, Johnson A (2001) Ductography: how to and what if? Radiographics 21:133–150, © RSNA
2. Tabár L, Tot T, Dean PB (2005) Breast cancer. The art and science of early detection with mammography: perception, interpretation, histopathologic correlation. Stuttgart; New York: Thieme
3. Tot T (2007a) Clinical relevance of the distribution of the lesions in 500 consecutive breast cancer cases documented in large–format histologic sections. Cancer 110:2551–2560
4. Tot T (2007b) The theory of the sick breast lobe and the possible consequences. Int J Surg Pathol 1:68–71
5. Ichihara S, Moritani S, Ohitake T, Ohuchi N (2005) Ductal carcinoma in situ of the breast: the pathological reason for the diversity of its clinical imaging. In: Research and development in breast ultrasound. Springer, Tokyo Ed, pp 104–113
6. Teboul M, Halliwell M (1995) Atlas of ultrasound and ductal echography of the breast. Ed. Blackwell Science Inc
7. Teboul M, Halliwell M (1995) Ductal echography: the correct ultrasonic approach to the breast. In: Teboul M, Halliwell M (eds) Atlas of ultrasound and ductal echography of the breast. Blackwell Scientific, Oxford, p 83
8. Teboul M (2003) Practical ductal echography: guide to intelligent and intelligible ultrasound imaging of the breast. Saned Editors, Madrid
9. Teboul M (2003) Advantages of ductal echography (DE). 13th International congress on the ultrasonic examination of the breast. Examination of the breast. International Breast Ultrasound School. The 10th meeting of Japan Association of Breast and Thyroid Sonology

10. Amy D (2003) Echo-anatomic comparison. 13th International congress on the ultrasonic examination of the breast. International Breast Ultrasound School. The 10th meeting of Japan Association of Breast and Thyroid Sonology
11. Amy D (2003) Sub-centimetric breast carcinoma. Echographic diagnosis. 13th International congress on the ultrasonic examination of the breast. International Breast Ultrasound School. The 10th meeting of Japan Association of Breast and Thyroid Sonology
12. Lee CC, Chen D-R, Chang R-F, Lee J-H, Jeng L-B (2003) Three-dimensional breast Ultrasound imaging in patient with nipple discharge: a pictorial review of 36 patients. 13th International congress on the ultrasonic examination of the breast. International Breast Ultrasound School. The 10th meeting of Japan Association of Breast and Thyroid Sonology
13. Georgescu AC, Enăchescu V, Simionescu C et al (2004) Ultrasound aspects of painful breast. In: Syllabus of the Euroson School Course Breast Ultrasound, Craiova, pp 64–69
14. Stewart W, Kleihues P (eds) (2005) Le cancer dans le monde. IARC Press, Centre International de Recherche sur le Cancer, OMS, Lyon, pp 190–195
15. Leconte I (2007) Breast ultrasound and screening. ECR, Vienna, A-127
16. Amy D (2000) Echographie mammaire: echoanatomie. JL mensuel d'echographie LUS 10:654–662

2 Breast Doppler Ductal Echography: Technique of Examination Related to the Breast Lobar Anatomy

2.1 General Technical Principles

Certain aspects of the sonographic technique are recommended when doing a breast examination related to the new engineering achievements:

- The dynamic focus capability of most modern equipments allows for high-resolution imaging of the breast from the superficial structures to the chest wall; therefore, for the evaluation of small lesions that are within 7 mm of the skin surface, an acoustic standoff with a gel pad approximately 1 cm thickness or less, or a mound of thick gel of equivalent depth, is recommended in the classical breast US. The best technique in DE necessitates a water-bag device adapted to a long linear transducer (nowadays, there are available transducers of ~9 cm in length of the sonographic surface), which is the most useful in the quick examination of the whole breast surface, while in the classical US, "the surface" technique is designated to characterize a small, precised area as a complementary method of examination. However, in the last years, we provided linear transducers with longer size of 8–9 cm and potential convex view, which are able to visualize almost the whole radius of a medium breast, with good resolution of the lobar structures and possibility of zooming or special software for increase penetration in large breasts.
- Adjustments of focal zone, overall gain, and time-gain-compensation curves should be a dynamic process during the examination, depending on the type of breast anatomy and the size and location of the region of interest (ROI).
- Tissue harmonic imaging (THI) has the ability to eliminate artifacts within cysts but also to improve contrast for the differentiation of low internal level echoes in solid tumors from the anechoic cysts; moreover, some hypoechoic fibroadenomas are better differentiated from the surrounding fatty tissue.
- Compound imaging better defines the margins of the masses, diminishing the lateral margin artifacts.
- Color and/or power Doppler is recommended to identify blood flow within a mass, the vascular pattern being useful in the positive and the differential diagnosis of the benign and of the malignant lesions, infected cysts, hyperprolactinemia, gynecomastia, precocious thelarche, and lymph node pathology.
- 3D and 4D acquisitions are suitable, and when they are not available, in minimum, the two orthogonal scanning planes in the radial and the antiradial axes must be analyzed for each lesion, to determine the volume and the ductal connections/spreading of the lesion.
- Sonoelastography will be indispensable for any equipment dedicated for breast US, as a complementary method for completing the differential diagnosis of the malignant lesions; the problem of cost will be justified by the reduction of unnecessary biopsies and the reduction of number of most expansive breast MRI examinations.
- Contrast-enhanced US (CEUS) is optional, due to its high costs; the improvement in the differential diagnosis of benign from malignant lesions in CEUS with the classical US is compensated by some advantages in the DE and sonoelastography, which are more easy to perform, are dedicated to the whole breast, are with high accuracy, and are cheaper.

Nowadays, these technical improvements are not widely available; however, the future will develop the US applications in the breast diagnosis and interventional therapeutics, by spreading the last technical acquisitions and facilitating the new anatomical breast ductal US especially by using the long linear transducers.

A. Colan-Georges, *Atlas of Full Breast Ultrasonography*, DOI 10.1007/978-3-319-31418-1_2

2.2 Ductal Echography: Radial US Technique of Scanning

2.2.1 Patient Positioning

All 2D and 3D US investigations should be performed with the patients in supine position with elevated ipsilateral arm. The examiner must sit on the right side of the patient, for a right-handed person, or on the left side, for a contrarily.

The patient is turned on the right side for the left breast examination, with the nipple oriented to the zenith, and turned on the left side for the right breast US. We can place a standoff under the elevated shoulder of the patient in the same position as in the surgical room, to allow a better localization of the lesion reproducible especially in large breasts [1]. The pelvis is oblique elevated, with the lower limb in flexion sustaining the body weight.

Although Amy recommends the alternative examination with the patient in sitting position, we think this is not good in large or elongated breasts, because of the distortion of the breast during examination, with difficulty in lesion localization, and insufficient opening of the axilla for the lymph node evaluation. Moreover, the examination in the sitting position is fatigable for the operator.

It is recommended to start with left breast examination, for a right-handed operator, because the patient may see the images at the beginning of the US and will be able to understand the technique of scanning and the normal and pathological findings (Fig. 2.1). This will result in physical and psychical comfort of the patient which are superior to all other imaging methods of the breast, increasing the confidence and cooperation.

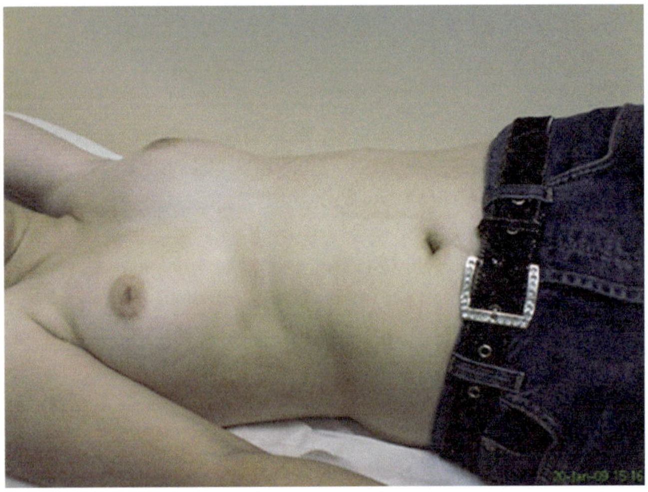

Fig. 2.1 The patient is turned to the right side for the left breast examination, with the nipple oriented to the zenith; the ipsilateral arm is elevated to expose the axilla, and the lower limb is set in flexion for a good sustention of the body. The breast has the nipple in the center, and the clockwise reporting of the findings is reproducible

2.2.2 Transducers

One of the main reasons for the unsatisfactory classical US approach of the breast was the manufacturing wrong transducers: usually, the linear high-frequency probes used till nowadays are too short, about 4.5 cm in length, and do not allow the scanning of a complete radius of the breast, so the images represented fragments of lobes in randomly scans [2]. For performing the anatomical, radial DE it is necessary a high frequency linear probe as long as possible to achieve the longest radial section of the mammary lobe, and thus to visualize as much as possible from a main duct, with a sufficient resolution to identify the ducts or lobules of diameter range 1 mm or less.

As a rule, the orientation of the transducer will be always in the necessary position to obtain the image of the nipple on the upper left side corner of the screen and the periphery of the lobe on the right side of the screen; the body mark will be used to precise the breast radius scan location, so the images will be interpreted by anyone [3].

As the probe's length is limited, being inversely proportional with the high frequency needed for a high resolution, there are few types of equipments with 8–9 cm-long linear probes of 7–9 MHz and good resolution, recommended for the first step examination (Fig. 2.2); the use of a 4–5 cm probe length of 9–14 MHz or even up to 18 MHz is recommended in the second step for the characterization of the lesion upon the US BI-RADS criteria, Doppler examination included, and in the third step of FBU, represented by the sonoelastography (see below).

In the case of the absence of a long linear probe, we must complete the length of the radial scan, making a composed image on a double screen, in the left half of the screen, the first half of the lobar radius, with the nipple oriented to the left, and in the right side of the screen, the second half of the radius, acquired by slipping the transducer in the radial centrifuge direction, as proceeded in the panoramic views [4]. Recently, new transducers came into the market, with 7–9 cm length and 14–18 MHz, which changed the vision of the breast and other small anatomical parts; the possibility of virtual convex scans allows a larger view of the glandular region of the breast, even with the loss of the peripheral regions of the skin and subcutaneous fatty tissues. Contrarily, the use of the panoramic views (type SieScape technique) offers us a spectacular image, but unuseful, because of the inconvenient:

- The image is not reproducible, because of the lateral slipping of the transducer on the skin and of the subjective speed of the transducer during the acquisition, so the radius length is not accurate.
- The image is not "anatomical," because the breast is randomly scanned, even when crossing a palpable mass, and is not reproducible, and there are no possible measurements in the horizontal axis, but only in the anterior-posterior axis.

2.2.3 Water-Bag Technique

The contour of the breast surface is not regular/plane, but spheroid, so it is difficult to follow-up its relief, without distortion of the internal architecture; especially on the nipple, we cannot perform a good examination in all cases, even using a lot of echo jelly; otherwise, the best resolution is obtained when the ductal axis is parallel to the probe surface.

To improve the quality of the images, it is recommended to use in the first step a water bag added to the transducer by an adaptor, recommended by Teboul and Amy [5], which will solve all the previous problems and will offer a better resolution in the superficial planes, especially for the skin and the fatty subcutaneous layer (Fig. 2.2).

2.2.4 Steps of Examination

1. *The first step is represented by the 2D gray-scale examination of the whole breast*, using radial scanning for DE, with a water-bag-long linear probe of the highest frequency possible (the frequency being limited by the probe length). Scanning in the plane of ductal anatomy can be achieved in the radial and antiradial axes (Fig. 2.3). The linear probes of about 6–7 cm length with virtual convex acquisitions may be useful in the absence of longer probe that could cover the radius.

Radial scanning is performed with the long axis of the transducer oriented along the long axis of the ductal and lobar anatomy (the nipple to the upper left screen corner, the periphery of the breast on the right screen side) and antiradial in the orthogonal planes to the radius. The transducer must be oriented to achieve the main duct in a horizontal plane, by changing the thickness of the water bag using balanced pressure of the hand.

It is recommended to always begin and finish the examination on the same radius, for exploring systematically the whole breast.

It seems to be useful to start with the left breast at 12:00 o'clock radius and continue on the clockwise sense, because we will identify for the beginning the anatomy of the upper-outer quadrant, which has better developed lobes and thus the anatomy is easier to recognize. Then, the lobar size progressively decreases towards 6 o'clock and will be the smallest in the inner quadrants with more fatty tissue between the glandular lobes which will be easier to recognize; other operators are trained with different starting positions. In large breasts and for the axillary prolongation of the mammary gland, it is necessary to slip to the periphery of

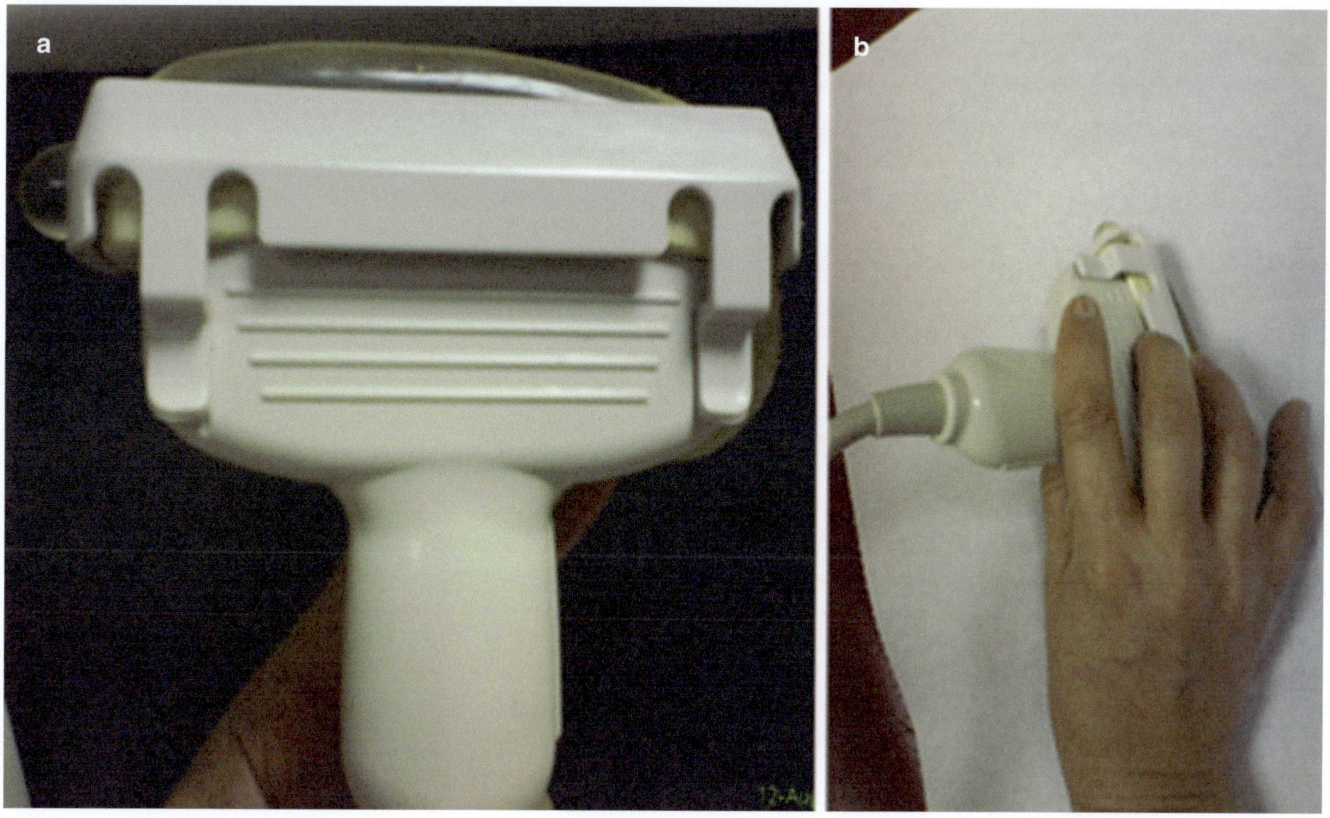

Fig. 2.2 A long probe of 8.5 cm with an adaptor for the water bag (**a**). The examination with rotation around the nipple for the radial scanning must be very gentle, without breast compression, and it is recommended to keep the fifth finger as a support on the skin

the radius, even when using a long probe, to cover the whole lobe, because omitting this area represents one reason for the false-negative exams of the US.

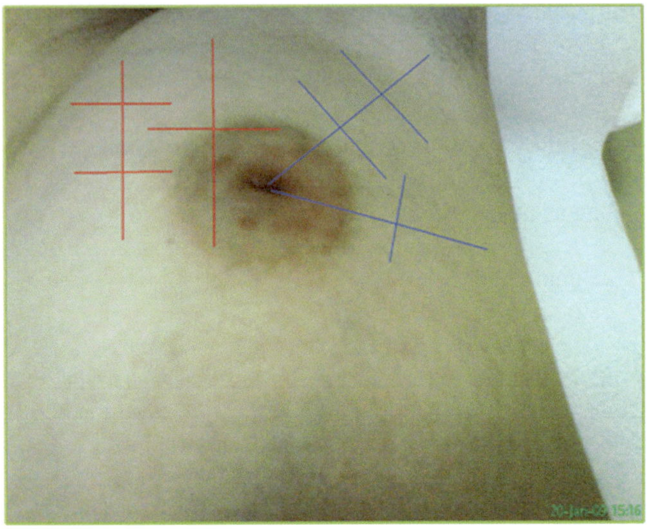

Fig. 2.3 DE will be performed following the model of the disposal of the mammary lobes, like a daisy petals, partially superposed. The radial scanning, in the main ductal axis of each lobe, completed with antiradial orthogonal scanning (*blue lines*), has the advantages of no "blind" areas and precise location upon the clockwise notation. The classical sagittal and transverse scanning (*red lines*) cannot be complete because the breast surface is not plane and there are various slipping of the transducer, and it is illogical because the breast anatomy is not corresponding to a chessboard or a random scan

Especially in the large breasts or when using short transducers, it is recommended to perform concentrically radial scanning, to cover the whole breast volume; any abnormality discovered implies the reconstruction of the complete radius for precise localization.

After identification of the normal structures, the abnormal findings are noted on a "map" noting the "hours" as the geographic "meridians" and precising the notations "R" for the right breast and "L" for the left breast. For example, "R6" represents a location at the 6:00 o'clock hour in the right breast; "L10:30" is the site in the left breast at 10:30H [6, 7]. We will mention the distances from the nipple to the lesions, equivalent to the globe's *parallels* or *circles of latitude*; thus, the precise location will be designated by standardized coordinates.

This reporting is useful both for the follow-up examinations, possibly performed by different sonographers and for a better location in the presumed therapeutic approaches (Figs. 2.4 and 2.5).

2. *In the second step will be performed a detailed ultrasonographic morphological analysis for each lesion noted on the map*, using the highest-frequency linear probe (transducer) available, in the radial and antiradial planes, for measuring the diameters and the volume of the lesion (Fig. 2.6). The demonstration of the connection of the lesion with the ductal-lobular tree is essential for the affirmation of a real mammary pathology, for the diagnosis of multicentric lesions and for the diagnosis of the "sick

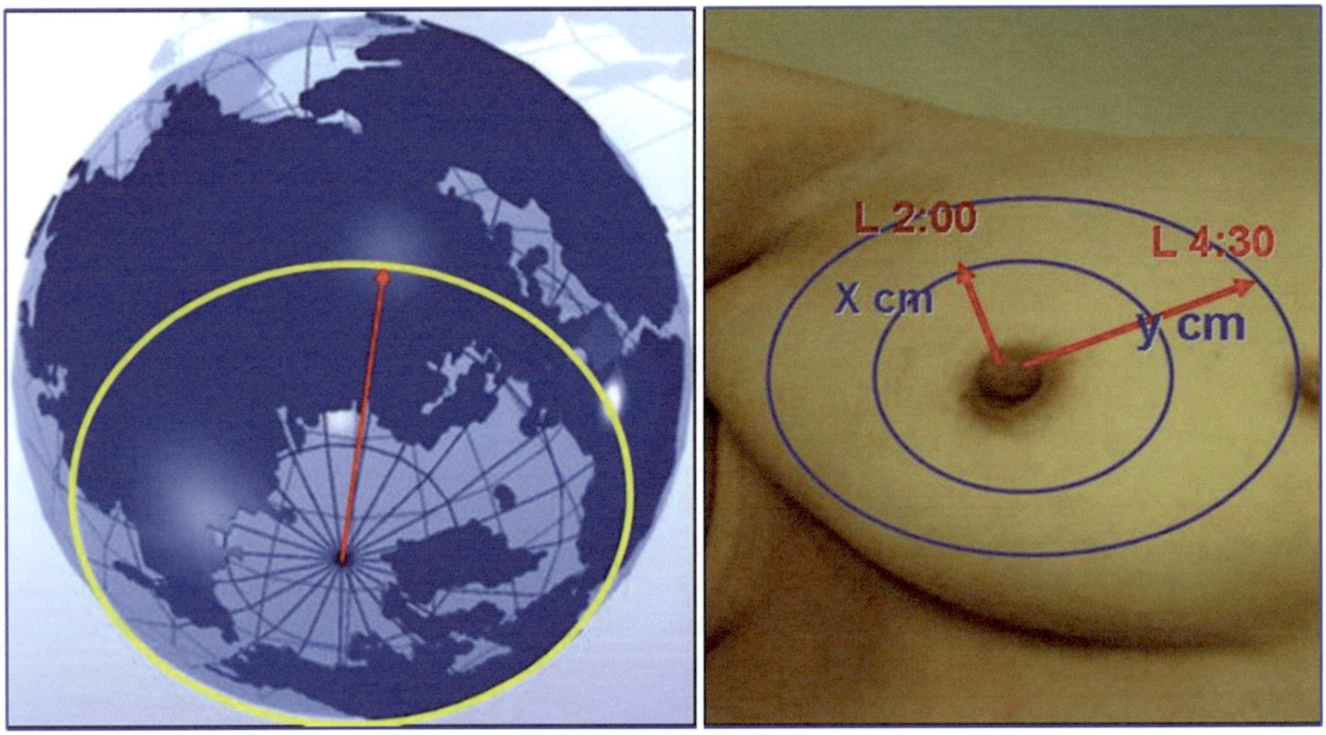

Fig. 2.4 Spatial coordinates: The horary marker represents "the meridian" and the distance nipple lesion represents "the parallel"

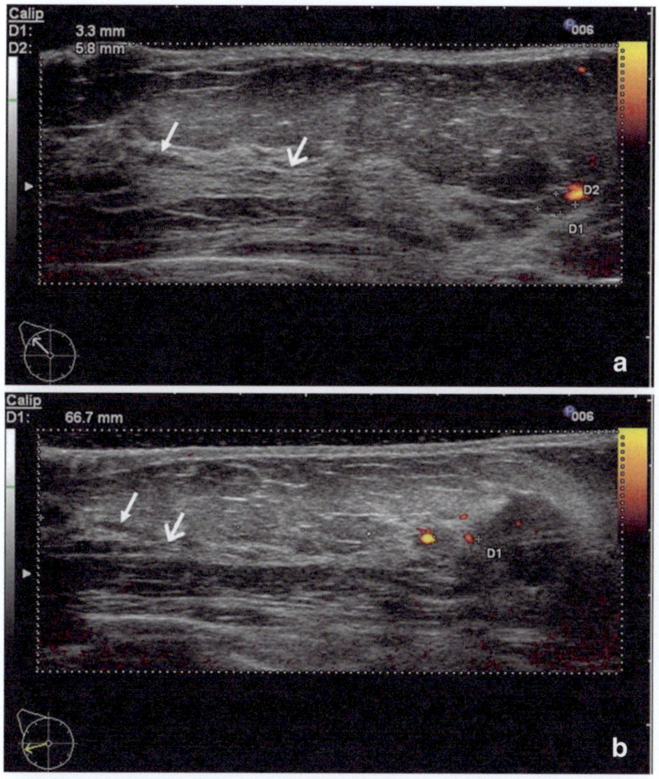

Fig. 2.5 The first step of the FBU: the whole breast exploring with DE is illustrated by R10:30 radial scan, with water-bag-long linear probe (**a**): the nipple is always on the *left side* of the image and the ducts and lobules are well-delimited by the surrounding hyperechoic stroma. In this case of a 56-year-old menopausal woman, there are thin, normal ducts (*open arrow*), hyperplasic ducts (*arrow*), and hyperplasic TDLUs (*calipers*). In R8:30 (**b**), the premalignant changes are associated with a peripheral suspect mass, at 67 mm distance from the nipple

lobe"; the volume is essential both for the treatment and for the follow-up of a "solid" mass or cyst. We can add 3D or 4D analyses for the volume and the relationships of the lesion; THI, Doppler, and eventually the CEUS are used for the characterization of the structure and of the vasculature of the lesion.

3. Finally, when possible, *in the third step, we will study the sonoelastography*, for the complete characterization of the risk of malignancy (Fig. 2.6).

The axillary and supra- and infraclavicular lymph nodes are always evaluated at the end of the examination of each breast, even in the case without suspect breast findings, and the 2D orthogonal planes, with Doppler and sonoelastography, should be performed. 3D/4D US could be valuable. Especially in suspect breast lesions located in the inner quadrants, the lymph nodes located along the intern mammary artery must be checked because the cartilaginous parts of the ribs are good sonographic "windows."

2.3 About 3D and 4D US Technique Related to DE

Two principal techniques and the combination of both exist to obtain 3D US information: manual or automatic scanner movement with echo data processing along the US beam. In about 3 s, the system obtains the entire 3D data volume set (about 10 MByte) and displays the information in a multiplanar image display mode (Fig. 2.7), while the 4D technique displays in real time the volume and the multiplanar orthogonal slices (Fig. 2.8).

The reasons for multiplanar examination in DE are the following [8, 9]:

- Measuring the lesion in three axes and calculating its volume, for short follow-up or therapeutically decision
- Establishing the basic anatomy of each breast, the size, the density, and the size of ducts and lobules, the thickness of the breast stroma, and the relationships of the TDLUs with the Cooper ligaments
- Establishing the breast architecture, for biopsy or surgical/postsurgical approach: lumpectomy or better lobectomy, breast reduction, and breast prosthesis

The multiplanar representation uses the 3D US information from the three planes (A, B, and C plane) that cut the voxel (the smallest box-shaped part of a three-dimensional image or scan) and are orthogonal to each other. In the classical US scanning, the planes A and B are random and so are irreproducible, and the C plane completing the information is usually parallel with the skin or the thoracic retromammary plane [2], without specific relation with the nipple's site.

Computer-aided diagnosis represented a false perspective for the improvement of the breast US by an objective analysis and standardization [10], because it was applied to the classical breast scan, which does not respect the anatomical architecture of the breast and thus does not analyze the normal ductal-lobular tree as base of the search for pathological findings. The advantage of DE is the standardization, with plane A being radial, following the ductal axis, allowing the measurement of the anterior-posterior and the longitudinal/radial diameters; plane B is antiradial and keeps the anterior-posterior diameter as reference, completing with the diameter antiradial orthogonal to the other two. Furthermore, the system allows the navigation through the entire acquired volume, conducting parallel interactive movement through the image slices and synchronous parallel image movement in all of the corresponding orthogonal planes.

The acquired US volume data allows a variety of three-dimensional rendering modes, and the most effective for visibility of the biopsy needle inside the 3D data set are transparency modes. Combined with an animated rotation of

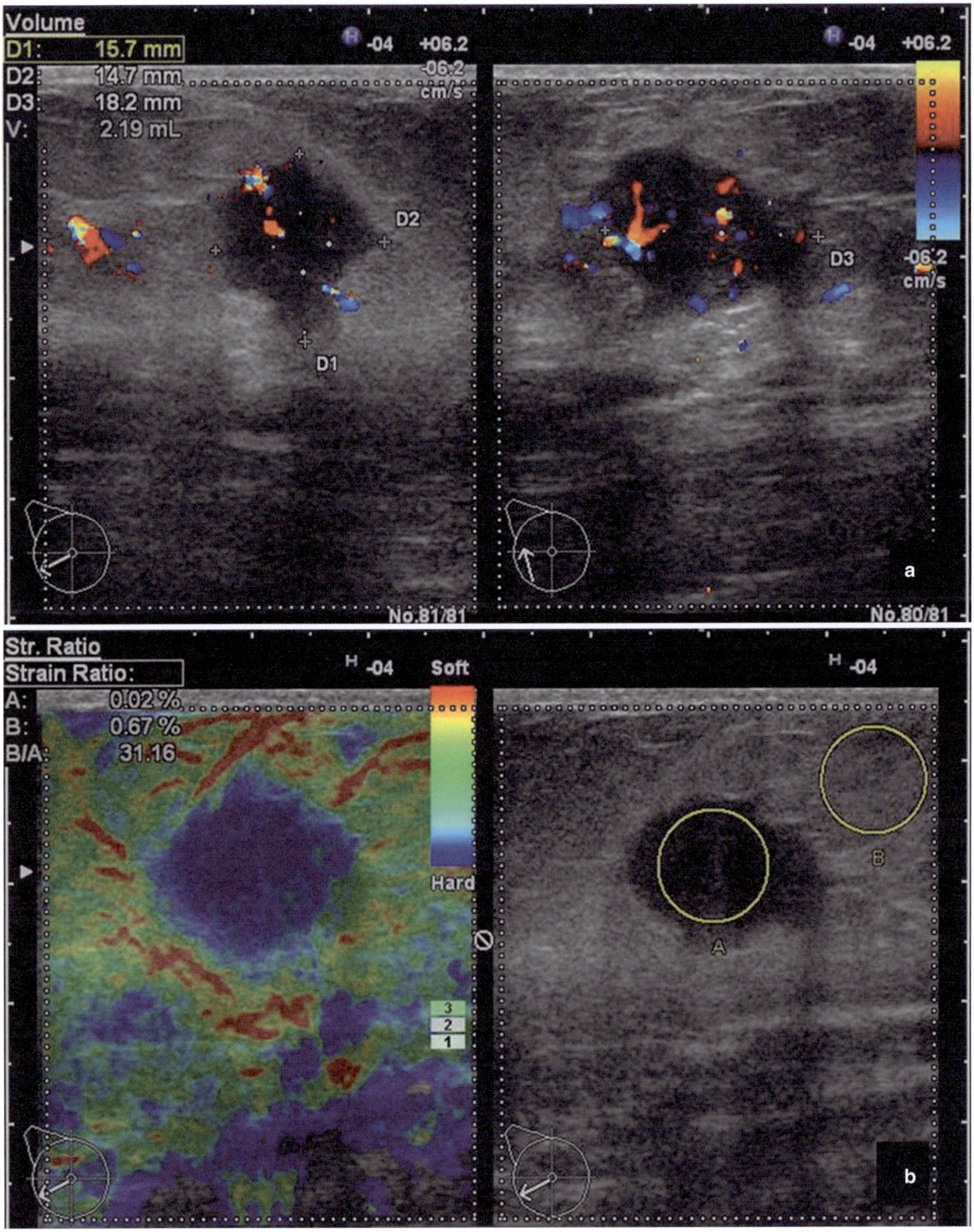

Fig. 2.6 The second step of examination in FBU (**a**), using a high-resolution "short" linear probe, in the radial and antiradial scans with Doppler research: the general features suggest malignancy, but without the halo of the desmoplastic reaction and without posterior shadowing. The third step (**b**) represented by sonoelastography for the characterization of the malignancy risk demonstrates a stiff lesion, scored 4 upon Ueno, with high FLR value, concordant with malignancy (US BI-RADS 5 category)

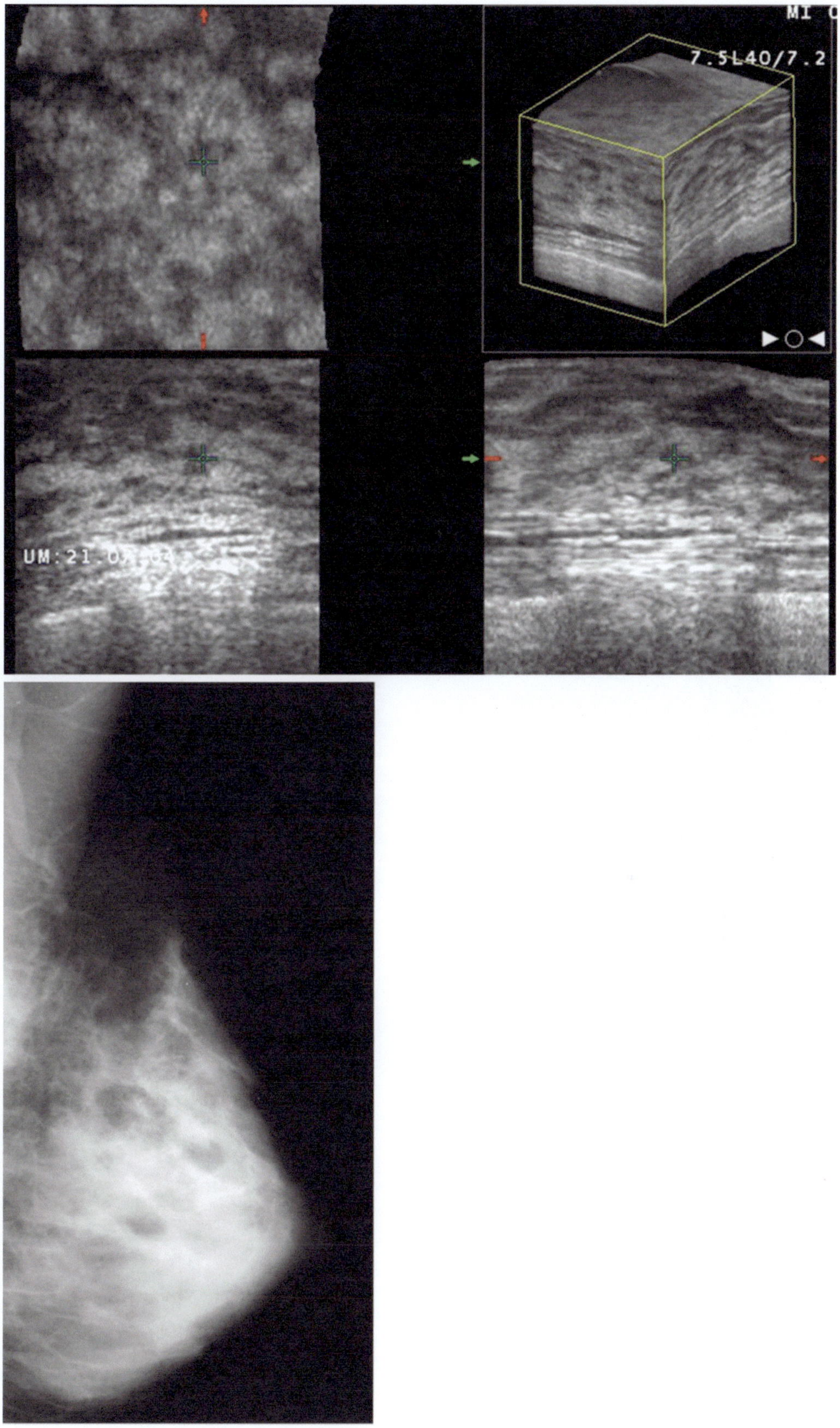

Fig. 2.7 The 3D technique, as a complementary method to the DE, better illustrates the architecture of the breast parenchyma, in this case of dense breast demonstrating clearly the lobules connected to the ducts (*calipers*). Despite the random scan in this 3D US, we are able to identify the real normal "architecture," and an eventually pathological distortion will be easy to discover and interpret, while on the mammogram of the same case, the analysis of the "breast architecture" is illusory

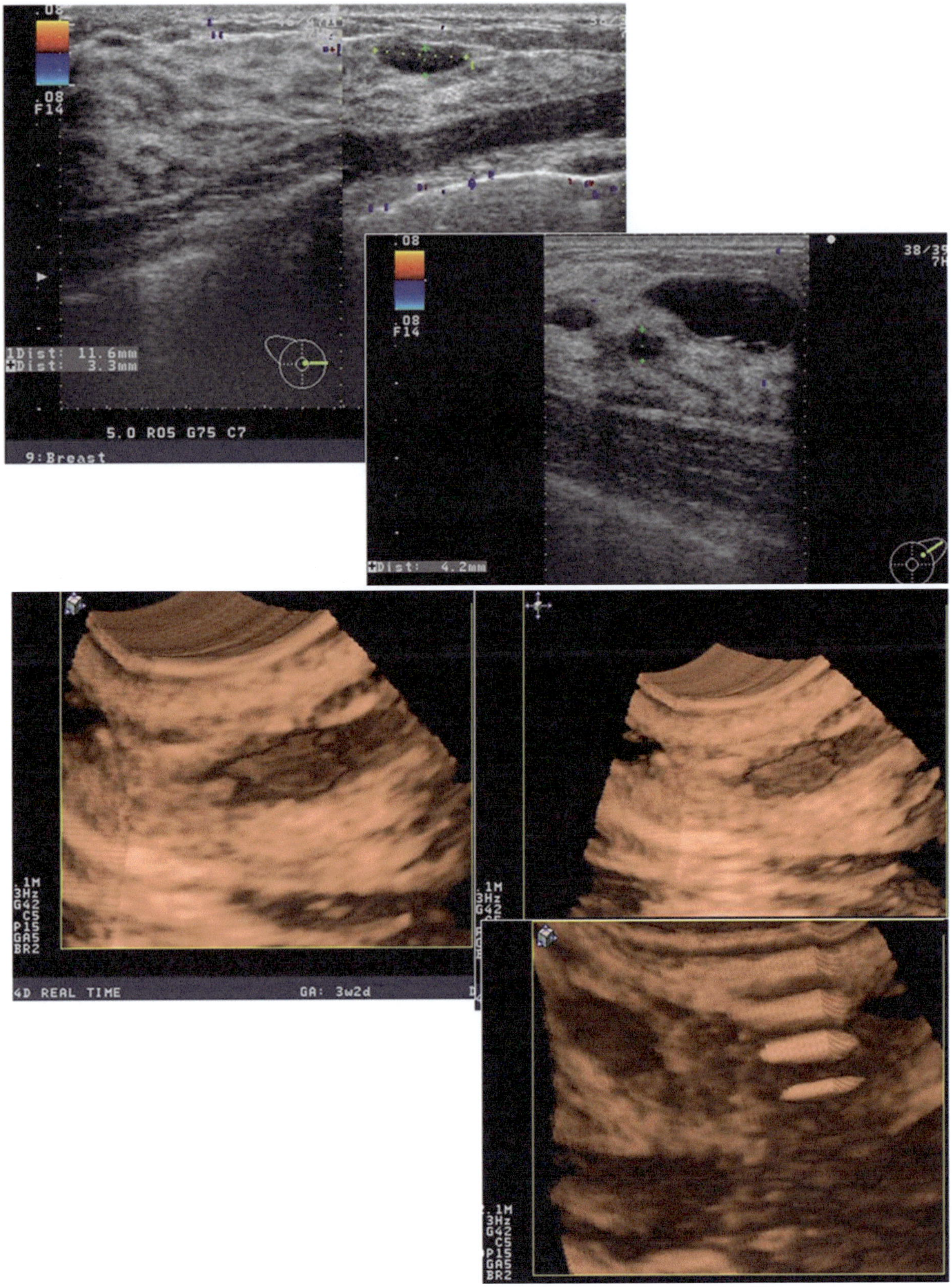

Fig. 2.8 The 4D utility as an additional tool to ductal US offers less precision of the lesions' location, but a good global representation of the breast; the lesions could be analyzed using different opacity levels, zooming, rotations, and angulations. These 4D/3D representations are impressive illustrations especially for the patients and for the clinicians, but the diagnosis has no significant improvements, such as in this case with cystic dysplasia

the transparent rendered tissue of the initially or virtually sectioned block, the position of the lesion or of the needle in relation to the lesion can also be better evaluated.

Up to date, few equipments are able to realize 3D power Doppler characterization of the lesion, much important than scanning 2D power Doppler technique [11].

3D result image is a constructed model of the lesion; the size and shape are operator dependent, especially related to the speed and the angulations of the transducer during the acquisition.

4D examination is better because the simultaneous acquisition of the entire volume allows accurate measurement and allows a better "navigation" for the surgical approach [12] or even for the targeted biopsy [13].

Another recent modality of spatial distribution is the parallel multislice rendering, similar to the sectional computed tomography, but his availability is restricted yet. After 2010 Siemens installed in many countries the automated breast volume scanner (ABVS), which accelerates breast examinations, reducing the required acquisition time to less than 15 min, offers the plan C in multislice rendering, and is intended to be operator independent. ABVS is not possible in large breasts, where we must perform automatic scanning of arbitrary denominated regions with indefinite limits, suitably superposed. For all breasts, only the coronal plane (plan C) offers the distance between the structures to be analyzed and the nipple; all the three plans are unuseful for the breast anatomy, because the lobar architecture and the main galactophorous duct are fragmental illustrated. As consequence, the "sick lobe" could never be demonstrated, because the multifocal lesions are less probable to be situated on the same plane whatever it could be; indeed, the ductal tree has an oblique orientation to all this ABVS planes. Moreover, the ABVS is intended to screening for the breast cancer, neglecting the benign or premalignant lesions.

2.4 Usefulness of the Panoramic Scans: SieScape-Type Technique Versus DE

Because the *field of view* (FOV) of the images acquired with former real-time ultrasound system was limited by the probe's size, it had sometimes difficulty in obtaining the whole image of the breast disease. Thus, it was imagined a panoramic view with automatic or freehand acquisition, which results in statically random scans of large regions of the breast (Fig. 2.9).

The panoramic view may be useful in large tumors, such as giant fibroadenoma or phyllodes tumor, in mastitis, or in the implant assessment. It could be useful for scanning continual intraductal structures, and thus, SieScape/panoramic view represents an important advancing technique in the anatomical study of the breast.

There are inherent limits of the panoramic scans: the lack of precision, the image resulted being a construction, depending on the speed of the transducer's movement (no any measurements in the horizontal plane, but only in the anterior-posterior plane); furthermore, this technique is imprecise as localization, rarely we will pass by the same route, thus the panoramic scan is not reproducible, the technique being operator and hazard dependent.

Additionally, as long is the SieScape scan, as much deformation by reconstruction we will obtain, inacceptable for a screening technique and incomparable with the precision and repeatability of DE with long probe; we can use only power Doppler in the panoramic technique, with motion artifacts, while in DE we can use any Doppler analysis and also the sonoelastography.

2.5 Reporting

Reporting data will include:

- *Clinical context* (notes about the familial or personal history related to the breast pathology, hormonal therapeutic or substitutive treatment, clinical signs and symptoms, last menstrual period, and other biological significant test results).
- *Analytical description of the breast architecture*:
  - Notation of the type of the anatomical-physiological structure (young-dense breast, adult dense breast, mixed or fatty breast, lactation breast)
  - General size of the ducts and lobules
  - Development of the breast glandular stroma (thin/less, medium/normal, thick/large) and evaluation of the general vascular aspect
  - Eventually changes of the skin, fatty tissue, or the thoracic wall
- *Analytical description of each lesion*: the site, the rapports with the ductal-lobular tree, the size/volume, and the characters upon Stavros included in the US BI-RADS assessment—the depth-to-width ratio, the shape, the contour, the internal echoes, the posterior effects, the vasculature (absent, increased by hyperemia or new vessels, number of vascular poles, their course arcuate or with incident plunging angle); the sonoelasticity should qualitatively and quantitatively complete the characterization of the lesion, and the final diagnosis will be the results of all descriptors.
- *Aspect of the lymph nodes*: axillary, subclavicular, and internal mammary, their location and number of pathological nodes "found," and the size, contour, internal structure, vasculature, and sonoelasticity.
- *Conclusion and the US BI-RADS category assessment.*
- *Recommendations.*

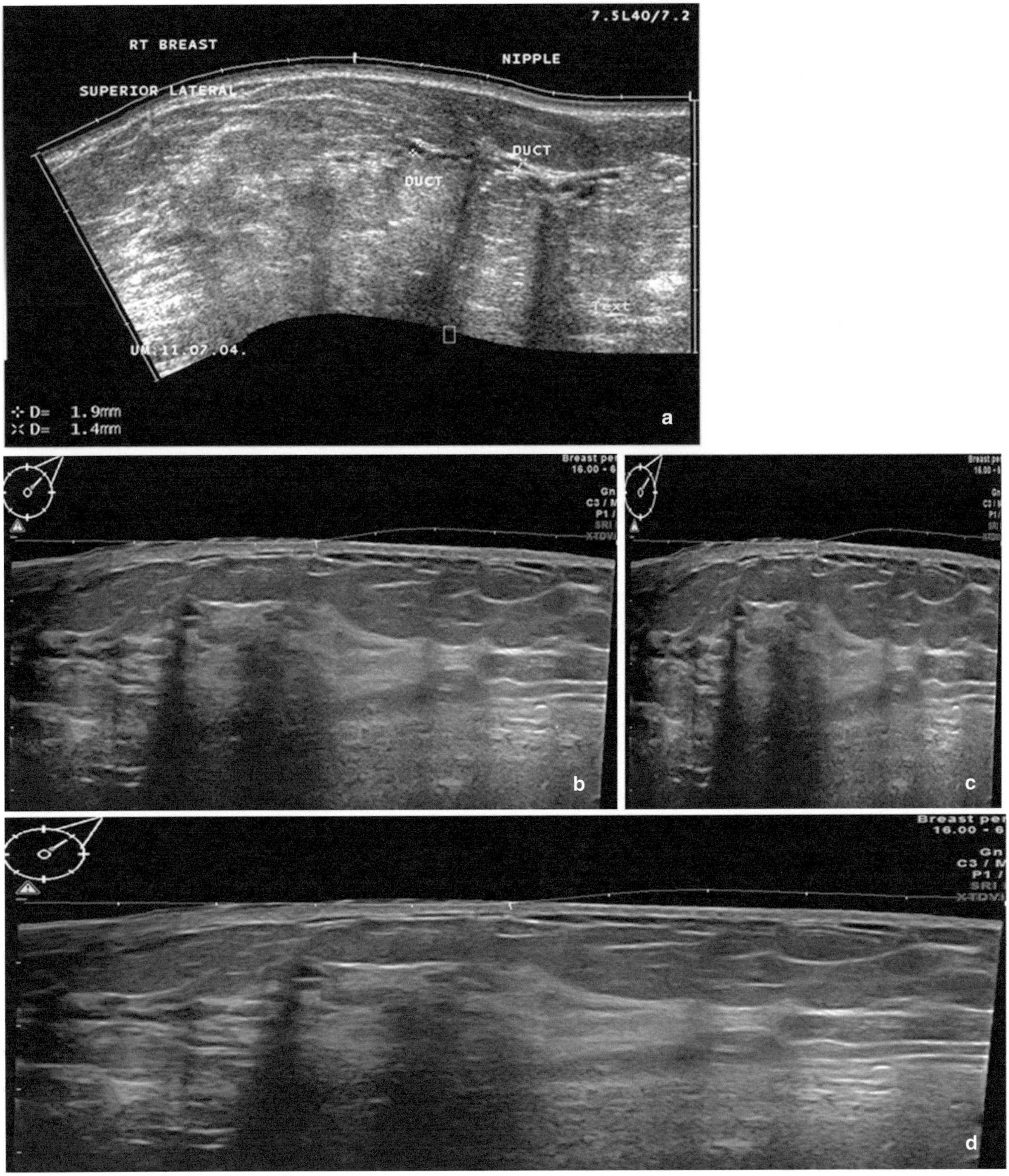

Fig. 2.9 The panoramic view in symptomatic breast with mastodynia revealed ductal ectasia; despite the large scan, when performed without any anatomical radial scanning, this type of acquisition is difficult to interpret, the location of a lesion is imprecise, and the image is irreproducible and thus is not useful in screening or as follow-up exam (**a**). When using the panoramic view with radial scanning, we better recognize the anatomy (**b**–**d**), but we can obtain different horizontal lengths according to the acquisition speed, as we imitate trying to reproduce the same anatomy (impossible in reality!) acquired with different speeds (**c**, **d**)

References

1. Teboul M, Halliwell M (1995) Ductal echography: the correct ultrasonic approach to the breast. In: Teboul M, Halliwell M (eds) Atlas of ultrasound and ductal echography of the breast. Blackwell Scientific, Oxford, p 83
2. Berg WA, Blume JD, Cormack JB, Mendelson EB (2006) Operator dependence of physician-performed whole-breast US: lesion detection and characterization © RSNA, 2007. Radiology 241:355–365, © RSNA, 2006
3. Teboul M (2003) Practical ductal echography: guide to intelligent and intelligible ultrasound imaging of the breast. Saned Editors, Madrid
4. Georgescu AC, Enachescu V, Bondari S (2010) The full breast ultrasonography: an anatomical standardized imaging approach of the benign and malignant breast lesions. doi:10.1594/ecr2010/C-0434
5. Amy D (2010) Lobar ultrasound of the breast. In: Breast cancer, 1.T. Tot (ed), © Springer, London Limited. doi:10.1007/978-1-84996-314-5_8
6. Amy D (2000) Echographie mammaire: echoanatomie. JL mensuel d'echographie LUS 10:654–662
7. Teboul M (2010) Advantages of Ductal Echography (DE) over Conventional Breast Investigation in the diagnosis of breast malignancies. Med Ultrason 12(1):32–42
8. Chang R-F, Huang SF, Chen D-R, Moon WK (2003) Detection of speculation in three-dimensional breast Ultrasound. 13th International congress on the ultrasonic examination of the breast. International Breast Ultrasound School. The 10th meeting of Japan Association of Breast and Thyroid Sonology
9. Rotten D, Levaillant J-M, Zerat L (1998) Use of three-dimensional ultrasound mammography to analyze normal breast tissue and solid breast masses. In: Merz E (ed) 3-D ultrasonography in obstetrics and gynecology. Lippincott Willams & Wilkins, Philadelphia, Chap. 11, pp 73–78
10. Chang R-F, Chen W-M, Chen D-R, Moon W-K (2003) Three-dimensional breast Ultrasound Computer Aided Diagnosis. 13th international congress on the ultrasonic examination of the breast. International Breast Ultrasound School. The 10th meeting of Japan Association of Breast and Thyroid Sonology
11. Moon WK, Chang R-F (2007) Solid breast masses: neural network analysis of 3-D power Doppler ultrasound image features for classification as benign or malignant. ECR, Vienna, B-278. http://www.myesr.org/html/img/pool/3_ECR_2007_Final_Programme_web.pdf
12. Tamaki Y, Inoue T, Tanji Y, Noguchi S (2003) 3D ultrasound navigation for breast cancer surgery. 13th international congress on the ultrasonic examination of the breast. International Breast Ultrasound School. The 10th meeting of Japan Association of Breast and Thyroid Sonology
13. Weismann CF, Forstner R, Prokop E et al (2000) Three-dimensional targeting: a new three-dimensional ultrasound technique to evaluate needle position during breast biopsy. Ultrasound Obstet Gynecol 16:359–364

3 Breast Development: Aspects of Doppler Ductal Ultrasonography of the Normal Breast

3.1 Breast Development

Breast development is not continuous, but has different stages in the intrauterine and extrauterine life. The precursor to the human breast originates in the "milk line," developed from some ectodermic elements and extended from the axillary area to the groin region, at about 6 weeks of the embryonic life. The middle and caudal portions of the milk line atrophy except in the region of the fourth intercostal space, from which the mammary bud develops [1]. When the appropriate portions of the milk line do not regress, accessory nipples with or without underlying breast tissue develop, decreasing in size as the distance from the normal nipple is longer (Fig. 3.1).

The presence of a mammary-specific bud in the newborn is certified by the hormonal mammary crisis in the first weeks of life, when a swollen bud and sometimes even a minimal lactiferous secretion appear.

The mammary bud rests unchanged after the newborn crisis for years during childhood. Breast development restarts in adolescence, with the surge of coordinated interactions of many hormones. Estrogen is the hormone primarily responsible for ductal development, while the progesterone is needed for lobular-alveolar development. This is the reason for ductal development in gynecomastia, associated with elevated estrogens and usually absence of the lobules because the progesterone is rarely elevated in men. Breast development is present, almost normal, in the Rokitansky-Küster-Hauser syndrome, characterized by the absence of the uterus because of the absence of development of the Müller ducts, but usually with the presence of the ovaries; otherwise, the breast is hypoplastic in Turner (45XO) syndrome, associated with amenorrhea.

Thelarche, the development of the breast bud, begins with the onset of puberty (mean age, 9.8 years). Premature thelarche is defined as breast development before the age of 8 years [2], while the lack of development before age 13 years is considered delayed.

The Tanner grading system is commonly used to describe the clinical stages of breast development:

- *Stage I, preadolescent*; the nipple elevates.
- *Stage II: the breast bud develops*; the breast tissue and nipple arise as a single mound of tissue.
- *Stage III: the single mound enlarges.*
- *Stage IV: a secondary mound develops*, with the nipple and areola projecting above the breast tissue.
- *Stage V: the areola regresses* to form a smooth contour with the rest of the breast tissue.

Adolescent patients may have a "breast mass" that represents the normal developing breast bud. Confounding the situation, especially in premature thelarche and because breast development may be asymmetrical and painful, the more developed side may be perceived as a "lump." Classical US examination over the palpable area shows "normal tissue" without a discrete mass lesion, but the anatomical correlation with the sonographic images is not

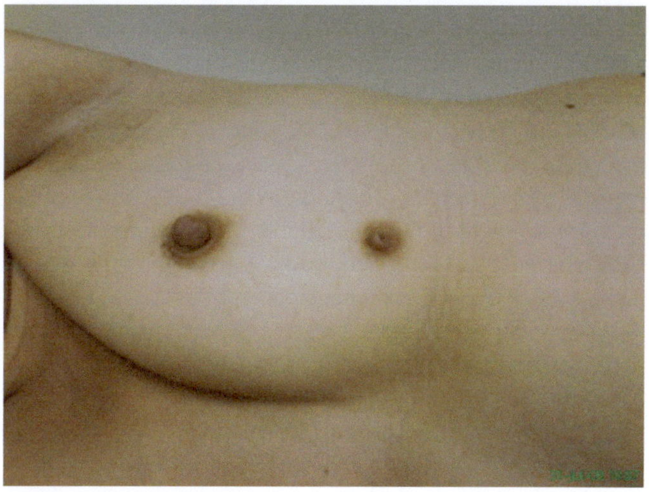

Fig. 3.1 Accessory nipple

A. Colan-Georges, *Atlas of Full Breast Ultrasonography*, DOI 10.1007/978-3-319-31418-1_3

well précised. Surgical excision must be avoided in these patients because iatrogenic amastia results if the breast bud is excised.

The normal DE aspect of the developing breast will be further described in this chapter.

3.2 Breast Anatomy and Ductal Echography

Classical US is less performing because of both wrong scanning and of the wrong interpretation of the imaging aspects with vague notions such as "breast tissue," "low echo area," "fibroglandular tissue," etc.

The DE is "intelligible" because the acquisition technique and the descriptive terms are necessarily anatomical and related to ducts (Figs. 3.2, 3.3, 3.4, 3.5, 3.6, 3.7, 3.8, 3.9, 3.10, 3.11, 3.12, 3.13, 3.14, 3.15, 3.16, 3.17, 3.18, 3.19, 3.20, 3.21, 3.22, 3.23, 3.24, 3.25, 3.26, 3.27, 3.28, 3.29, and 3.30).

The Skin It appears as a brightly echogenic complex, which can have a laminar appearance and usually is less than 3 mm thickness. The areolar tissue, represented by a loose network of fibrous tissue and elastic fiber that connect the skin to the underlying structures and the nipple, is quite thicker and hypoechoic in adult and may present irregularities because of the Montgomery's glands.

Cutaneous and subcutaneous palpable lumps such as sebaceous cysts are common, and it is therefore important to image the skin layer well, using a standoff or better using a water bag. The areola changes in diameters and thickens by reflex contraction of some smooth muscular fibers, and this reversible aspect must not be considered as pathological. Rarely, some pores of the ductal-ampullary systems have aberrant openings in the areolar surface, outside the nipple.

The Fatty Lobules Elliptical lobules of medium-gray echogenicity contain characteristic linear and punctate echogenic foci. Medium-gray echogenicity of the subcutaneous fatty layer is the standard against which the echogenicity of any masses in the breast is compared, because this layer is more constant; moreover, the elasticity of the breast structures is reported to the fatty tissue elasticity ("fat-to-lesion ratio"—FLR), because the fat is "the softest" tissue and the malignant lesions have always more stiffness.

The aspect of the fatty tissue is depending on the age, nutrition, and hormonal status including physiological and pathological changes. The typical aspect is a continuous braiding fashion without abrupt margination, divided by *fascia superficialis* into a subcutaneous, uniform layer (hypoderm) and a subfascial, deep pre- and retromammary layer (Fig. 3.2). The subfascial fatty tissue has the characteristic aspect in *gothic arcs* or *tents* at the limit with the mammary lobe, where the Cooper ligaments intersect. The superficial fatty tissue is absent in the retroareolar area, where the ductal ampullae/sinuses are located superficially, convergent to the nipple. Fatty lobules may intermix equally with glandular mammary lobes or between different branches of a lobe, producing an overall heterogeneous appearance of the mammary scan on classical US, which is responsible for many misinterpreting images. This mixed structure is better analyzed in DE, where the continuity of the ducts equally hypoechoic but surrounded by the hyperechoic glandular stroma offers the overall image of the distinct compact or branching glandular lobe.

The disposition and the quantity of the fatty lobes are different according to the breast quadrants: less fatty tissue in the outer quadrants, more peripheral with fewer fats between the mammary lobes, justifying the dense aspect on mammography of the upper-outer quadrants, and progressively smaller mammary glandular lobes with much more interlobar fat in the inner quadrants, with a radiolucent aspect on mammography.

In the young breast or in cases with hyperestrogenism or malnutrition, the glandular mammary lobes present areas in contact with the skin, on the sites of lack of fatty layer, determining a pseudonodular aspect on palpation because of differences in tissues consistency. Otherwise, in obese patients, physiological glandular atrophy in menopause, or pathological atrophy in ovarian insufficiency, the fat is dominant in all quadrants, while the mammary lobes are thin, with few amount of glandular hyperechoic stroma and linear, submillimetric galactophorous ducts without visible lobules. The fatty breasts present longer apparent Cooper ligaments. The regions in the vicinity of the Cooper ligaments include the atrophic TDLUs, the site of the developing of the most benign and malignant breast lesions. In the classical US, some cancers apparently are surrounded by fatty tissue, but they are located along the Cooper ligaments and are developed from remnants of the TDLUs; these aspects are difficult to detect without DE because both fat and cancer are hypoechoic.

In the literature, the general opinion is that in fatty breast, malignancies are less visible on US because of their hypoechogenicity, similar to those of the adipose tissue. Moreover, some authors were surprised that fatty tissue was found to be more hypoechoic in breast than elsewhere, and fantasy was used to present explanations [3]. In fact, fatty tissue in the breast is not delineated from the subcutaneous fatty tissue of the surrounding regions, but there is a continuous layer from the breast hypoderm to the axillary, thoracic, abdominal, or upper and lower limb regions. The misunderstanding of the fatty tissue on the classical US images can be explained by the small areas visualized using short linear transducers, and consequently by neglecting the anatomy of the whole segment explored. In fact, the superficial fatty tissue of the body is hypoechoic because of the high-frequency probe used, which has better resolution and can magnify the tissular structures, while the abdominal probes have usually lower frequency and so less resolution; moreover, the subcutaneous fat is represented by larger cells, with fewer interface echoes, which thus results to hypoechogenicity, while the deeper fat, for example, the retroperitoneal fat, is usually hyperechoic due to the smaller cells with a higher number of interfaces (internal echoes of the tissue). Even the retroperitoneal fat, in obese patients, presents a relative hypoechogenicity, with the internal echoes similar to the subcutaneous adipose tissue. The same explanation is for breast lipomas, which are usually hyperechoic, because of the greater number of smaller cells (adipocytes) than in the normal hypoderm.

Moreover, with the probes of more than 7 MHz, we can see two layers of the superficial fat of the breast: the hypodermal layer separated by *fascia superficialis corpora* from the second fatty layer that cover the true mammary structures; fascia superficialis appears on a scan as thin, undulated hyperechoic line, composed of the superficial part of the Cooper ligaments, which change their oblique direction, fuse together, and become parallel with the skin.

The True Breast Parenchyma: Galactophorous Ducts and Lobules As defined, the breast comprises a branching system of ducts leading down from the nipple (Figs. 3.4 and 3.5) and ending in acini aggregated into lobules, which have the potential to secrete milk. The subdivisions of the lactiferous ducts form regular and simple to complex branching breast segments and are different from one woman to another. One lobe contains 1–3 main ducts, with their secondary and tertiary branching ducts ending with lobules; even the lobes are thought to be distinct/discrete anatomically and physiologically, and they may interdigitate with each other at their boundaries without connection between the ductal branches. The ducts branching ultimately are giving rise to the TDLUs.

The breast parenchyma is better interpreted in US in relationship with the nipple, the ductal-ampullary units being better visualized when they are fulfilled with fluid contents. Despite that the radiological galactography offered a range of the main ductal size and of their branches, whose lumen has limits from few millimeters to less 0.5 mm, and despite that the high resolution of the highest-frequency transducers allows accurate measurements of 0.4 mm, there are still opinions that US cannot visualize the main ducts and the lobules described by Teboul. In fact, breast MRI that has a lower resolution demonstrates the images of ductal segments and of lobules. The negation of visibility of mammary ducts in US is the translation of the impossibility to visualize the breast parenchyma in mammography, due to the X-ray low absorption. The pathological ducts, even with peripheral location, are enlarged/thicker than the normal surrounding thin branches and are well identified in US because either hyperplasia or duct ectasia is more hypoechoic. The lobules are usually up to double the size of the nearby ducts and isolated or contiguous and may be unapparent in glandular atrophy.

It is unanimously accepted that one breast ("the complex mammary gland") contains 14–20–25 lobes/segments ("simple mammary gland") arranged radially around the nipple as daisy petals. Each lobe is based on a branching ductal system, with one or more main ducts, collecting from segmental and subsegmental ducts that end with terminal lobules containing alveoli/acini. There is theoretical and practical assessment that lobes are distinct, without interlobar anastomosing, in concordance with the *sick lobe theory* [4]. Some authors noted some rare presence of intersegmental anastomoses, without clinical significance [5]. The distinct lobes are proved by galactography, despite the absence of a "capsule" or other anatomical boundaries, with difficulties in their histological delimitation in random small section; the gross section upon Tibor Tot [4] in a radial axis may better illustrate the lobar anatomy, but cannot delineate its boundaries.

In the classical approach, the amount of "glandular tissue" in the breast is dependent on the hormonal activity and fluctuates with the menstrual cycle. This aspect determines the schedule of the mammograms for the first week of the menstrual cycle, because in the luteal and premenstrual phase, the intensity of the breast glandular opacity increases and needs increasing of the radiation dose with less contrast or anatomical details on the radiological film. It was not clear which anatomical component is responsible for the cyclical menstrual changes in "breast tissue," but almost all ultrasonographers are neglecting this relationship because the US images are less influenced. US observations of the ductal and lobular thickness during the menstrual cycle did not reveal any significant changes, but it is possible that the glandular stroma increases its volume in the premenstrual phase by fluid imbibitions, thus determining the higher attenuation on mammography. Another argument for the hormonal involvement of the glandular stroma in determining the radiological attenuation is obtained by comparing the breast radiologically increased densities in cases with large amount of stroma in US and the "radiotransparency" of the breast parenchyma (ducts and lobules) in cases with less stroma but with parenchymal hyperplasia demonstrated by DE.

The ducts and alveoli are lined by two layers of epithelium (one layer of continuous, secretor epithelium with milk-secreting cuboidal cells, surrounded by a discontinuous peripheral layer of myoepithelial cells with receptors for oxytocin), supported by a basement membrane. Most diseases of the breast affect ducts and lobules, and carcinomas (cancers) arise from the epithelial cells lining these branching structures. Because in the young the ductal epithelium is folded, the ducts are thicker and may mimic hyperplasias; in adulthood, the walls are smooth, and US demonstrates the walls delineated by the interfaces with the virtual lumen as a couple of regular, less than 1 mm each, hypoechoic lines with a central hyperechoic line. A small amount of intraductal fluid determines the "double line sign" with two interfaces of wall/fluid. That demonstrates the ductal visibility in US, of the same size such as MRI presentation. Sonoelastography of the normal ducts shows parallel soft lines in green upon the Ueno/Tsukuba scale, represented by the ductal walls, with central band in red for the fluid in small ectasias, while the largest ones appear with a BGR (blue-green-red) score similar to the cysts.

There are different models of a breast lobe in the modern approach. The simplest, but representing the key of the DE, is the model of Teboul (1995), also sustained by Amy [6, 7]. In this model, a lobe has an ovoidal shape and is arranged radial around the nipple as a daisy petal. The main duct(s) is (are) oriented with the longitudinal axis from the nipple to the periphery of the breast radius and it branches in ductules ended by lobules aligned each side as the roadside trees, one row of lobules superficial, oriented to the transducer, another one deeper, posterior from the main duct, usually of smaller size. The lobules are oblique-perpendicularly oriented to the duct, so the early fibroadenoma originating in the lobule has initially the long axis perpendicular to the skin, an inverse deep/wide range than is known for benign masses; in time, the growing lobule becomes oblique until lies on the horizontal plane and appears as a typical fibroadenoma. The intersection of the Cooper ligament axis with the ductal-lobular axis represents the site of the TDLUs, considered the initiation site of the most benign or malignant lesions (Fig. 3.8).

There are other radial models more complex of the mammary lobe. In 1984, Ohuchi et al. described the beginning site of different malignancies; then in 2001 and in 2005, Ichihara and Ohitake et al. imagined a complete three-dimensional network model, with individual duct systems (lobes) arranged radially, with irregular branching pattern and a sector-shaped overall distribution [5]. This model explains that several duct systems overlap one another in the same region of the breast, in different planes superposed on the radial scan, but separated by the interlobar fatty lobes. The branching lobes based on branching ducts offer the explanation for multicentric distant cancers apparently located in different lobes; we can prove the same lobar location "*following the duct*," as Teboul says, up to finding the ductal confluence, confirming the *sick lobe* theory. Practically, the two models are concordant, and technically, following the ducts, we will find all spreading ductal tumors, which seem to have a centripetal/centrifugal evolution upon the minimal intraductal pressure; some malignancies are connected to the nipple by duct ectasia, even when there is not present nipple surge.

In conclusion, in DE, the main ducts extend radially from the nipple, where they begin in the ampullae/sinus with the dilated lumen and then course parallel to the chest wall in the supine patient position. The main ducts present as hypo- to isoechoic linear structures ranging in size generally on few millimeters in diameter, usually 1–2.5 mm. The ductal lumen can be visible in a collapsed duct as a thin central echogenic line, better illustrated when incident US wave is applied (*the sign of the central hyperechoic line*) (Fig. 3.6). The central hyperechoic line is useful as differential diagnosis between ductal cylindrical hyperplasia and intraductal papilloma or ductal carcinoma in situ of the *comedo* or the *cribriform* type (*the central hyperechoic line sign* is absent). The ductal lumen can contain a small amount of fluid determining the presence of a couple of parallel intraductal hyperechoic lines representing the interfaces of the wall epithelium with the ductal fluid (*the double line sign*). Some cases present intraductal vegetations, easier to visualize in the presence of ductal fluid. Radial and antiradial scanning allows better evaluation of ductal lumen and allows the differential diagnosis of ductal ectasia from the microcysts.

The TDLUs can be identified in some patients as a globular-shaped, blunt-ending projection of the duct running in an oblique-perpendicular orientation. In DE, we can observe, mainly in young breasts and in lobular hyperplasia, the lobules which are blunt-ending isoechoic ovoidal structures, with the long axis oblique-perpendicular to the draining duct, of 2–4 mm in size, and the short axis a bit larger than those of the connecting ductal diameter. With actual up to 14 MHz probes, the vasculature of the normal lobules is not detectable on Doppler, so any micronodule less 6 mm diameter connected to the ductal-lobular tree, with lobular appearance, without any malignant sign on 2D US but with a salient vascular pole is suspect (Fig. 3.7).

The appearance of ducts and lobules (composed of the microscopic acini) within each breast, and even into the same breast, is variable. Appearance is considered within normal limits as long as in DE the ducts and lobules appear normally oriented, of uniform shape and dimension in the same lobe, with gradual changes from a quadrant to another, and with no areas of focal dilatation of the lumen, thickening of the walls, or demonstrated increasing vasculature. Some rare cases present abnormal helical ductal orientation together with the whole breast lobe, with a pseudonodular shape named "breast within a breast" malformation (Figs. 3.9 and 3.10).

The Cooper ligaments as they are described in anatomy are fibrous bands connecting the pectoralis fascia with the deep dermal surface, with an arcaded orientation, running across the retromammary fatty tissue, the lobar structures, and subcutaneous fatty tissue up to the deep dermal surface. These thin hyperechoic septae serve as supportive fibrous septae of the breast. They can produce an appearance of segmental echogenic arcs, which scallop fatty lobules in the superficial mammary layer, sometimes with pseudotumoral palpable aspect, especially in obese patients. In fact, we visualize only thin scans of the Cooper ligaments that are curved surfaces with antiradial disposal intersecting as really tents, discontinuous in the lobar spaces traversed by the main ducts with radial orientation (Fig. 3.11).

As a characteristic appearance, neglected in the classical US but well demonstrated on mammography, the arcs of the Cooper ligaments are crossing in couples just at the limit of the lobar anterior or posterior surface with the limit of the fatty perimammary layer that results an appearance of "tent" or "gothic arcs." These "tents" are better visible in DE, their size is bigger on the superficial side of the lobe, and they are important for the location of the TDLUs [6, 7].

Another importance of the Cooper ligaments is related to the technical acquisition of the images in DE: the focal shadowing of the Cooper ligaments when scanning in the orthogonal plane could mimic a malignant lesion or a calcification; in such cases, we must differentiate the Cooper ligament from the pathological shadows by changing the angle of the US beam wave, and the shadow will change the size and location.

Moreover, the anatomy of the Cooper ligaments include thin vessels, which are not visible on Doppler examinations in normal breast but become larger and visible in the vicinity of a TDLUs cancer; the Cooper vessels become large with the increasing thickening of the ligament, demonstrating the way the cancer spreads and justifying the hyperthermia and the orange skin aspect in the developed stages.

The fibrous tissue of the breast is a wrong descriptor represented in the classical US by the echogenic component of the mammary layer that is composed of "fibroglandular tissue" and is believed that its appearance is related to hormonal status and age.

In breast imaging, stroma is interpreted worldwide as an amount of connective tissues, with fibrous collagen and elastic elements, vessels, lymphatics, and nerves. In cell biology, the stroma of any organ is a supportive tissue of the specific parenchymal tissue, and it contains a variable number of stromal cells, such as fibroblasts and pericytes. The interaction between stromal cells and tumor cells is generally known in cancer growth and progression, and for the breast cancer, it is illustrated by the desmoplastic reaction. Stromal cells are thought to not become cancerous, but in the breast, there were described stromal cancers. Moreover, a report of the 2006 *California Breast Cancer Research Program* showed that nearby cancer cells can significantly influence the stroma to change its gene expression and the amount of stroma alters the amount of protein secreted; this relationship will better explain the development of the breast cancer and is expected to allow the future diagnosis of the premalignant lesions [8].

The relationship between the hosts' cancer-associated fibroblasts (CAFs) and the epithelial malignant cells changed the understanding of the breast cancer as a systemic disease; CAFs are changing the tumor cells' microenvironment promoting cancer initiation, angiogenesis, invasion, and therapeutic resistance [9]. Other stromal components such as endothelial cells, macrophages, or adipocytes seem to play a role in the microenvironment of the parenchymal susceptible cells.

Another important aspect when studying breast stroma is the possibility to find a primary stromal sarcoma (malignant fibrous histiocytoma, spindle cell tumor, etc.), which is a rare malignancy, and usually it is diagnosed by biopsy; indeed, there are few studies presenting the imaging differential diagnosis with breast parenchymal cancer. The importance of the noninvasive diagnosis is related to the possibility to cure these sarcomas by wide excisions [10], and the future investigations should facilitate the imaging differential diagnosis from other breast cancers.

In the DE, as in the classical US, the hyperechogenic component of a mammary lobe is *corresponding to the glandular stroma*. It seems there are no connections between the ductal-lobular trees of the different lobes, so the lobe is a morphofunctional unit and the pathology of the lobar stroma will spread to the neighbor lobes only in the advanced stages of the disease.

The amount of lobar stroma is generally correlated with the hormonal status, that is, the young breasts or the lactation breasts will present a large stroma, which justifies the high opacity of the breast on mammography and defines the "dense breast"; indeed, the normal ductal-lobular tree is not obvious at the mammography, as well as at tomosynthesis.

In the pathological cases, the hyperestrogenism and/or hyperandrogenism determines the thickening of stroma, while physiological or pathological breast lobar atrophy may induce an extreme reduction of stroma, with thin hyperechoic linear aspect at US and thin linear opacities at mammography. Some cases with only parenchymal, ductal-lobular atrophy and stromal preservation appear as a dense breast at mammography, justifying the above affirmations. The FBU aspect of the stroma is completed by sonoelastography, which presents a higher stromal stiffness than the ductal-lobular parenchyma, especially in young dense breasts or in cases with "simple" mastodynia. The response of the breast to the hormonal status seems to be related to the estrogen receptor-beta that is expressed in stromal cells, being proved the high receptor density in fibroadenomas and benign phyllodes tumors [11].

The Chest Wall Pectoralis muscles and underlying serratus anterior muscle overlie the ribs and the intercostal muscles. Muscles appear as medium-gray horizontally oriented fibrillary structures containing linear echogenic bands. The pectorals must be identified when checking the tumoral peripheral infiltration and when assessing the location and the pathology of the breast implants. A special attention must be accorded to the pectoral layer in radical breast surgery, because some surgical benign findings (suture granuloma, seromas, and scars) or malignant findings (intramuscular metastasis) may be identified. The axillary lymph nodes could be located under the lateral edge of the major pectoral muscle and sometimes may be found as remnant nodes post lymphadenectomy.

Ribs appear as focal ovalar hypoechoic homogeneous or heterogeneous structures, without or with posterior shadowing, respectively, when scanning a cartilaginous or a bony segment, respectively, in the short axis; a hypoechoic band appears when turning the transducer into the long axis of the costal cartilage, with posterior hyperechoic line of the pleura, and the aspect becomes an arcuate/linear hyperechoic structure, with accentuate shadowing effect when scanning the osseous part of the rib, either in the longitudinal or in the orthogonal plane. It is important to adjust focal zones to include the posterior mammary layer and chest wall to reassure the complete scanning of the whole breast structures.

The sonolucency of the cartilaginous parasternal ribs is useful in the visualization of the internal mammary vessels and of their eventually pathological satellite lymph nodes. The US is the only available technique of examination that can replace the breast MRI for the internal mammary vessels, and Doppler technique is cheaper than MRI contrast agents.

The Lymph Nodes Lymph nodes may be located throughout the breast, but intramammary findings are rarely, usually located in the peripheral regions of the outer quadrants and usually as unique and unilateral finding; normal intramammary lymph nodes are usually less than 0.5 cm in their short diameter. Their normal particular structure can be easily recognized in US (see below), mammography, CT, or MRI, while nodes with pathological changes (inflammatory or tumoral) are extremely rare findings for this location (Figs. 3.15, 3.16 and 3.17).

In breast US, the lymph nodes must be systematically researched in the axillary, supraclavicular, subclavicular, and internal mammary regions.

One of the best imaging techniques of diagnosis of the lymph nodes is US. The lymph node can be demonstrated on US as an ovoid-shaped mass with an echogenic center, representing the medullary/sinus, and a peripheral, hypoechogenic cortical region, interrupted on the hilum, which give a reniform shape. A hilar notch or a fatty hilum should be visible to make the diagnosis. The shape, size, and appearance of normal lymph nodes are variable for different patients, for the same patients are different for different regions and for the same nodes are for different scanning planes. For the axillary lymph nodes, a normal value for the transverse/short axis measures 4–8 mm, with a longitudinal axis up to 25 mm; the lymph node cortical is normally thin, without salient vasculature, and the normal fatty hilum is hyperechoic, with or without small vessels in the hilum. The sonoelastography demonstrates a score 2 Ueno, with normal FLR up to 3.00 (Figs. 3.12, 3.13 and 3.14).

The heterogeneous echotexture of the small, normal lymph nodes can appear indistinguishable from the surrounding breast fatty tissue or the surrounding axillary fatty tissue. Usually, the number of the normal lymph nodes identified on US or other imaging techniques is smaller than those of the lymph nodes identified on the pathological exam following a lymphadenectomy. The benign lymph node never has any capsular or cortical visible vasculature, because the normal cortex receives only the small afferent lymphatic vessels with centripetal orientation toward the hilum, while the sinus receives the artery and releases the vein and the large efferent lymphatic pole. The normal lymph vessels may not be visible on Doppler due to the small velocity.

Subclavicular and internal mammary normal lymph nodes are less visible than the pathological ones. The internal mammary satellite lymph nodes are researched using color Doppler technique, easily to perform parallel with the lateral board of the sternum, the cartilaginous costal arches being sonolucent, and the internal mammary artery signal well visible (Figs. 3.18 and 3.19).

The benign inflammatory changes in lymphadenitis may enlarge the node but with preservation of the ovoidal shape with the ratio of the short axis to the long axis $l/L < 0.5$ and preservation of the ratio cortical/medullary thickness < 1.0; the vasculature could be increased, normal, or absent according to the acute, subacute, or chronic stage. The central part of the medullary lymph node appears hypoechoic in the chronic lymphadenitis, corresponding to the benign histiocytosis on pathology (Fig. 3.20).

Malignant metastatic or infiltrated nodes are more salient than the normal ones as they become larger, rounder, and more uniformly hypoechoic due to the regularly/irregularly thickening of the cortical zone with progressive restriction of the hyperechogenic medullar area. The Doppler exam demonstrates in the metastatic lymph nodes the new vasculature in the thickened cortex, while the acute lymphadenitis presents increasing vasculature/hyperemia in the hilum with centrifuge development toward the cortex. The last noninvasive method of diagnosis of the type of lymph node is represented by the sonoelastography, which depicts a score 4 or 5 Ueno for the thickened nodal cortex or for the whole lymph node in suspect cases (see Chap. 4 and Sect. 8.5.1).

The size of the lymph node is less significant for the assessment of malignancy, but the short axis over 1.0 cm becomes suspect; whatever, the thickening of the cortical with new peripheral vasculature and the high stiffness are more significant for a breast cancer sentinel node, while voluminous lymph nodes without these abnormalities in Doppler and sonoelastography could be either normal variant or chronic inflammation such as nonspecific lymphadenitis, sarcoidosis, etc. The malignant aspect for the axillary lymph nodes may be related to a known breast lesion, but there are difficulties of differential diagnosis when the breast suspect lesion is not obvious (see Sect. 8.5.2).

The diagnosis of the adenopathy is based usually on a subjective qualitative analysis, responsible for the discordant results in the literature, which recommend biopsy as a rule in any suspect or detectable lymph node. The CAD develops applications for US, especially for breast US, and the complete characterization of a breast lesion must include the analysis of the satellite lymph node appearance. Because of the large variability of the measures, shape, and cortical-to-medullary ratio, lymph nodes could be considered as a *fuzzy shape*, and specialized software are developed to make possible the CAD in the future applications and especially in the screening of the breast cancer, either in mammography or US [12].

Vessels Blood vessels are identified in the axillary region and throughout the breast with the aid of color Doppler. Power Doppler is more sensitive in detecting small vessels and represents the reference tool in 3D acquisitions with vascular analysis [13].

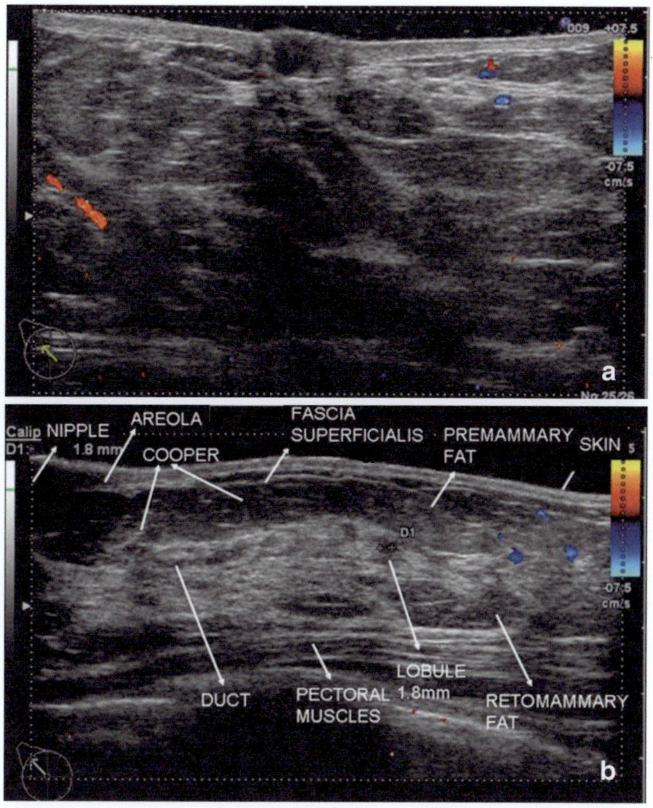

Fig. 3.2 The nipple and the retroareolar convergent atrophic lobes separated by fatty tissue are well visualized using a water-bag probe (**a**). Radial scan at R10:30 illustrates detailed anatomical rapports inside and outside the mammary lobe, performed with a long-linear probe provided with a water bag, with respect to breast relief (**b**)

Usually, there are few vessels visible on Doppler exam of the normal breast, commonly the periareolary circle and incidentally small vessels located in the fatty layers or in the glandular stroma (extraductal always!) in the rest of the breast; the largest vessels may mimic duct ectasia in 2D US, but they are usually oriented in nonradial axes, usually in the sagittal plan. The periareolary circle is visible in most cases, and some vessels may be followed up to the axilla or up to the internal mammary artery, especially in pathological breasts. The actual sonographic devices have not developed the 3D/4D acquisitions with Doppler for the small parts with good resolution, but the future technical development will allow a better understanding of the physiology and pathology of the breast vasculature.

In the physiologically developing breast, such as the thelarche and the lactating breast, or in the pathological development such as florid gynecomastia, there is always a hyper-/new vasculature present, which is a useful sign in the differential diagnosis.

The diffuse increase of the salient vessel density in the breast may be benign, of functional type, either physiological in the lactating breast or pathological in the hyperprolactinemia associated to galactorrhea; in acute mastitis, frequently in lactating breasts, the hyperemia is due to combined factors, hormonal and infectious. The chronic galactophoritis (duct ectasia, chronic plasma cell mastitis) even with proved bacterial overinfection have no salient changes in the breast vasculature.

The most important pathological diffuse increasing vasculature is visible in the carcinomatous mastitis, which has no specific characteristic in the absence of localized suspect mass or malignant-type satellite lymph nodes but has pathological findings in sonoelastography, inverse to the benign-type mastitis (see Sect. 8.4.1).

Any mass in the mammary region with detectable vasculature is pathological, and the smallest less than 5 mm solid-type lesions connected to the ducts that present Doppler signal are suspect for angiogenesis and thus are suspect for malignancy. That corresponds to the breast MRI diagnosis criteria (Fig. 3.3), the contrast enhancement curves being the most important differential diagnostic criterion; moreover, some authors recommended in suspect cases repeated mammography or tomosynthesis after injection of iodinated contrast agent.

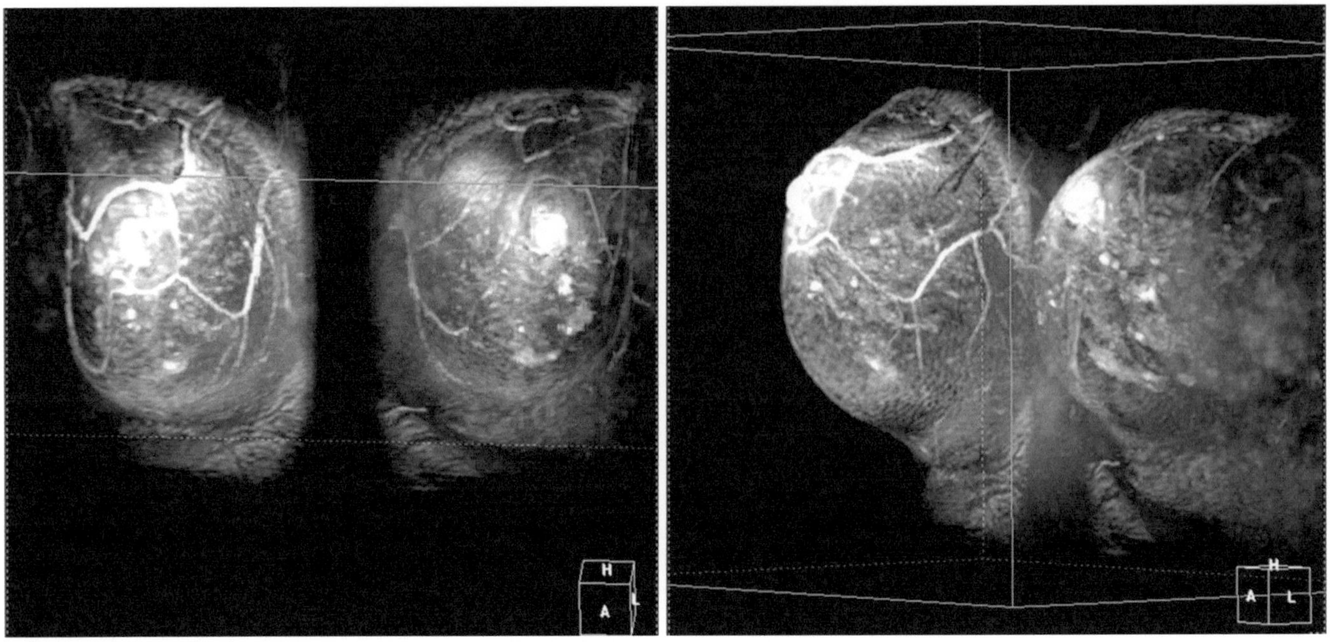

Fig. 3.3 The 3D IRM reconstruction demonstrates the periareolary vascular ring and the affluent vessels from the axillary, subclavicular, and internal mammary artery

3.3 Types of Normal Breast Anatomy on DE

3.3.1 Thelarche (Mammary Bud)

Thelarche represents the developing breast early in the pubertal age. DE is useful in the differential diagnosis of normal bud from pathological mammary lesions. The water-bag probe or an amount of echo jelly is suitable for better visualization of the superficial structures in the small breasts.

Normal developing bud is illustrated on DE/FBU related to the clinical stages of breast development, presented in the beginning of this chapter. In the initial stages upon Tanner, the elevated nipple is accompanied by an amount of small retroareolar hypoechoic parenchymal tissue, with discrete irregular borders and a thin peripheral hyperechoic specific breast stromal component. As the developing breast is usually asymmetrical, the presence of the smaller contralateral bud, usually without clinical complaint, is useful in the positive diagnosis.

In stage III, when the nipple-areolar complex is more elevated, the retroareolar bud enlarges; the peripheral boards present ductal branching with the characteristic central hyperechoic line of the virtual lumen, all separated and surrounded by the hyperechoic stroma, which represents a useful component in the differential diagnosis with the pathological pubertal breast. As the parenchyma enlarges, the branching continues and the ductal tree develops, with a lobar radius more elongated and with more complex range of ducts, and finally can be identified with the presence of the lobules. As a characteristic sign, stroma seems to precede the parenchyma, so the peripheral hyperechoic area is larger. The developing breast is an active process, so the vasculature appears initially in the retroareolar area, then develops radially during puberty, and finally reduces its appearance, in the nonactive breast, until the lactate stage reactivation (Fig. 3.21).

3.3.2 Young Dense Breast (Figs. 3.22 and 3.23)

Young dense breast is the worst examined breast on mammography, but is the most "clear," the most "anatomical," and so the easiest to interpret in DE. The layer of subcutaneous fatty tissue separated by the superficial *corporis fascia* from the premammary fat are both thin, while the retromammary fat and the interlobar fat are almost absent, while the mammary lobes are large, with well-differentiated isoechoic parenchyma. The ductal distribution may be not uniform, some areas containing dense ductal-lobular structures, while other areas illustrate large stromal apparently "unpopulated areas." The young breast is the model type with the most visible lobules, up to 3–4 mm diameter, and with ducts up to 2–3 mm diameter. Where superficial fat is absent, dense breast lobes are palpable as pseudotumoral masses, identified by DE as normal glandular anatomy. In the dense breast, the vasculature is normal; usually, we can identify the periareolary circle, and with the usual actual machines, we can rarely visualize the largest vessels, without connection to a particular area or to the parenchymal structures.

Some women present dense breast late in their lifetime and sometimes even in postmenopause, frequently after using hormonal therapy (birth control pills or substitution hormonal therapy); therefore, in these cases, the stroma is well developed, and there may be numerous visible ducts, but they are thinner than in young breast, usually less than 1.5 mm, and the lobules are almost not visible or present various types of dysplasias. That results when using hormonal substitution therapy or birth control pills, women will present dense breasts uncorrelated with the age, with increased risk of developing breast cancer than in cases of mixed or fatty menopausal breasts; the screening by FBU in these cases of risk will be suitable, because of the poor results of mammographic screening in dense breast.

3.3.3 Mixed Adult Breast

The normal adult breast has usually a mixed asymmetrical structure, which means that the upper-outer quadrant contains the largest and the longest lobes, which progressively decrease in the clockwise, being separated by interposed fatty tissue. The smallest lobes are visualized in the lower-inner quadrant, and then they begin to increase progressively toward the 12:00 ray. The diameters of the ducts are the largest in the outer quadrants; the lobules are usually small, sometimes not visible. The axillary breast glandular prolongation contains usually rich glandular parenchyma, so this can explain the mastodynia in this area. The decreasing lobar volume due to reduced glandular stroma appears as a lobar "contraction" along the main ducts, consequently accompanied by the apparent prolongation of the glandular structures along the Cooper ligaments, which may appear falsely elongated and falsely thickened, because they are surrounded by the remnants of the atrophic TDLUs [14]; this aspect is physiological and must be differentiated from the real Cooper ligaments pathology, with tumoral thickening by epithelial proliferation or desmoplastic stromal reaction.

3.3.4 Fatty Breast

Fatty breast represents a physiological involution of the lobes, with progressively increasing fatty tissue in the premenopausal and the menopausal woman. The remnant parenchyma is located retroareolarly and in the upper-outer quadrant, while the other quadrants have only some thin hyperechoic bands with lobar distribution, containing atrophic linear ducts surrounded by minimal stroma [15].

As the lobes retract, the prolongations of the glandular structure around the Cooper ligaments apparently increase, so there are long segments of thin secondary ducts and remnant lobular cells which are usually unapparent; these lobar structures immersed into the fatty tissue are real challenges for the DE, which can demonstrate the ductal continuity, but they represent the principal source of mistaken diagnosis in the classical US where the intralobar anatomy is neglected. These cases are better examined by mammography because the fatty breast is radiolucent and offers the best contrast for detecting any abnormal opacity.

In cases with dishormonal pathology related to ovarian hypofunction (amenorrhea, bradimenorrhea, hypomenorrhea) or prolonged hormonal birth control pill treatment, fatty breasts with abnormal glandular atrophy in women less than 40 or even less than 30 years old are usually observed. These changes are reversed during pregnancy, but in most cases, their lactation is reduced (Figs. 3.24, 3.25 and 3.26).

3.3.5 Lactating Breast

As a physiological transformation, the lactating breast presents clinical and US changes during pregnancy, with early debuting in the first trimester and progressive developing in the second and in the last trimester; the physiological lactation has some almost specific findings similar to the pathological galactorrhea, which may be found both in women and men with hyperprolactinemia.

The characteristic finding in Doppler DE of the lactating breast is an increasing of the size of ducts and lobules, reducing of the stromal volume but increasing of the periductal vasculature; the ductal-ampullary ectasias are variable with the pregnancy age and with the breast-feeding horary; the ductal content is usually transonic, but in the peripheral ducts the fluid may be isoechoic or simply the central hyperechoic line become doubled.

It is very difficult to make a differential diagnosis of a diffuse acute mastitis from a normal lactating engorged breast: usually mastitis presents supplementary skin edema. Doppler DE is the most useful method in the detection of the deep galactocele, of the previous cysts, and of the solid masses, because in the lactating breast, mammography is avoided or inefficient due to the high breast density; the clinical exam by inspection and palpation has a poor sensitivity.

The galactorrhea presents similar changes with less expression than the physiological lactating breast, and the increased breast vasculature helps us to differentiate the hormonal etiology from other factors determining the ductal ectasia and the nipple surge (Figs. 3.27, 3.28, 3.29 and 3.30).

In cases with large amount of axillary fatty tissue, normal lymph nodes may be obscured on 2D US, but Doppler scans and sonoelastograms of the whole axilla are useful in locating them (Figs. 3.12, 3.13, 3.14, 3.15, 3.16, and 3.17)

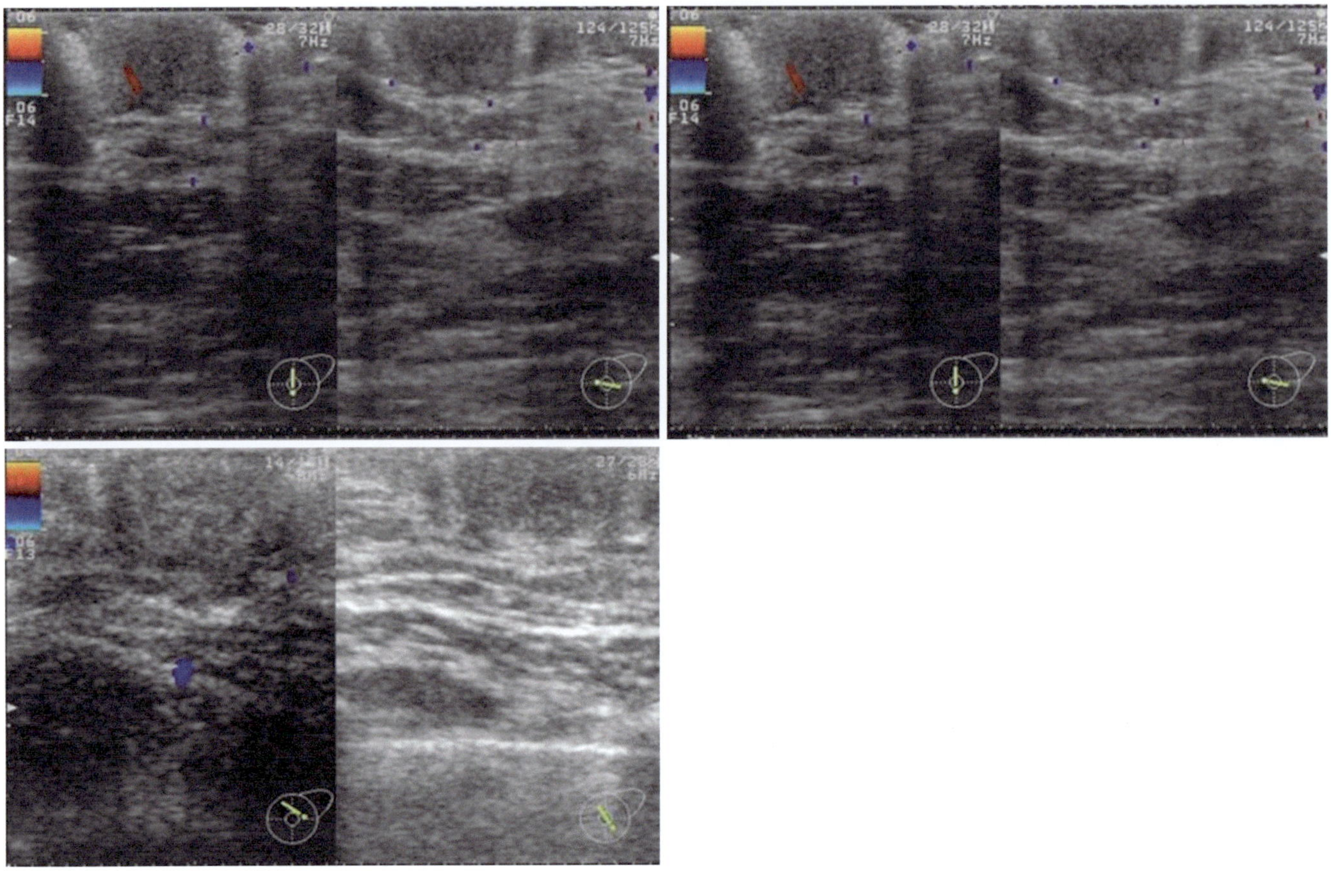

Fig. 3.4 The nipple and its parenchymal connections by the ampoules which may be emptied, dilated, or atrophied; the nipple has no salient vasculature, and in SE, its hardness corresponds to the score 4 Ueno. The correct US examination may be performed with an amount of echo jelly in the sagittal and axial plans

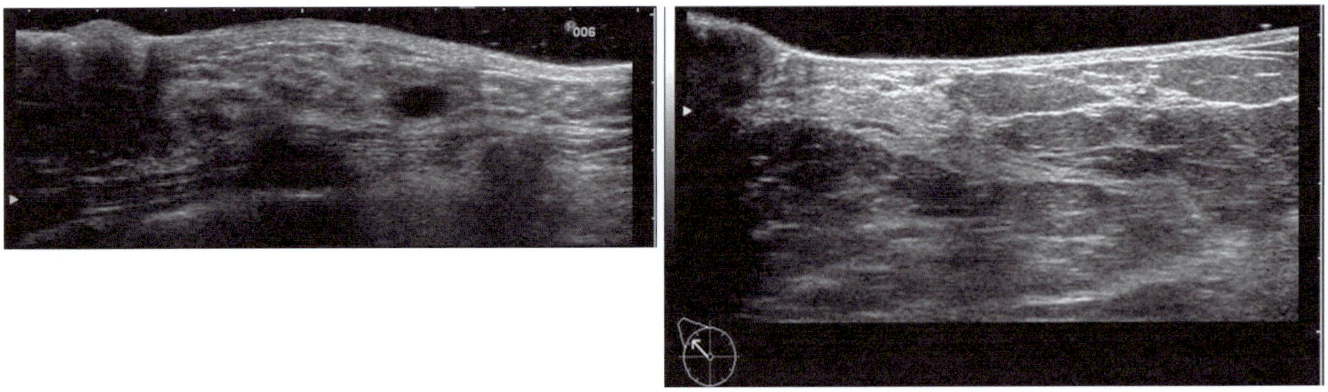

Fig. 3.5 The nipple and areola are well illustrated with a water-bag probe, with respect to the relief and good assessment of the retroareolar structures, both in dense breast and in mixed or fatty breasts; the standardized DE illustrates the nipple in the upper-left corner of the scan

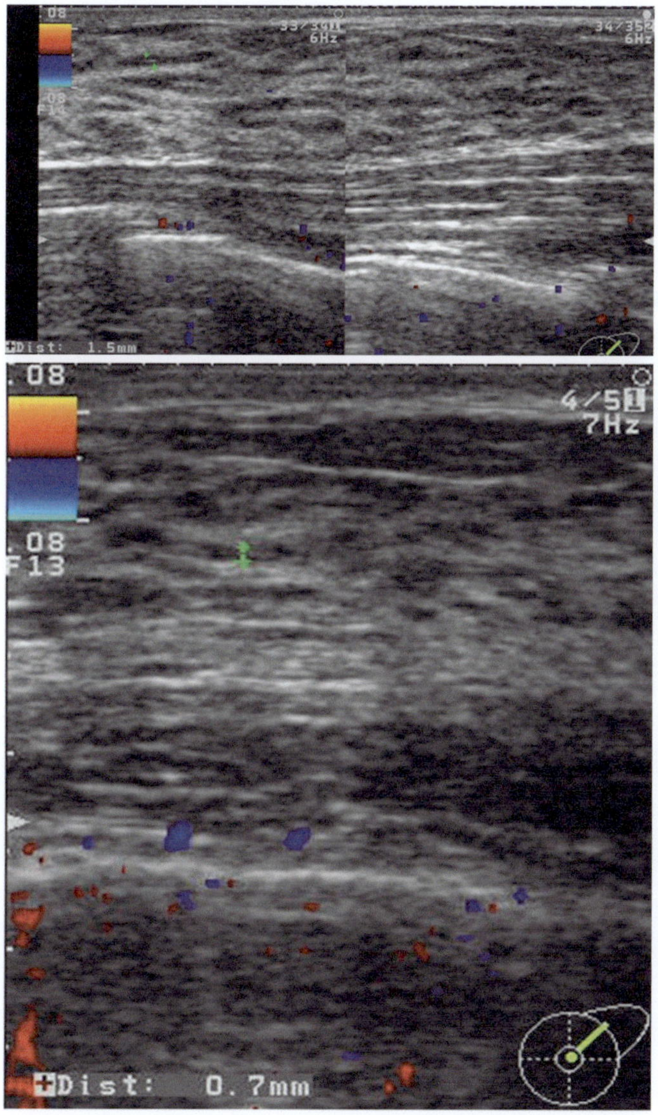

Fig. 3.6 The galactophorous ducts present a hyperechoic central line that is significant for the virtual lumen and represents the interface between the ductal walls, the pathognomonic sign for normal ducts. The transverse diameter of the duct is measured including the lumen, and its range is 0.5–2.5 mm, according to the age and the physiological changes

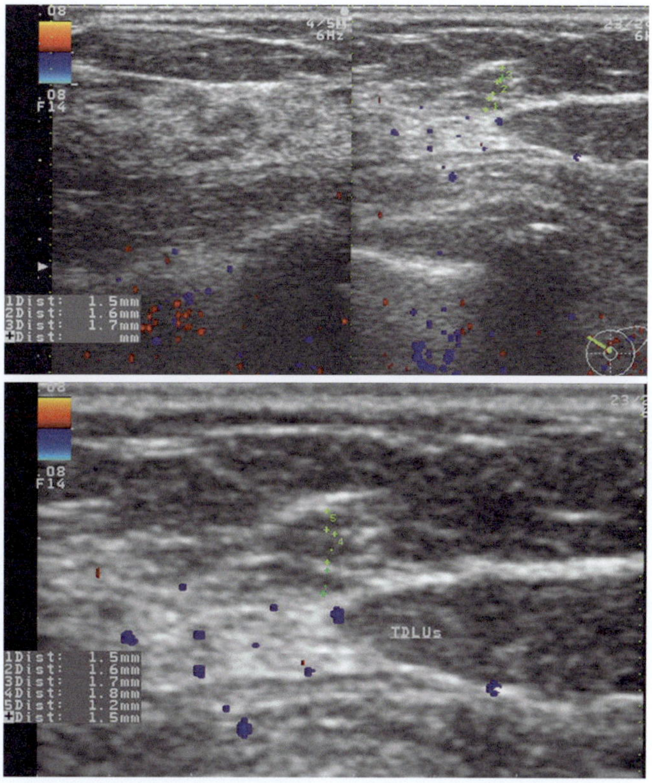

Fig. 3.7 The terminal ductal-lobular specific unit (TDLUs) is located at the vault of the crossing lines of the Cooper ligaments, and it groups a number of lobules connected to the duct, better delimited on a zoomed scan. The anterior TDLUs are greater than the posterior ones, and this is believed to justify the most frequent anterior location of the initiating site of breast cancer

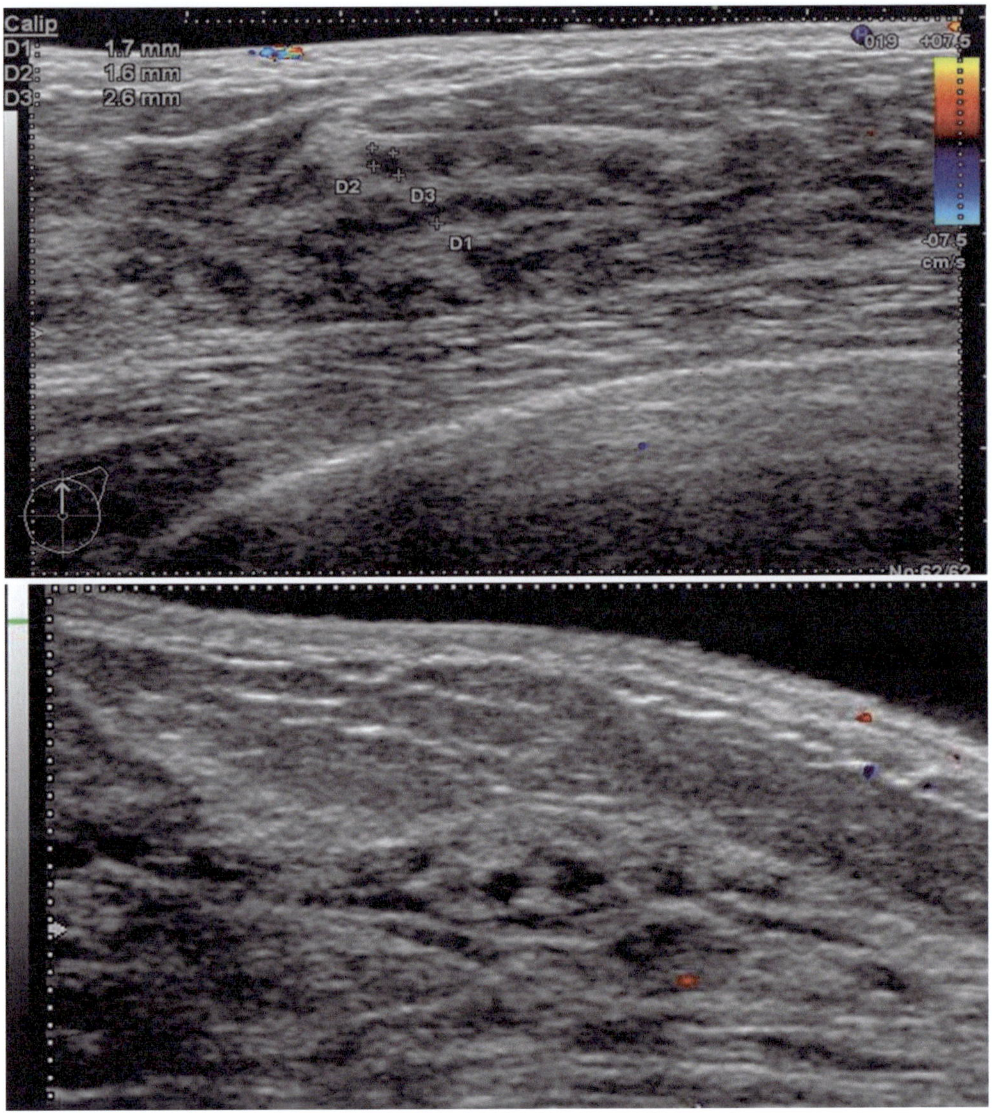

Fig. 3.8 The lobar anatomy upon the model of Teboul and his promoters: the main duct is bordered by the lobules like a "roadside trees." The normal architecture is better visible when there is some physiological or pathological thickening of the parenchyma and a significant amount of hyperechoic stroma

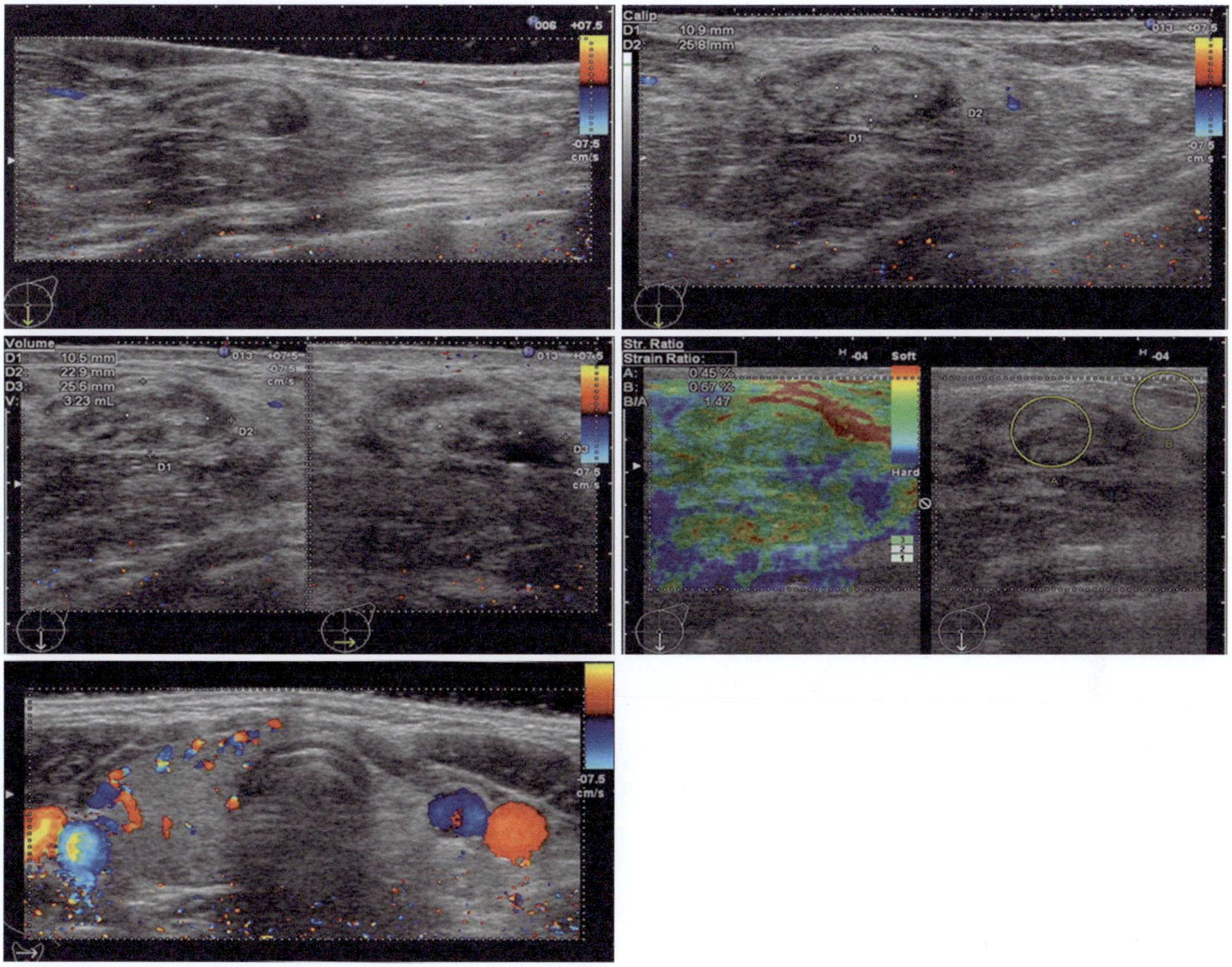

Fig. 3.9 A 50-year-old patient presents a lump at L6:00, with a benign mass appearance; on FBU, a spiral orientation of a mammary lobe with ductal and stromal architecture similar to those of the surrounding glandular structures illustrates a "breast within a breast" anomaly. As a curiosity, the same patient had congenital left thyroidal lobe hypoplasia, associated with the left breast congenital pathology

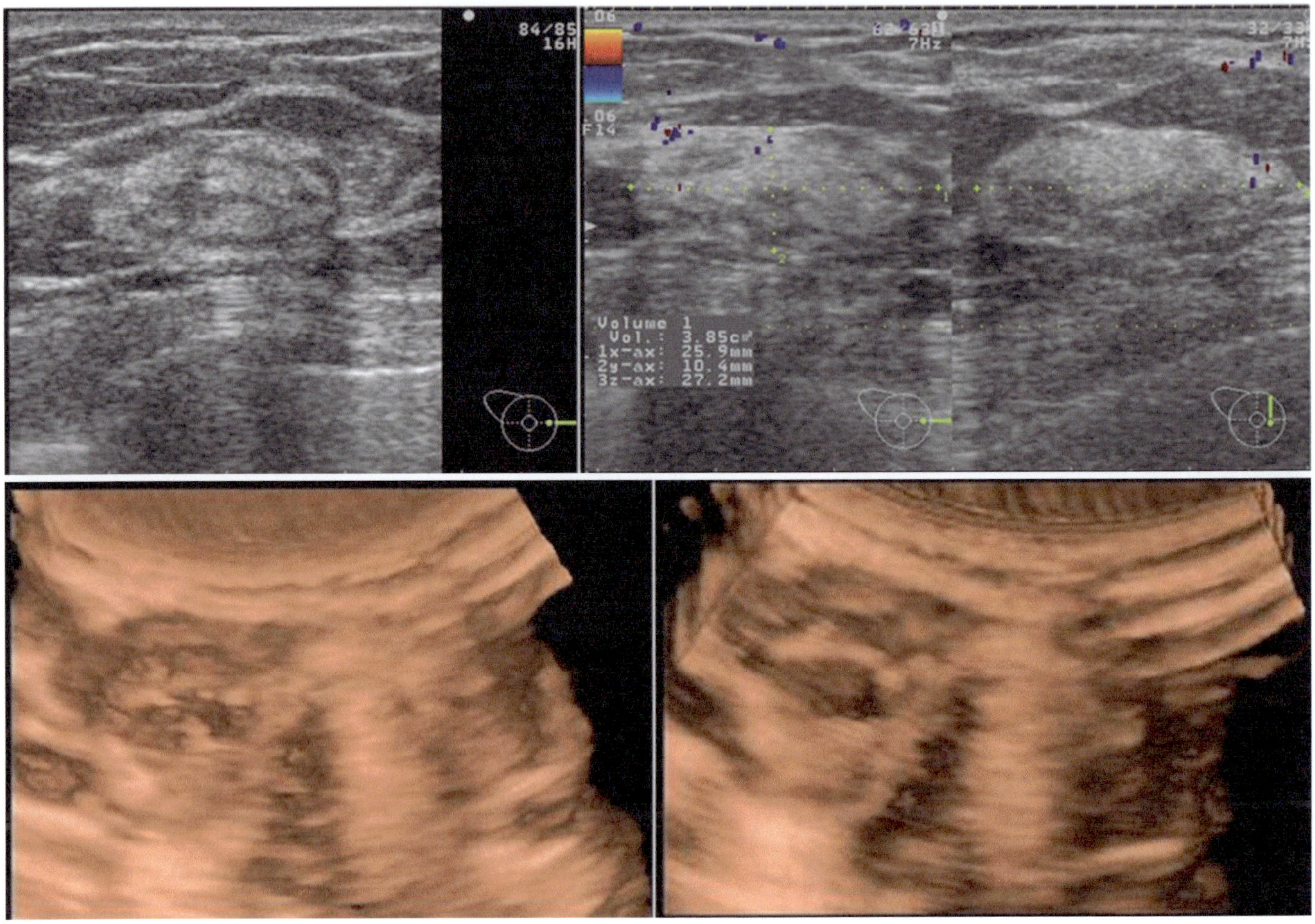

Fig. 3.10 A 52-year-old patient with "breast within a breast" anomaly at R 3:00; the helicoidal orientation of the ducts and the overall benign aspect are visible in both 2D radial and antiradial scans and in the 4D acquisitions

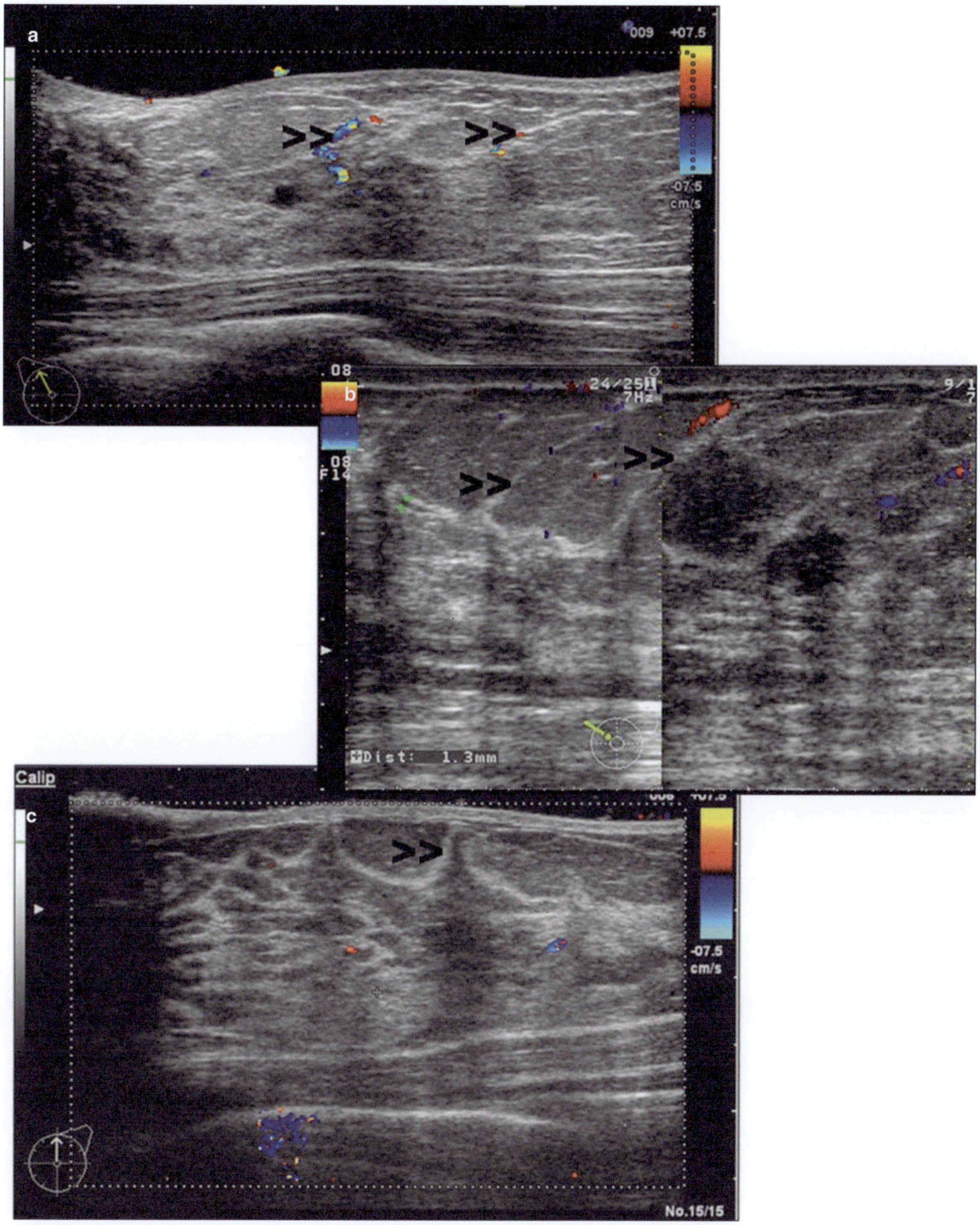

Fig. 3.11 Cooper ligaments (>>) in mixed breast containing vessels (**a**); the fatty breast presents global lobar atrophy, longer Cooper ligaments surrounded by lobar remnants with reliquary of ducts and lobules explaining the start points of the breast carcinoma (**b**); the dense breast illustrates normal thickened Cooper ligaments containing TDLUs (**c**)

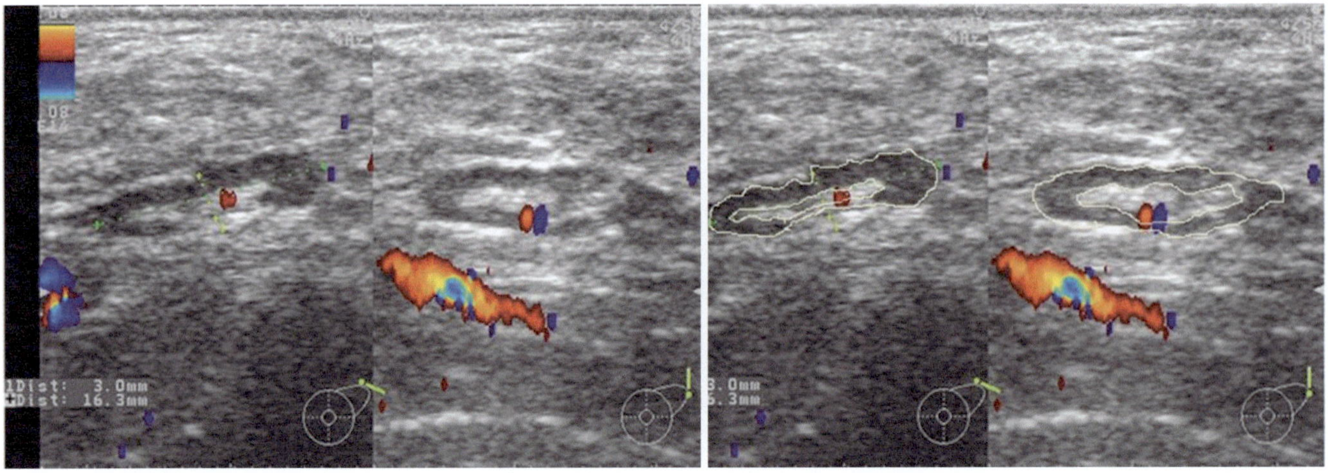

Fig. 3.12 Typical axillary lymph nodes with normal features: an ovoid kidney-shaped, homogeneous hyperechoic medullary, peripheral thin cortical interrupted at the hilum level that presents characteristic vessels; color Doppler in this case presents the artery arising to the lymph node toward the transducer, colored in red, and the vein flowing away colored in *blue*. Few blue spot artifacts are accepted at the lowest limit of the gain velocity necessary to detect the node's hilum

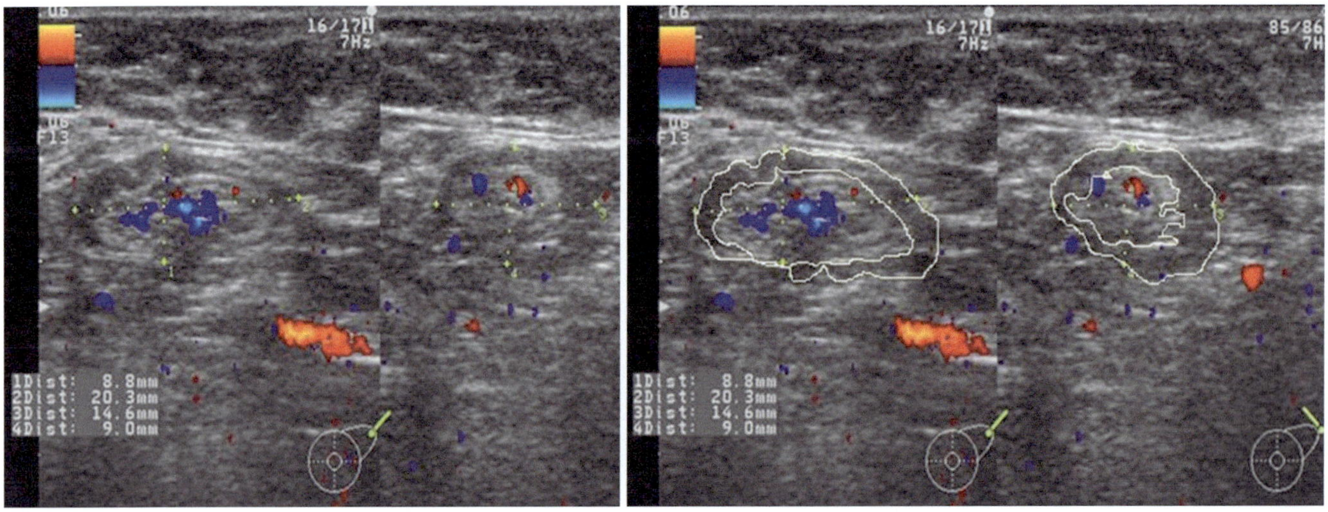

Fig. 3.13 Axillary lymph nodes with benign appearance, kidney-shaped, the short axes less 10 mm, a normal cortical area, but a hypoechoic medullary (hilum) that presents increased vasculature, suggesting chronic inflammation (benign histiocytosis)

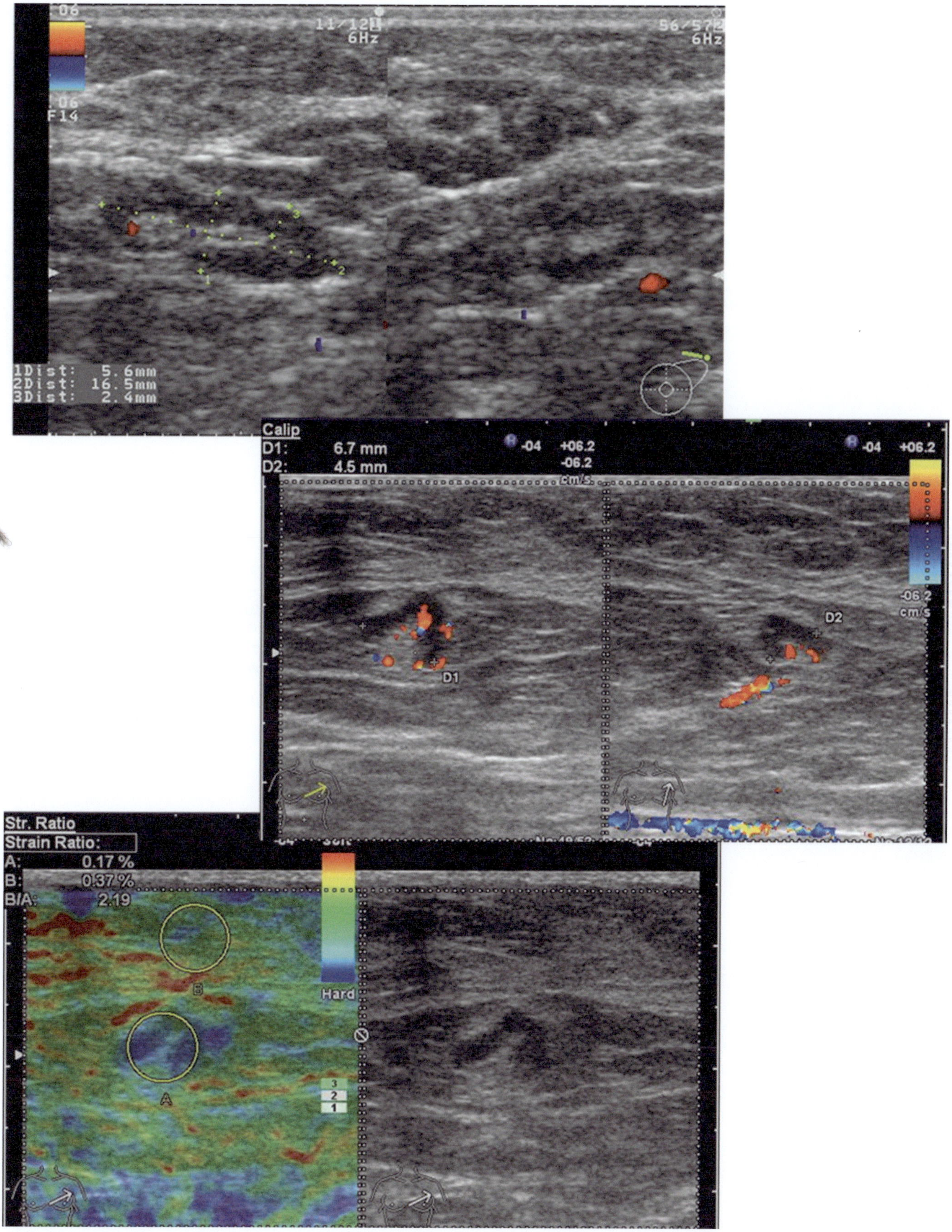

Fig. 3.14 Axillary normal lymph nodes: usually the short axis is less 10 mm, the thin cortex has more or less regular ovoid shape or with polycyclic contour, the hyperechoic hilum has normal centrifuge vasculature, and the benign strain presents a score 2 Ueno with low FLR

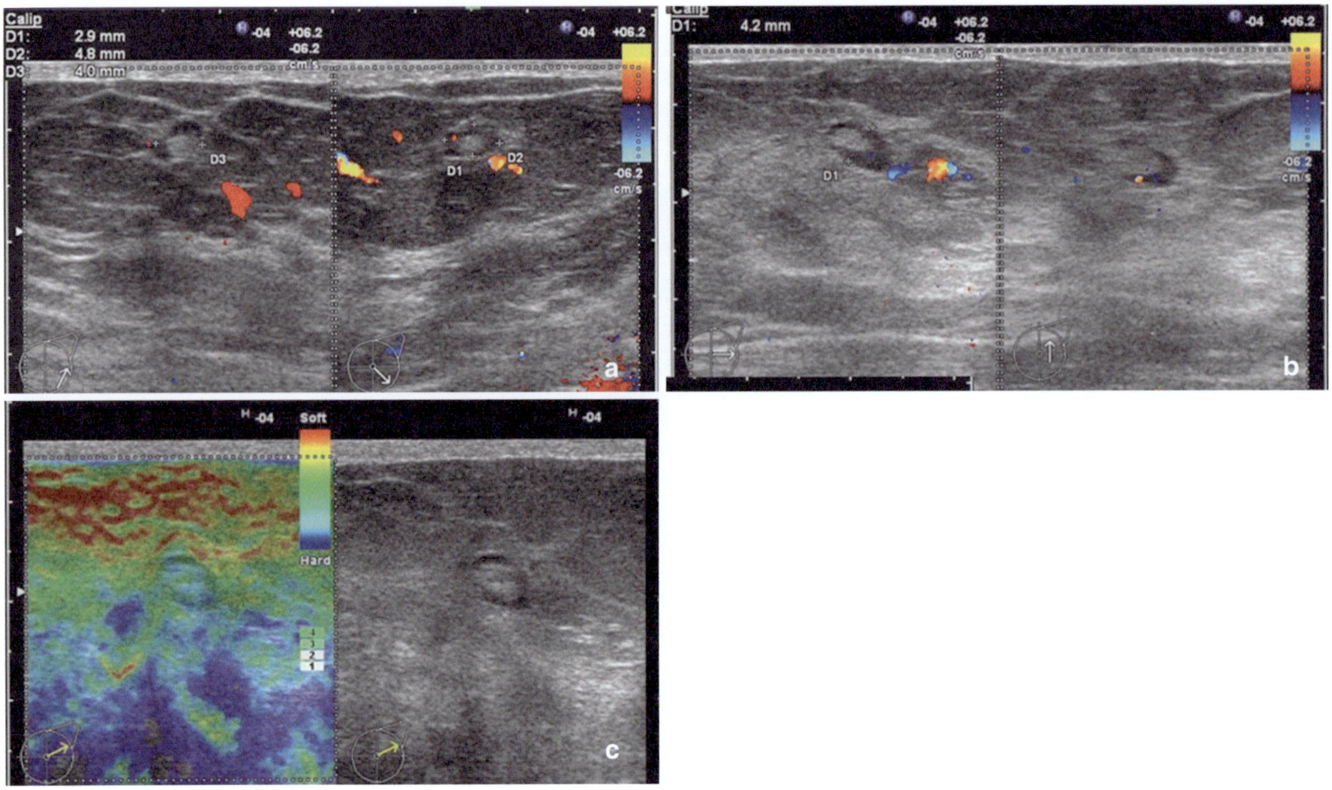

Fig. 3.15 Intramammary normal lymph nodes, located inside the preglandular fatty tissue along a Cooper ligament (*upper scan*) or inside the mammary lobe in a TDLUs (*middle and lower scans*): the nodes are usually small, with the short axis in the first 5 mm, the dedifferentiation of the cortex from the medullary area is present, a minimal eccentric vasculature could be visible, and "benign"-type elasticity is demonstrated, in this case of score 2 Ueno (*lower scan*). In the absence of any breast abnormality, intramammary lymph nodes could be assessed by US BI-RADS 1 category. The fatty echoes of the lymph node hilum/medullary is corresponding to the radiolucent structure on mammography and of the fatty signal on the MRI acquisition, but FBU is the most complete examination without any contrast agent use and without risk of irradiation

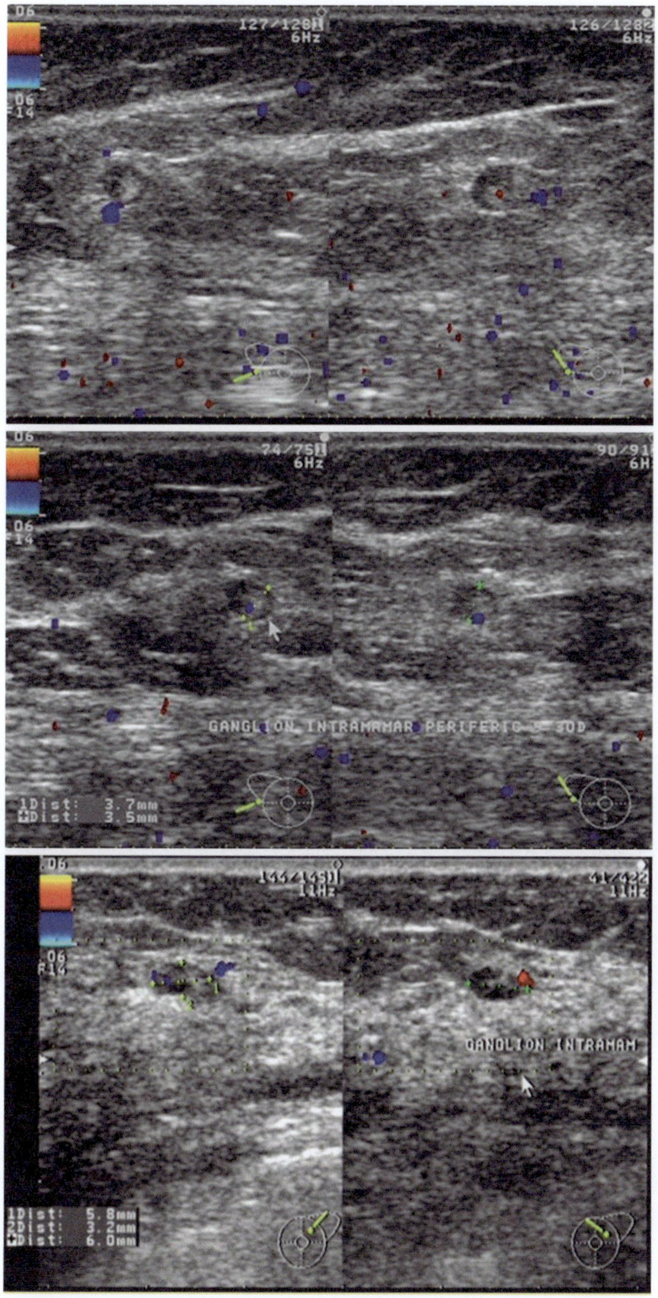

Fig. 3.16 Intramammary kidney-shaped normal lymph nodes: they are usually peripheral and infracentimetric, and color Doppler is useful in detecting and characterizing their hilum, as a pathognomonic sign which excludes other breast masses

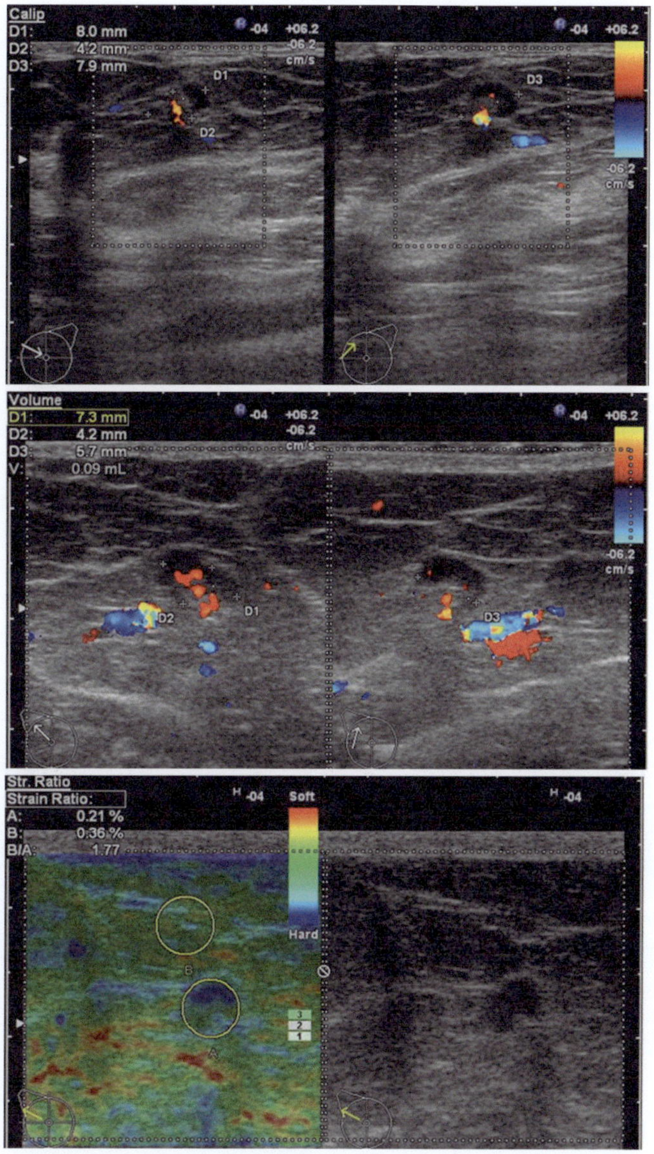

Fig. 3.17 Intramammary lymph node in an upper-inner quadrant, rare findings; despite the cortical thickening with hypoechoic texture, easy to detect in this fatty breast, the vasculature is of "benign" type and SE has score 2 Ueno with low FLR, according to a benign node. Note the eccentric location with respect to the main ductal (lobar) axis

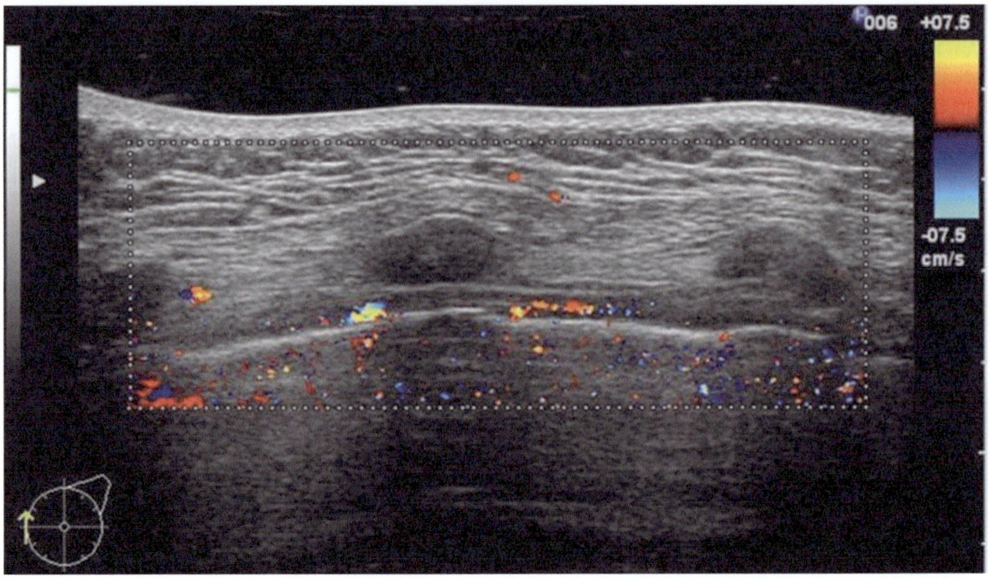

Fig. 3.18 The right internal mammary artery is easy to visualize because the cartilaginous parts of the ribs are permissive to the sonographic wave; the normal internal mammary lymph nodes are not distinguishable, but the pathological ones, rare, become visible especially in cases of inner quadrant breast cancer

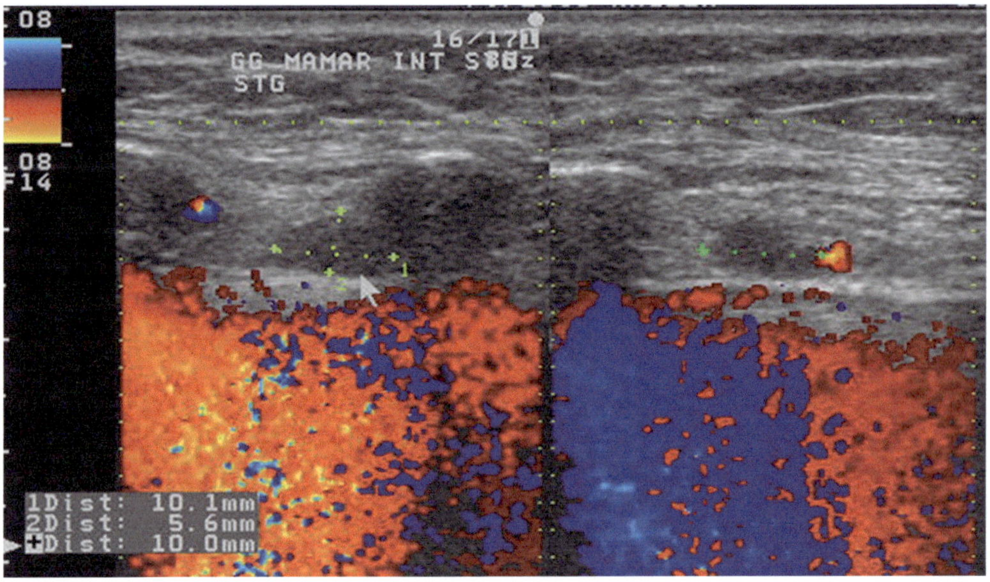

Fig. 3.19 Left internal mammary lymph node enlargement in a patient with L 8:30 ILC (see Chap. 8)

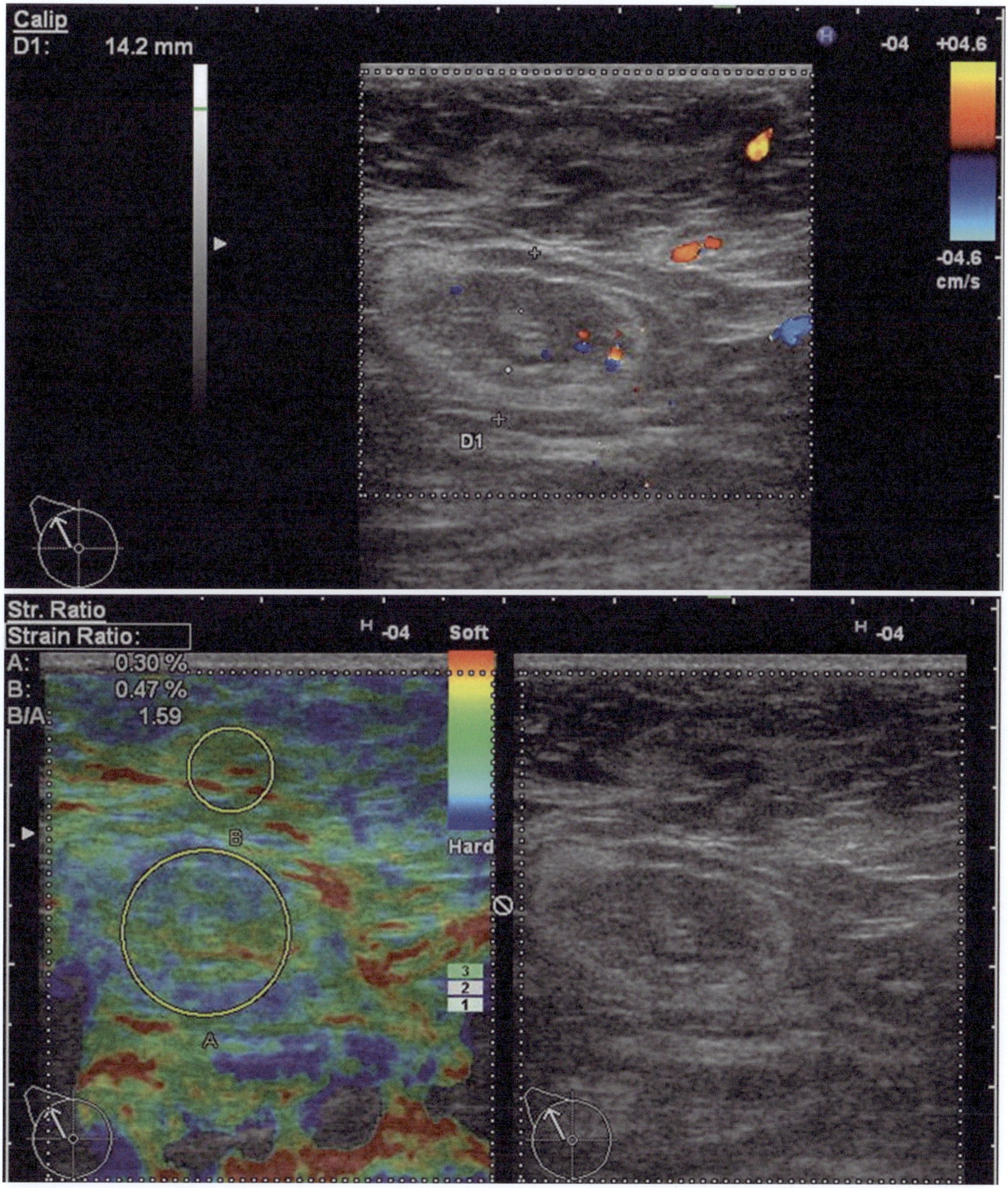

Fig. 3.20 Enlarged lymph node of the basis of the axilla, with thin cortex, less vasculature, but a large hypoechoic core of the sinus (medullary), a usual aspect of benign histiocytosis

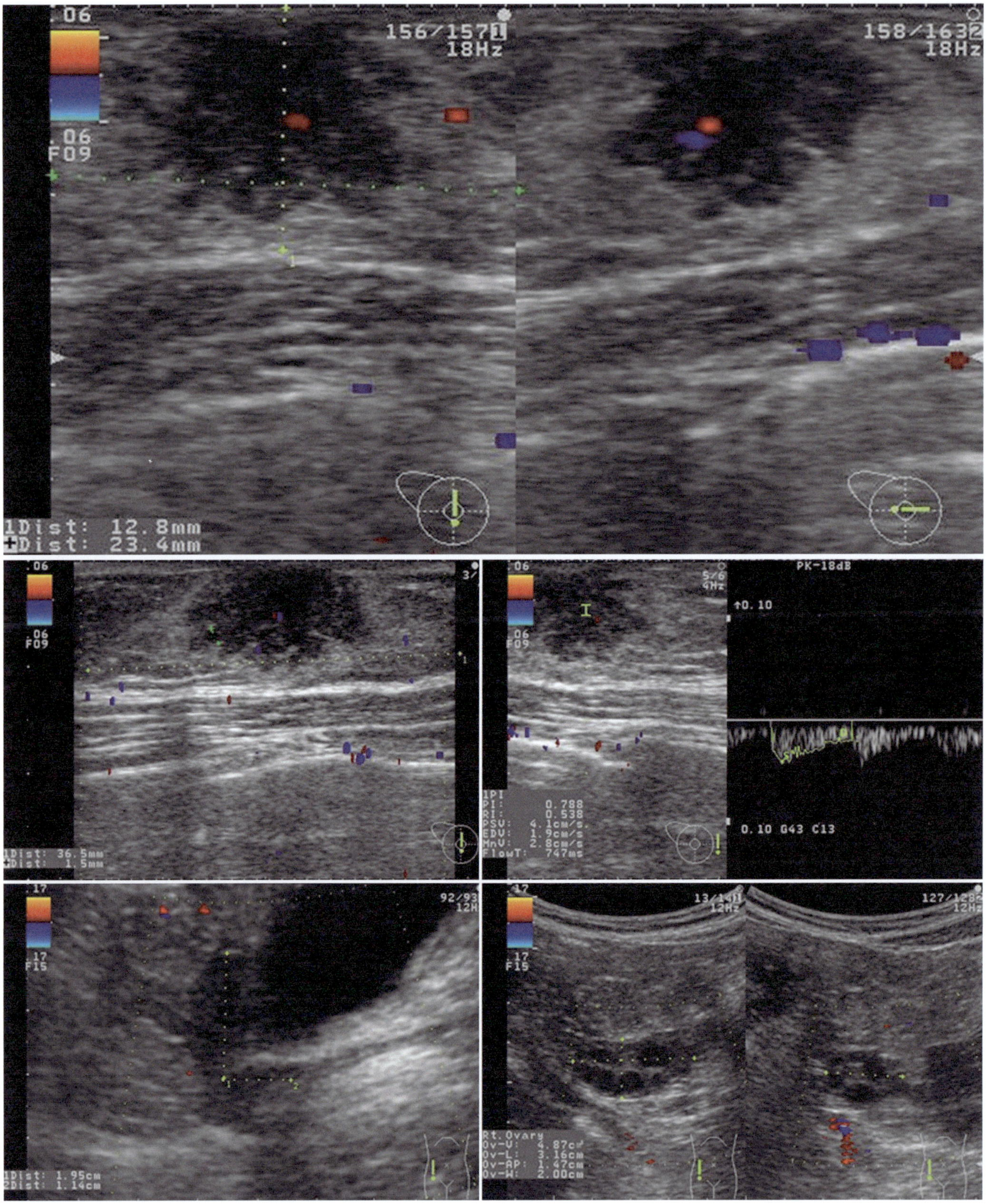

Fig. 3.21 A 9-year-old girl: Thelarche presenting hypoechoic mammary bud with ductal branches, surrounded by hyperechoic glandular stromal component and a new vasculature characterized by low Doppler velocity indices (significant for low blood flow resistance). The inversed corporeal/cervical uterine ratio and the presence of the antral ovarian follicles are the proof of the beginning puberty

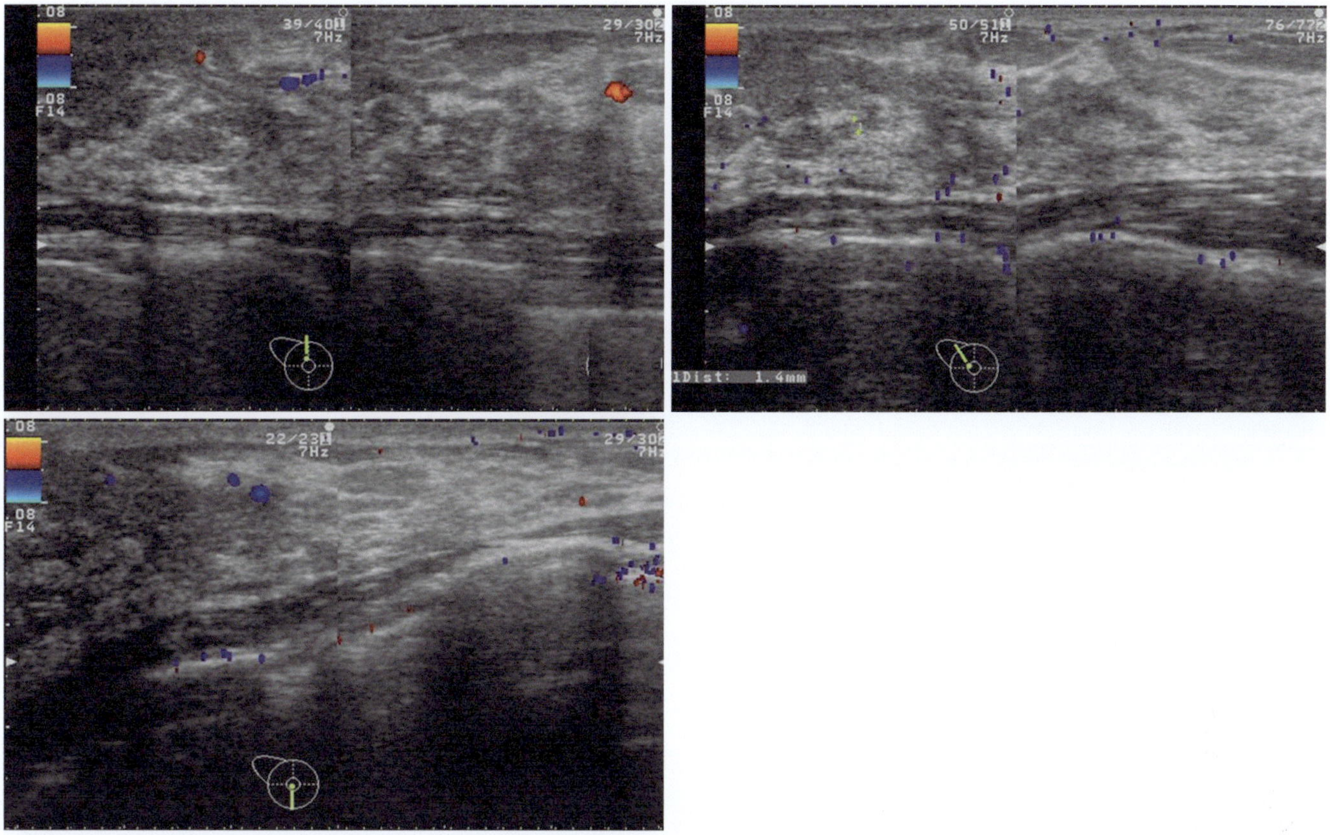

Fig. 3.22 A 27-year-old patient: Dense breast with contiguous back-to-back ducts and lobules especially in the central part of the mammary lobes, with less stromal component, mimicking infiltrative carcinoma; normal vasculature and normal elasticity on sonoelastography confirm the DE aspect of young-adult breast, but a diffuse hyperplasia and hyperestrogenism could be discussed at this age

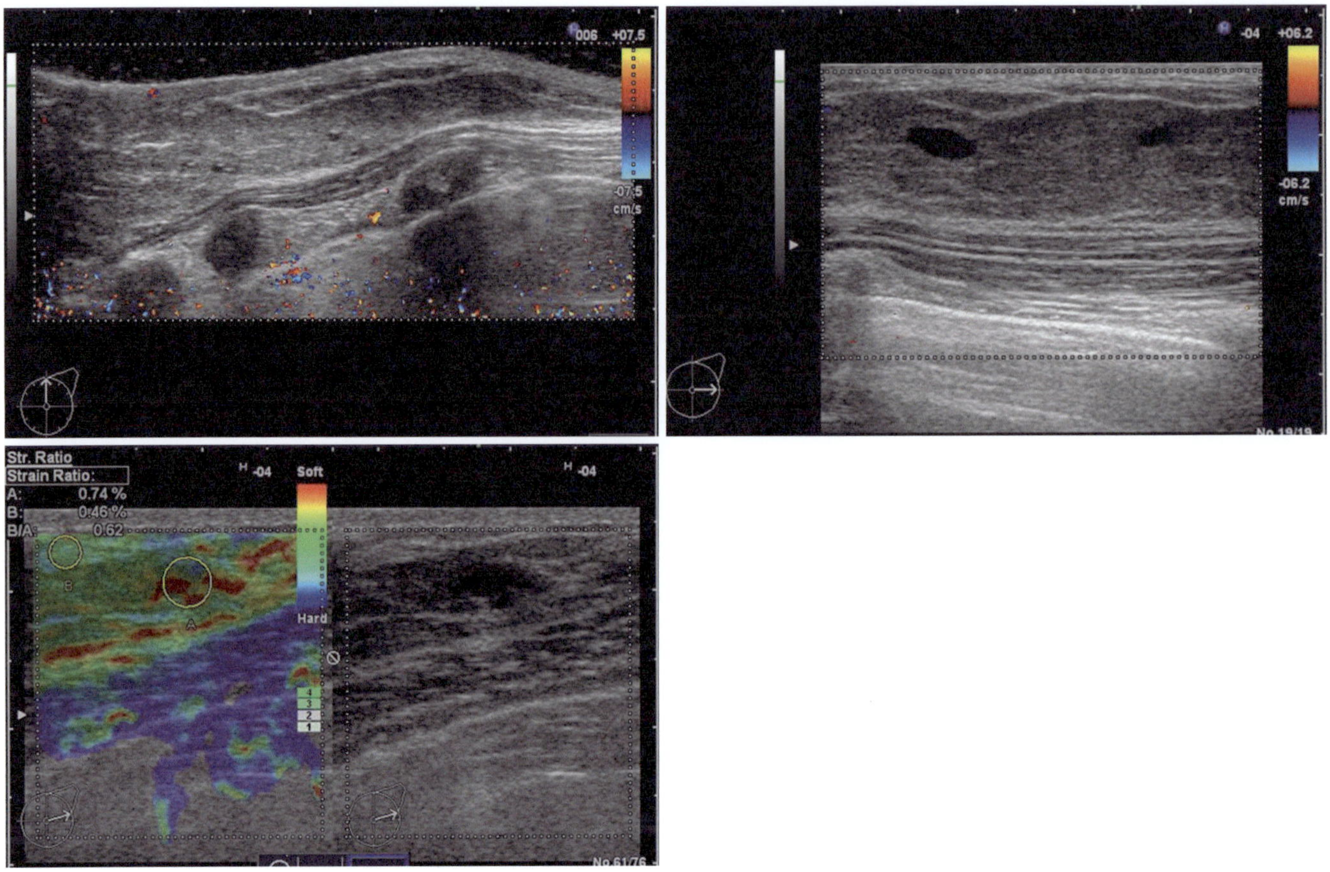

Fig. 3.23 A 40-year-old patient: Dense parenchymal breast with minimal glandular stroma and contiguous "back-to-back" ducts, associated with cystic dysplasia

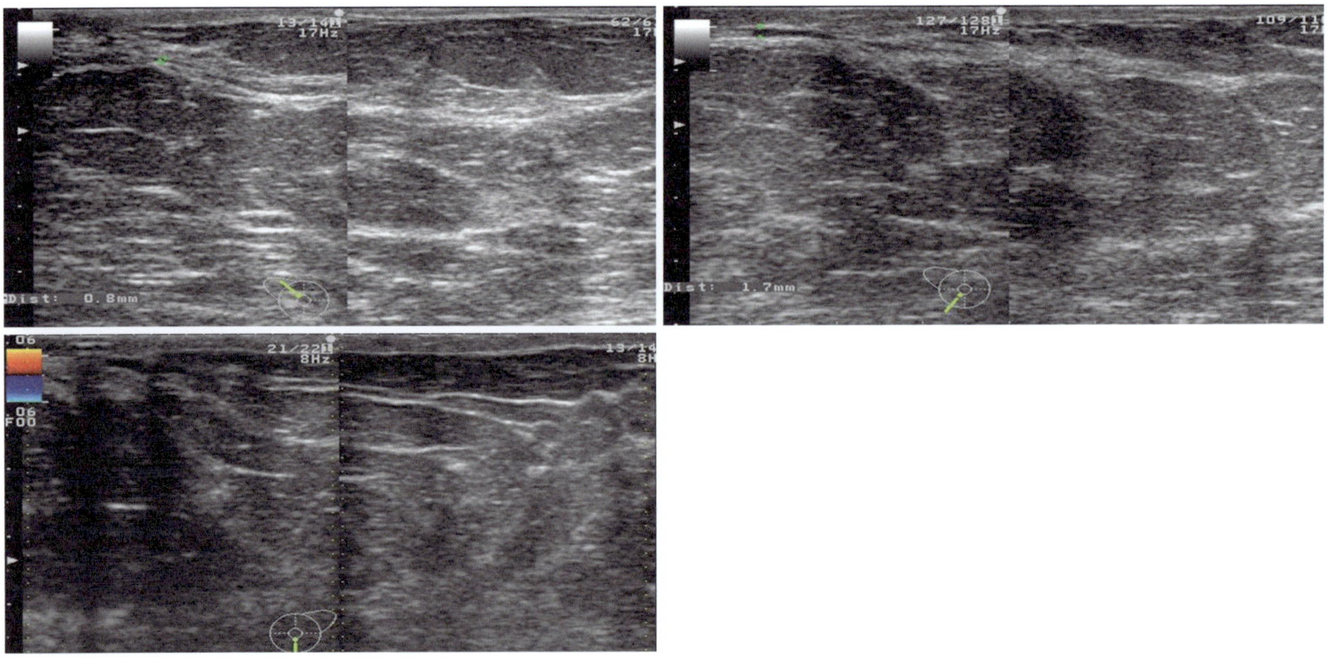

Fig. 3.24 A 39-year-old patient: Fatty breast with global lobar atrophy (stroma and parenchyma); few small ductal ectasias could explain the reduced nipple discharge and the discomfort self-described by the patient as "stings"

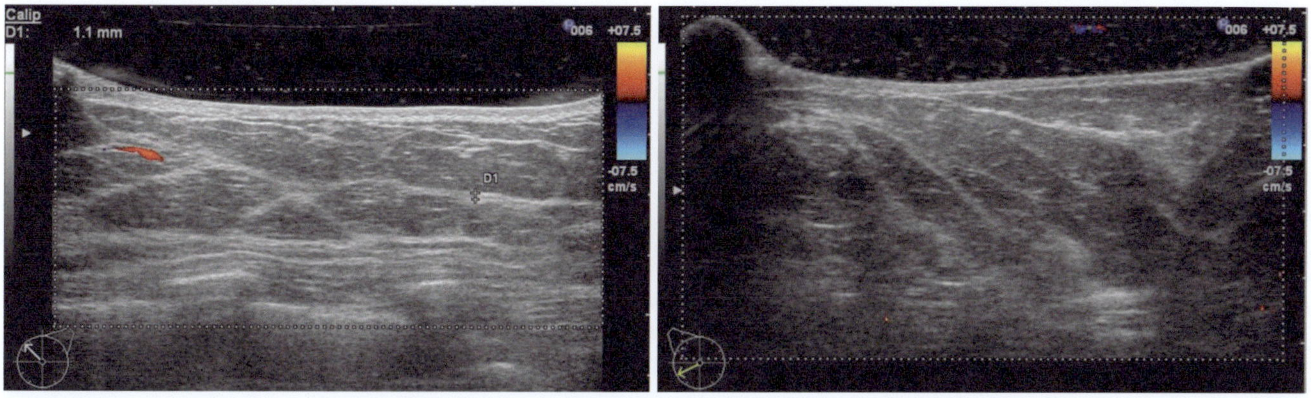

Fig. 3.25 A 52-year-old patient: Fatty breast with global lobar atrophy, but with clear limits of the lobe toward the premammary and the retromammary fatty tissues segmented by the Cooper ligaments; the still visible main duct certify a lobar anatomy

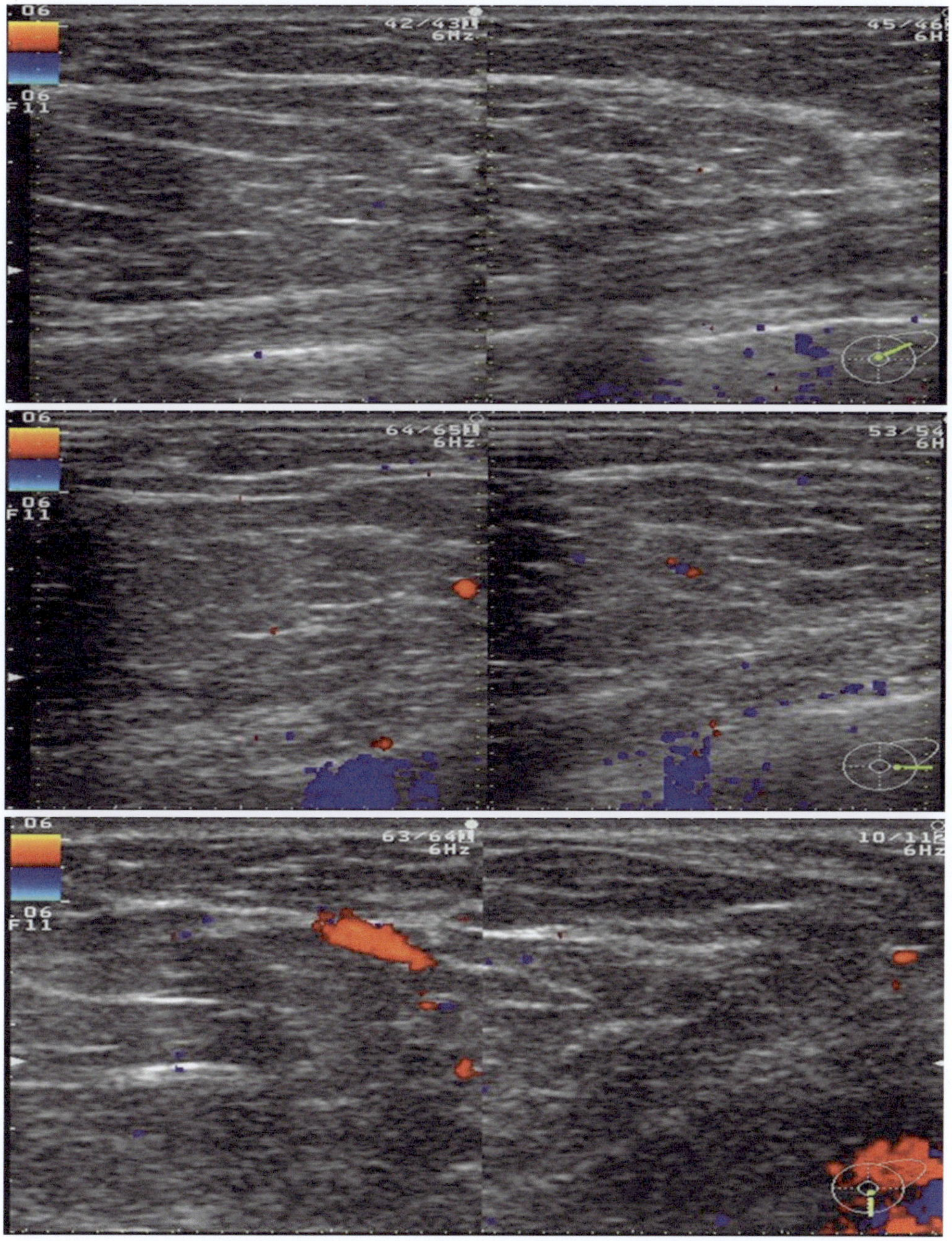

Fig. 3.26 A 45-year-old patient: Mastodynia with mammary atrophy following hysterectomy and ovariectomy for hemorrhagic uterine leiomyofibroma

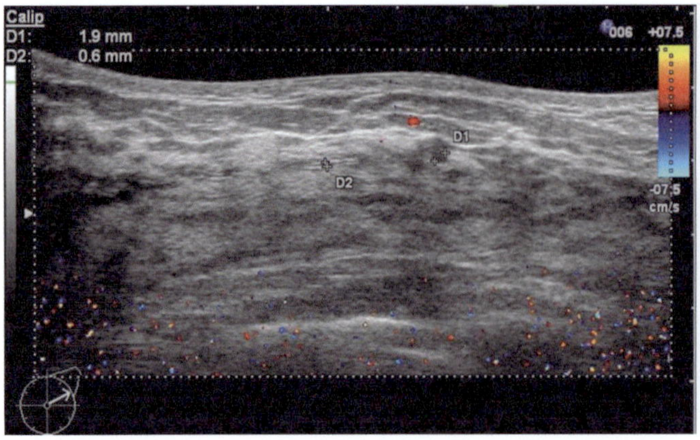

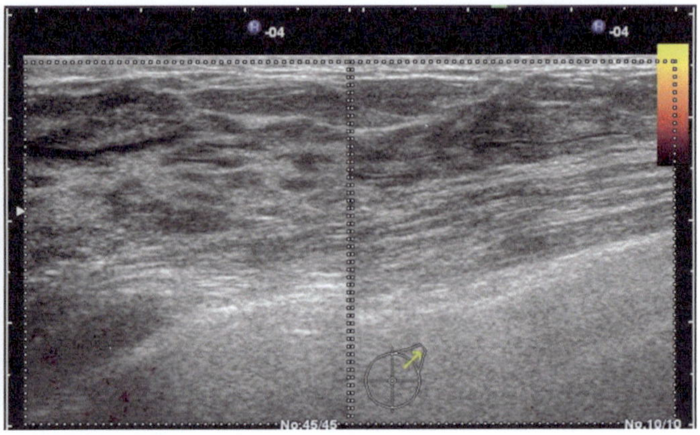

Fig. 3.27 Small ductal ectasia presents *the double central line sign*; in fact, the interfaces of the ductal walls with the fluid that may be represented by serous surge, milk, bloody surge, or pus, with corresponding density from transonic to hypoechoic or isoechoic aspect. The *double line sign* is pathognomonic for the ductal lumen and demonstrates the noninvasive imaging of the ductal contents and allows the measuring of the ductal wall thickness

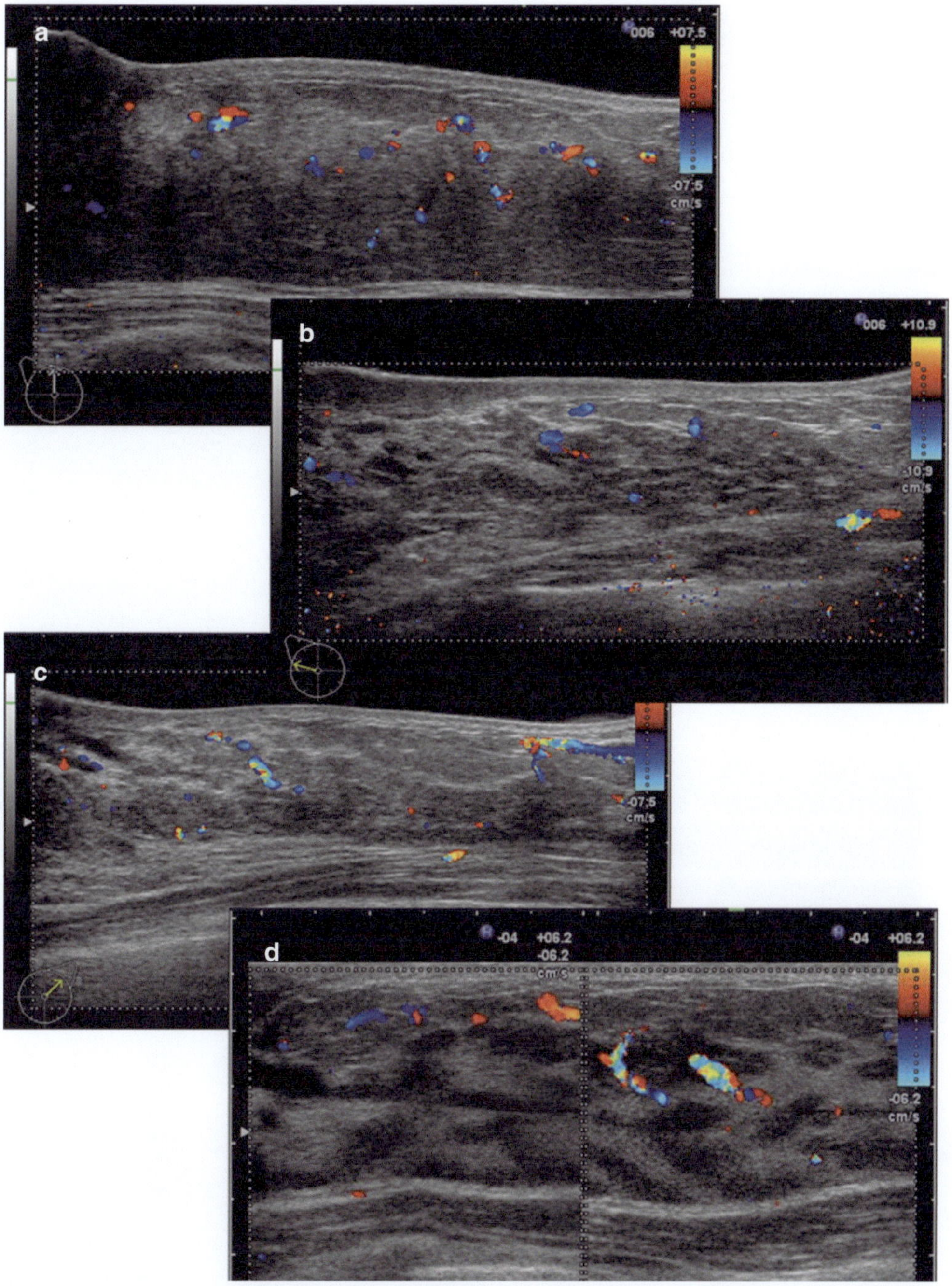

Fig. 3.28 Lactating breast of puerperium of a 29-year-old (**a**) and a 35-year-old (**b**) or during pregnancy at 21 years old (**c, d**) demonstrate the thickening of the lobules and of the lactiferous ducts that may contain some fluid (milk), with reducing of the glandular hyperechoic stroma and with diffuse increasing of the vasculature by hyperemia

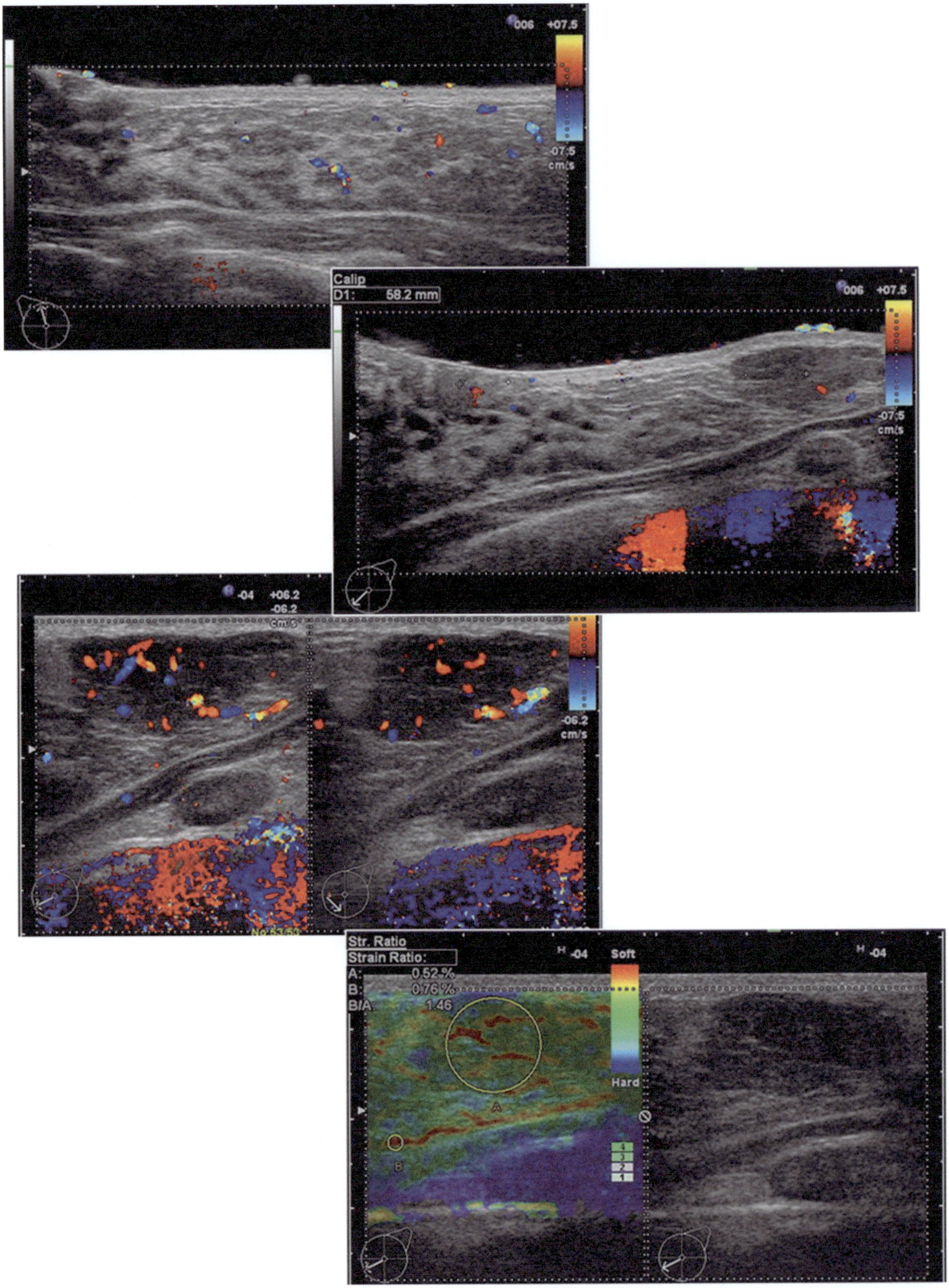
006 +07.5
-07.5
cm/s
Calip
D1: 58.2 mm
006 +07.5
-07.5
cm/s
-04 +06.2
-06.2
cm/s
-06.2
cm/s
Str. Ratio
Strain Ratio:
A: 0.52 %
B: 0.76 %
B/A: 1.46
Soft
Hard
A
B

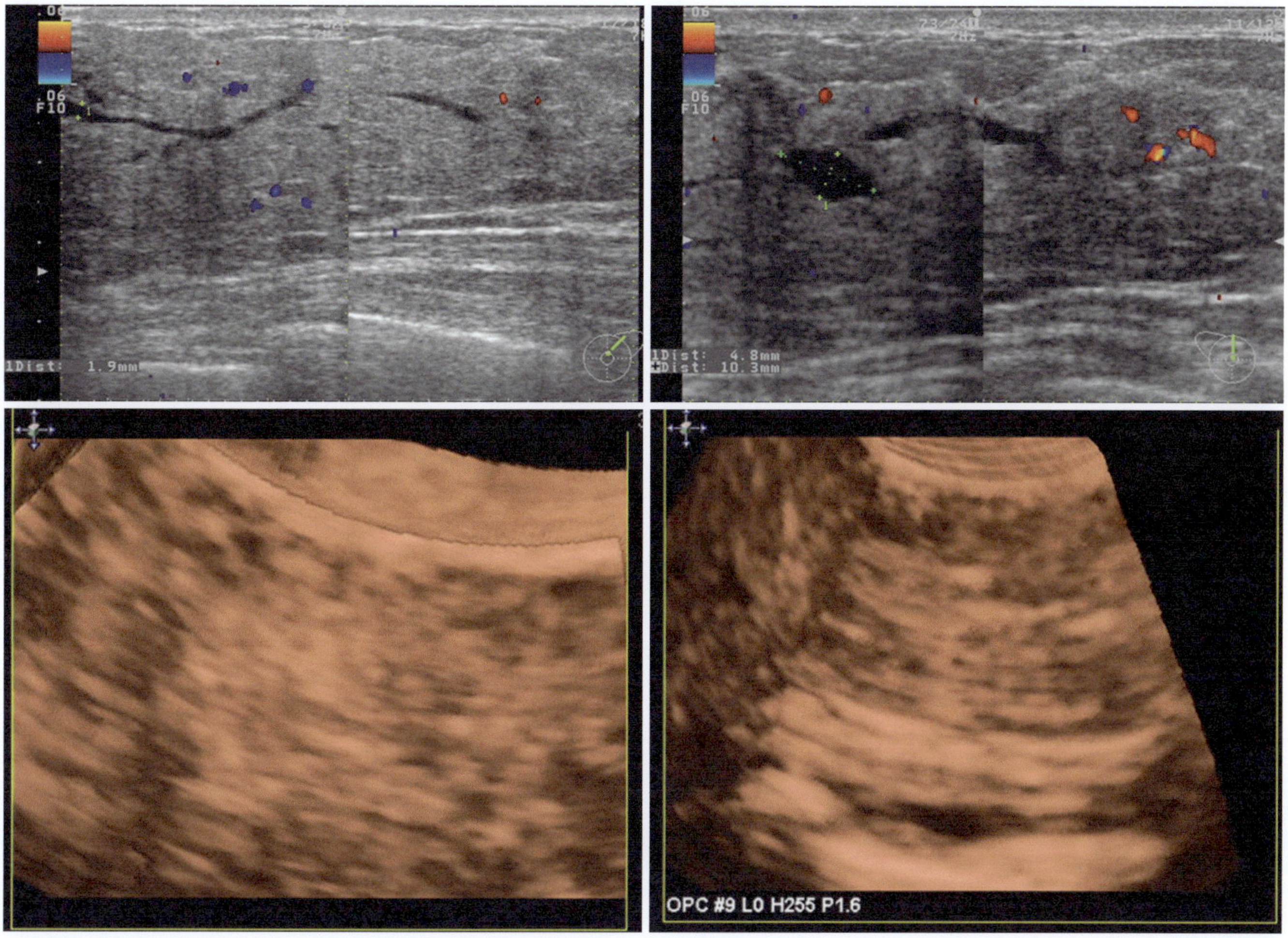

Fig. 3.30 Dense breast-feeding with reduced fatty tissue and glandular stroma and increased amount of the lobules and mammary thin ducts; the main ducts are fulfilled with fluid (milk), and some reversible cystic dilatations may mimic pathological aspects, but are transient; the 4D reconstructions are useful for illustrating the dense breast parenchyma

Fig. 3.29 A 21-year-old patient: Doppler DE suggests a pseudomalignant mass at R8:00, but the complementary SE confirms a benign lobular hyperplasia with physiological hyper vasculature in a young woman with lactation breast

References

1. Osborne M (1996) Breast development and anatomy. In: Harris JR, Lippman ME, Morrow M, Hellman S (eds) Diseases of the breast, 2nd edn. Lippincott-Raven, Philadelphia, pp 1–14
2. Stanhope R (2000) Premature Thelarche: clinical follow up and indication for treatment. J Pediatr Endocr Metab 13:827–830
3. Kopans DB (2006) Breast imaging, 3rd edn. Lippincott Williams & Wilkins. Philadelphia, p 121
4. Tot T (2007b) The theory of the sick breast lobe and the possible consequences. Int J Surg Pathol 1:68–71
5. Ichihara S, Moritani S, Ohitake T, Ohuchi N (2005) Ductal carcinoma in situ of the breast: the pathological reason for the diversity of its clinical imaging. In: Research and development in breast ultrasound. Springer, Tokyo Ed, pp 104–113
6. Teboul M, Halliwell M (1995) Atlas of ultrasound and ductal echography of the breast. Ed. Blackwell Science Inc
7. Amy D (2000) Echographie mammaire: echoanatomie. JL mensuel d'echographie LUS 10:654–662
8. Stefanie J, Thea T (2006) Breast stromal genes act as early markers of malignancy. Grant#:8EB-0106, http://cbcrp.org.127.seekdotnet.com/research/ByAwardType1.asp?mechanism_id=38
9. Mao Y, Keller ET, Garfield DH, Shen K, Wang J (2013) Stromal cells in tumor microenvironment and breast cancer. Cancer Metastasis Rev 32(1-2):303–315. doi:10.1007/s10555-012-9415-3
10. Miliaras D, Konstantinides E (2012) Malignant fibrous histiocytoma of the breast: a case report. Case Rep Pathol 2012:579245. doi:10.1155/2012/579245
11. Sapino A, Bosco M, Cassoni P et al (2006) Estrogen receptor – beta is expressed in stromal cells of fibroadenoma and phyllodes tumors of the breast. Mod Pathol 19(4):599–606
12. Georgescu V (2009) Clustering of fuzzy shapes by integrating procrustean metrics and full mean shape estimation into K-Means Algorithm. In: Proceedings of the joint 2009 international fuzzy system association world congress and 2009 European Society of fuzzy logic and technology conference, Lisbon, July 20–24; available: psu.edu
13. Moon WK, Chang R-F (2007) Solid breast masses: neural network analysis of 3-D power Doppler ultrasound image features for classification as benign or malignant. Vienna, B-278, p.285. http://www.myesr.org/html/img/pool/3_ECR_2007_Final_Programme_web.pdf
14. Teboul M (2003) Practical ductal echography: guide to intelligent and intelligible ultrasound imaging of the breast. Saned Editors, Madrid
15. Amy D (2014) Lobar ultrasonic breast anatomy. In: Francescatti DS, Silverstein MJ (eds) Breast cancer: a new era in management. © Springer Science+Business Media, New York. doi:10.1007/978-1-4614-8063-1_4

4 Sonoelastography in Addition to Doppler Ductal Echography: Full Breast Ultrasonography

4.1 Definition of the Sonoelastography: Systems of Acquisition

Elastography refers to the measurement of the elastic properties of the tissues, based on the well-established principle that malignant tissue is harder than benign tissue. The standard medical practice of soft tissue palpation is based on qualitative, low-resolution assessment of the static elastic modulus of tissues. Pathological changes are generally correlated with changes in tissues' elastic modulus, and breast palpation is the first diagnostic method, early used by Hippocrates, with an accuracy evaluated to 60–65 %. The different response to the compression with the transducer of the benign or malignant lesions was early published in 1977 on statically images by Kobayashi, which presented the deformation of the tissues with increasing posterior enhancement effect and of the lateral shadows for benign masses, while the malignant ones presented less compressibility but increasing shadowing [1, 2].

We agree in general that a lesion may not possess echogenic properties which could make it ultrasonically detectable, such as prostatic tumor or hepatic cirrhosis or breast tumor in classical US [3, 4], but we deny this affirmation for Doppler DE, because there are no cases of breast tumor undetectable on DE, confirming the opinion of the promoters of this method [5]. When adding sonoelastography, we are able both to better visualize the differences between the suspect abnormality and the surrounding breast tissues and to characterize its risk of malignancy.

To assess the elasticity, it is necessary to apply an external mechanical stimulus to the tissues and to observe the response in terms of local internal deformations. In principle, any high-resolution imaging modality may be used for such observations. The use of ultrasound for this purpose, however, has several important advantages such as real-time imaging capabilities, very high resolution in motion estimation (~1 μm), simplicity, noninvasiveness, and relative low cost, as compared with MRI elastography.

In clinical practice, sonoelastography was used by some authors as a single method of diagnosis, with doubtful accuracy as compared with US alone [6], but we recommend combining sonoelastography with the ductal, even with the conventional, ultrasound, using them as complementary diagnostic tools, similar to Doppler used in addition to US B-mode examination. *Elastography is only another descriptor of a tissue/tumor* such as margins, echo texture, and posterior effects, and it is illogical to compare its performance with US alone, while nobody compared Doppler exam with 2D US alone.

Conventional elastography, i.e., the process of imaging the axial strain in tissues that occurs in response to a known external displacement, ignores many properties of the tissue's response to an applied stress. Elastography uses raw ultrasound obtained before and after a slight compression of tissues, typically achieved with a transducer. Compression may also be performed using vibrations in a technique known as real-time sonoelastography (RTSE). Elastography measures and displays strain represented by the change in the dimension of tissue elements at various locations in the region of interest. It is known that substantial strain contrast is due to the stress distribution that is specific to the boundary conditions of the experiment, rendering strain images non-quantitative. Moreover, it seems that such elastogram is influenced by, and sometimes contains information about tissue properties (viscosity, porosity, anisotropy, nonlinearity of the stress-strain relationship). In clinical applications, quantitative imaging may improve ability to distinguish benign from malignant tumors and may open up new applications such as monitoring the effects of and response to treatment; it is also expected to improve lesion visibility and imaging understanding, by reducing image artifacts, such as the retroareolar shadowing or false microcalcifications in nodular fibro-micro-cystic dysplasia.

Different approaches on the elasticity imaging have been investigated, and at present some are at the stage of developing the practical system. In clinical measurement, a

A. Colan-Georges, *Atlas of Full Breast Ultrasonography*, DOI 10.1007/978-3-319-31418-1_4

high-speed processing is required for real-time diagnosis, and freehand manipulation of ultrasonic probe like the usual ultrasonic diagnosis is desirable for simple operation. The American achievements concerning 15 years of research about tissues' elasticity were presented justly to the *2006 ECR* by Ophir et al., from Texas, who have constructed a device based on a Philips imaging system designated to produce elastography of the breast in vivo [4], while at the *2005 RSNA* meeting, tomosynthesis was the most important breast imaging development. Elastography was earlier developed in Japan by Shiina and Ueno, which at the beginning of the nineteenth century conceived a real-time tissue elasticity imaging system (consisting of an ultrasonic 7.5 MHz probe, an ultrasonic scanner, and a personal computer Intel Pentium IV), with freehand tissue compression based on the extended combined autocorrelation method [7], and the results were presented in 2003 [8]. Furthermore, their method was implemented and developed on the Hitachi devices.

Nowadays, there are two available types of equipments for sonoelastography:

a. The equipment from Hitachi Medical Corporation, completed in 2003 and commercialized and marketed since 2004, which uses mechanical external or better freehand compression of tissues, *HI-RTSE (Hitachi Real-time Tissue Elastography)* with two rendering methods: a qualitative and a quantitative sonoelastography. The *qualitative method* uses a color scale from red for the soft, normal structures to blue, for stiff, malignant lesions. This scale comports a classification named *Ueno* (promoter) or *Tsukuba* (the University), which will be presented on what follows and used as the best scoring system. Hitachi equipments include a *quantitative* sonoelastography too, which is more accurate and calculates the *strain ratio* or *fat-to-lesion ratio (FLR)*, with a cutoff established at 4.7 (5.0 as maximum), that means lower FLR is found in most probable benign conditions and higher is found in the malignant lesions. It is recommended by the manufacturer to select the ROI for the pathological area ("B" area) and for the normal fatty tissue area ("A" area) for the calculation of the strain ratio (B/A) on the 2D grayscale display, because some benign lesions may be not visible on the color display; other sonographers recommend to select the ROI on the color display, because the pathological area is better delineated especially in the malignant lesions [9]. Practically, both methods are used together and offer similar results, because the HI-RTE is easy to perform, fast, accurate, and reproducible.
b. The equipment from Siemens, experimented mainly by British and Italian radiologists and promoted by American researchers from Texas, *eSie Touch™ elasticity imaging*, which uses a specialized software for imaging the relative tissue compression; practically the tissue elasticity is investigated using an "internal palpation" produced by the ultrasonic wave front compression and ultrafast measuring of their displacements. Rendering the elasticity, elastograms were presented in both *a 2D log grayscale* less used because of less sensibility and less resolution and in a *color scale*, initially with inversed colors as compared with HI-RTE, from violet for normal/benign structures to red for stiff/malignant ones. Nowadays, there are optional color scales with less popularity.

Initial studies of English researchers demonstrate a significant reduction of benign unnecessary biopsies; moreover, because elastography overestimates the size of many malignant tumors because the peritumoral stromal reaction is best delimitated, it was considered useful for guiding surgery, with re-excision rates being reduced. Using comparative freehand strain imaging of the Siemens equipment, it is possible to halve the benign biopsy rate when using a strain/B-mode ratio of 75 % as the cutoff point [10]. Unfortunately, the system has not been widely promoted in the USA, and it is being used only at a handful of research facilities, because in the USA there is a greater tendency to biopsy breast lesions and the manufacturer development is mainly oriented to breast MRI or the improvement of full-filed digital mammography, CAD, PET-CT, and tomosynthesis, which are more operator independent but are more expansive, less available, and do not have completely less side effects (even MRI could have some side effects of the paramagnetic contrast agents or directly on the nervous system).

Therefore, there are new developments of the techniques of elastography, such as *ShearWaveTM Elastography* presented at the ECR 2009 by The Theragnostic CompanyTM on a platform named the AixplorerTM Ultrasound System, which measure the quantitative elasticity in kilopascals, offering user-skill-independent and reproducible results with a remarkable image quality.

While manufacturers have patent disputes, the two main sonoelastographic systems coexist; therefore, the color scale from Hitachi with the scoring system of the tissues' elasticity, superposed on the BI-RADS classification, named upon the University of Tsukuba or upon the main promoter Professor Ei Ueno, is already more familiar, and many researches confirmed its viability, so this method will be mainly presented and illustrated in this volume. Many manufacturers implemented in the last years this scale and the strain ratio upon Hitachi (such as Aloka, Toshiba, General Electric), resulting to an almost standardized technique of examination.

4.2 Accuracy of the SE

There are not yet many published studies with sonoelastography applied to DE, except for a few works of their promoters and other disciples [5, 9, 11, 12], so the most published results represent the applications on classical breast US. Even with the classical US, which is itself less performing, the results of sonoelastography revealed a revolutionary technique, relatively cheap, noninvasive, available, without side effects, and with reduced emotional burden, thus being repeatable and suitable for screening and the best recommendable for the differential diagnosis of benign from the malignant masses in soft tissues, such as the breast, thyroid, musculoskeletal US, or in deep organs, such as the prostate, liver, uterine cervix, or kidney.

For lesions of all sizes, classical breast US elastography using Hitachi technique achieved sensitivity of 80 %, specificity of 93 %, positive predictive value of 85.3 %, and negative predictive value of 90.3 %, in a French report in 2006 consisting of elastography applied in classical US [13]. Sensitivity was the best for lesions less than 5 mm (90 %), while specificity was the best for lesions over 10 mm (95 %). Researchers also reported false positives with elastography (such as fibrous mastopathy and sclerosis adenosis) and false-negative findings (such as DCIS). Other results are in favor of sonoelastography, avoiding unnecessary biopsies, with accuracy between 95 and 99 % [14]. There are yet doubts about the ability of sonoelastography to prove definitely if a lesion is benign or malignant, and there are opinions that even if elastography indicates a lesion as benign, if another feature looks suspicious, the biopsy might still go ahead. The doubts are partially justified, in our opinion, on one hand because of the yet no standardized technique of examination in elastography, with two systems, two scales, less trained operators, and less known method by the clinicians, and on the other hand because of the irrational, classical, non-anatomical approach of the breast in classical US, resulting to false limits of sonoelastography.

In fact, a good anatomical US technique of examination of the breast, combined with Doppler characterization of the lesions and sonoelastography, results in an accurate prediction of the malignancy of the breast lesions. None technique was proved to be sufficient to assess the malignancy risk, but the Doppler features combined with sonoelastography are able to increase the performance up to 100 %; as consequence, this duality of Doppler-sonoelastography applied to DE represents the trinity named the full breast ductal Doppler ultrasonography or briefly full breast ultrasonography (FBU). The major fault of the previous reports is the lack of correlation between Doppler and sonoelastography. For instance, the false-positive fibrous mastopathy, fibrous-micro-cystic dysplasia, and sclerosis adenosis may mimic a breast cancer on classical US with sonoelastography, but in DE they have different aspects; moreover, usually these dysplasias have less/absent salient vasculature, while cancers have new formation vasculature visible in Doppler as well as in contrast MRI (where vasculature determines the enhancement curves characterizing the malignancy risk). Contrarily, the false-negative DCIS/LCIS on classical US with sonoelastography appears in FBU as a lesion less than 5 mm in diameter with ductal localization/connection and with detectable increased focal vasculature, which is suspect for malignancy. In all cases, we recommend the use of the quantitative FLR for sonoelastography, because the results are more specific for cancer than with the qualitative elastography alone.

4.3 Technique of Sonoelastography: Integration in FBU

There are few steps recommended in the FBU examination:

I. *Detection*: A radial scanning of the entire breast (DE) with the long probe, using a water-bag adaptor and noticing all the abnormalities (L3:00, R12:00); usually 7–10 MHz probes of 7–9 cm length are the best available, resulting a compromise between the length radial scan and the frequency related to the image resolution.

   This technique is standardized by Teboul et al. and is recommended in screening, with better sensibility than that of the mammography.

II. *Characterization of US BI-RADS applied to DE:* A reexamination of the solid or suspect lesions concerning all criteria of the Stavros in 2D and 3D/4D US, using DE (the radial technique), is performed with a very high-frequency probe, usually of 4–5 cm in length and up to 16 MHz, which offers a better resolution; the high resolution in DE is the key for better characterization of the ductal-lobular "tree" and of the abnormal ultrasound findings.

   This examination includes the characterization of the vasculature on Doppler imaging, using especially the qualitative analysis of the vessels, in the radial, antiradial, and 3D acquisitions.

   This step is standardized for DE and the US BI-RADS assessment; it maximizes the sensibility and offers a high specificity of breast US for benign and malignant lesions. Some manufacturers produced linear transducers of intermediate length of approximately 6–7 cm, multifrequency, with good resolution for all depths and with possibility of virtual radial scanning, which can be used instead of the two types successively as described above; that results in good evaluation of the mammary lobar radius and good assessment of the vasculature and of the tissue stiffness.

III. *Characterization of the stiffness*: The third step is represented by sonoelastography applied to each lesion found before and to the retroareolar structures. Every lesion must be initially characterized in B-mode and color Doppler, because on the real-time dual image display sonoelastography (with elastogram and B-mode image), the internal echoes and the marginal regions of the lesion cannot be evaluated properly, because the pressure given with the probe is too weak for a good US image. The qualitative sonoelastogram is standardized basing on the Ueno/Tsukuba score, and the quantitative sonoelastography is referring to the fatty tissue strain (FLR), being less operator dependant and increasing the specificity of the FBU over 90 %. The examination will be accomplished with the assessment of the satellite lymph nodes, with the high-frequency transducer, including the Doppler and sonoelastography applications.

According to most authors and our experience, a FLR less than 4.70 (5.00) at repeated measurements is high, predicting for a benign breast structure, and is correlated with the scores 1, 2, and 3 Ueno and BGR; when FLR is around 5.00 (4.50–6.00), a borderline structure may be affirmed; malignancies with score 4 or 5 Ueno present usually a high FLR value, usually over 10.00, and its value is as high as the lesion that may contain (unapparent in US!) malignant microcalcifications or strong desmoplastic reaction. It is recommended to assess FLR better as interval or the superior limits for benign findings and the most inferior values for the malignant-type lesions, and to avoid affirming a precise value for FLR.

This sequence is the most performed examination, and its efficacy was proved by Amy and other promoters [9, 15, 16]; in fact, this sequence is logical, and any other sequence could be incomplete and will increase the risk of misdiagnosis or will impose supplementary tests (i.e., biopsies or breast MRI). The first step will explore the whole breast; the second and the third will characterize each lesion with complementary findings for the final diagnosis. The whole examination of both breasts, for trained operators, takes about 30 min, and the patient is informed immediately and without any harmful procedure about the diagnosis and about the recommendations, without any waiting stress and supplementary expenses.

For the best accuracy of sonoelastography, it is recommended to use the highest-frequency available transducer, without water bag. We can perform this exam in any plan of the breast volume, but it is logical to initiate it in the same radial plan that realize the detection and the establishment of the rapports of the lesion. A small compression pad could be attached to the probe/transducer, so that stable tissue compression is attained and the stress field is more uniformly transmitted. The compression with a stepping motor could be better because the compression direction is the same as the axial direction of the ultrasonic beam, the best for strain estimation. However, the freehand technique is preferred as in the usual ultrasonic diagnosis, and a good training and the use of the combined autocorrelation method of Shiina and Ueno can suppress the lateral slip. When applying freehand technique, a light pressure with a soft touch is preferable, because a strong pressure produces strain even in hard tissue, providing erroneous information.

There are two possibilities of achieving freehand elastograms [7]:

- Making a small compression on the region of interest, with uniform release, this technique is more difficult to train to the operators and somewhat subjective.
- Making fine, 1 mm movement in normal breast, up to 2 mm for deeper lesions or for large breasts; the movement consists in quick series/cycles of 2–3 s of compressions, obtaining a real-time elastogram. This method is easy to perform and to train, and the results are reproducible.

Because the level of the strain changes while compressing or relaxing the tissues, Shiina and Ueno calculated the mean of strain distribution within a ROI, with a maximum range set of 2.5 times the mean value and the minimum set of 0, so the stable strain image is no more depending on the level of compression.

After selecting the elastography mode, we must set up elastography ROI according to the size of the lesion and thickness of the mammary grand. The elastogram shows the distribution of the relative strain, so adjacent normal breast tissue must be included in the ROI:

1. In the depth direction: from subcutaneous tissue to pectoralis major muscle
2. In the width direction: full range of the screen

The display will be adjusted so that the lesion occupies a quarter of the screen width or less. If the lesion is larger than a quarter, we must change to a smaller cross section. When selecting a wrong ROI, the same lesion might appear different depending on ROI size, for instance, for a too small wrong ROI, the lesion may appear as benign (score 2 Ueno), but for a good large ROI, the lesion may be typically malignant (score 4 or 5 Ueno). If the tumor size is large, the recommendation of the manufacturer is to move tumor position from the center to the edge of the ROI, and then we will be able to compare it clearly with the normal surrounding tissues.

Training the operators is essential, because a wrong technique may result misdiagnosis. The probe is placed on the breast so it is not deformed and the movement of 1–2 mm up and down is made from this position, with an optimal frequency of 2 Hz (2cycles/second). If the initial compression is too strong, when performing sonoelastography, the normal tissues are in tension, their elasticity is reduced in that position, and the eventually stiff tumor has similar score, so the result is false negative. The probe must be fixed to not laterally sliding, and it is useful to anchor the operator's hand by resting the fifth fingers on the breast skin. The acquisition is accomplished when reproducible elastogram is obtained.

4.4 Rendering Sonoelastogram

The ultrasonic echo signals from the inside of a tissue, before and after deformation during the compression and the relaxation made with the transducer, are measured simultaneously, and a displacement distribution of each point is estimated. Then, the spatial displacement distribution is visualized as an elasticity image. Using a base algorithm of the combined autocorrelation method, the system can estimate the strain distribution accurately and at a high speed, supporting a large dynamic range of strain, with a lateral slip to about 4 mm. Tissue hardness is displayed in color tone, with increasing hardness presented in descending order of red, yellow, green, and blue on the Hitachi model, or optional in the inversed order on other platforms.

Because the area and the boundary of the tumor in a strain image and B-mode image are not necessarily the same, for recognition, the corresponding area in the two images was imagined in a way to display both images simultaneously: a strain image is superimposed on the B-mode image with a translucent color scale, where, for example, red indicates that the tissue is soft and blue indicates that the tissue is hard/stiff. In the dual elastographic mode, we have on the left side of the screen the B-mode display and on the right side the strain image for the ROI superimposed on the B-mode image. The system allows us to verify the range of stream and repeat the acquisition if it is not optimally situated in the manufacturer recommendations. That results an operator-independent technique, without significant differences between different compressions ranges. For each ultrasound machine with a particular patent of sonoelastography, there is a specific modality to display the level of the pressure applied during the acquisition; the manufacturers offer the possibility to self-control the compression intensity and to immediately correct when it is out of recommended limits. Obviously, only the correct acquisitions must be interpreted and reported.

4.5 Interpretation of the Elastogram

The color-coded elastograms are similar, but not entirely superposing images to B-mode achievements, because they measure not only the elasticity of the researched mass but the effect of the mass to the surrounding tissues. For example, for the fibroadenoma, the area on strain display is either absent/indistinct and if a small lesion, either smaller than in B-mode or equal. Inversely, for the malignant masses, the strain image is either equal (if there aren't surrounding infiltration produced by the desmoplastic reaction) or larger, the central tumoral dark blue area being surrounded by a boundary light blue or halo, corresponding to the peritumoral malignant infiltration or to the peritumoral desmoplastic reaction.

When analyzing the real-time dual image display during the exam, it is recommended to look at the elastogram image, because when looking on the grayscale image, the resolution is not very good and there is tendency to push too hard with the probe, which can produce false-negative images. Another key is to review the record of the dynamic acquisitions: if the scores vary, the initial pressure may be too high or compression movement too large, and the sonoelastography must be repeated. If the acquired breast images have the same score during compression in the dynamic image, the operator's performance is validated, and the elastogram will have high diagnostic value.

The classification system developed by Ei Ueno is already largely accepted, because it is practically easy to recognize and especially because it is pathologically correlated, almost superimposable on the US BI-RADS classification. The Italian score is a variant less utilized, where the score 1 is represented by the cystic aspect and some small differences are presented for the other scores, but without significant diagnostic improvements.

4.5.1 The Elasticity Score Named Upon Ueno/Tsukuba University: Benign

Score 1: Entire area is evenly shaded green, as is surrounding tissue (Figs. 4.1, 4.2, and 4.3). DE presents the normal ducts and lobules in green yellow and interprets the score 1 Ueno, while the small ectasias have the ductal walls in green and the content of the lumen colored in red, with the same score 1.

Score 2: Lesion area shows a mosaic pattern of green, blue, and red (Figs. 4.4, 4.5, and 4.6). The DE illustrates for the different ROI of a mammary lobe including parenchyma and glandular stroma, a score 2 Ueno, which is considered as normal. The normal satellite lymph node sonoelastogram may appear as score 1 or 2 Ueno.

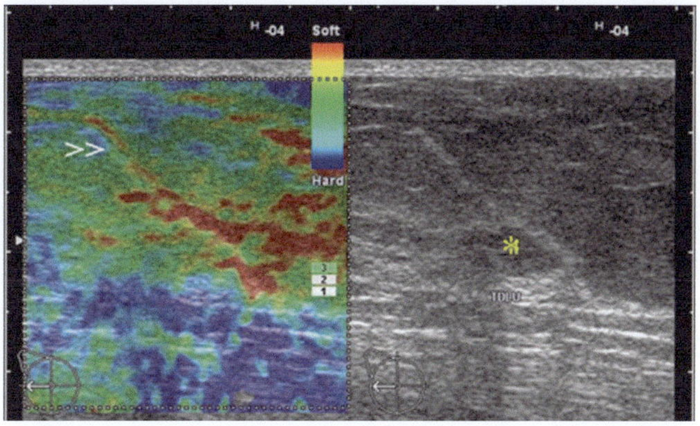

Fig. 4.1 Sonoelastography in fatty breast with ductal atrophy, difficult to differentiate from the fatty tissue, with the score 1 Ueno; there are some salient remnant glandular structures in a TDLU (*) and along the Cooper ligament, which appears "elongated" (>>). The pectoral muscles are normally stiff (US BI-RADS 1 category)

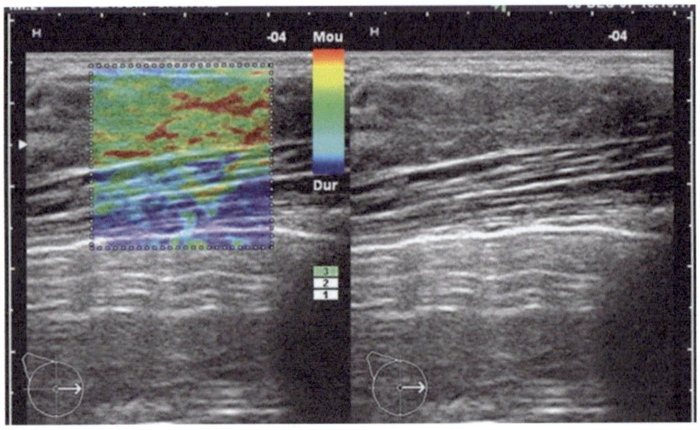

Fig. 4.2 Sonoelastography in dense glandular breast dystrophy in a thin woman, with almost absence of subcutaneous and retromammary fatty tissue, reduced glandular stroma with contiguous "back-to-back" ducts and lobules on DE, presenting normal architecture on the elastogram—score 1 Ueno for normal parenchyma (US BI-RADS 1 category)

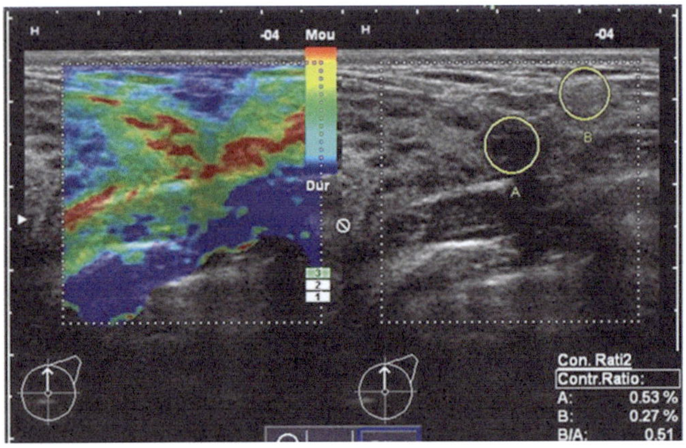

Fig. 4.3 Sonoelastography is the best choice in the pseudomalignant US findings: DE shows a suspect lesion, based on the classical US features; in this case an US lesion type BI-RADS 4–5 category presents an elastogram score 1–2 Ueno and a very low FLR, high suggesting for benign lesion, avoiding unnecessary biopsy (US BI-RADS 2 category)

Score 3: Central part of the area is blue (stiff), and peripheral part is green (soft), so the lesions appear smaller on the elastogram than in the grayscale display. Score 3 is a state in which malignancy cannot be ruled out, but it is usually applied for some fibroadenomas (Fig. 4.7).

4.5.2 Malignant

Score 4: The entire area is blue (stiff), with the same size as the area on the grayscale; the malignant lesion is well delineated, usually noninvasive small cancer or particular types such as mucinous or medullary cancer (Fig. 4.8). The intracystic or intraductal carcinoma is typical for the score 4 Ueno, but very aggressive, undifferentiated invasive cancers with rapid growth that do not allow the desmoplastic reaction to develop may equally present the score 4 Ueno.

Score 5: The entire area and its surrounding area are blue (stiff), so the lesion appears larger on the elastogram. This corresponds to the typical scirrhous carcinoma with peripheral desmoplastic reaction that shows a light-blue halo, corresponding in B-mode to the hyperechoic signal at the border determined by the malignant halo and to the attenuated echo on the posterior side (shadowing) (Fig. 4.9). Score 5 is not specific for malignancy, but for any hardness of the tissues, such as scars, fibro-micro-cystic disease especially the nodular form, chronic inflammation, or fibrosis related to the implant pathology.

However, these scores can be considered to correspond to the assessment category of BI-RADS [17], but we must be precise for the final diagnosis of the sonoelastography and must rely to the Doppler characterization.

In addition, for the cysts larger than 5 mm, a special score was described, a composed image with two internal level-level structures, represented by *blue/green/red (BGR) complex* that is characteristic for the liquid, and the same aspect appears in abscess, hematoma, seroma, and implants, as well as in the cross section of the large vessels (Fig. 4.10). In cases of nodular fibro-micro-cystic dysplasia, the fluid content of the immeasurable cysts on US determines the BGR-summation score, with the unique elastogram BGR being equivalent to those of a cyst of equal size as the sum of the cluster of microcysts (Fig. 4.11). In other cases, there is a complex of BGR-summation score (Fig. 4.12), either in a large dysplasia or in a multiloculated hematoma, area of edema, recent large scar, infected cysts or galactoceles, and other benign conditions. It is remarkable that mucinous carcinoma appears always as malignant, without BGR score. By consequence, the proper use of sonoelastography as a complementary method allows a better interpretation of the Doppler DE or of the Doppler classical US.

Observation The Ueno score classification system was conceived in classical US, despite the group of researchers that the coordinates are familiar with in the ductal US approach. That means some terms such as *surrounding tissue* adopted by the practitioners of the classical US which represent in fact the surrounding stromal components, while the breast parenchyma may appear green or red; especially ductal-lobular benign hyperplasia is green yellow, while small ductal ectasia appears in red in the central luminal area, due to the presence of the liquid, bordered by the ductal walls in green yellow. Nevertheless, the largest duct ectasias will illustrate a similar BGR scoring as the cysts with a ribbon shape.

The value of sonoelastography is revealed in such conditions by confirming the malignancy in hyperechoic breast cancer (when it is surrounded by fatty tissue, which is

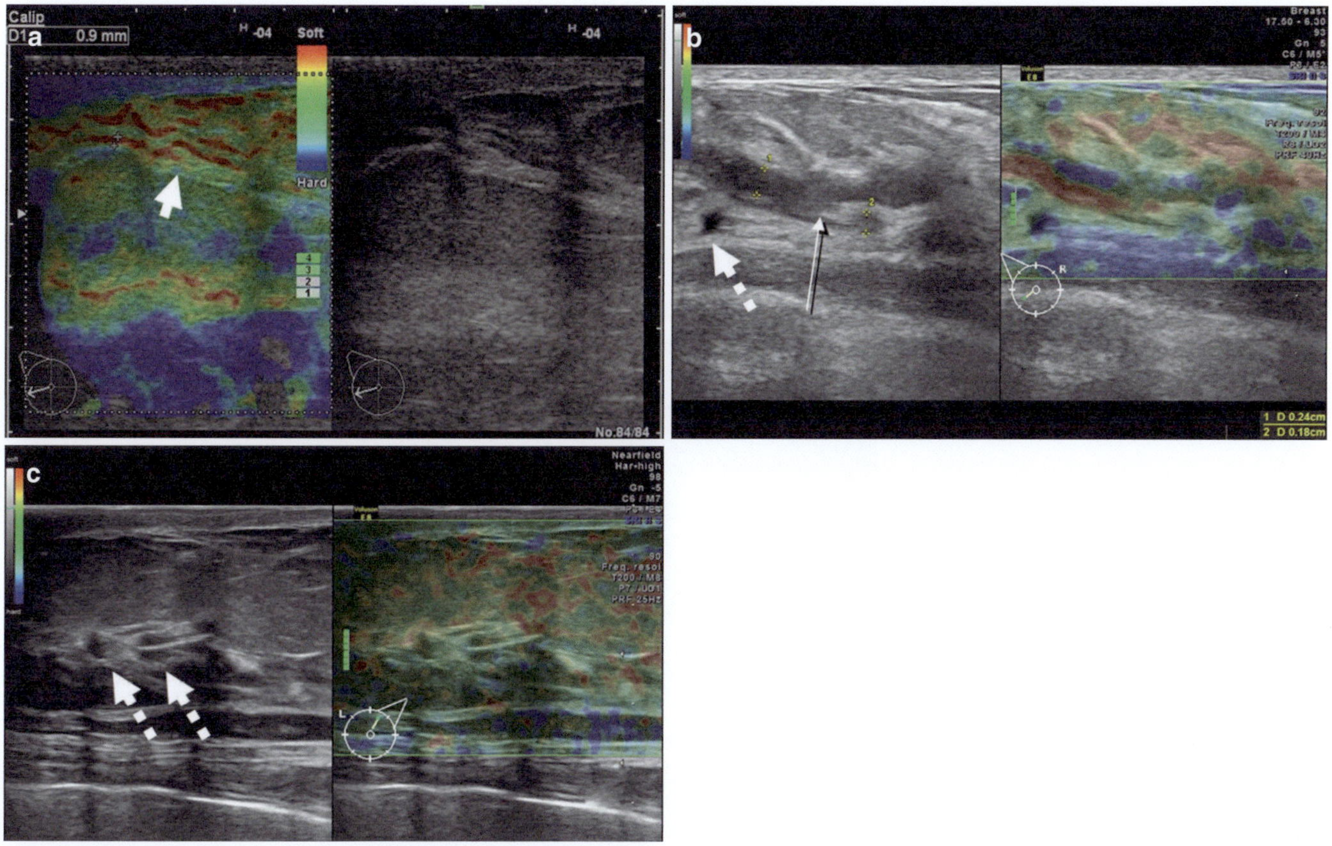

Fig. 4.4 Sonoelastography of normal heterogeneous breast (**a**), with thin, less than 1 mm in diameter ducts, scored 1 Ueno; duct ectasia of 2.4 mm in diameter (**b**) with BGR score (*long arrow*). Lobules may be visible usually in young, adult dense breast or in adenosis (**c**), with global sonoelastography of the mammary lobe score 2 Ueno (*square dot arrows*)

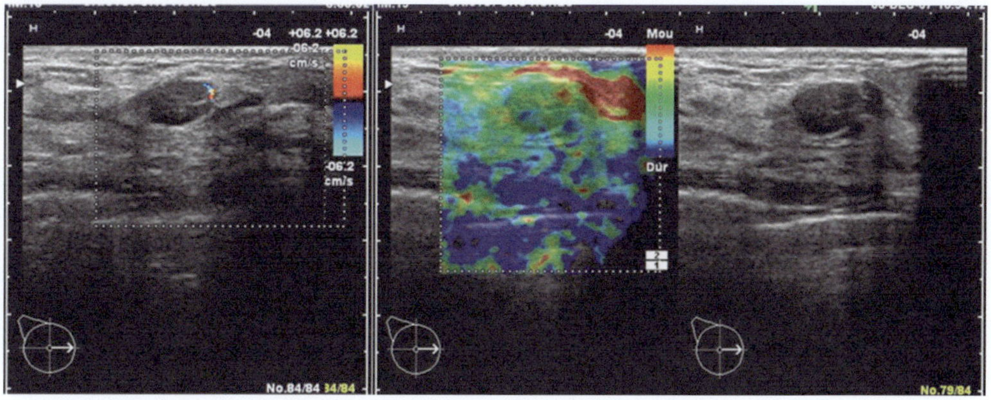

Fig. 4.5 FBU: benign 2D appearances, peripheral unipolar new vasculature, and sonoelastography with the score 2 Ueno for this mass connected to the ductal tree on DE could be considered highly predictive for fibroadenoma (US BI-RADS 2 category). The tumoral development is demonstrated on these scans as a combined process of internal growths (concretion) and accretion of the neighboring lobules

hypoechoic) or by the possibility to differentiate the nonmalignant simple postoperative scar from the local recurrence. Moreover, the most relevant utility of sonoelastography presented by Ueno is the precise visualization in blue color of the nonpalpable intraductal breast carcinoma, which represents unexpected finding. This is the same for the early-stage breast cancer detected by mammography, based only on the visualization of the microcalcifications, without any salient tumoral mass; astonishingly, less than 5 mm dimension tumoral proliferation is easily diagnosed by sonoelastography.

Another important advantage of sonoelastography is the possibility to better visualize the nondefined malignant masses, such as heterogeneous hyperechoic ill-defined infiltrative carcinomas or postoperative local recurrences after breast-conserving surgery, which are difficult to differentiate from the benign extensive scar at mammography or at MRI with enhancement curve analysis.

The most important aspect is that sonoelastography is able to detect the nonpalpable noninvasive carcinomas,

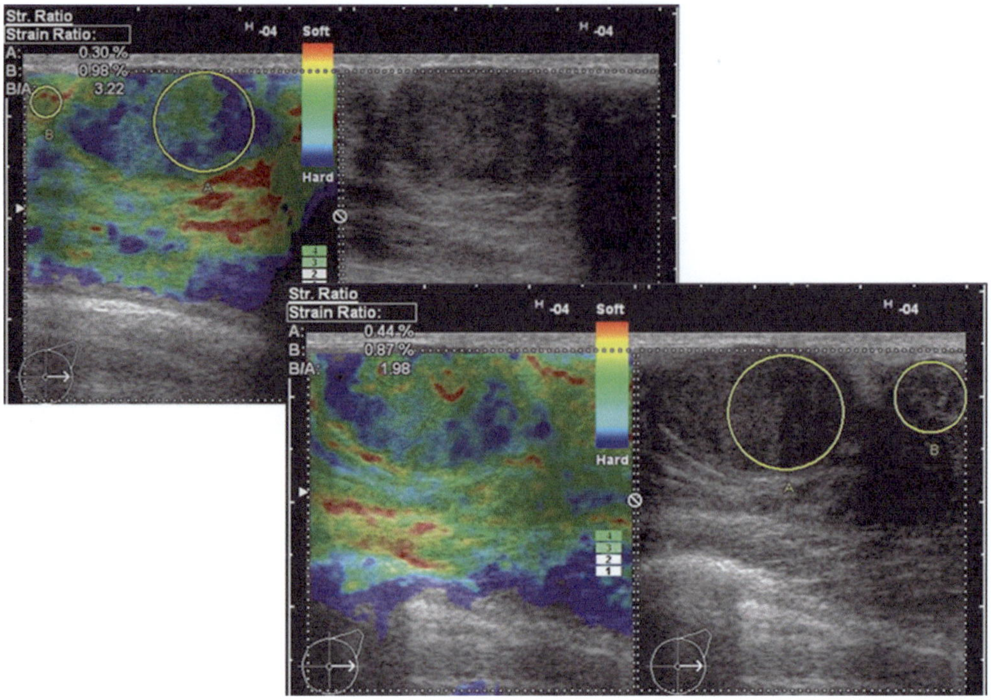

Fig. 4.6 Sonoelastography in the case of a fibroadenoma demonstrates in both elastograms the score 2 Ueno, with low (but different!) FLR, which is due to the different tissue samples

which are difficult to characterize in classical US and difficult and painful to localize by mammographic guidance with harpoon planting or by MRI guidance.

There are some important score assessment rules established by the manufacturer:

1. For scores 3, 4, and 5, we have to make the assessment over the width of the lesion and not its depth.
2. Score 2 is the image that shows mosaic shapes of green within a large area of the lesion.
3. It is hard for the pressure to penetrate deep into the lesion and difficult to extract the signal in the case of poor penetration. In this case, we must not overestimate the elasticity score (but we can change the acoustic window).
4. Blurring in the direction of depth: the faster the compression speed, the more blurring occurs:
   - At the upper part of lesion near the subcutaneous fat
   - At a deeper position at the back of the lesion near to the retromammary fat

   The elastogram must be repeated with the correct technique, to avoid the overestimation diagnosis.
5. Tumor in deep layer of mammary gland must be carefully examined because:
   - It is hard to get sufficient compression for elastography.
   - It is harder to get a good signal (only light pressure should be used).

In this case, the sensitivity of the elastography score is low, and it must be interpreted according to the grayscale and Doppler imaging; most cases from the classical ultrasound are easily interpreted in DE. Sometimes, it is useful to change the acoustic window and to repeat the elastogram in a nonconventional scan, but with the lesion in a more superficial position.

4.6 Role of SE in Nonpalpable Breast Lesions

A real challenge was to evaluate the diagnostic utility of sonoelastography in differentiating benign from malignant nonpalpable breast lesions.

An interesting study by Scaperrotta et al. evaluated 293 BI-RADS 3–5 impalpable breast lesions up to 2 cm in diameter in 278 women, which were examined with B-mode US and with sonoelastography before performing US-guided biopsy. Their conclusion was that the overall performance of sonoelastography was lower than that of US, with sensitivity and specificity of 80 % and 80.9 %, respectively, and 87.4 % for US. Their statistical analysis showed no improvement in the joint use of sonoelastography and US over the use of US alone, whose performance, however, was very high in their study.

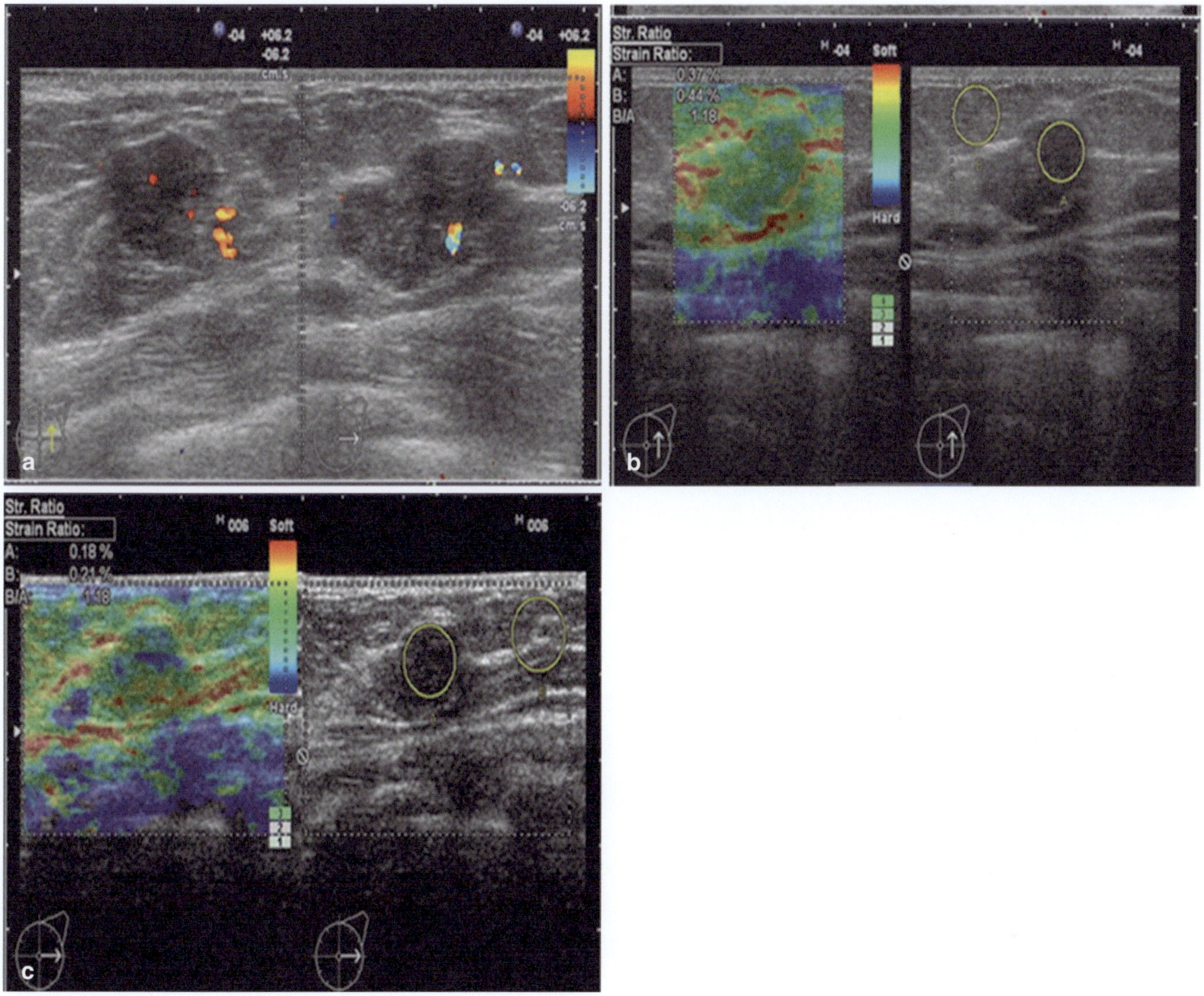

Fig. 4.7 Doppler US illustrates a borderline mass: multilobulated contour and moderate new vasculature with incident angle; however, sonoelastography performed on radial and antiradial scans scored 2 Ueno with low FLR suggesting benign lesion. The final assessment was US BI-RADS 3 category (nodular fibro-micro-cystic dysplasia)

Wherever, they recommend sonoelastography as a simple, fast, and noninvasive diagnostic method that may be a useful aid to US for less experienced radiologists in the assessment of solid nonpalpable breast lesions, especially BI-RADS 3, where specificity was higher (88.7 %) [6]. What should we learn from this study? The authors compared the results of the B-mode US and SE as different methods of imaging diagnosis, while they are parts of a unique technique, we mean the complete US. In the US diagnosis of a lesion, we must combine all the disposable information: the morphological criteria of Stavros and BI-RADS classification on B-mode US, the vasculature assessment of Doppler investigation, and the strain characterization of sonoelastography, all of them being necessary to finalize the diagnosis. The full examination in US is logical, similar to using all the procedures on the mammography, completing the standard examination with complementary views or magnification films. The same full action is achieved in breast MRI, which is not complete without adding the contrast paramagnetic agents and curve enhancement analysis.

The wrong application of sonoelastography is responsible for the discordant published reports and the lack of confidence in some countries with rich technologies; it is expected further that training operators will improve the quality of the examinations and their results. Contrarily to the

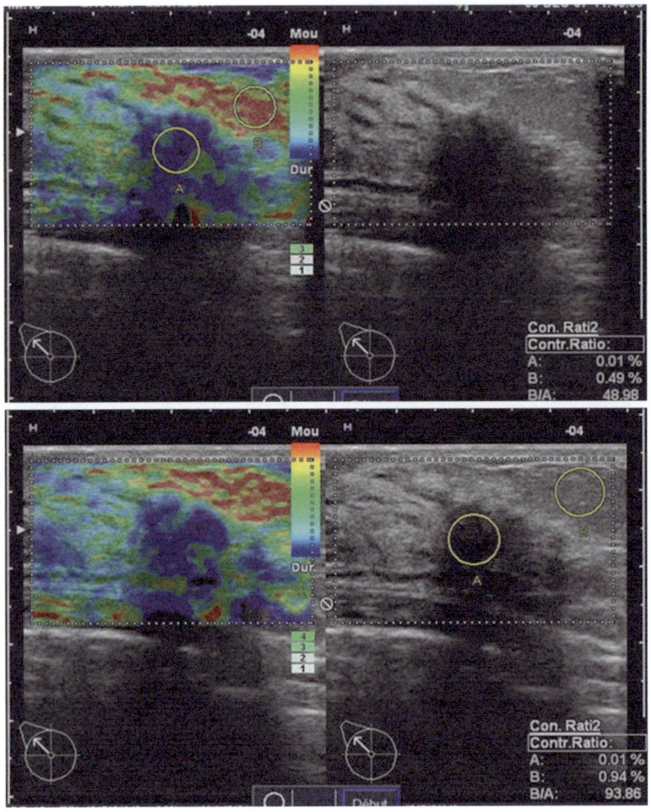

Fig. 4.8 Sonoelastography of a typical malignant lesion at R 10:30 on DE, with large hypoechoic area, irregularly shaped, taller than wide, with angular borders, connected to the ductal tree, and with intense acoustic shadowing. The corresponding area presents a heterogeneous elastogram, predominantly blue colored of score 4 Ueno, with high values on repeated determinations of the FLR 48.98–93.86, concordant for the diagnosis of malignancy (US BI-RADS 4 category if Doppler signal of malignant-type)

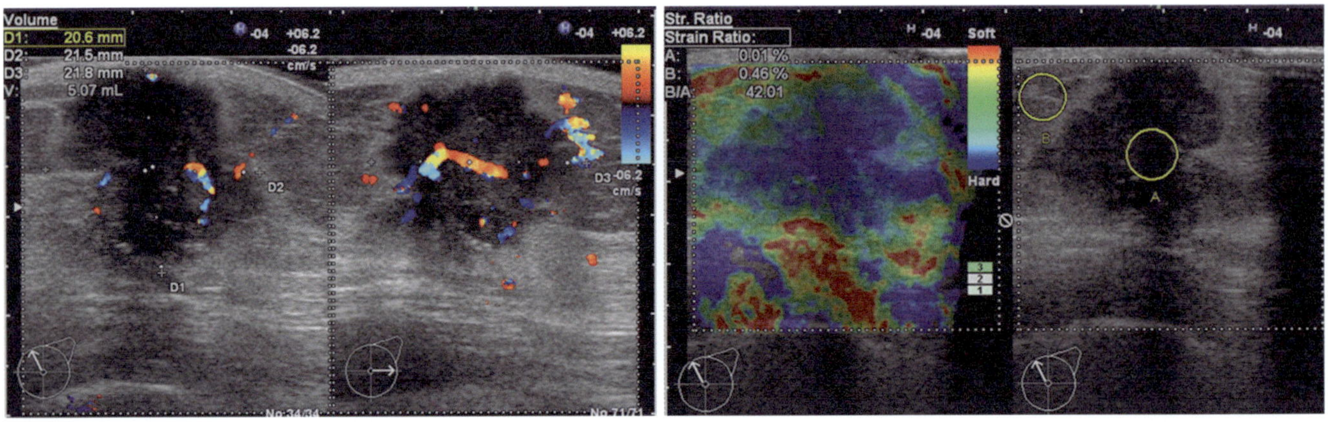

Fig. 4.9 Sonoelastography of typical malignant lesion at Doppler US: low elasticity, mostly intratumoral (*dark blue*) and peritumoral (*light blue*), the halo representing the desmoplastic reaction. The score 5 Ueno is correlated with the US BI-RADS 5 category, the final assessment in FBU

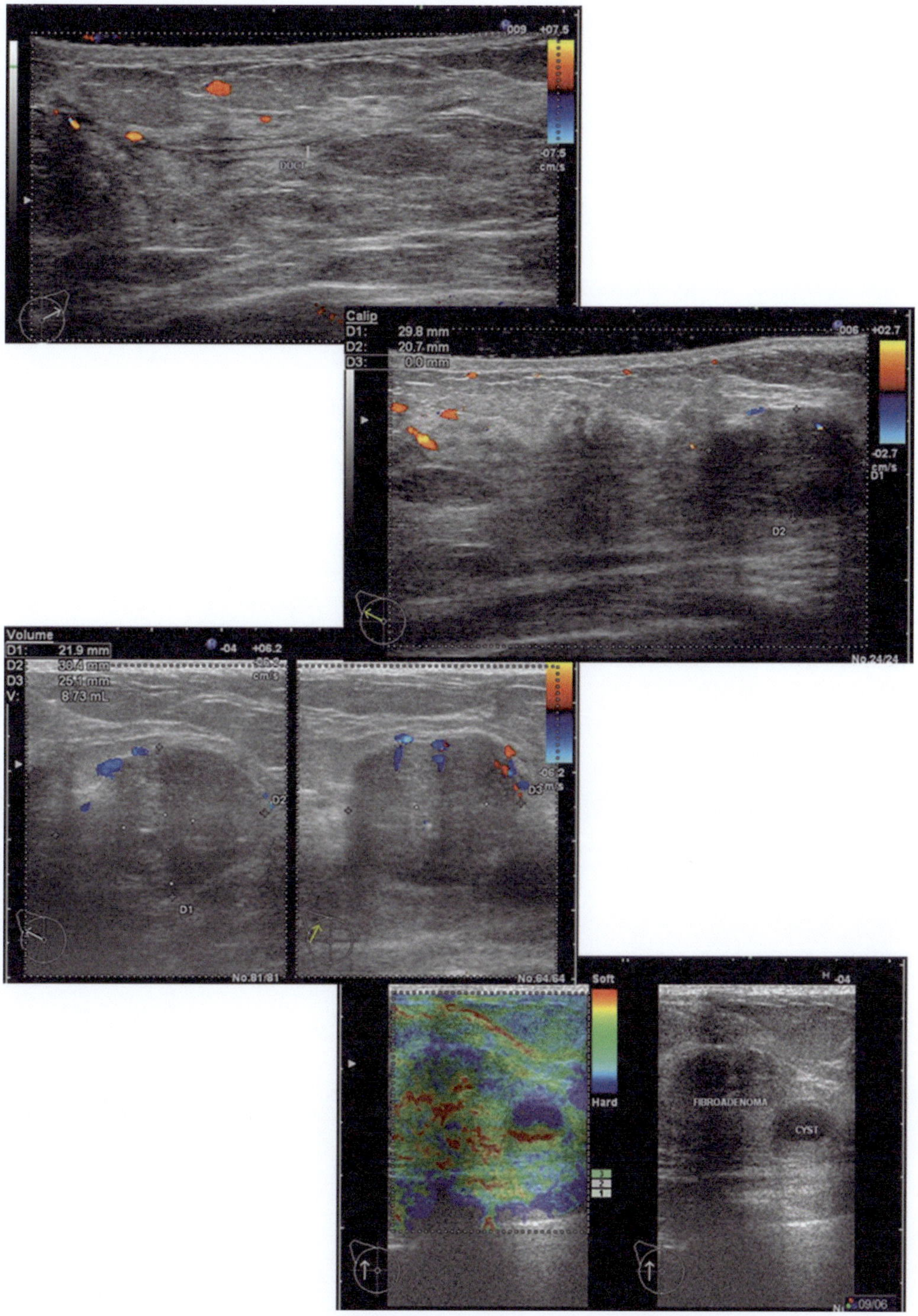

Fig. 4.10 Lactating the breast, with ductal ectasias and hypervascularity: at R 9:30, there is a solid lesion (Stavros criteria) with color Doppler of benign type, suggesting fibroadenoma; the elastogram presents a score 2 Ueno for the solid lesion, associated with a BGR score corresponding to a neighboring cyst. Both lesions are better characterized using all the available tools of US, representing FBU

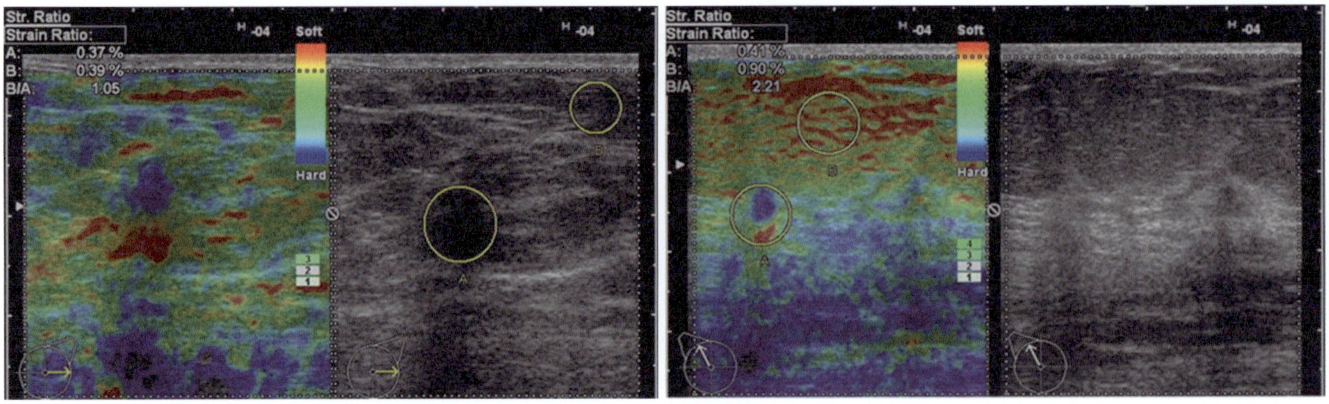

Fig. 4.11 Sonoelastography of pseudomalignant lesions at 2D US, hypoechoic, taller than wide, with irregular borders, and with acoustic shadowing; the elastograms are changing the assessment from 4 to 5 US BI-RADS categories in BI-RADS 2 category. The BGR-summation score is suggesting for fluid content, and the overall FBU diagnosis is fibro-micro-cystic dysplasia located in TDLUs

Fig. 4.12 Pseudomalignant aspect at US of this scar in a patient after conservative surgery, but without suspect Doppler signal and with complex BGR score; FBU certifies a benign scar (US BI-RADS 2/3 category), difficult to characterize by mammography, and more expansive examination by MRI

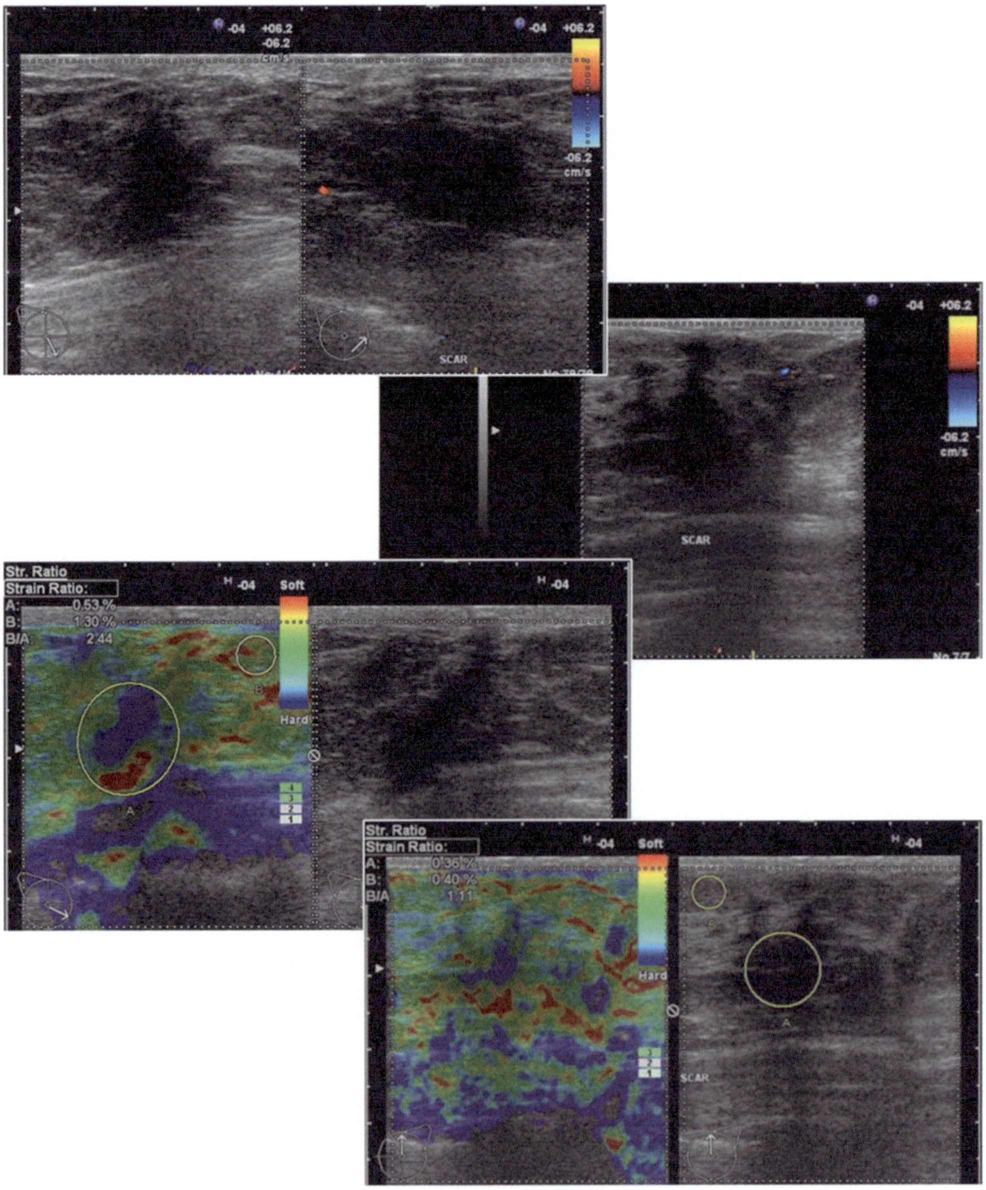

above-presented study, we think sonoelastography is a useful tool in the hand of trained and experienced operators.

Conclusions

Sonoelastography will reduce the diagnostic biopsies in suspect lesions, especially for the BI-RADS 4 category, and the publications estimate that this technique will avoid unnecessary biopsies for 25–40 % cases. The benefit is especially due to the absence of side effects, as compared with vacuum-assisted breast biopsy, which is followed by hematoma in up to 94 % cases after a week and 55 % after three weeks, or fine-needle aspiration biopsy (FNAB) with up to 60 % hematomas or fat necrosis [18].

Sonoelastography alone has low specificity for benign lesions such as fibro-micro-cystic dysplasia and for the scars and chronic inflammatory lesions, but FBU offers a better accuracy compared with MRI. The new concept of FBU will improve the overall results of breast US and of sonoelastography; this is a challenge recommended in diagnosis, screening, and guiding interventional procedures. Sonoelastography presents smaller areas of some benign lesions as compared with grayscale imaging (score 3 Ueno) or greater area in the score 5 Ueno, so it should not be used as a single method of diagnosis.

Moreover, for the malignant lesions with a score 5 Ueno, where sonoelastogram presents larger area including the transitional zone/the halo, there are implications in the conservative surgery, for the correct excision with "safe tumoral margins"; as a benefit, the presence of the light-blue halo avoid false-negative biopsies that omit the center/core of the lesion.

Despite the beginning age of sonoelastography, when there are some criticisms due to the misunderstanding of the technique and heterogeneous devices and techniques of acquisition, the method proved its value and some international guidelines were published [19], with recommendation to correlate this technique with the BI-RADS malignancy probability scale [20]; moreover, it seems sonoelastography is more useful in characterizing the risk of malignancy than the more expansive CEUS.

References

1. Kobayashy T (1977) Gray-scale echography for breast cancer. Radiology 122:207–214. doi:10.1148/122.1.207
2. Hashimoto H, Masuda S, Mizutani M, Morishima I et al (2003) Lexicon for breast lesions posterior echoes. In 13th international congress on the ultrasonic examination of the breast. International Breast Ultrasound School. The 10th Meeting of Japan Association of Breast and Thyroid Sonology
3. Ophir J et al (1991) Elastography: a quantitative method for imaging the elasticity of biological tissues. Ultrason Imaging 13:111–134
4. Ophir JA (2005) Review of theoretical and experimental aspects of imaging the elastic attributes of tissues in vivo. In Research and development in breast ultrasound. Springer, Tokyo Ed, pp 3–6
5. Teboul M (2010) Advantages of Ductal Echography (DE) over Conventional Breast Investigation in the diagnosis of breast malignancies. Med Ultrason 12(1):32–42
6. Scaperrotta G, Ferranti C, Costa C et al (2008) Role of sonoelastography in non-palpable breast lesions. Eur Radiol 18:2381–2389
7. Shiina T et al (2002) Real-time tissue elasticity imaging using the combined autocorrelation method. J Med Ultrasonics 29:119–128
8. Shiina T, Ueno E (2003) In vivo breast examination by real-time freehand elasticity imaging system. In 13th international congress on the ultrasonic examination of the breast. International Breast Ultrasound School. The 10th Meeting of Japan Association of Breast and Thyroid Sonology. In Research and development in breast ultrasound, Springer, Tokyo Ed, pp 7–15
9. Amy D (2007) Introduction & principal of elastography, In 6th Biennale Meeting of the Asian Breast Cancer Society, Hong Kong
10. Svensson WE, Amiras DG, Shousha S et al (2006) Elasticity imaging on 234 breast lesions shows that it could halve biopsy rates of benign lesions. Eur Radiol 16(supp 1):213–214
11. Georgescu AC, Enachescu V, Bondari A, Bondari S, Manda A, Simionescu C (2011) A new concept: the Full Breast Ultrasound in avoiding false negative and false-positive sonographic errors. doi:10.1594/ecr2011/C-0449
12. Georgescu AC, Enachescu V (2010) The diagnosis of gynecomastia by Doppler ductal ultrasonography: Etiopathogenic, endocrine and imaging correlations. doi:10.1594/ecr2010/C-0420
13. Tardivon A, Deloqnette A, Lemery S et al (2006) Ultrasound elastography: results of a French multicentric prospective study about 345 breast lesions. ECR; B-344 [online].http://posters.webges.com/e-Poster/poster.php?id=1057&step=2
14. Locatelli M, Rizzatto G, Aliani L et al (2007) Characterization of breast lesions with real-time Sonoelastography: Results from the Italian multicenter clinical trial. ECR B-271, Vienna, p.285. http://www.myesr.org/html/img/pool/3_ECR_2007_Final_Programme_web.pdf
15. Amy D (2010) Lobar ultrasound of the breast. In: Tot T (ed) Breast cancer. © Springer, London Limited. doi:10.1007/978-1-84996-314-5_8
16. Georgescu A, Bondari S, Manda A, Andrei E-M (2012) The differential diagnosis between breast cancer and fibro-micro-cystic dysplasia by full breast ultrasonography – a new approach. ECR Viena, EPOS ™. doi:10.1594/ecr2012/C-0167, Control Nr #4281
17. American College of Radiology (2003) Illustrated breast imaging reporting and data system (BI-RADS): ultrasound. American College of Radiology, Reston, http://www.acr.org/departments/stand_accred/birads/us_assess
18. Hertl K, Marolt-Musik M, Kocijancic I et al (2007) Haematomas after percutaneous vacuum-assisted breast biopsy. Ultraschall Med 30:33–36
19. Bamber J, Cosgrove D, Dietrich CF et al (2013) EFSUMB guidelines and recommendations on the clinical use of ultrasound elastography. Part 1: Basic principles and technology. Ultraschall in der Medizin34:169–184.doi:http://dx.doi.org/10.1055/s-0033-1335205
20. Barr GR, Nakashima K, Amy D et al (2015) WFUMB guidelines and recommendations for clinical use of ultrasound elastography: Part 2: Breast. Ultrasound Med Biol 41(5):1148–1160

Full Breast Ultrasonography and the Ultrasound: BI-RADS Assessment

5

5.1 Importance of the Ultrasound BI-RADS Assessment

The necessity of standardization of the reporting and of the management of the mammogram findings for screening and diagnosis determined the issue of guidelines. The mammographic Breast Imaging Reporting and Data System (BI-RADS®) assessment improved the characterization of the opacities as masses, distortion of the architecture or calcifications, and the final recommendations were included in the American standards since 1992 (MQSA, Mammography Quality Standards Act). BI-RADS® for mammography is published and trademarked by the American College of Radiology (ACR); it has been used widely in the USA, nowadays being accepted worldwide and becoming the principal tool for the classification and the management of the screening programs. Actually, the fourth edition is in use since 2003.

There is some confusion created by the French lexicon named the "Classification ACR," adopted by the *French Haute Autorité de Santé* and the *National Committee for Breast Cancer Screening*, which is adapted from BI-RADS but influenced by the French national screening program, with the aim to limit undesirable risks of screening (false positives and overdiagnosis).

The actually in use BI-RADS Atlas from 2003 (updated in 2013) includes new sections for US (ACR BI-RADS–US) and MRI (ACR BI-RADS–MRI). ACR BI-RADS–US (2003) may help standardize the terms used for characterizing and reporting lesions, thereby facilitating patient care, the characterization of lesions, and the development of possible screening applications [1]. It opened the way for the screening US, without solving the problem of standardization of the technique of US acquisition even after the lexicon of 2013 [2], which was developed independently by Teboul and his collaborators under the name of ductal echography.

The classical US was growing importance in providing specificity to mammographically observed lesions for avoiding unnecessary biopsies; moreover, US had to detect occult carcinomas in dense breasts where mammography was inefficient, and to guiding procedures, easier for the patient and for the operator than by the mammographically guidance. All these tasks for US determined its complementary position in the diagnosis of breast cancer, neglecting the differential diagnosis between benign lesions and completely ignoring the possibility of using US as first-intention technique of imaging diagnosis in symptomatic cases or screening. However, the development of a standardized group of descriptors and an assessment and management scheme for US became necessary, and inevitably, it was created similar to those for mammography; this wrong approach was presented despite of the different physical principles of image acquisition (X-ray absorption laws and ultrasound-wave reflection imaging) which logically result in some different descriptors of the breast findings. Moreover, there were neglected differences between volumic radiological projections in complementary planes of the whole breast by one side and the sectional imaging acquisition in US, with different sizes, shapes, resolutions, and precise anatomical locations of the breast's normal and abnormal structures.

The contradiction between the applicability of the mammographic BI-RADS assessment, which refers to the management of the diagnosis of *whole breast*, and the US BI-RADS assessment in the classical examination, which refers to the *visualized lesion*, neglecting the rest of the breast volume, is the main criticism for its use in the classical US, as it is in present.

The lexicon of the breast was designated by an expert group from the USA and international representatives, in 1998, which was oriented to a breast US screening, to a better differentiation of benign from malignant, and to the use of US as a therapeutic agent or the US-guided therapy. Other groups, in particular Japanese researchers, have contributed to the definition of the US lexicon. By the introduction of the US lexicon and of a standardized protocol of US examination (despite being illogical and inefficient in the variant of the classical US) and by using the US BI-RADS assessment, it was intended to reduce the operator-dependent limit of US;

A. Colan-Georges, *Atlas of Full Breast Ultrasonography*, DOI 10.1007/978-3-319-31418-1_5

multicentric studies presented promising results both for the experts and for the beginning operators.

Where possible, the same descriptors used for mammography have been transferred to US; these two different methods of diagnosis, based on different laws of physics and addressed to different targets (volume and slice of tissue), were gifted with some similar descriptors of diagnosis, and the confusion will be perpetuated until a new US lexicon will be learned and accepted worldwide. Indeed, the aims of the US BI-RADS lexicon were unsatisfactory, and the fault was attributed to US, as less accurate method of diagnosis, not to the wrong interpreting by using the wrong descriptors. In the following, we will present the values and the limits of this lexicon.

The BI-RADS assessment recognizes some categories unique to the technique of radiology or sonography, however, like echogenicity for US and density for mammography. For US, the main categories for masses are (1) shape; (2) margin; (3) orientation; (4) echo pattern (5); posterior acoustic features; (6) breast calcifications; (7) associated features including architectural distortion, duct changes, vascularity, and elasticity (8); and (9) special cases. These descriptors were evaluated for usage agreement by radiologists at the Society of Breast Imaging 2001 meeting, with good agreement as determined by the kappa statistic [3]; that explains the "radiological" point of view about the ultrasonographic method even in 1003 and 2013 BI-RADS edition and the lack of contribution of independent ultrasonographers.

In the followings, the descriptors, their categories, and associated assessment and management recommendations of the US BI-RADS® fourth edition will be presented and completed with the Japanese guidelines and the FBU interpretations that highlight the value of the duality vasculature (by Doppler evaluation) and strain (by sonoelastography).

Nevertheless, US BI-RADS is useful and could be improved, and its correlation with sonoelastography was recommended by the World Federation for Ultrasound in Medicine and Biology (WFUMB) [4].

5.2 Ultrasound Diagnostic Criteria

Diagnostic Criteria has been removed by some Japanese authors, and the term *Guideline of Ultrasonic Diagnosis* is recommended. As a rule, no single feature can be predictive of benign or malignant etiology. Analysis of multiple features together is more accurate in arriving at an assessment.

Classically, the most important descriptors in determining the likelihood of malignancy are the margins and the shape and, secondarily, the orientation, the posterior features, and the echo pattern [5–7]. The microcalcifications, essential in mammography, are mentioned as descriptors in US, but even in the classical US, they are not mentioned in the above list.

In FBU, the most important in determining the likelihood of malignancy are the qualitative Doppler characterization and the sonoelastography, individually (Doppler) or combined. The vascular aspect is neglected in the classical approach, despite its value demonstrated on the pathological reports and on the breast MRI that analyzes the curves of enhancement of the paramagnetic intravenous contrast agents for the final assessment. Sonoelastography was officially launched in 2006, at ECR in Vienna, and the different manufacturers with different techniques of acquisitions and different scoring systems determined an initial discordance of opinions between the specialists about its diagnostic value.

The criteria for assessing breast lesions continue to be validated. For mammography, the "probably benign" lesion, with a reliable management recommendation of short-interval follow-up, has a <2 % likelihood of malignancy.

A similar category for US, the prototype of a fibroadenoma, remains to be validated across multiple centers for US, but the results are significant improved when using the DE.

The new concept that unifies the DE, Doppler, and sonoelastography is not yet very well known, but the complete characterization by US of a lesion, in breast or elsewhere, will not be complete without an anatomical US approach, combined with vascular study and the evaluation of tissues elasticity.

5.3 Lexicon for Breast Lesions

In the lexicon of the US BI-RADS assessment, the classification of the breast diseases in mass image-forming lesions and non-mass image-forming lesions was taken over from mammography [8], but in FBU, we will never find cases from the last category.

For reasons of systematic analysis, we will present the two groups of lesions.

5.3.1 Diagnostic Guidelines for Mass Image-Forming Lesions

5.3.1.1 Shape

Definition: This refers to the impression of shape given from the whole image of a tumor. This is assessed for classification by tumor cross sections [9]:

Classification: *round/oval*, *polygonal*, *lobulated*, and *irregular*

Observations: The impression of shape given from the whole tumor only depends on a judge's subjectivity, but judging must be more objective referring to a criterion, and the Japanese authors proposed *constriction* and *angularity*. Even malignancy can sometimes show a round or oval shape, while benignity can sometimes appear irregular. The major inconvenience of this classification in classical breast US is that there is no correlation of the abnormal US finding with the normal breast parenchyma, ducts, and lobules, and so the eventual imaging lesion may not be a true breast lesion, but a constructed one; that means we are not sure we are seeing a true lesion because we cannot localize it, referring to the lobar anatomy, and we must perform a biopsy. As results in the classical US, either we cannot characterize all lesions or we are characterizing mass "outside" the mammary lobe, or we are missing some, and this is why US accuracy is denied.

5.3.1.2 Margin/Border

Margins are characterized by multiple aspects:

1. Definition: *well-defined* (*benign*) *or not clear* (*malignant*)
2. Irregularity: *smooth* (*benign*) *or rough* (*malignant*)
3. Halo: *none* (*benign*) *or existent* (*malignant*, better seen on sonoelastography)
4. Gland surface: *continuous* (*benign*) *or interrupted* (*malignant*)

These aspects are not really specific as they are assumed, except the halo corresponding to the score 5 Ueno.

5.3.1.3 Internal Echoes

Internal echoes, that is, the echoes from the inside of the mass, are analyzed for judging a lesion and for characterizing it as solid or complex liquid, eventually cysts with fluid-fluid level, with more or less benign or malignant appearance. Internal echoes are analyzed for:

1. *Intensity* (*echo level*): The echo level of the mass is graded, comparing with that of subcutaneous fatty layer as the standard tissue, having five levels:
   - *Echo free* (cyst)
   - *Very low* (sclerosing adenosis, highly homogenous, such as medullary carcinoma and malignant lymphoma; scirrhous carcinoma)
   - *Low* (fibroadenoma, papilloma, scirrhous carcinoma)
   - *Equal* (fibroadenoma, mucinous carcinoma, and lipoma)
   - *High* (mucinous carcinoma, panniculitis, and lipoma)
2. *Homogeneity*: Internal echoes are assessed to be *homogeneous* (*benign*) or *heterogeneous/inhomogeneous* (*malignant*) according mainly to the regularity in echo distribution or texture.

As a particular aspect, there are described *high echo spots*, usually representing calcification and divided into three types according to the size: fine (malignant), small (malignant), and coarse (benign) [10]. We agree with Teboul and Amy that in US the microcalcifications are not important for characterizing breast tumors, but they are very important in mammography. US and MRI must not repeat the same descriptors as mammography, but the diagnostic may have different criteria; nevertheless, MRI could not differentiate the calcifications in general from other hyposignals, and the microcalcifications with their inframillimetric size are too small for the MRI scans of more than 1 mm in thickness. In fact FBU has much sensitive signs than the eventually visible "microcalcifications," which are too large when visible in US for malignant-type calcifications. Indeed, when visualized in US, the microcalcifications are more than 0.5 mm in size, and usually they have no acoustic shadowing, so the images are not specific; frequently, the images judged as microcalcifications in US, which is used as the first technique of examination, appearing as hyperechoic spots, are not seen on mammography, but they could represent the tiny posterior hyperechoic enhancements of microcysts, sometimes completed with lateral shadowing. Inversely, if we analyze a mammogram as the first examination that presents true microcalcifications and then we perform a complementary US, we are tented to "recognize" them (see Chap. 7).

5.3.1.4 Posterior Echoes/Effects

Posterior echoes are one of the findings that indirectly reveal the tissue characteristics inside the mass and depend on the attenuation of the lesions. The intensity of the posterior effects is classified into four levels by means of comparing the surrounding echo intensity at the same depth:

1. *Accentuating*: cyst, fibroadenoma, papilloma, phyllodes tumor, invasive ductal carcinoma (solid-tubular type), medullary carcinoma, mucinous carcinoma, malignant lymphoma, and intracystic carcinoma
2. *No change*: fibroadenoma, adenosis, and invasive ductal carcinoma (papillary-tubular type)
3. *Attenuating*: scar, sclerosing adenosis, invasive ductal carcinoma (scirrhous type), and invasive lobular carcinoma
4. *Deficient*: calcification, old fibroadenoma (with calcification), and silicon granuloma

The mass with high cellularity and cystic lesion tends to accentuate, but mass with abundant fibrous tissue or calcifications tends to attenuate or become deficient [11].

We think that the surrounding tissue has great importance for the intensity of the posterior echoes. For instance, if the hyperechoic glandular stroma is thick, the posterior effects are better visible than in cases with fatty involution of the breast; in such cases, the relation of the lesion with the duct or the TDLUs is the key of diagnosis, and the FBU is the best method to demonstrate it. If the posterior changes are not very well visible, we recommend either a moderate increase of the compression with the transducer on the skin or better the complementary use of THI, which will increase the posterior echo effect.

5.3.1.5 Compressibility

It is admitted that the lesions which are easily deformed are benign, while those incompressible are malignant; this subjective characterization was described by Kobayashi [12, 13] and was recently confirmed by sonoelastography. It is unclear why the subjective compressibility was accepted as descriptor of masses, and sonoelastography was denied by many authors, despite its more objective character.

5.3.1.6 Vascularity

Qualitative color Doppler or equivalents (color flow mode) and power Doppler (uniflow or dual energy) are the unanimous recommendation for the vascular lesion characterization in the breast; there are no vascular or just a hypovascular mapping in benign and a hypervascular mapping in malignant lesions. Quantitative indices of velocimetry are less useful in breast US, compared with other localizations of tumors or tissues, such as the endometrium, ovary, uterine arteries, or musculoskeletal tumors. More important is the vascular orientation toward the tumor, with a peripheral, arcuate course with few centripetal vessels (1–2 vascular poles) in the benign lesions and with multipolar, large, and tortuous vessels, with incident angle of the plunging artery, in the malignant masses [14]. Any less than 5 mm lesions with visible vasculature of any type are suspect for malignancy with the actual US technology.

Labeling of Breast Ultrasonographic Images

In the classical US as in FBU, breast sonographic examination can show the existence of breast lesions three-dimensionally. Therefore, precise labeling for sonographic images becomes very important and is systematized, in favor of another technique of screening than mammography and of surgical referring. We will present the labeling of those systematized by a Japan group of authors, which is largely accepted [15]:

I. *Labeling for the breast lesion location* is made following four attributes:
   1. *Breast laterality*: right or left.
   2. *Breast quadrant*: Inner high/superior, inner low/inferior, outer high/superior.
      Outer low/inferior, beneath the nipple
   3. *Axis* is indicated by o'clock designation (the "meridian/longitude").
   4. *Distance* of the tumor/lesion from the nipple ("the parallel/latitude").

II. *Quantitative evaluation of the lesion* is made by measurement of the following items:

$$\text{Tumor Size} = a \times b \times c(\text{mm;cm}) \qquad (5.1)$$

In the classical ultrasonographic images, measurement is made in the plane which shows the largest diameter of the lesion: (*LDP = largest diameter plane, section A*) and a plane perpendicular to LDP (*section B*).

The detailed process of the measurement is as follows:

(i) Measure the largest diameter in the section A—*line a*.
(ii) Measure the largest diameter perpendicular to line a—*line c*.
(iii) Measure the largest diameter in B—*line b*.

This tumor size is labeled as

$$V = a \times b \times c$$

In FBU, we will scan logically the lesion first in a radial plane, we will measure the anterior-posterior diameter, which is perpendicular to the thoracic plane (sometimes we cannot use a horizontal plane for the skin), and then we will measure the radial diameter, in the same plan; afterward, we will obtain the section in a antiradial plane, which is perpendicular to the previous described, and we will measure the antiradial diameter, which is orthogonal on the two others achieved. This technique is logical and better standardized, so it can be reproducible and is useful as a follow-up measurement. The volume is automatically calculated by almost all modern machines if there are three orthogonal diameters:

$$\text{Depth / Width Ratio}(D / W) \qquad (5.2)$$

In classical US, depth-to-width ratio is measured on the LDP (section A) of the breast lesion. Measurement should be made only for the hypoechoic tumor area, excluding the hyperechoic boundaries. This technique is relatively imprecise and is not reproducible: we can appreciate the largest section of the tumor with inherent subjective errors (slipping hand transducer, different compression because of the different position of the breast against the thoracic wall, etc.).

In FBU we propose the depth-to-width ratio measured either in the radial or in the antiradial plane, with precise mentioning of the plane using the body mark for the breast. We will use the largest diameters, without compression as possible, and we will mention the relation with the ductal axis. *D*/*W* is rather <1 in benign lesions and usually ≥ 1 in the malignant tumors, except for the small fibroadenomas developing from hyperplasic lobules, which have initially a vertical orientation, orthogonal to the skin and to the main duct; then becoming more large, they will change the orientation in an oblique position; and finally, when they have developed sufficiently, their long axis will course parallel to the skin.

5.3.2 Diagnostic Guidelines for Non-mass Image-Forming Lesions

There is also a diagnostic guideline for non-mass image-forming lesions by the Japan Association of Breast and Thyroid Sonology (JABTS) and Japan Society of Ultrasonics in Medicine, which is concordant with the American guidelines and refers to "the lesions that are difficult to recognize as 'mass image-forming lesions'," which may exist separately or may associate with them [8]. These guidelines offer few characterizations about these so-called non-mass image-forming lesion, but they suggest that in classical US, similar to mammography, there are cancers not visualized per primam; therefore, it is proved that after breast MRI lesion identification and localization, US is useful in the characterization of its risk of malignity, so the initial "not-mass image-forming" lesion becomes visible on US, which means that it is not the US that is unable to visualize some lesions but the classical technique unsatisfactory in detecting them. We agree with Amy that in FBU, we never had a "not-mass image-forming" lesion, because the interpreting is better, so if a small abnormality, equal or larger than a duct or lobule, is present, FBU is able to detect by everyone. The problem remains in DE in the diagnosis of lobar carcinoma and of carcinomatous mastitis, but sonoelastography added supplementary information that could differentiate them from diffuse hyperplasia or infectious mastitis (see Chap. 8).

However, this last guideline is useful because it describes some lesions such as duct thickening, duct ectasia (contains plasma cell mastitis), intraductal papilloma, and others; unfortunately, it still multiplies the mammographic incertitudes, such as *architectural distortion, which is the distortion and/or retraction of the normal tissue inside and/or outside of the breast tissue, low echo area whose character is different from surrounding gland or suitable area in the opposite breast*, and *geographical low echo area*. All these descriptions and more others are tentative to eliminate the false-negative results in classical breast US, but they are unsuccessful because of a nonanatomical approach and thus a non-understanding of the breast structure. For instance, it is not explained what the *normal tissue* and the *breast tissue* mean; the term *surrounding gland* is vague, as well as *geographical low echo area*, because there is no correlation with the mammary lobe or with the ductal-lobular tree, so the location of these *non-mass image-forming* lesions is imprecise. Moreover, these lesions are still forming some images, but without mass aspect, that means without tridimensional coordinates; these suspect lesions are visualized only as representations in a plane, which is obtained arbitrarily in classical US examination; then how could it be compared with a *suitable area in the opposite breast*?

By using FBU, the interpretation of the breast will allow an anatomical analysis:

- *The description of the type of the normal breast*: young, adult, fatty, mixed, and lactating/secretory; glandular stroma and global vasculature must be mentioned.
- *The description of the normal ducts and lobules* for each case, related to the age, menstrual cycle or substitution hormonal therapy, constitutional factors, nutrition, etc.
- *The description of the abnormal findings* related to the breast parenchyma or other structures: *localization* type in o'clock completed with the distance from the nipple (the "coordinates"), *number* (multifocality), *rapports* with the surrounding structures (Cooper ligaments, fatty layers, pectoral muscles, skin—the description of the rapports is missing in the classical US guidelines), and all the known descriptors of a lesion (*shape, border, internal echoes, posterior echoes, vascularity, elasticity*).

In FBU we will use only anatomical or pathological terms, and we will never use confusing terms such as *low echo area with indistinct margin*, because they are not useful for the clinicians, surgeons, or oncologists and especially because these images are not reproducible for different operators.

5.3.3 Ultrasound BI-RADS Assessment

ACR BI-RADS–US describes seven assessment categories of lesions. One category is for lesions that are incompletely characterized, and for which, further imaging is needed for final assessment. The six other assessment categories have implications on patient care.

Because the dense breast is difficult to diagnose on mammography, there is a classification of the glandular density that is important for the dose of radiation and for the quality of the images, implied in the accuracy of diagnosis. This model was transferred in US diagnosis, but we mention that in US, the anatomy and the pathological findings in the "dense breast" (improper term for the "predominantly glandular breast") are better viewed than in the fatty breast, because the malignancies and most of the benign lesions are izo- or hypoechoic and thus are difficult to differentiate from the fatty layers.

There may be two methods of *US BI-RADS density categorization*:

1. *Qualitative-descriptive*:
   - *Predominantly fat*
   - *Fat with some fibroglandular tissue*
   - *Heterogeneously dense*
   - *Extremely dense*

2. *Quantitative, fraction of volume occupied by fibroglandular density*:
   - *0–25 %*
   - *26–50 %*
   - *51–75 %*
   - *76–100 %*

In both categorizations, the evaluation is subjective and operator dependent; the so-called quantitative evaluation is not the result of some measurements, neither an evaluation specific to the US, because the scans may overlap some areas and omit other regions of the breast; in all cases, the scans are different according to the quadrant, asymmetry, and heterogeneity, the inner ones being more fatty and the outer more glandular in texture. In fact, the US breast density categorization is an imitation of the mammographic assessment that is justified by the whole breast standardized projection and by reasons of technical and electrical parameters of acquisitions and of radiological interpreting of mammograms.

5.3.3.1 US BI-RADS Assessment by the ACR (2013)

Incomplete Characterization

Category 0—Supplementary imagistic evaluation required

Examples: Supplementary mammography when suspect FBU (for microcalcifications); MRI when US is inconclusive for the differentiation of the local recurrence from a scar following conservative breast surgery or radiotherapy; MRI in suspect multifocal/multicentric or diffuse lobar cancer.

Complete Characterization

Category 1—Negative

ACR: Normal breast US, without any abnormalities such as masses, architectural distortions, skin alterations, microcalcifications, and pathological lymph nodes

FBU: Normal breast US, without any abnormalities such as masses, ductal ectasias, ductal or lobular hyperplasias, pathological vasculature or pathological strain, skin alterations, scars, and pathological lymph nodes

Category 2—Benign aspects

ACR, US without any suspect lesions, but benign findings: follow-up after conservative surgery, intramammary lymph nodes (they could be included in the category 1), mammary implants, architectural distortions, oil cysts, lipomas, galactoceles, and hamartomas.

In FBU we can add ductal and lobular hyperplasia without suspect vasculature, ductal ectasia, and ductal and lobular precocious atrophy (Fig. 5.1).

Category 3—Probable benign findings

ACR: A short-interval control is recommended rather than biopsy; there is a malignancy risk less than 2 %. The following are included: solid masses with circumscribed limits, ovoid shaped with the great horizontal axes, suggestive for fibroadenoma, but inhomogeneous or with more than three microlobulations; less complicated cysts or the grouped microcysts (cluster).

In FBU we can add intraductal and intracystic papillomas, ductal-lobular hyperplasia in postmenopausal women or after hormonal therapy, ductal ectasia with bloody nipple discharge, and nodular fibro-micro-cystic dysplasia with less vasculature but increased strain.

Category 4—Suspicious abnormalities

ACR: Biopsy is largely recommended; there is a variable risk for cancer, between 4–94 %. The large interval of risk requires a subdivision in low, moderate, and high risk, corresponding to *4a*, *4b*, and *4c categories*. The following are included: the US masses without all criteria of benignity/malignity, the phyllodes tumor, and other suspected findings. In case of one or two criteria of malignancy, the biopsy is classically recommended [16].

FBU: The suspect lesions will present suspect/malignant-type vasculature, with borderline or suspect sonoelastography of score 3 or 4 Ueno and FLR around 4.00–6.00. The satellite lymph nodes are still of "benign" aspect.

Category 5—Highly suggestive of malignancy

ACR: The risk of malignity is evaluated over 95 %; the Stavros criteria in the classical US are demonstrated, or there is a vasculature with malignant characters. The biopsy and immediate treatment is recommended.

More accurate, the FBU combines the classical features of malignity with Doppler malignant-type new vasculature and sonoelastography, with the score 5 Ueno and FLR over 4.70 (5.00); the satellite lymph nodes could be still of "benign" aspect or suggesting for metastases. The intraductal dissemination with multifocal lesions, the multicentric suspect findings, the lobar cancer, and the malignant mastitis are assessed as US BI-RADS 5 category. FBU is more accurate, and the biopsy could be avoided for the BI-RADS 4 and 5 categories when surgical biopsy is recommended in small lesions, with extemporaneous pathological examination; in large lesions, the immunohistochemical and hormonal tests are suitable for the treatment protocol.

Category 6—Biopsy is performed; malignancy is demonstrated.

An immediate therapeutic action is recommended. The US examination can be requested for a follow-up evaluation of an initial chemotherapy or neoadjuvant radiotherapy or after incomplete excision (Fig. 5.2)

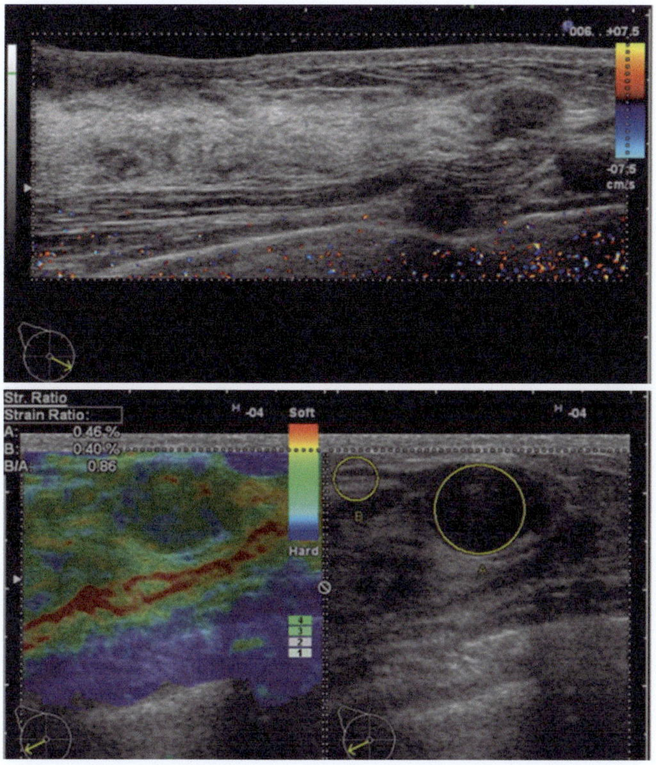

Fig. 5.1 Benign-type breast lump in a 25-year-old patient, with less salient vasculature and SE of score 2 Ueno; the US BI-RADS assessment is category 2

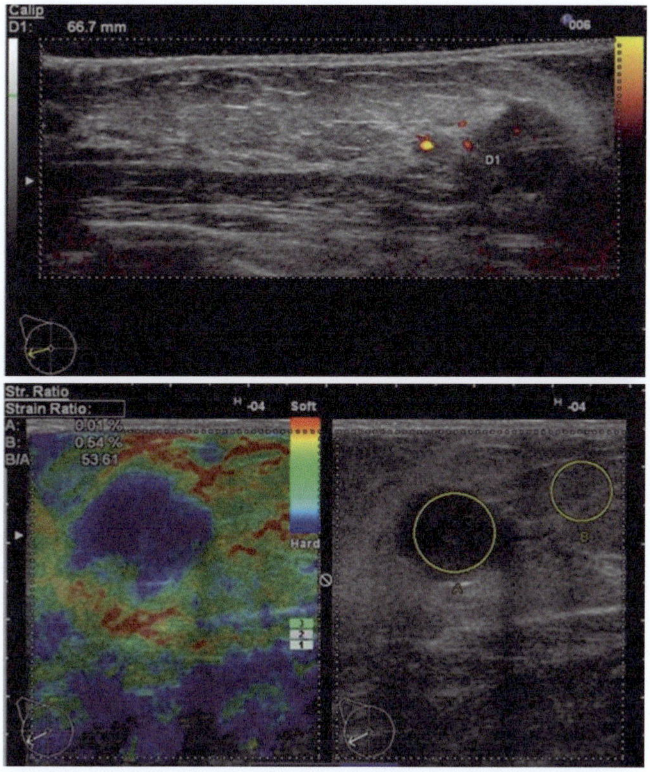

Fig. 5.2 Malignant-type lump in a 56-year-old patient, with similar features in 2D US, but with salient new formation vasculature in medium-resolution (7 MHz) transducer and with score 5 Ueno, assessed as US BI-RADS 5 category

References

1. American College of Radiology (2003) Illustrated breast imaging reporting and data system (BI-RADS): ultrasound. American College of Radiology, Reston, http://www.acr.org/deparments/stand_accred/birads/us_assess.pdf
2. D'Orsi CJ, Sickles EA, Mendelson EB, Morvis EA et al (2013) ACR BI-RADS ® atlas, breast imaging reporting and data system. American College of Radiology, Reston
3. Mendelson EB, Berg WA, Merritt CR (2001) Toward a standardized breast ultrasound lexicon, BI-RADS: ultrasound. Semin Roentgenol 36(3):217–225
4. Barr GR, Nakashima K, Amy D et al (2015) WFUMB guidelines and recommendations for clinical use of ultrasound elastography: part 2: breast. Ultrasound Med Biol 41(5):1148–1160
5. Mendelson EB (2003) BI-RADS® for Ultrasound. 13th international congress on the ultrasonic examination of the breast. International Breast Ultrasound School. The 10th meeting of Japan Association of Breast and Thyroid Sonology
6. Mendelson EB (2003) Ultrasonic diagnostic criteria. 13th international congress on the ultrasonic examination of the breast. International Breast Ultrasound School. The 10th meeting of Japan Association of Breast and Thyroid Sonology
7. Mendelson EB, Baum JK, Berg WA et al (2003) Breast imaging reporting and data system BI-RADS: ultrasound, 1st edn. American College of Radiology, Reston
8. Diagnostic guidelines for non-mass image forming lesions by Japan Association of Breast and Thyroid Sonology (JABTS) and Japan Society of Ultrasonics in Medicine (Draft) (2003) 13th international congress on the ultrasonic examination of the breast. International Breast Ultrasound School. The 10th meeting of Japan Association of Breast and Thyroid Sonology
9. Watanabe T, Ueno E, Endo T, Kubota M, Konishi T et al (2003) Lexicon for breast lesions. Shape. 13th International Congress on the Ultrasonic Examination of the Breast. International Breast Ultrasound School. The 10th meeting of Japan Association of Breast and Thyroid Sonology
10. Kubota M (2003) Lexicon for breast lesions. Internal echoes. 13th international congress on the ultrasonic examination of the breast. International Breast Ultrasound School. The 10th meeting of Japan Association of Breast and Thyroid Sonology
11. Hashimoto H, Masuda S, Mizutani M, Morishima I et al (2003) Lexicon for breast lesions posterior echoes. 13th international congress on the ultrasonic examination of the breast. International Breast Ultrasound School. The 10th meeting of Japan Association of Breast and Thyroid Sonology
12. Kobayashi T (1978) Clinical ultrasound of the breast. Springer, New York
13. Kobayashi T (1979) Diagnostic ultrasound in breast cancer: analysis of retrotumorous echo pattern correlated with sonic attenuation by cancerous connective tissues. J Clin Ultrasound 7(6):471–479
14. Kujiraoka Y, Ueno E, Yohno E, Morishima I, Tsunoda-Shimizu H (2005) Incident angle of the plunging artery of breast tumors. In: Research and development in breast ultrasound. Springer, Tokyo, pp 72–75
15. Mizutani M, Morishima I, Yasuda H, Watanabe T, Ueno E et al (2003) Lexicon for breast lesions labeling of breast ultrasonographic images. 13th international congress on the ultrasonic examination of the breast. International Breast Ultrasound School. The 10th meeting of Japan Association of Breast and Thyroid Sonology
16. Madjar H, Ohlinger R, Mundinger A et al (2006) BI-RADS analogue DEGUM Kriterien von Ultraschallbefunden der Brust – Konsensus des Arbeitskreises Mammasonographie der DEGUM. Ultraschall Med 27:374–379

6 Full Breast Ultrasonography of the Benign Lesions

6.1 Classification of the Masses in Benign, Indeterminate, and Malignant Based on Stavros Criteria

The well-known landmark study published in 1995 by Stavros et al. established US criteria for characterizing solid breast masses [1]. This work was facilitated by evolving technical improvements in US equipment that provided better resolution and images. They demonstrated that US may be used to accurately classify some solid lesions as benign, allowing follow-up by imaging rather than biopsy. Stavros used high-resolution transducers, state of the art at that time, and performed examinations using the nonanatomical technique, with sagittal and transversal scans completed by radial and antiradial targeted planes; the wrong scans and the short linear transducers available did not visualize the lobar architecture of the breast, as did the DE of Teboul, a technique simultaneously published but rested almost unknown for more than 15 years. Thus, ultrasonography as it was used from the beginning has focused mainly on the evaluation of suspected areas, conventionally scanned in the transverse, longitudinal, and random planes. Stavros et al. proposed a US scheme for prospectively classifying breast nodules into one of three categories: benign, indeterminate, or malignant.

Of the 424 lesions that Stavros et al. (1995) prospectively classified as benign by means of US, only 2 were found to be malignant at biopsy, resulting in a negative predictive value of 99.5 % in a population with a cancer prevalence of 16.7 %. Of the 125 lesions found to be malignant at biopsy, 123 were classified as malignant or indeterminate with US, yielding a sensitivity of 98.4 %. Biopsy was preserved for nodules that were classified on US as either malignant or indeterminate. This study demonstrated the value of breast US in an era when Doppler technique had no good supporting technology and its value was widely neglected.

However, nowadays it is not acceptable why, after approximately 20 years, US is still considered inferior to other methods of breast diagnosis, less performing, and it is used mainly as a second method of examination. As we will illustrate, the indeterminate masses are rare in the FBU, which added supplementary descriptors of the lesions to the valuable Stavros criteria that are actually in use [2] and represent the base of the US BI-RADS assessment.

6.2 Characteristics of the Benign Breast Lesions in FBU

Many masses that are demonstrated on mammograms require biopsy to determine whether they are benign or malignant. Taylor et al. (2002) reported that the use of US in conjunction with mammography increases specificity from 51 to 66 % in a population with a malignancy prevalence of 31 % [3]. This improvement could significantly reduce the biopsy rate of benign lesions.

To be classified as benign based on Stavros, a nodule had to have no malignant characteristics; in addition, one of the following three combinations of benign characteristics had to be demonstrated:

1. Intense uniform hyperechogenicity
2. Ellipsoid or wider-than-tall (parallel) orientation, along with a thin, echogenic capsule
3. Two or three gentle lobulations and a thin, echogenic capsule

A nodule was classified as indeterminate by default if it had no malignant characteristics and none of the three benign characteristic combinations listed above.

To be classified as malignant, a mass needed to have any of the following characteristics based on Stavros:

- Spiculated contour
- Taller-than-wide (not parallel) orientation
- Marked hypoechogenicity

A. Colan-Georges, *Atlas of Full Breast Ultrasonography*, DOI 10.1007/978-3-319-31418-1_6

- Angular margins
- Posterior acoustic shadowing
- Punctate calcifications
- Ductal extension
- Branch pattern
- Microlobulations

Many benign breast conditions have a nonspecific appearance on US. However, some masses, such as simple cysts, sebaceous cysts, and intramammary lymph nodes, have a characteristic appearance that suggests a specific diagnosis. Almost all highly echogenic masses are benign.

If color Doppler imaging demonstrates blood flow within the contents of a complex cyst or dilated duct, then these contents consist of solid tissue rather than just debris or blood clots. However, we have seen solid tumors that lack demonstrable blood flow on color Doppler imaging; in these cases, we assume benign masses, but the sensibility of the US machine and the high frequency of the transducers may change the degree of vasculature detection. Several investigators reviewed the ability of color Doppler US or contrast-enhanced Doppler to distinguish benign from malignant lesions. The results were variable; unfortunately, Doppler US is not generally used to distinguish benign from malignant solid breast masses. If we judge the findings are fortuitous chance in classical US technique, the masses are less correlated with the lobar anatomy, Doppler characterization of the structures is not systematically applied, and the sonoelastography is yet unavailable for large majority of sonographers, the sensibility and specificity of the breast US are unfortunately discordant between different centers and countries.

In the following, we will present the well-known characteristics of the benign lesions based on the classical criteria (Stavros completed by BI-RADS), but applied to the ductal (radial) echography combined with Doppler techniques and sonoelastography (FBU).

6.3 Mammary Cysts and Fibrocystic Dysplasia

Cysts may occur in any age group, although they most commonly occur between the ages of 30 and 50 years. US is an ideal noninvasive method for differentiating solid from cystic masses.

There are two etiologic types of cysts:

(a) Cysts may arise from the lobule caused by dilation of the lobular acini, with a round to ovoid shape on the scan, which is believed to result either from an obstruction of the duct leading to the lobule or from an imbalance of fluid secretion and resorption; the second explanations seem to us as more believable, because the dimension and the local sensibility (mastodynia) are dependent on the menstrual cycle (increasing premenstrually) and on the hormonal substitution therapy. Some lobular cysts could communicate, with some remnant walls mimicking incomplete septae, or groups of microcysts of less than 1 mm in diameter are surrounded by fibrous tissue mimicking solid nodule.

(b) Other cysts occur from the ducts themselves, and they attaint large dimensions with a more ovoidal shape, the long axis parallel to the skin and continuing a visible galactophorous duct. A particular type is represented by the cystic dilatation of the galactophorous ampullae/sinuses, with a specific retroareolar location and sometimes with ductal visible connection. The most valuable argument is that after an FNA puncture under DE guidance, the not complicated ductal cysts collapse during the evacuation of the content with the recovery of its canalaire shape.

The classical appearance of a cyst is a well-circumscribed mass, having a peripheral sharp, well-circumscribed echoic rim, usually anechoic avascular content, with posterior medial enhancement bordered by lateral shadowings, known as the benign Kobayashi sign [4].

If the cyst contain protein debris, it may have an echoic appearance, mimicking a “solid” lesion, especially when infected or in the presence of galactorrhea; in chronic infections, there is no salient local vasculature, but in acute cystic mastitis, it could be present an incomplete peripheral ring of blood vessels, eventually associated with an inflammatory halo and skin edema.

Some cysts present intracystic proliferations as echogenic structures, eventually with visible axial vasculature, represented by intracystic papilloma; other cysts may contain incomplete septations due to the incomplete fusion of a number of lobular cysts. Larger cysts develop by a “running together” of the acini, with concomitant dissolution of the lobular specialized stroma, so the incomplete septations represent in fact non-neoformation tissue, but incomplete tissue resorption; these formations and their septations are delineated by benign epithelium, despite the unjustified denomination of “complicated cysts” usually attributed to them (somewhat influenced from the description of the ovarian cysts).

The true complex cystic masses presenting thickened, echogenic walls, indistinct margins or evaginations into the surrounding parenchyma, heterogeneous low-level echoes, thick septations, or an intracystic solid component raise suspicion for malignancy. Intervention with aspiration or biopsy is widely recommended in these cases, but we think unnecessary biopsies can be avoided in DE adding the study of the vessels of the solid component by Doppler US and/or by sonographic contrast agent enhancement; moreover, evaluating the stiffness by sonoelastography can differentiate an infected cyst with a complex BGR score from an intracystic carcinoma with a score 4 or 5 Ueno. The dense content of the cyst may represent chronic infection of the milky secretion, usually determined by saprophytes or pathogenic staphylococcus or streptococcus or by other germs such as *Escherichia coli*, *Candida albicans*, and combinations [5]. These chronic infections are underestimated, but cystic aspirate demonstrates usually pathological cytology with final unnecessary surgical treatment; therefore, if the infection is treated according to the antibiogram, the results demonstrate the outcome of a benign lesion. Moreover, many cases present both cysts and ductal ectasia and nipple surge with the same pathogenic bacteria (see Sect. 6.9).

In the FBU technique, the cysts are located either in the periphery of the lobe, usually in TDLU area, originated in the lobular acini, or in the central area of the lobe, formed by a segmental dilatation of a duct or directly by a dilatation of a ductal ampulla. The location of a cyst is very important, because if we find a peripheral cyst, we must check the entire lobe to find other cysts, based on the theory of the *sick lobe* of T. Tot [6]. Even if the lesions are located in different radial planes, we can easily demonstrate the connections between cysts by thin branches of the ductal tree, draining in the central axial main duct that is taking its course towards the nipple. There are many cases presenting cysts associated with ductal ectasia in the same lobe or in different lobes, without salient vasculature and usually associated with chronic galactophoritis (see Sect. 6.9).

Ultrasound can diagnose uncomplicated cysts with nearly 100 % accuracy. The posterior effects described by Kobayashi, represented by the posterior enhancement with marginal shadowings, are proportional with the size, the intracystic content, and the plentitude degree. Posterior acoustic enhancement may be weak if the mass is only a few millimeters in size or deep in location, particularly next to the chest wall, but the contrast enhancement by using THI technique is useful. The tinny cysts, especially in the nodular form of the fibrocystic disease, appear as small hyperechoic foci of 0.5–1.0 mm without significant posterior effects, misdiagnosed in US as calcifications. Moreover, the microcalcifications seen in US are too large for malignancy, but too small for posterior real acoustic shadowing. For such cases, a good resolution of high-frequency transducers and the FBU with sonoelastography, THI techniques, and 4D techniques could make the differential diagnosis (see Chap. 7).

One particular cystic dysplasia is the Reclus disease, presenting extended lesions and considered by some authors with malignant risk. This dysplasia represents a genetic disorder, with probably associated acquired etiologic-pathogenic factors, and the risk for malignancy is similar to the non-Reclus cases. In fact, the cysts are not true premalignant lesions. The risk was erroneously attributed because the cystic disease is the most frequent dysplasia, found in about 2/3 of cases [7], and its association with the breast cancer is by consequence the most frequent at all (according to a statistical weighted mean).

The nodular form of the fibro-micro-cystic disease may mimic a breast cancer on mammography, on DE, and even on sonoelastography, but it has a hypovascular aspect suggesting slow evolution, and the follow-up examinations may avoid unnecessary biopsies. For the nodular form of fibro-micro-cystic dysplasia, the scoring of the sonoelastography must be completed with the summation-BGR score that represent a similar elastogram to a simple larger cyst or with the complex BGR score, which is represented by composed, multiple, and unequal small BGR grouped on the lesion, similar to complex cysts, hematomas, necrosis, etc. [7].

The calcified cysts appear as eggshell lesions, with or without acoustic shadowing, according to the wall thickness and to their size; however, the tinny calcifications of the acini, seen on the mammography, could be omitted in FBU.

The peripheral new formation vasculature of benign type is discordant with the score 4 Ueno, and the middle-high FLR (3.20–11.57) is suspect of malignancy. The mammographic aspect is corresponding to BI-RADS 4 classification. The discordance between Doppler and RTSE is the characteristic sign for fibro-micro-cystic dysplasia (Figs. 6.1, 6.2, 6.3, 6.4, 6.5, 6.6, 6.7, 6.8, 6.9, 6.10, 6.11, 6.12, 6.13, 6.14, 6.15, 6.16, 6.17, 6.18, 6.19, 6.20, 6.21, 6.22, 6.23, 6.24, 6.25, 6.26, 6.27, and 6.28).

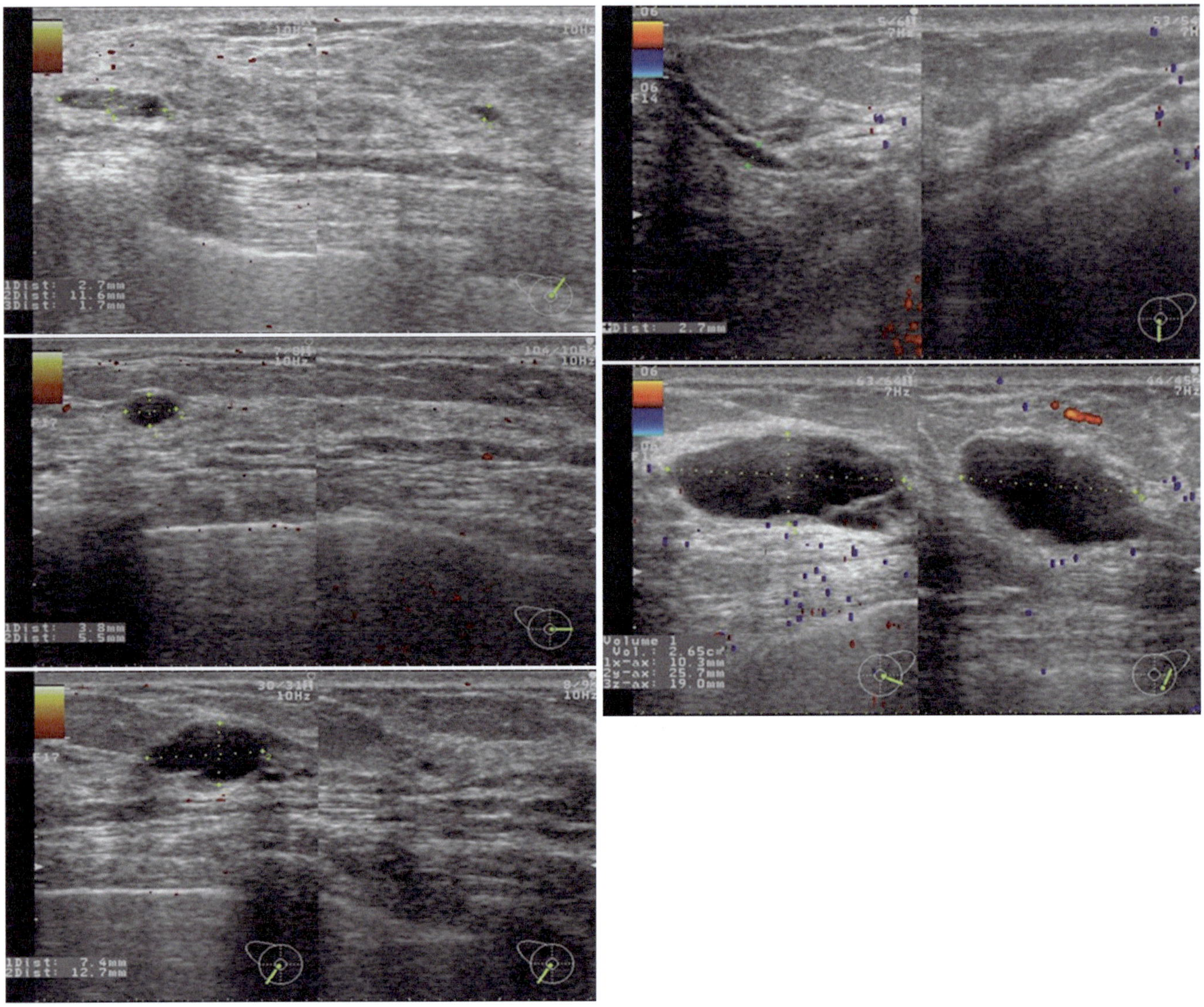

Fig. 6.1 Fibrocystic dysplasia in this case is a continuous disease from ductal ectasia and lobular microcysts to large, pseudo-septated cysts. No vascular abnormalities are seen and the lobar architecture is preserved. The disease usually is bilaterally asymmetrical and may be associated with ductal ectasia or ductal or lobular hyperplasia. Cysts are larger in the premenstrual days and could develop mastodynia, while postmenstrual could be impalpable, the so-called ghost tumors

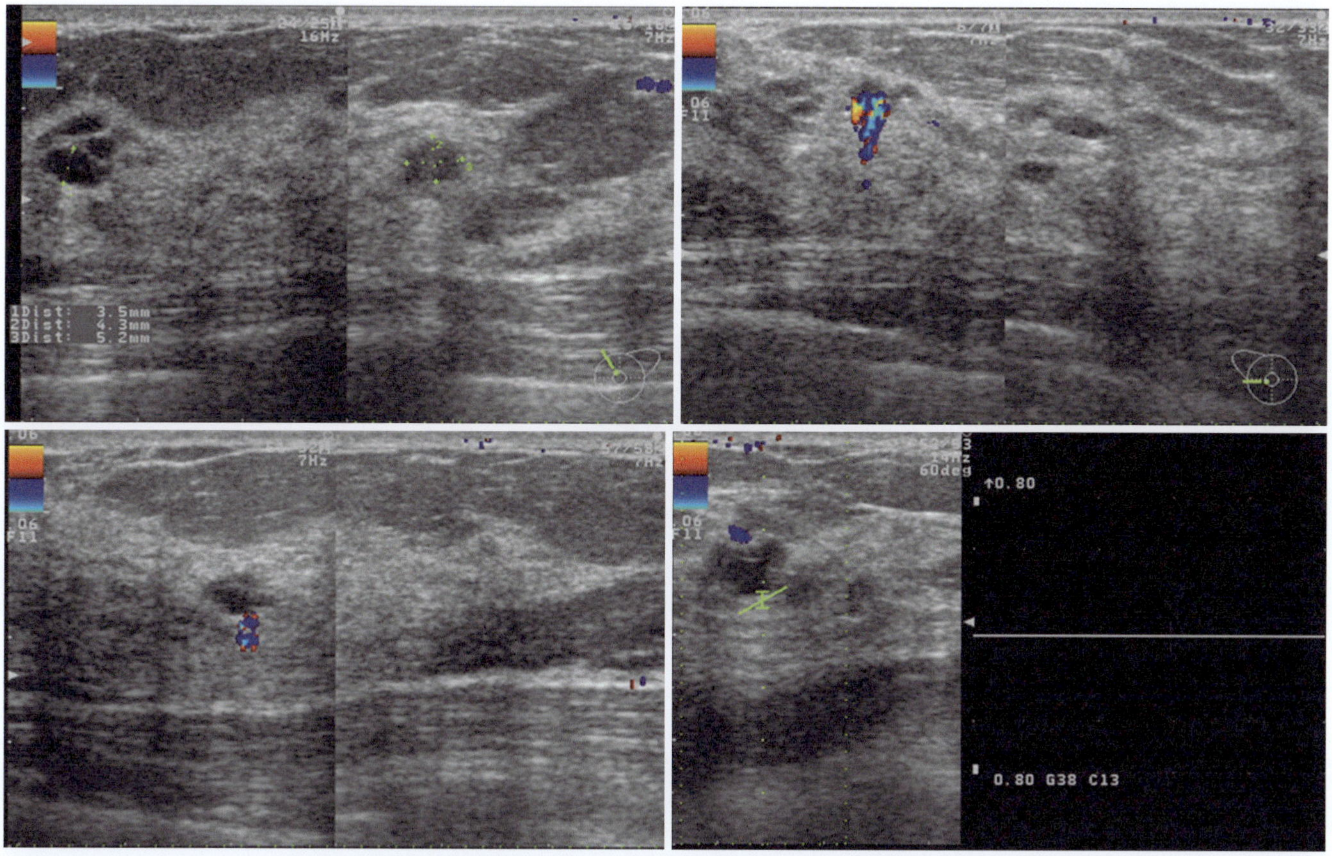

Fig. 6.2 DE in a 38-year-old patient: cluster of fibro-micro-cystic dysplasia and posterior twinkling artifact with aliasing on color Doppler. The differential diagnosis with real vessels is important

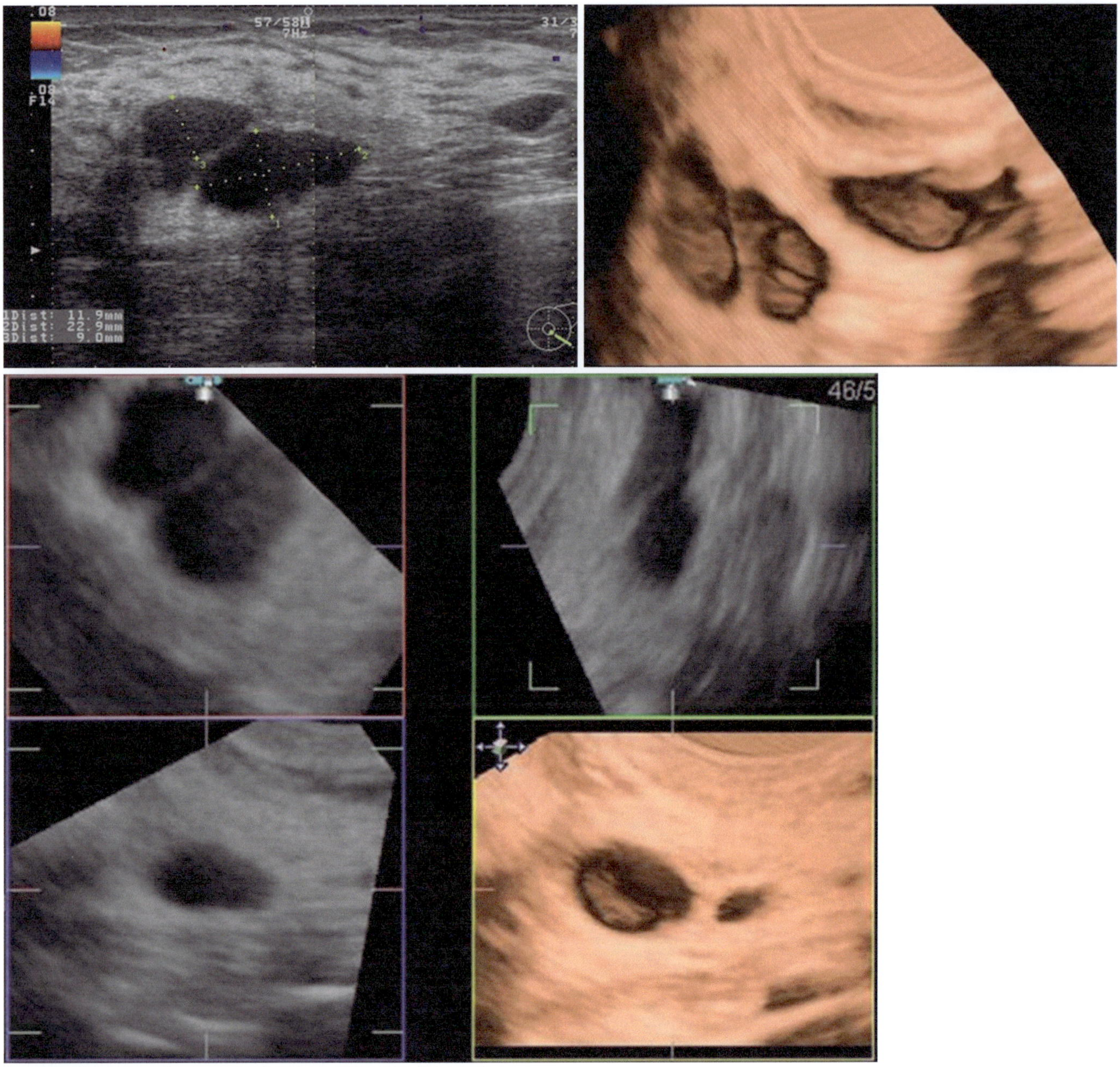

Fig. 6.3 DE in a 28-year-old, with dense breast: different size and shape of the cysts, with internal pseudo-septae in the largest ones, representing true cystic walls of the smaller tangent lesions. 3D/4D US is useful for the differential diagnosis with the complicated suspect cysts. Real-time Doppler could demonstrate *the snowstorm sign/the raining sign* in the presence of small floating particles

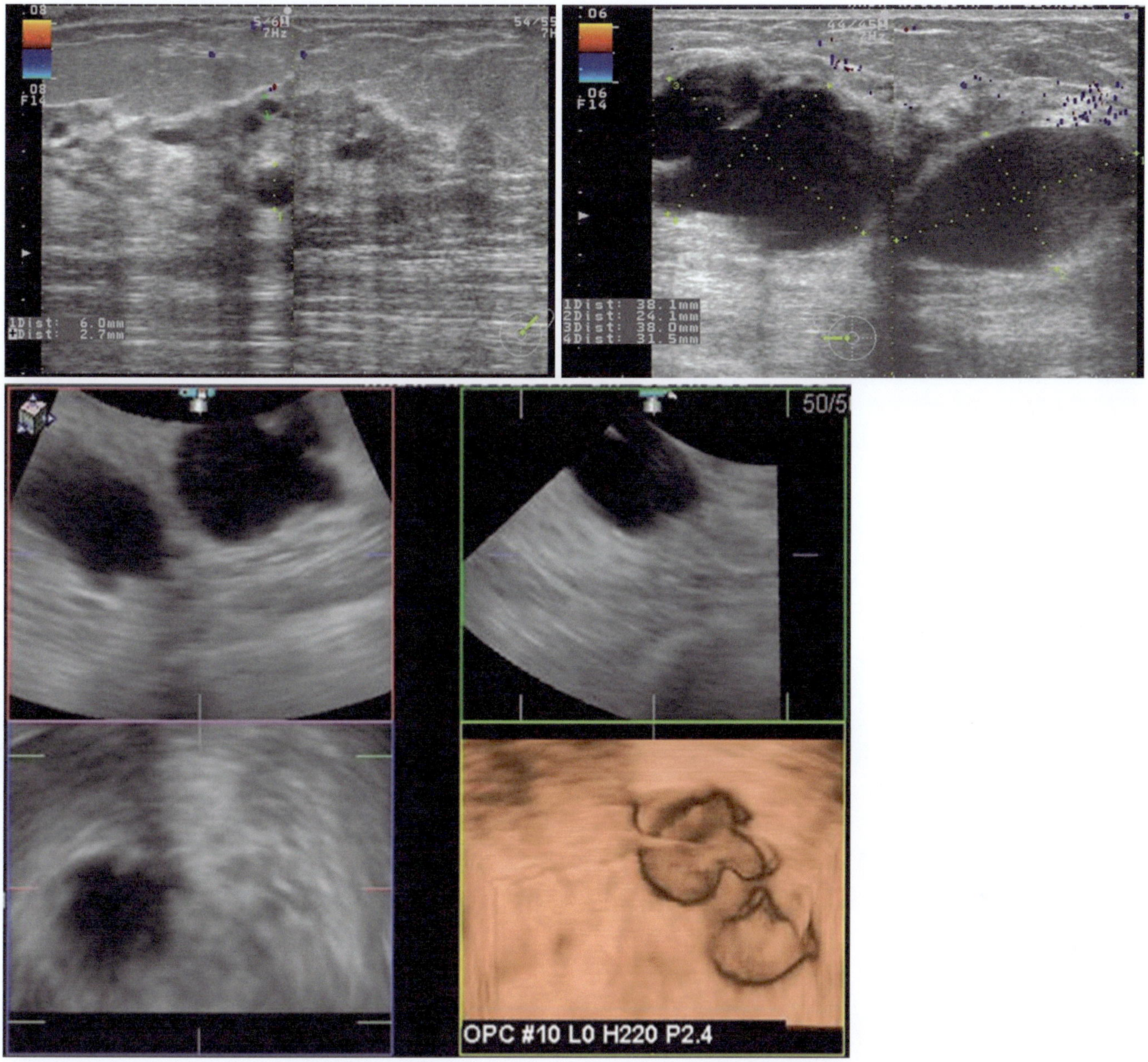

Fig. 6.4 The same case: The cystic walls mimicking septae could be demonstrated in 2D and 4D by the shape "of the number 3" at the edges of a cystic couple

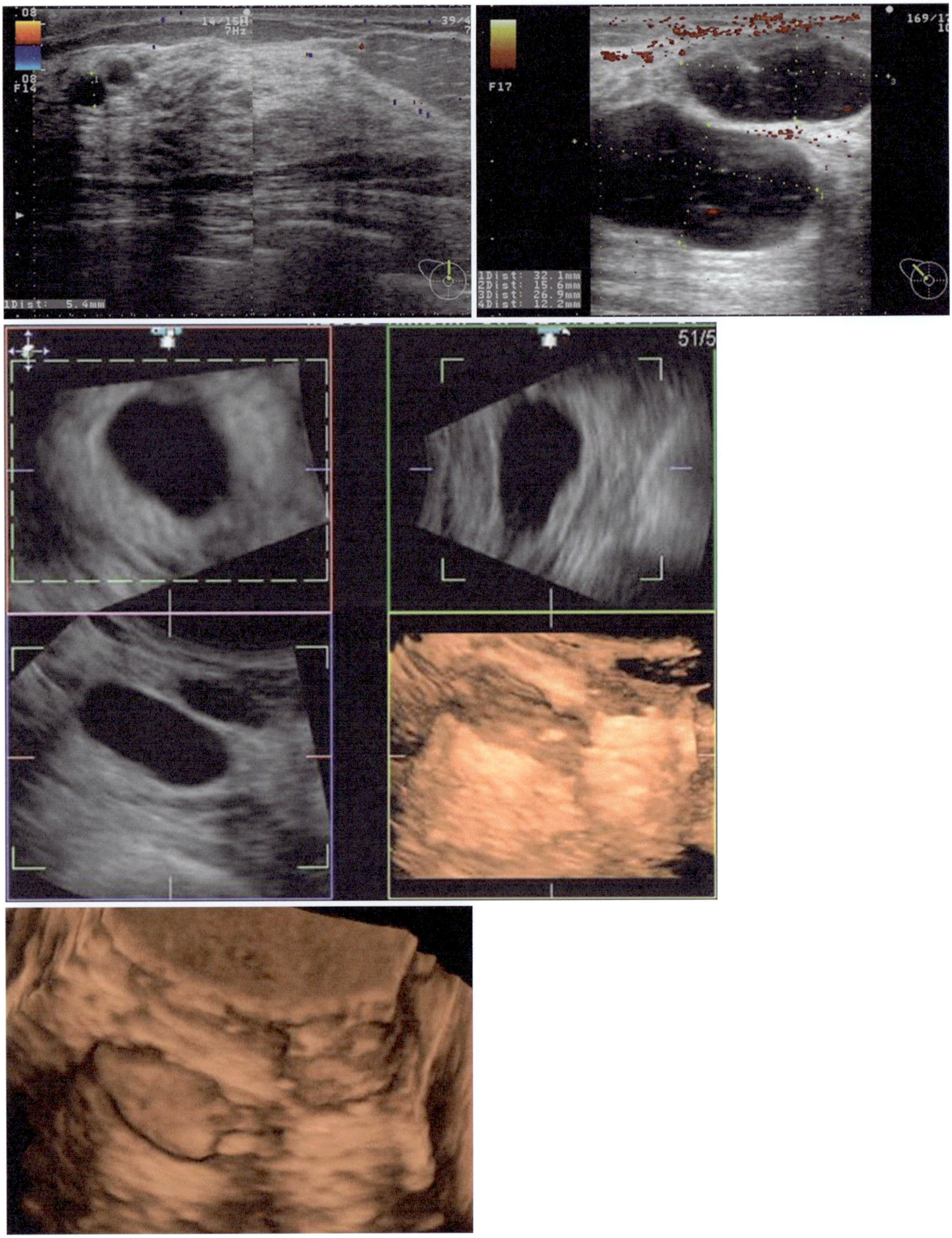

Fig. 6.5 DE in a 44-year-old with mixte breast: fibrocystic dysplasia, with 4D representations that demonstrate the polycyclic contour and incomplete remnant walls as pseudo-septae

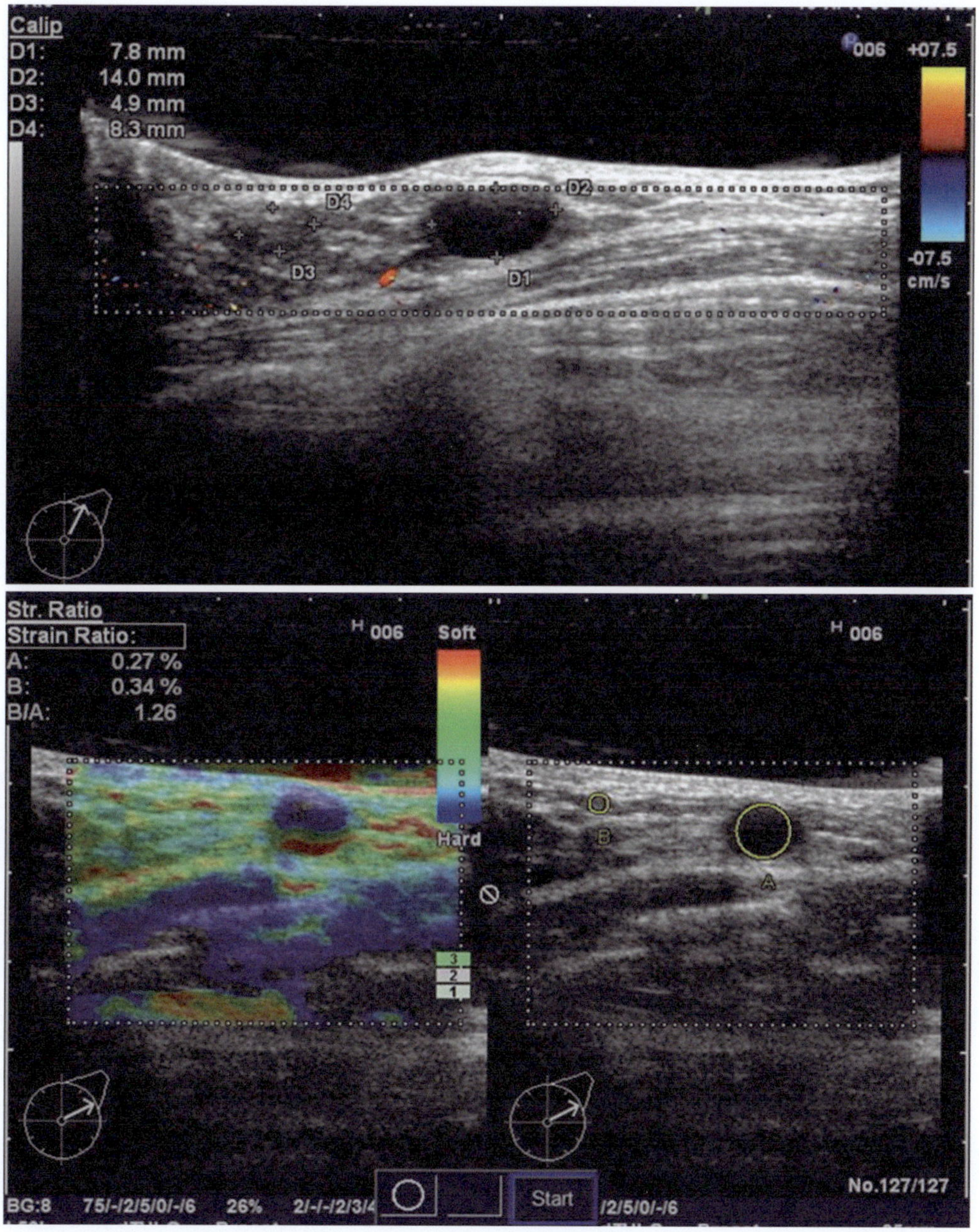

Fig. 6.6 FBU in a 38-year-old patient: fibrocystic dysplasia in a thin, dense breast; the sonoelastography is recommended to be achieved with water-bag long probe, because otherwise the fatty tissue is insufficient for a good estimation of the relative breast stiffness

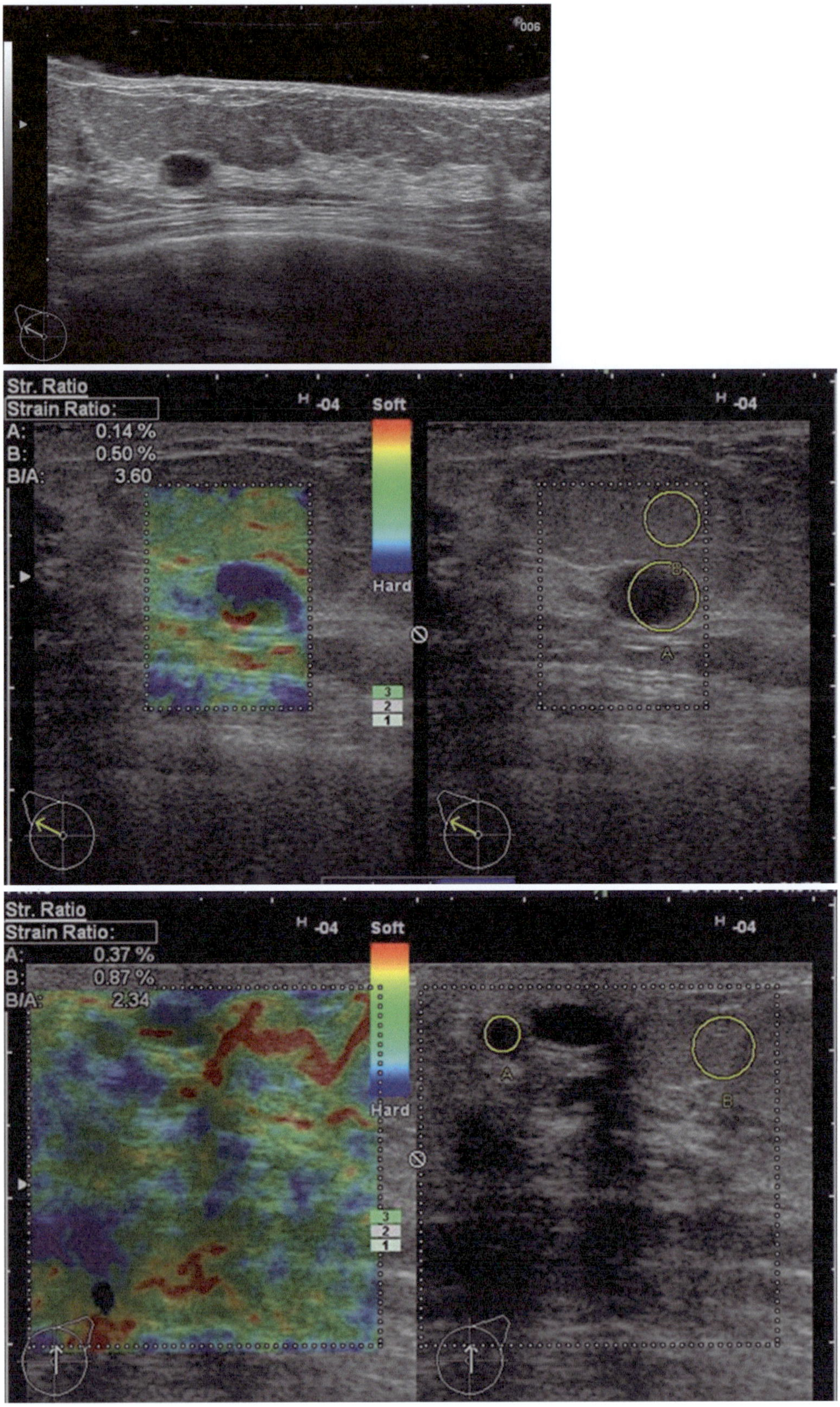

Fig. 6.7 A 41-year-old patient: fibrocystic dysplasia with cystic wall thickening and typical BGR aspect on sonoelastography; low FLR (fat-to-lesion ratio) is suggesting benign lesion; small cysts have just green-red elastogram, as the "solid" benign lesions

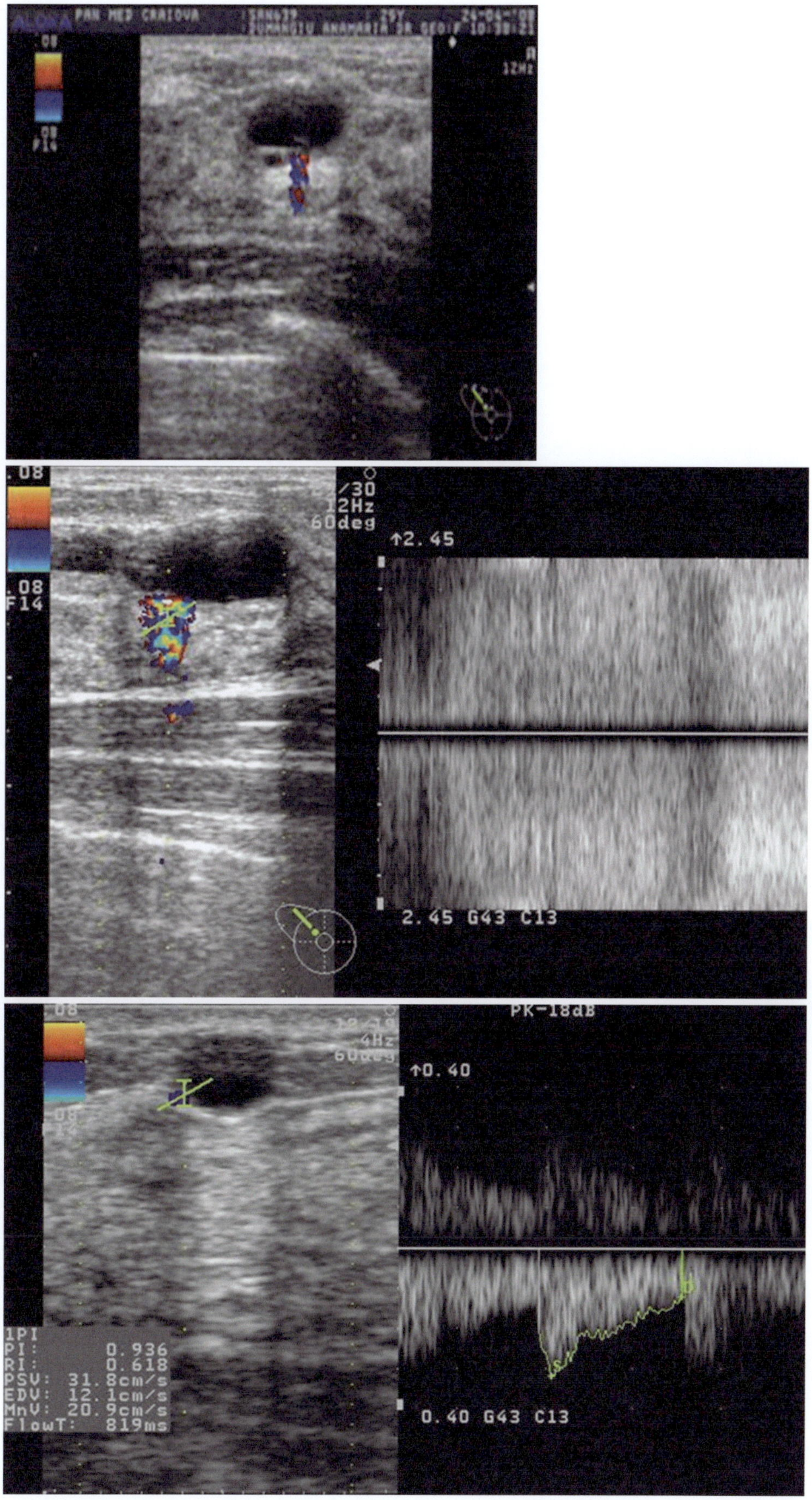

Fig. 6.8 The twinkling artifact posterior to a cyst, in color Doppler and spectral mode, as compared with the normal vascular signal even in small vessels

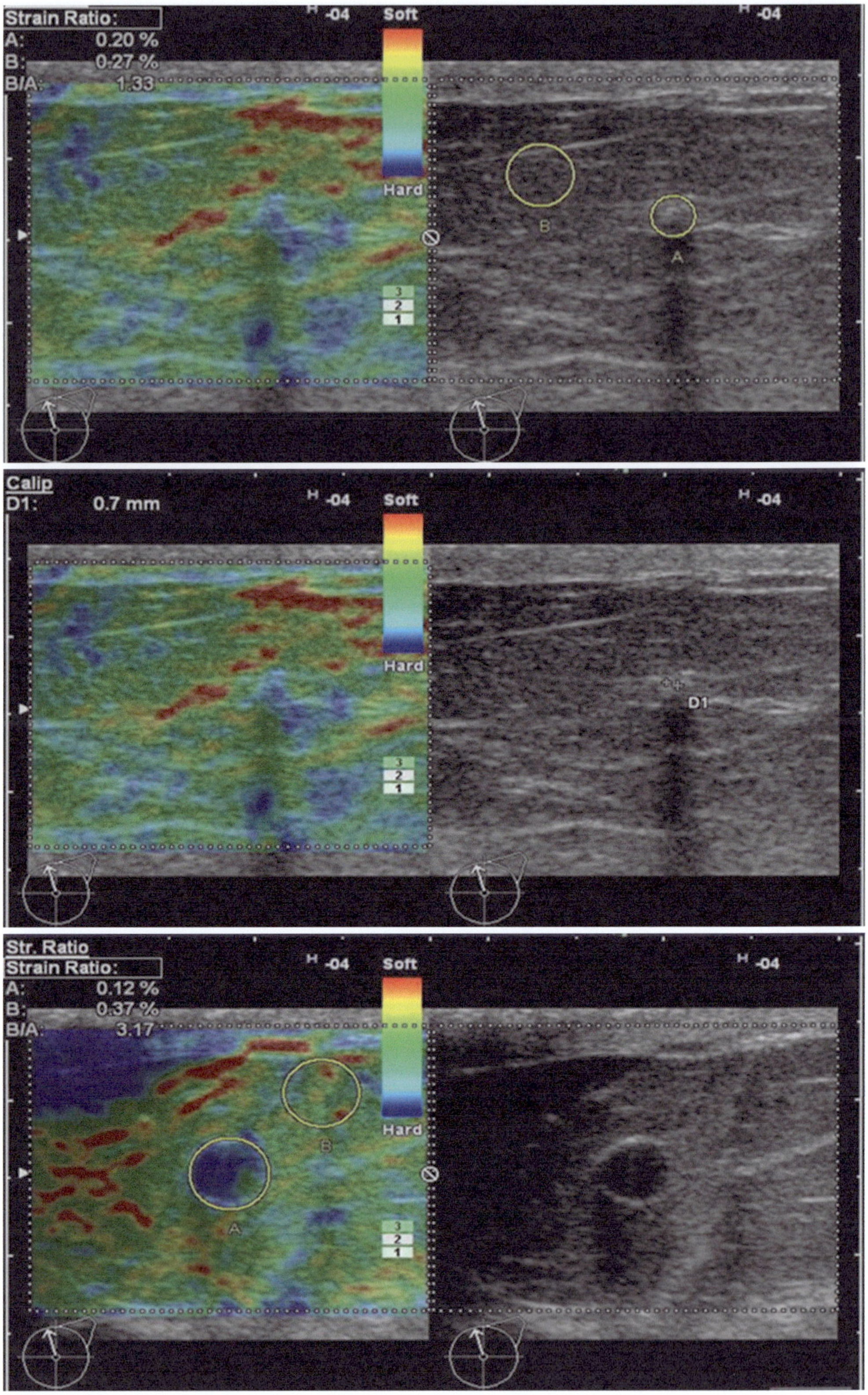

Fig. 6.9 Benign calcifications on US with RTSE: lobular clustered microcalcifications over 0.5 mm, with low FLR of 1.33, and calcified small cyst, with higher but benign FLR of 3.17

Fig. 6.9 (continued)

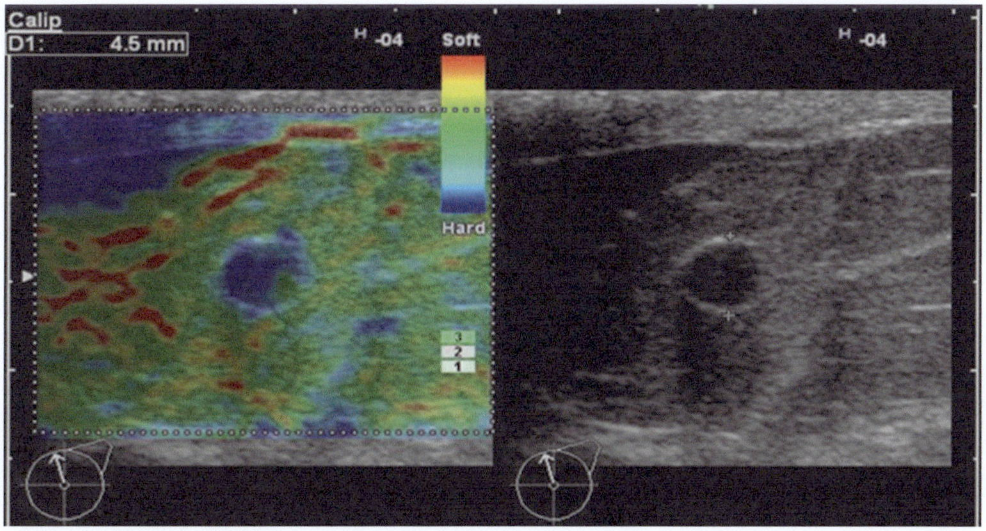

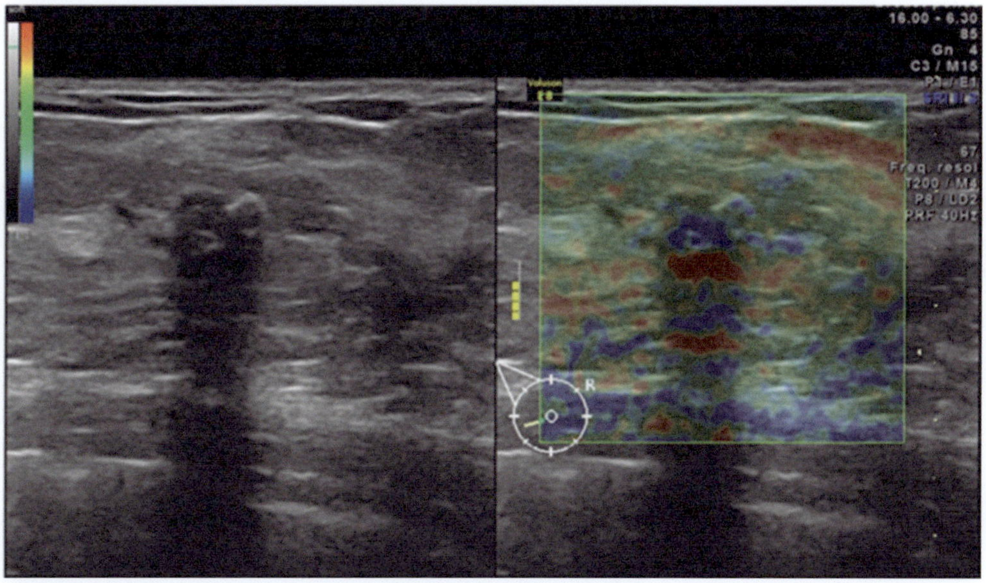

Fig. 6.10 Nodular type of fibro-micro-cystic dysplasia, with pseudomalignant aspect; the calcified cyst and the BGR score of the hypoechoic adjacent mass allow the differential diagnosis and avoid the unnecessary biopsy

Fig. 6.11 An 83-year-old patient presents a large mammary cyst of ductal type, with polycyclic contour suggesting a branching ductal cyst. The water-bag device allows a better evaluation of the cyst and of the surroundings, without any distortion: the volume can be estimated based on 3 axes, while the mammographic size is always overestimated because of the reduction of the diameter in the sense of the compression of tissues with projection of the lesion in the largest false diameters

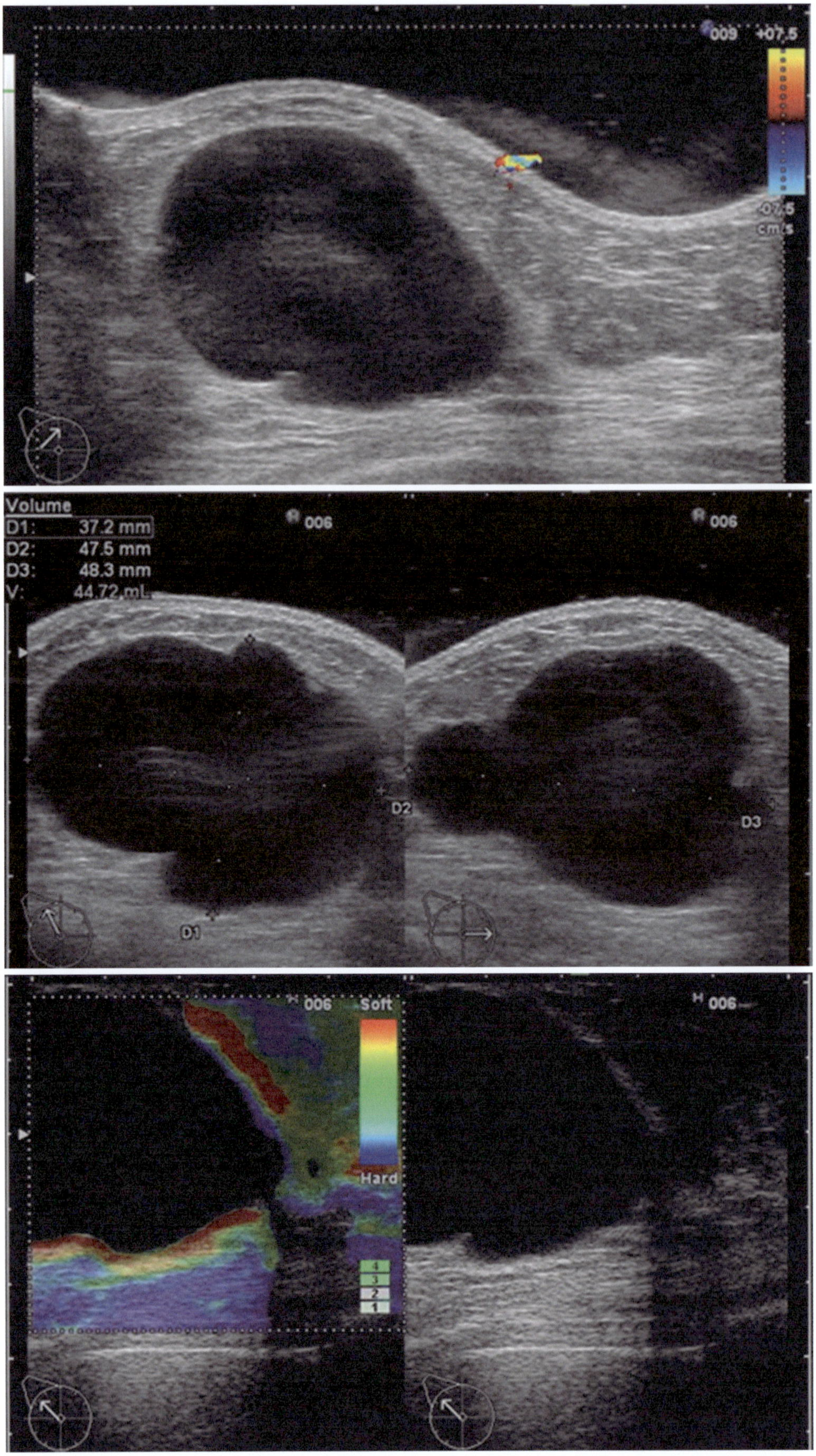

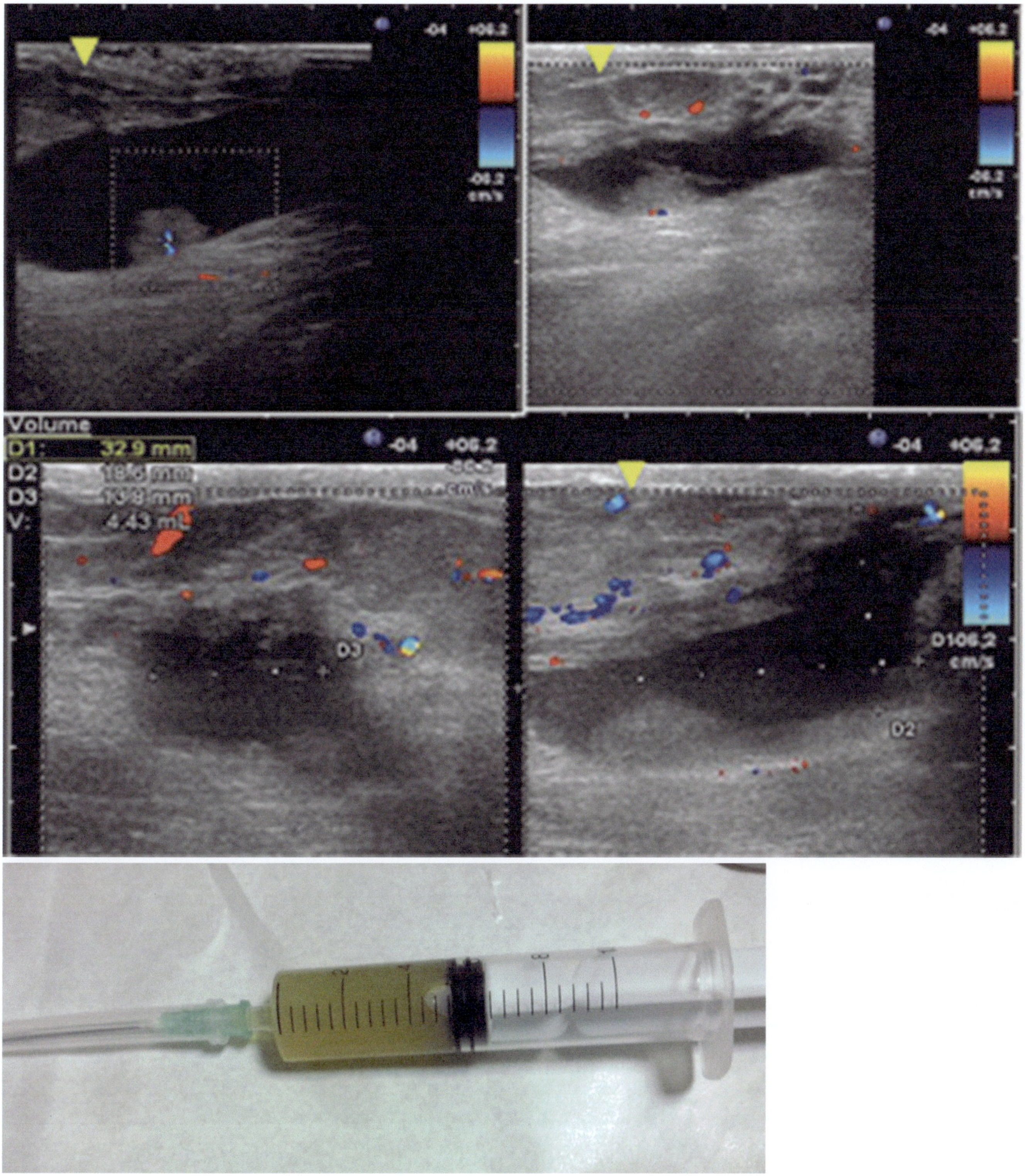

Fig. 6.12 US-guided puncture (▼) evacuated 85 ml gray-citrine fluid, with benign cytology despite of the intracystic papilloma; a bacteriological test identified a *Staphylococcus aureus*, whom sensibility to antibiotics was determined and oriented the treatment. The 1-year follow-up exam illustrated a residual cyst of 1 ml volume, without any proliferation. An ordinary syringe may be used for local anesthesia, and by the same puncture with the needle in place, a small pressure penetrates the cystic wall and the fluid is aspirated

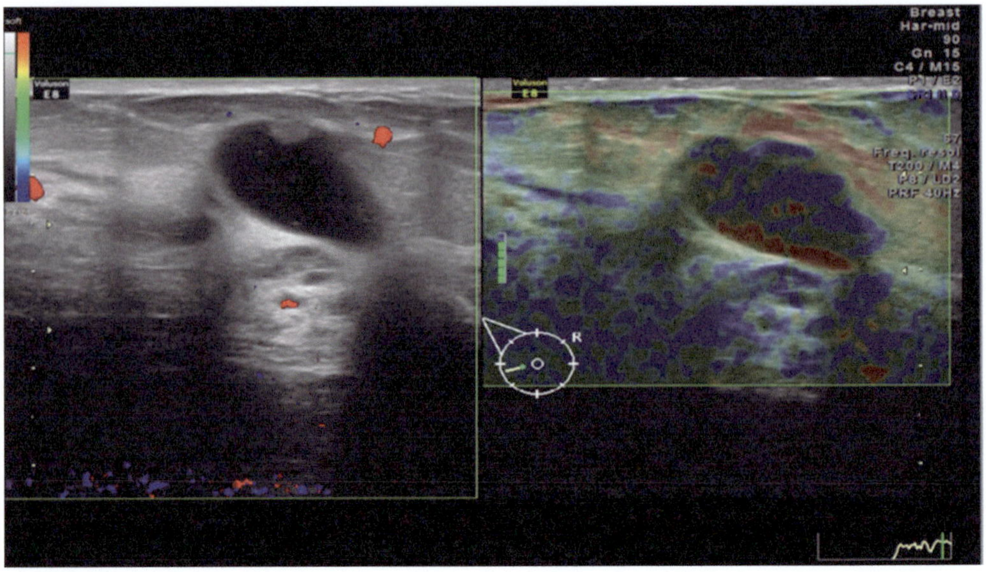

Fig. 6.13 Sonoelastography of a complex cyst: small intracystic papilloma with benign strain and floating echoes suggesting a proteic content corresponding to a complex BGR score

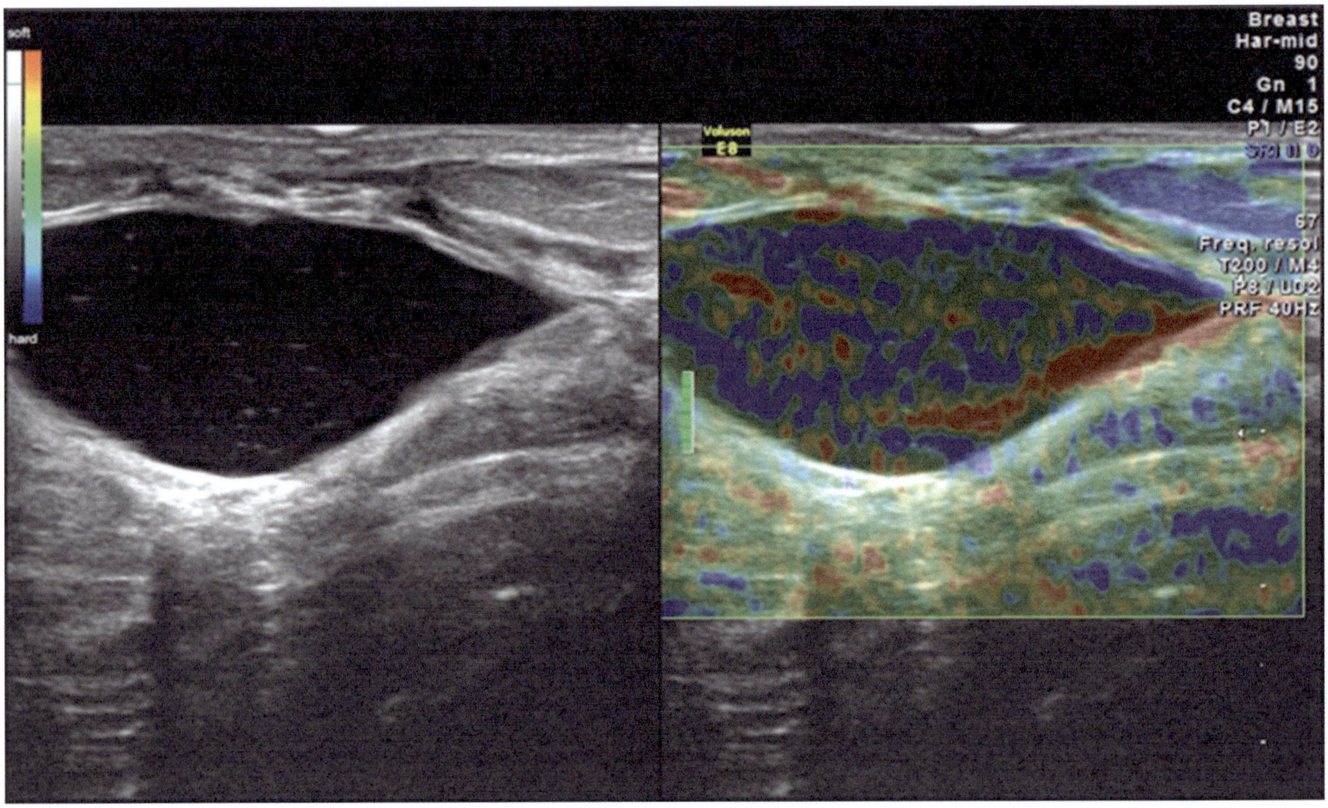

Fig. 6.14 Sonoelastography of a large cyst with inhomogeneous content, the floating debris demonstrating complex BGR score

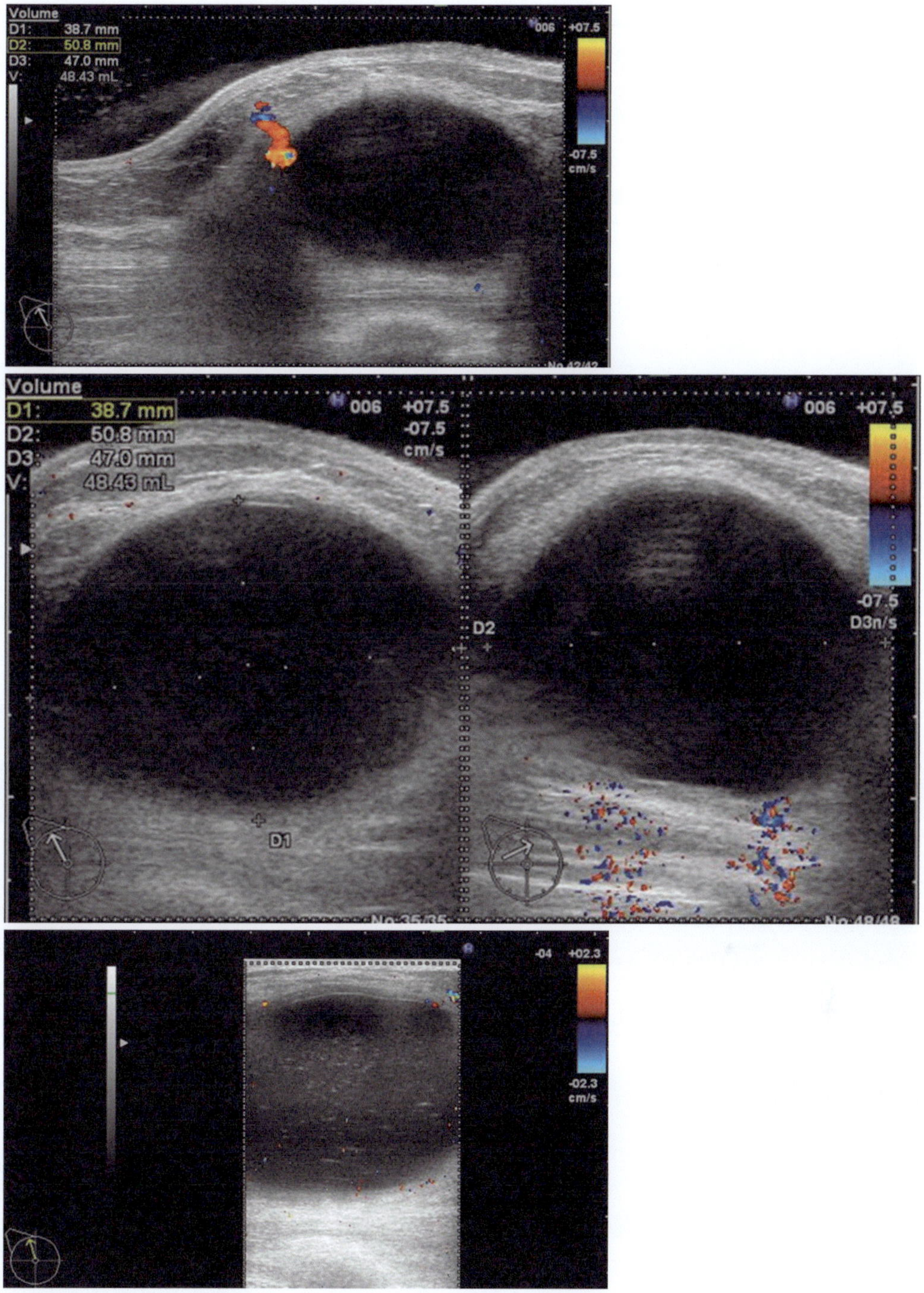

Fig. 6.15 Huge cyst of 48.4 ml, with echogenic particles floating in the content, without peripheral Doppler signal, proved infected with *Staphylococcus aureus*; after aspiration-drainage and antibiotherapy evolution with complete healing without recidivism

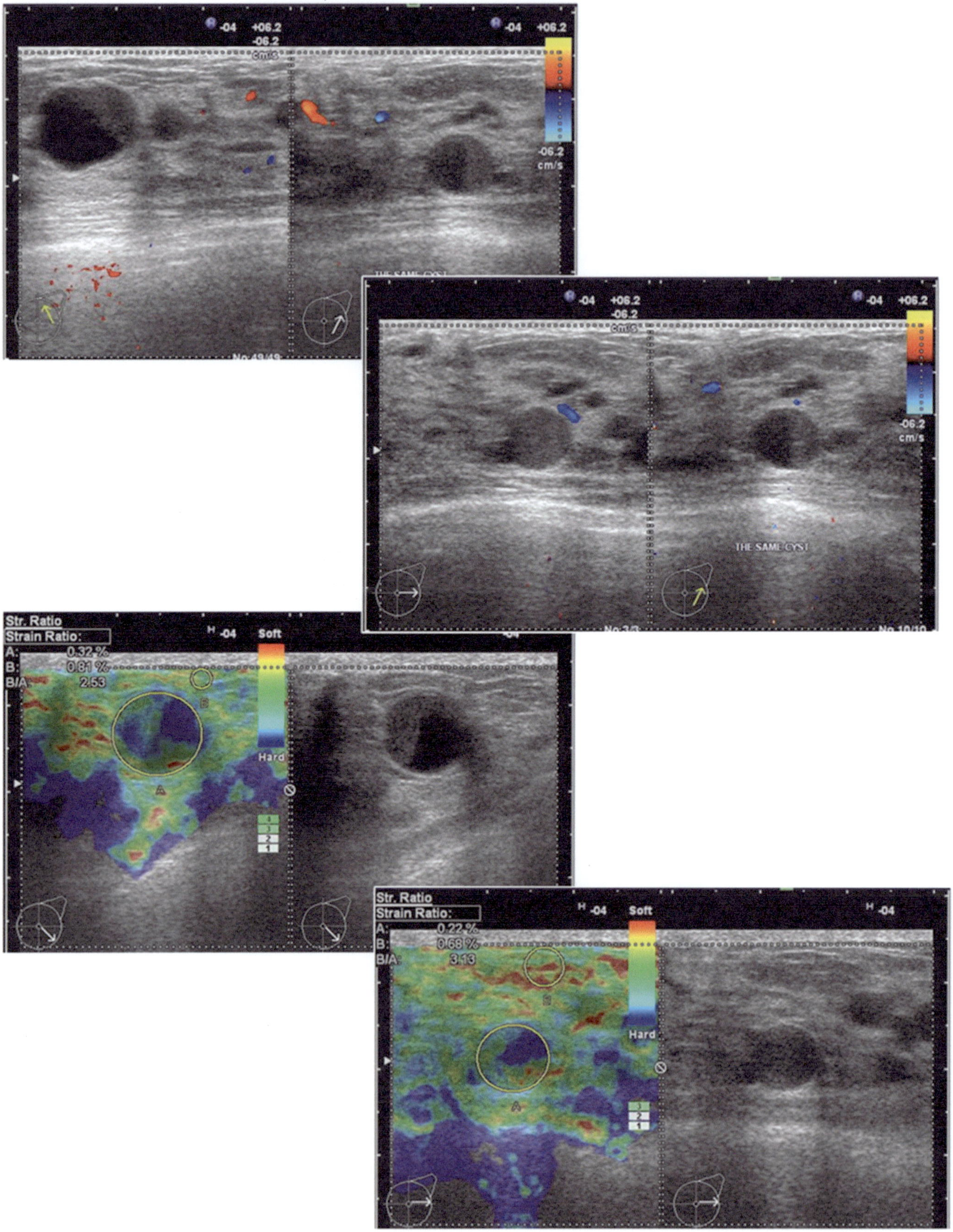

Fig. 6.16 FBU in fibrocystic dysplasia, with fluid/debris level, mimicking "solid" lesions but with BGR score variants; the level could have a vertical or oblique orientation on the echogram, according to the orientation of the lobe against the gravitational forces (clockwise scanning radius of the DE)

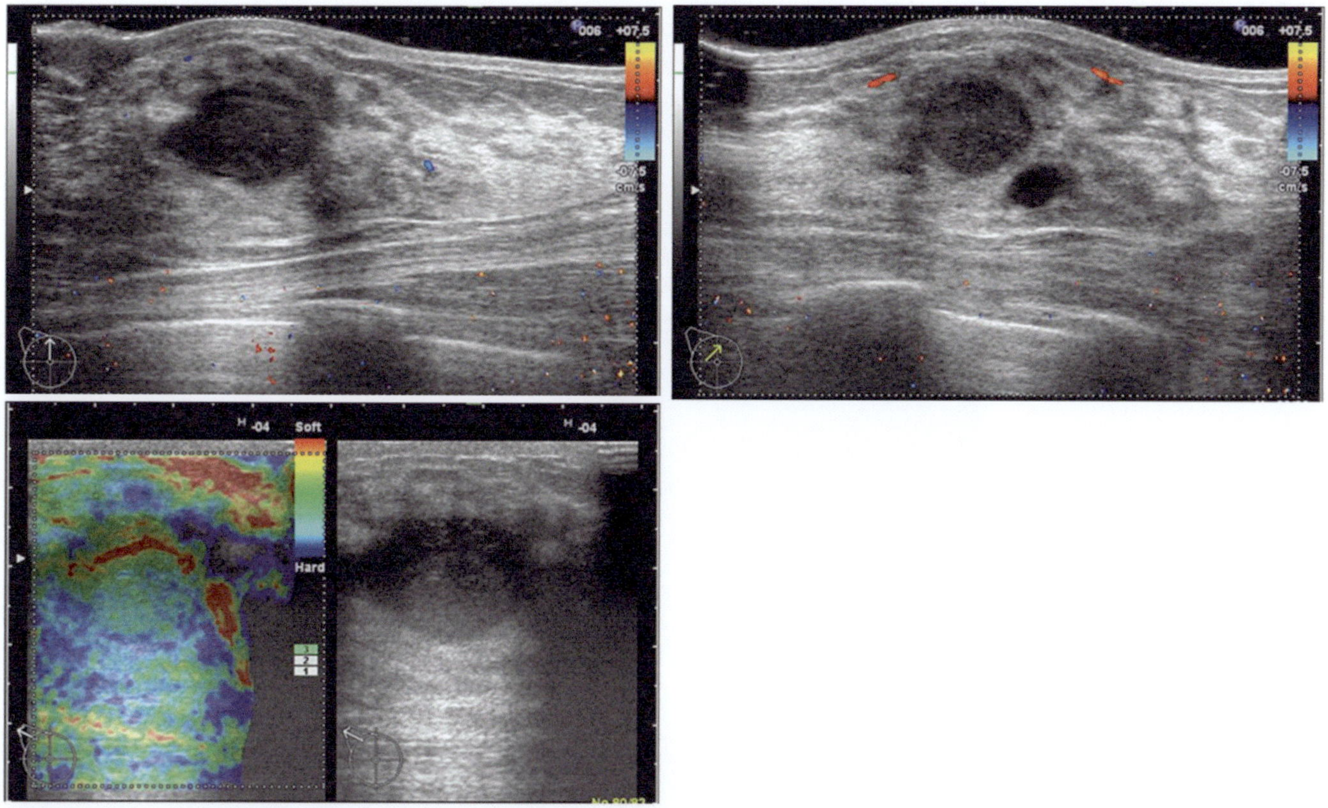

Fig. 6.17 FBU of an inspissated cyst, mimicking a solid-type lesion both at DE and RTSE, but without internal new formation vasculature and with benign Kobayashi findings of the posterior effects

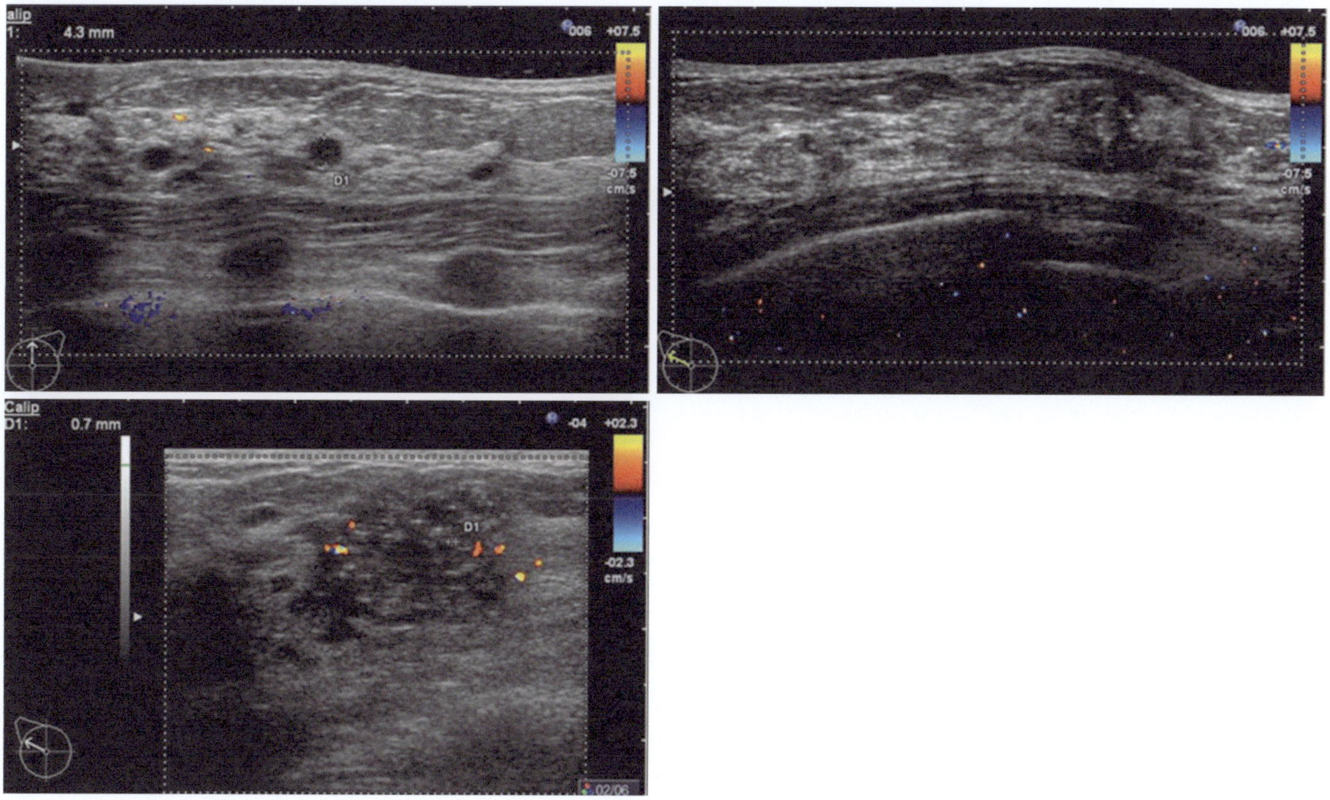

Fig. 6.18 A 49-year-old patient with previous lumpectomy for fibrocystic dysplasia; actually she demonstrates multiple bilateral infracentimetric cysts and a lump at R 9:30, with ill-defined borders, benign Kobayashi posterior effects, heterogeneous structure with small cysts, and many hyperechoic, less than 1 mm in size, horizontal artifacts mimicking calcifications

Fig. 6.18 (continued)

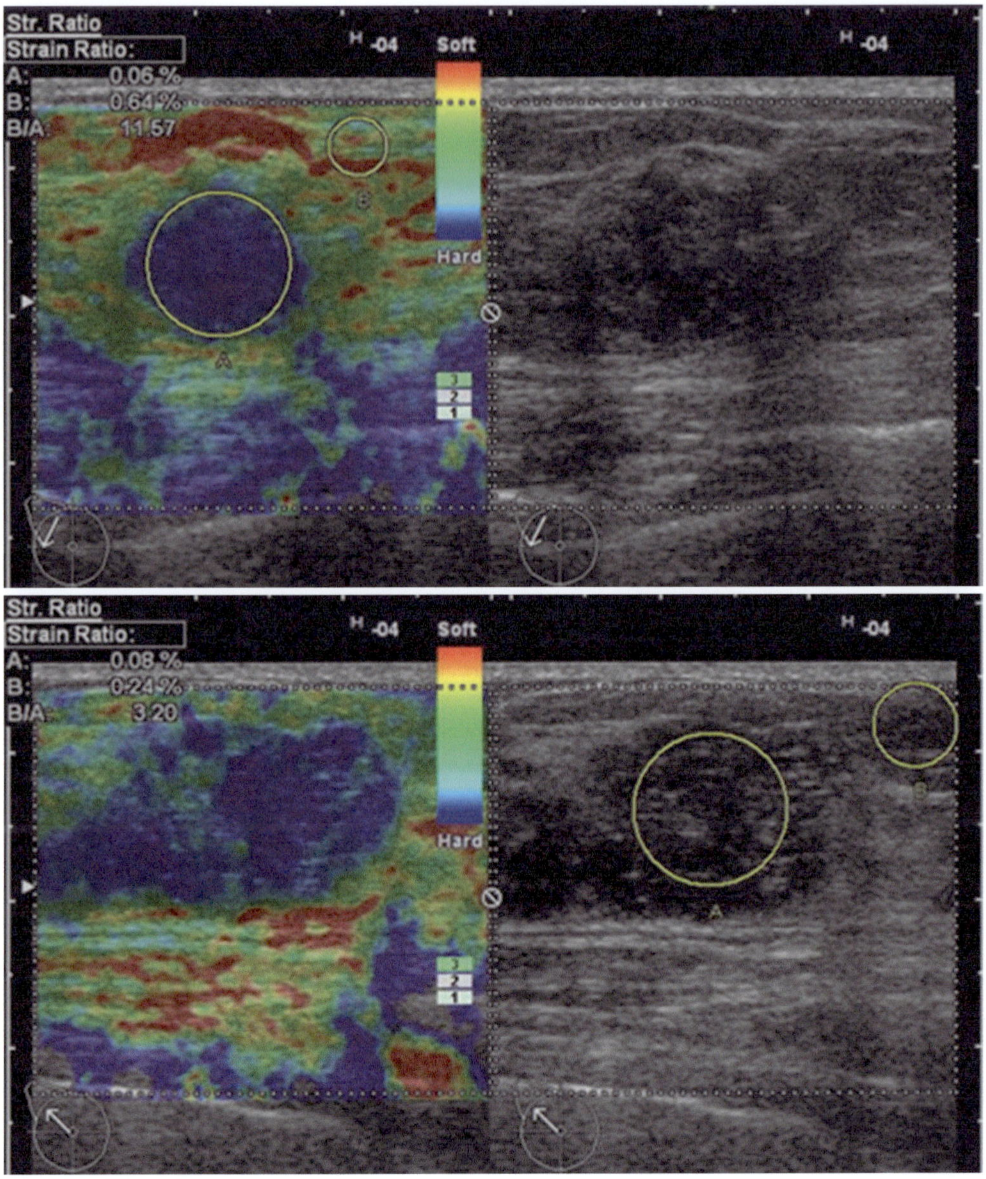

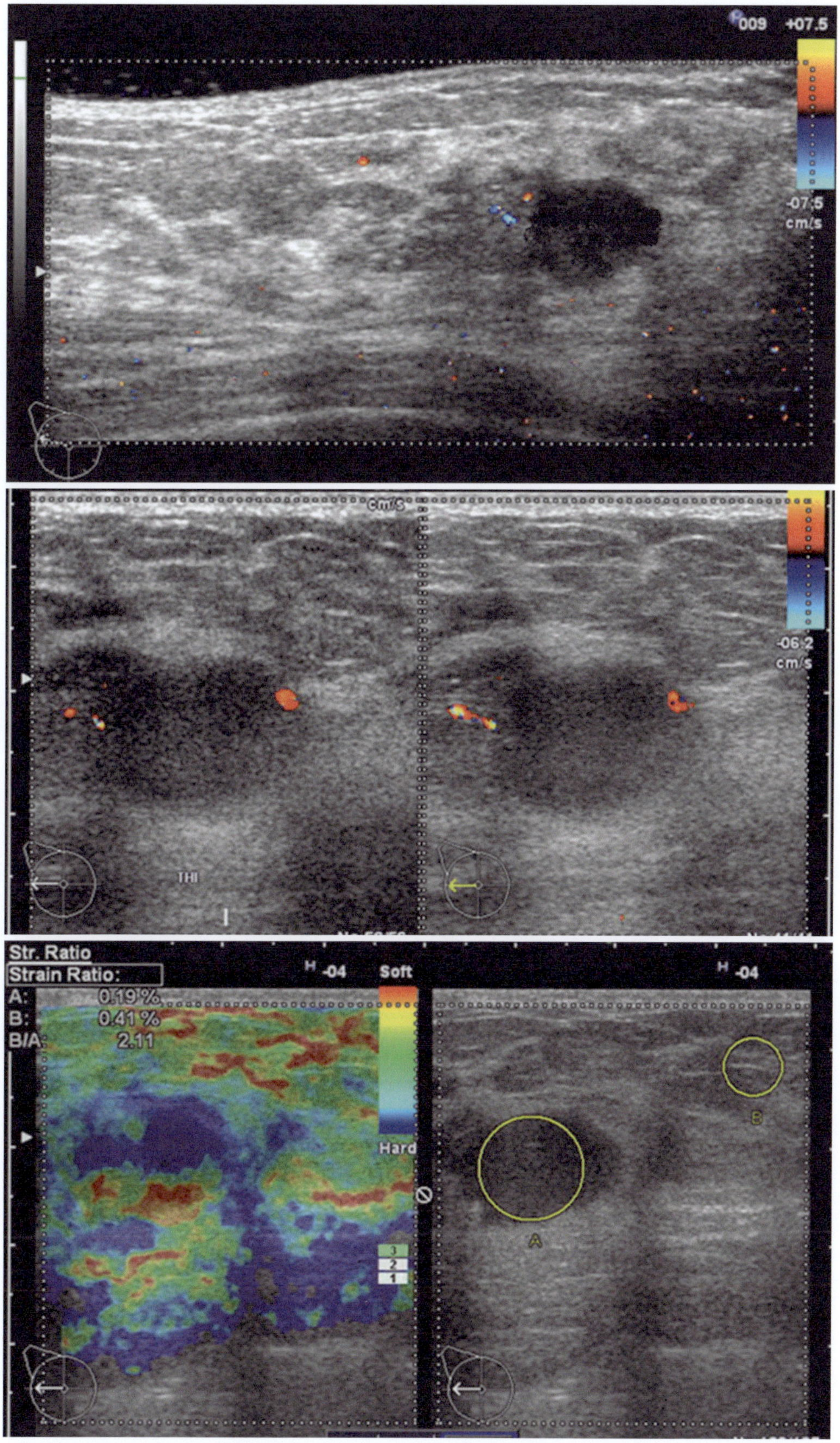

Fig. 6.19 FBU of an infected cyst, with pseudonodular aspect: ill-defined borders, surrounding edema, perilesional enhanced vasculature, and hypoechoic content; high-resolution scans reveal debris/debris level and a thick cystic wall, confirmed by the BGR score on sonoelastography

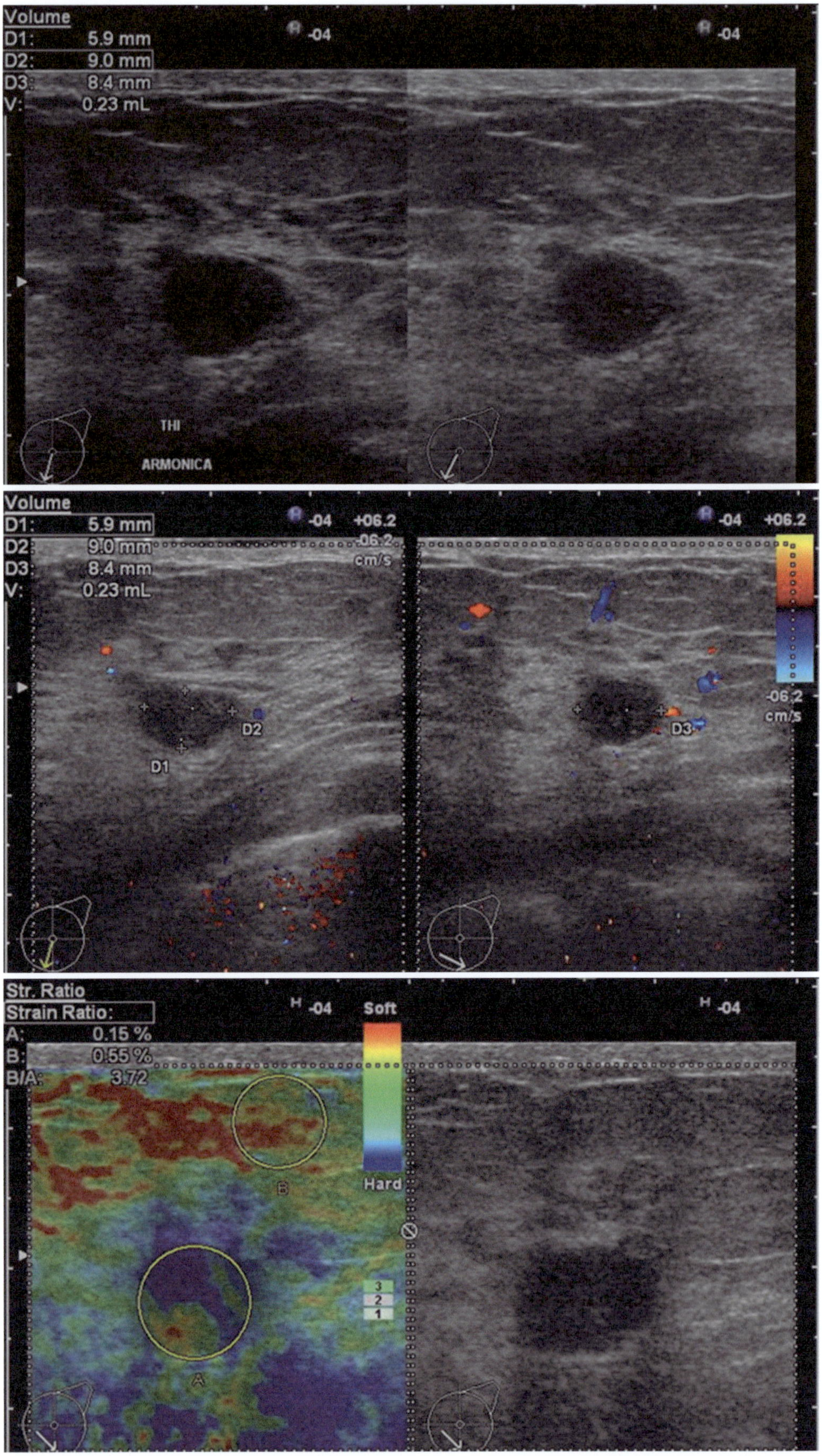

Fig. 6.20 Illustration of FBU as the best tool in the differential diagnosis of an infected cyst from a pseudonodular, ill-defined lesion

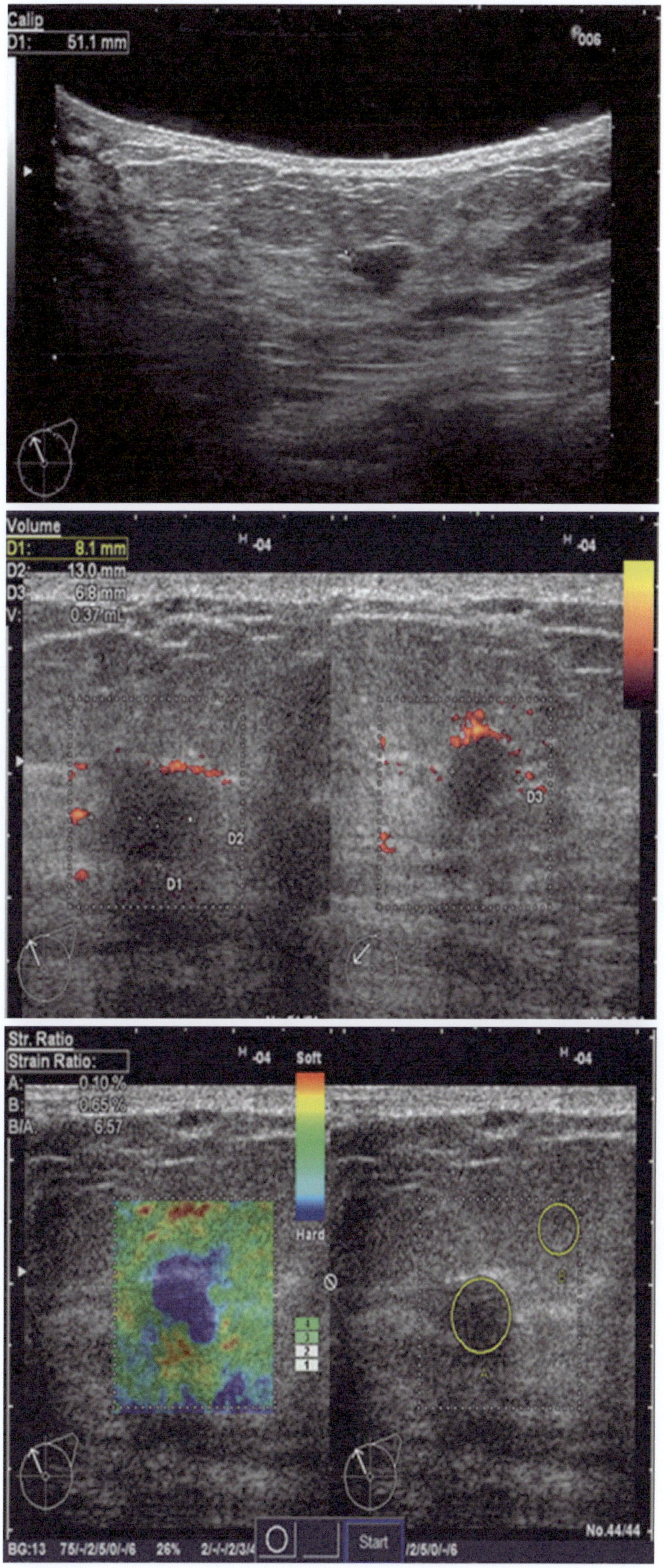

Fig. 6.21 FBU in infected cyst at L 6:30, with pseudotumoral aspect, demonstrates debris, local salient vasculature, and complex BGR score

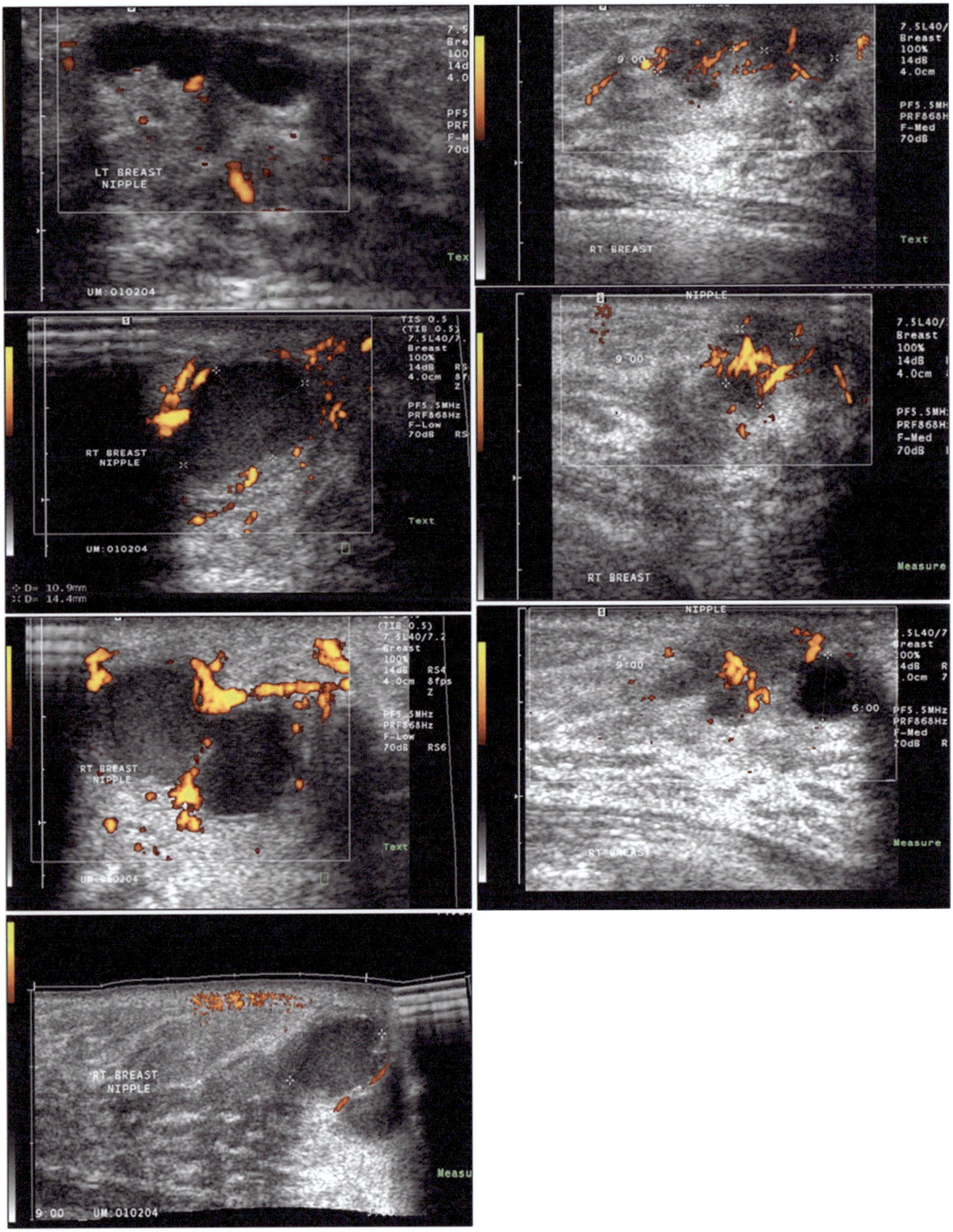

Fig. 6.22 Acute mastitis with some infected cysts presenting hypoechoic content and inflammatory peripheral hyper-vasculature, associated with transonic lesions (*left*). 10 days after antibiotherapy, the evolution showed resorption almost complete of the infected cysts and unchanged aspect of the simple, clear ones (*right*)

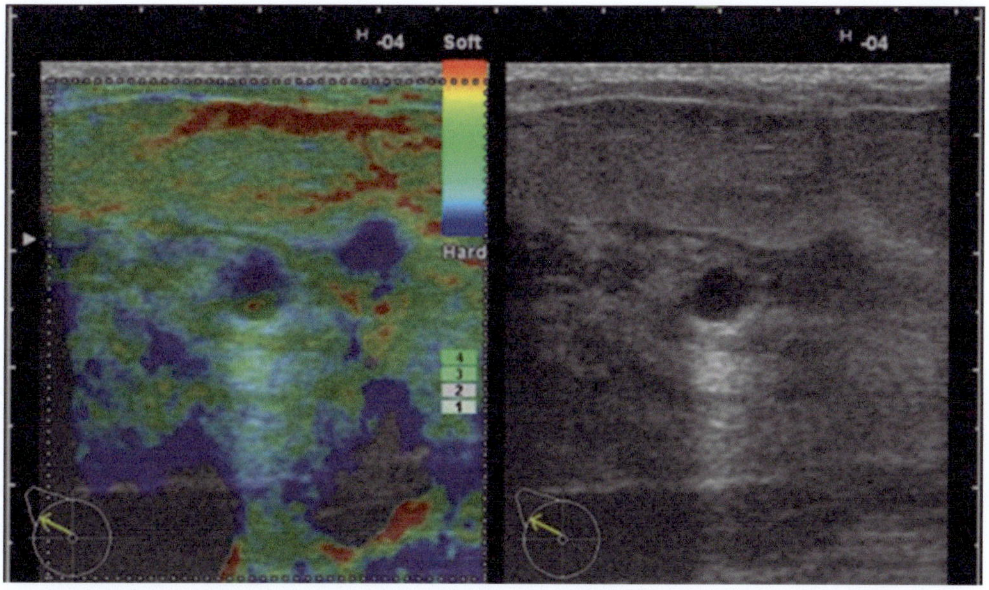

Fig. 6.23 Sonoelastography in fibrocystic dysplasia demonstrates a couple of BGR score, corresponding to a measurable unique cyst and to a nodular form of fibro-micro-cystic aspect in a TDLU location, respectively

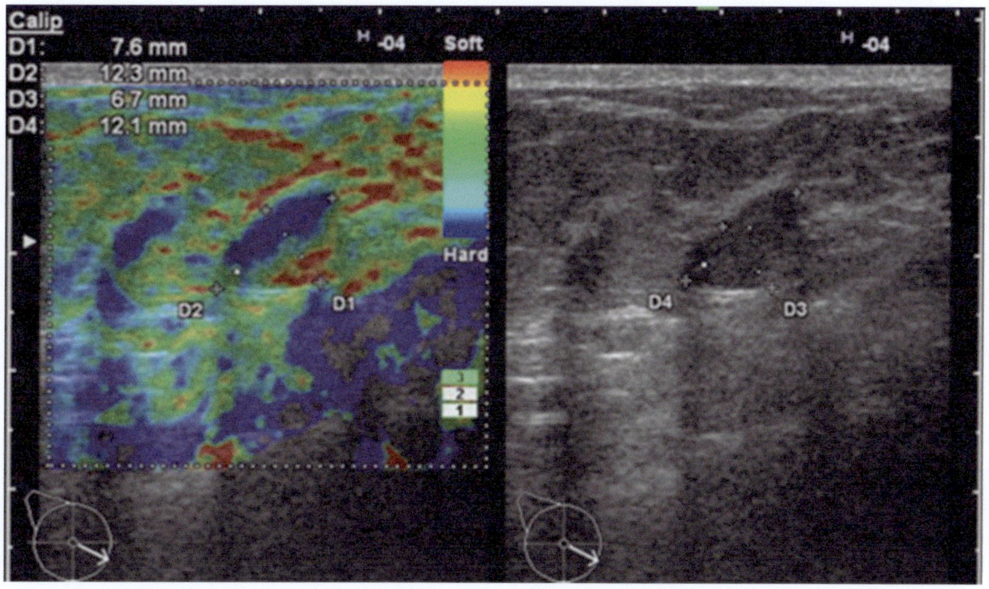

Fig. 6.24 Fibro-micro-cystic dysplasia with pseudonodular aspect in TDLU location, presenting oblique-triangular shape, posterior acoustic enhancement with marginal shadowings and the BGR score of summation type; the TDLU site is logically for a cluster of lobular microcysts immeasurable by US

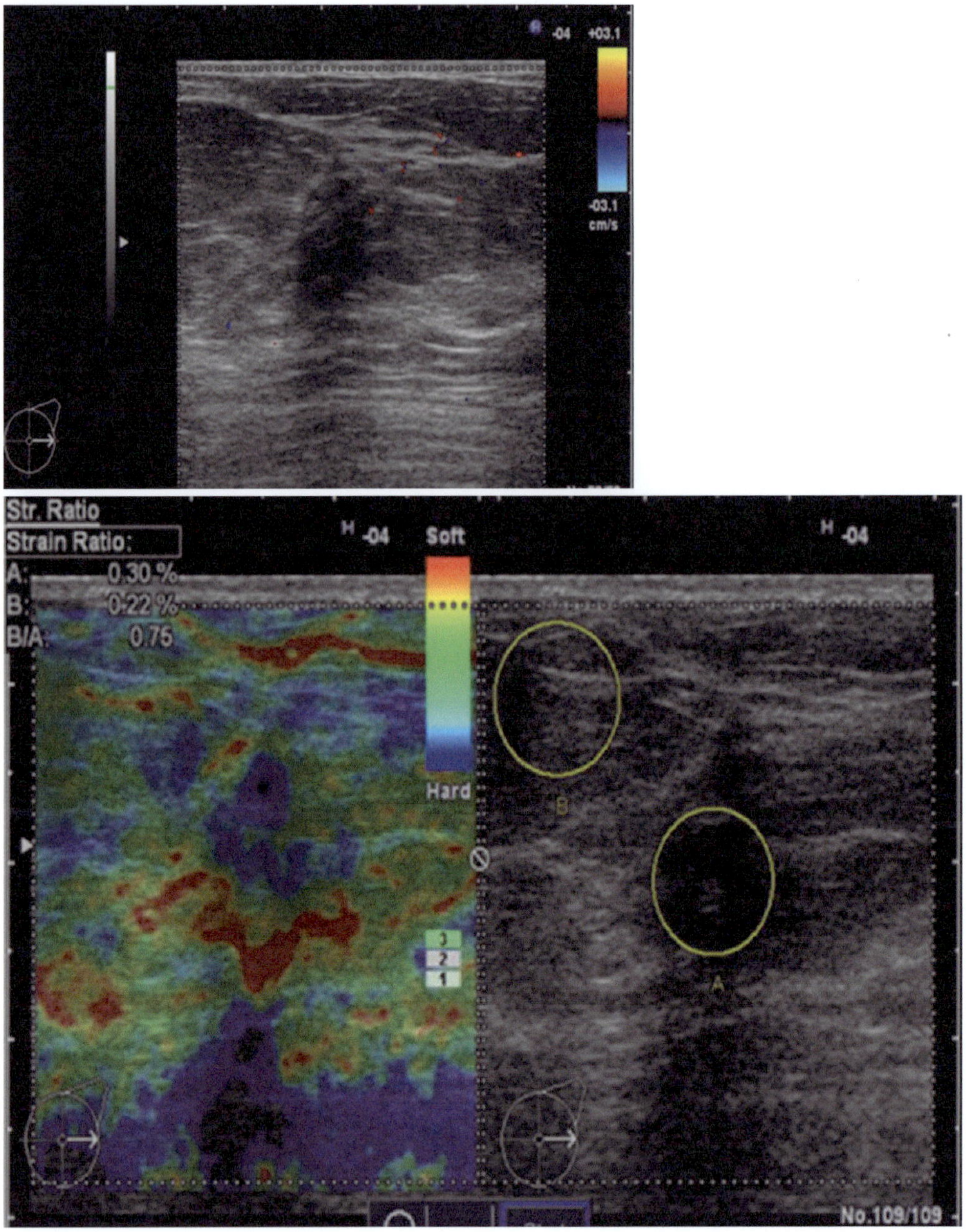

Fig. 6.25 Pseudomalignant area in a TDLU site, hypoechoic, taller than wide, with acoustic shadow and ill-defined contour, but with no suspected vascular signs on Doppler and few tinny cysts, no greater than 1 mm; the SE is concluding for BGR of summation type, and the unnecessary biopsy is avoided, despite the mammographically suspect feature

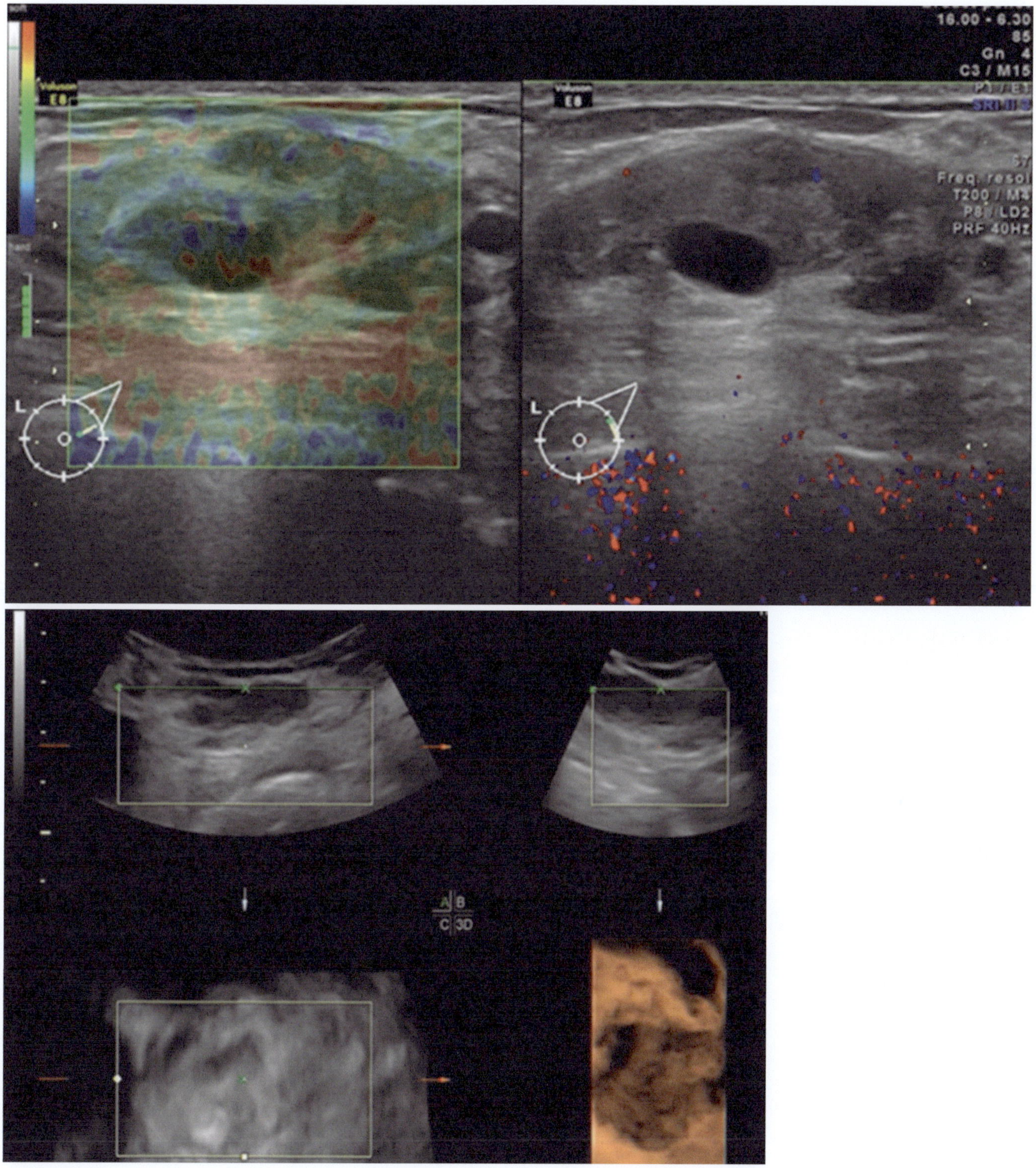

Fig. 6.26 For the ultrasonographic devices not yet provided with performing sonoelastography, the nodular form of the fibro-micro-cystic dysplasia is salient in the 4D acquisitions, because of the better contrast of the microcysts from the "solid" fibrous tissue

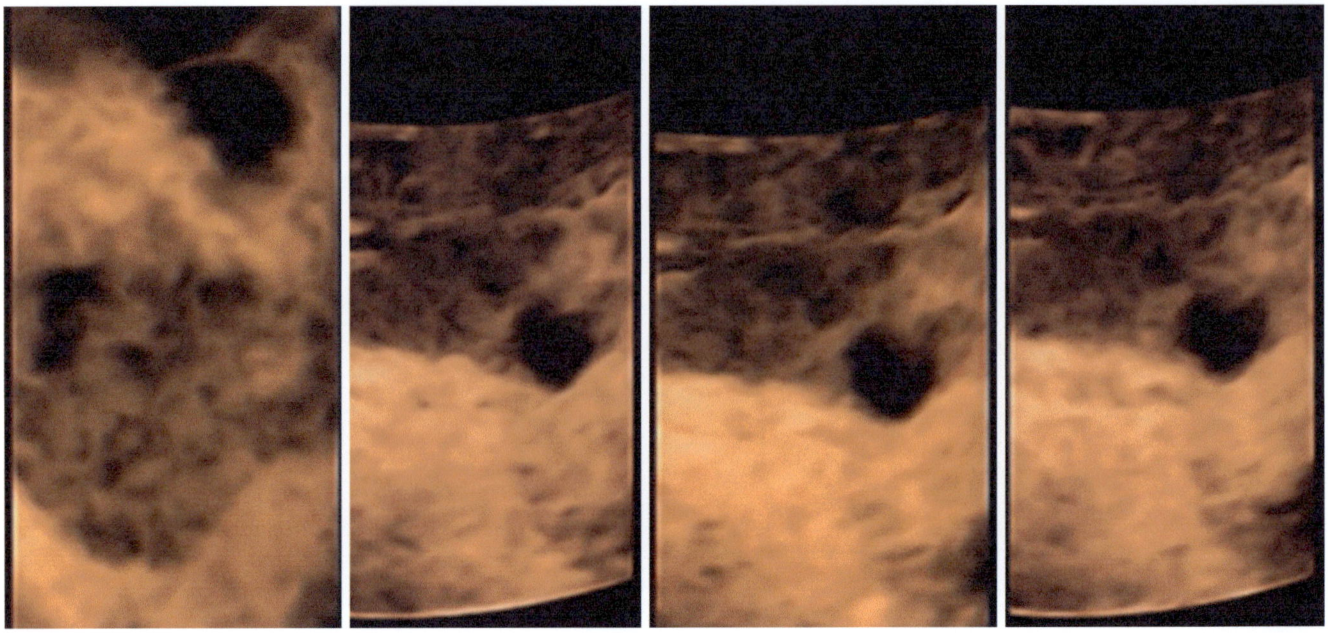

Fig. 6.26 (continued)

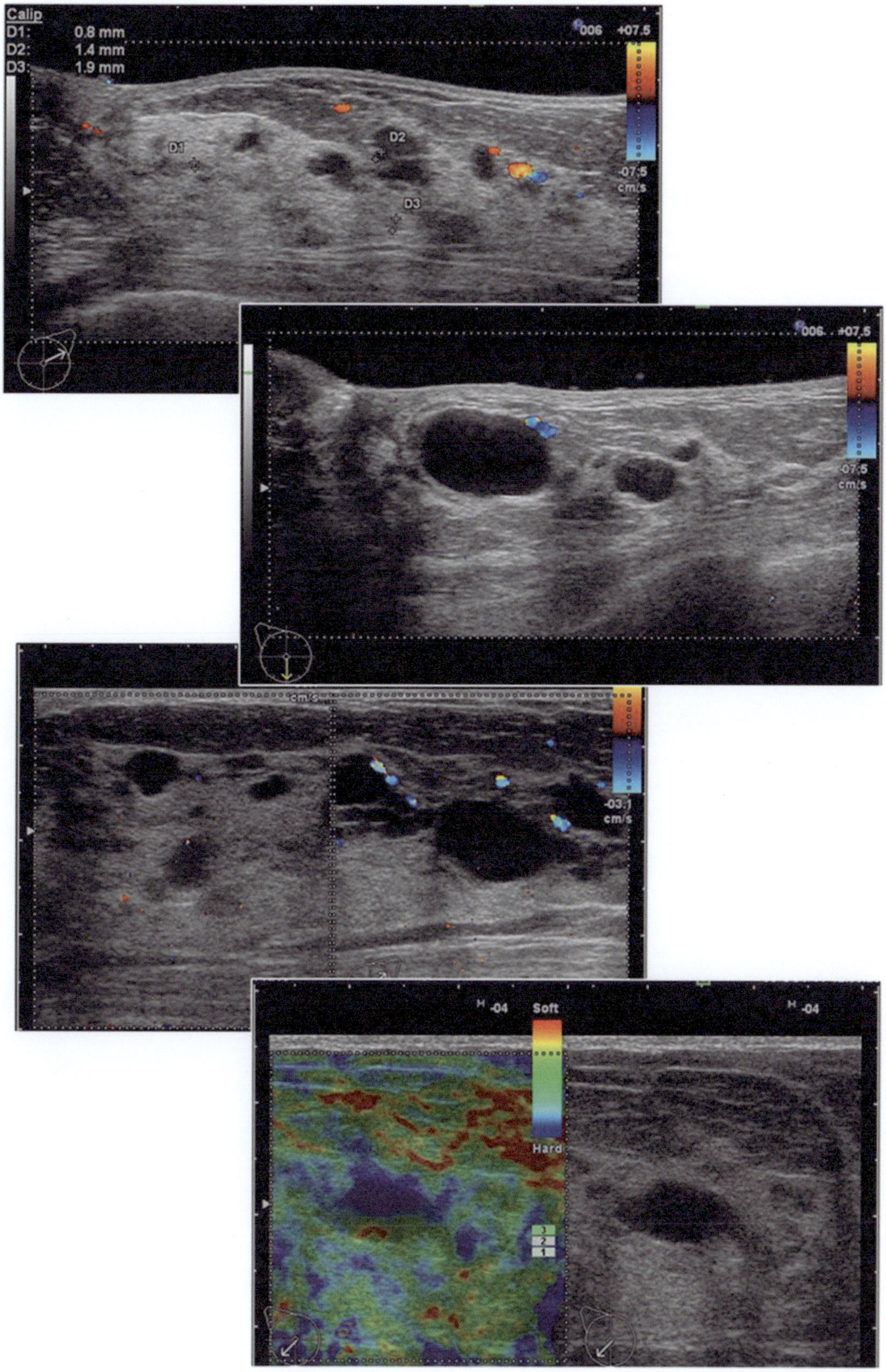

Fig. 6.27 FBU in generalized fibrocystic dysplasia, the Reclus disease, presenting multiple cysts of various sizes and small ductal ectasias; the salient breast vasculature in this case is due to a hyperprolactinemia

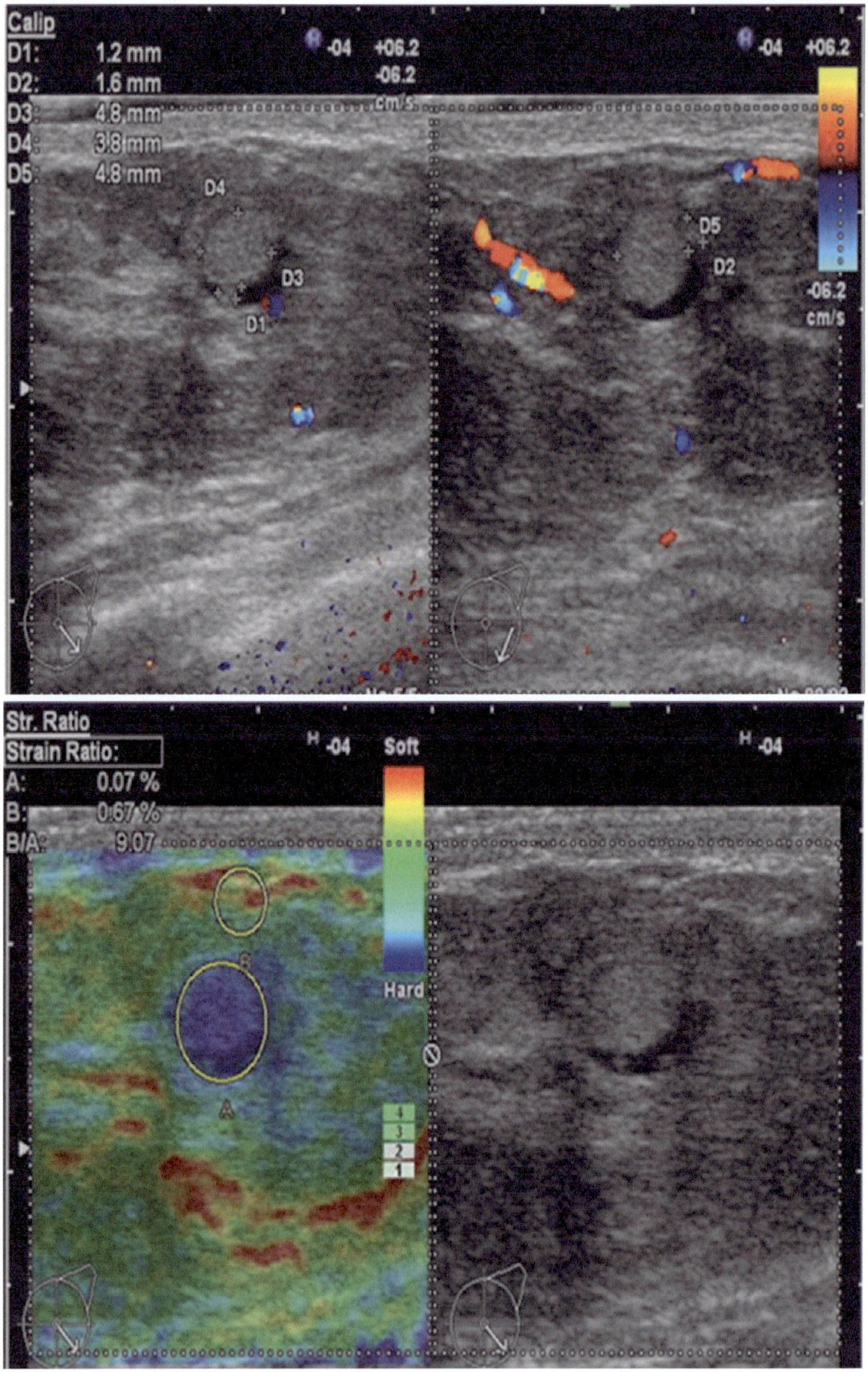

Fig. 6.28 FBU illustrates at L 4:30 less than 5 mm intracystic nodular proliferation with solid appearance, peripheral increased Doppler signal, and score 5 Ueno, with elevated strain ratio; this lesion is highly suspected for intracystic carcinoma, otherwise with benign mammographic appearance due to the smooth cystic wall

6.4 Adenosis and Ductal Hyperplasia in FBU

Adenosis represents a mammary proliferative dysplasia, located in the TDLUs, resulting both in an enlargement of the lobules and in an increasing of their number. Some authors consider adenosis as premalignant lesion, especially sclerosing adenosis which is thought to have the risk of developing breast cancer increased about 1½–2-folds as compared with the risk of women without lobular dysplasia.

Adenosis is related to dense breasts, with clinical symptoms represented by painful breast related or not to the premenstrual syndrome (mastodynia). The hormonal tests often reveal hormonal disturbances, mainly hyperestrogenism; other cases relate history of substitution hormonal therapy, either in active women, usually for ovarian functional pathology, or in postmenopausal for avoiding precocious osteoporosis; in other cases, there are histories of hormonal therapy in assisted fertilization techniques. It is possible that the estrogen-like increased amounts of food contaminants, which are almost ignored or insufficiently mentioned on the products, are responsible for breast proliferations in the so-called unexplained cases.

Pathologically, there are described multiple types of adenosis: *apocrine adenosis*, *microglandular adenosis*, *sclerosing adenosis* (in postmenopausal), *simple adenosis*, or *tubular adenosis*. Adenosis and sclerosing adenosis maintain the lobular architecture, but it becomes exaggerated and distorted.

Some cases present a mass (tumor adenosis) or unspecific calcifications on imaging. Both on mammography and US, tumor adenosis presents relatively low density in the center, despite of a huge surrounding spiculated response as in breast cancer; with classical US and mammography being in general unspecific, the biopsy is usually required. It is estimated that over one million American women have a benign breast biopsy annually, and a study published in 2014 found sclerosing adenosis in 27.8 % cases, where 62.4 % of biopsies coexisted with proliferative disease without atypia and 55.1 % of biopsies with atypical hyperplasia [8].

The importance of *adenosis* is higher than those of the fibrocystic dysplasia, because (sclerosing) adenosis can be seen as a component of other proliferative lesions and can coexist with other proliferative lesions such as intraductal and/or sclerosing papilloma, complex sclerosing lesion, fibroadenomas, and up to both in situ and invasive cancers [9].

In *sclerosing adenosis*, which usually occurs from adenosis in menopausal women, the lesion acquires infiltrative margins; the enlarged lobules become distorted by scar-like fibrous tissue and may be associated with DCIS. Pathologically, the sclerosing adenosis of the breast is defined as a benign lobular-centric lesion of disordered acinar, myoepithelial, and connective tissue elements, which can mimic infiltrating carcinoma both grossly and microscopically.

The classical clinical and radiological/imaging diagnosis is difficult because normal lobules are not visualized on mammography or breast MRI, and as a consequence, it results to the abnormal initial enlargement of lobules as in adenosis which cannot be diagnosed; moreover, in the classical US, the lobules are not studied despite their visibility, because of the neglecting of the ductal-lobar architecture of the breast parenchyma. In addition, adenosis is strongly associated with various proliferative lesions, including epithelial hyperplasias, intraductal or sclerosing papilloma, complex sclerosing lesion, calcification, and apocrine changes, up to both invasive and in situ cancers. By consequence, the final diagnosis is classically represented by the FNA, the core biopsy, or the surgical biopsy in suspected lesions. In such cases, the disadvantages added to these invasive methods of diagnosis, with possible errors or side effects, are increased costs and possible scars in nonsurgical cases, with supplementary difficulties of diagnosis in the follow-up exams.

A particular pathological form is the *microglandular adenosis*, characterized by a proliferation of round, small glands distributed irregularly within dense fibrous and/or adipose tissue; they may contain open lumina with eosinophilic content, and usually it may lack the outer myoepithelial layer seen in other types of adenosis, mimicking the tubular carcinoma. Although microglandular adenosis is considered benign, it is thought with potential development risk for invasive carcinoma, and it has a tendency to recur if not completely excised.

Apocrine (*adenomyoepithelial*) *adenosis* and *tubular adenosis* are rare variants of microglandular adenosis that should be distinguished from tubular carcinoma. The importance in the managing of the lobular hyperplasia is the nonspecific imaging appearance of the benign and premalignant lesions; moreover, both typical lobular hyperplasia and lobular carcinoma in situ, collectively termed lobular neoplasia, present very similar histological appearances, the only difference being the extent and degree of epithelial proliferation.

The clinical and the mammographic aspect of adenosis are unspecific; there may be either diffuse increased consistency on palpation, or localized area mimicking a lump with mammographically aspect of a diffuse heterogeneous opacity or respective a pseudotumoral aspect (architectural distortion, mass with/without microcalcifications in 40–55 % of cases [10], asymmetrical density, malignant-type mass mimicking invasive breast carcinoma [11]).

Sclerosing adenosis can be found on US as focal or diffuse, while clinically it is not palpable in 80 % of the cases; in rare cases, it might determine skin retraction.

There are few descriptors for adenosis in the classical US, usually without any characteristic appearances, something borrowed from mammography.

Based on the incidental histological findings, it was believed that lobular hyperplasia/lobular neoplasia is a rare condition, most prevalent in menopausal women. It does not determine significant clinic abnormalities, despite the mastodynia usually present. In fact, due to the hormonal substitution therapy or to the techniques of assisted fertility, the lobular hyperplasia is more often proven on the FBU. This technique demonstrates the multifocal (in the same lobe, the lesions connected to the same main duct) and/or multicentric (in different mammary lobes, located in the same or in different quadrants) lobular involvement.

FBU is recommended both in the characterization of the adenosis and in the detection of infracentimetric associated malignancies when occurred. DE illustrates adenosis by the presence of multiple lobules of micronodular shape, connected to the ducts and enlarged usually up to 4 mm in their short axis. Their aspect is isoechoic or hypoechoic, with round-oval shape and distinct regular/irregular borders; the enlarged lobules are distinct or joined, without any salient vasculature at less than 14 MHz transducers. The characteristic features are the ductal connection of these multiple pseudonodules, located in the TDLUs or arranged on both sides of the ducts as roadside trees. Sonoelastography will illustrate a score 1 Ueno for the simple adenosis or scores 2–3 Ueno for sclerosing adenosis.

Monitoring the lobular size allows the detection of the issue of suspect pathological findings, such as local new vessel formation or heterogeneous shadowing, which are high predictive for malignancy.

In detecting adenosis, 3D or 4D techniques are useful in the demonstration of the multiplanar micronodular shape and in the differential diagnosis with the galactophorous ducts, which are tubular structures presenting long and short axes.

In young dense breast type, there is frequently an identified "physiological" adenosis, with large amount of lobules, with distinct or contiguous in the TDLUs, and at the periphery of the mammary lobes, characterized by uniform enlargement up to 3.5–4 mm diameter, connected to the ductal tree, but without any pathological vasculature and with low stiffness to sonoelastography, score 1 or 2 Ueno.

Adenosis may regress spontaneously or following a therapy; usually it is associated with other proliferative lesions, such as multiple fibroadenomas or breast cancer. Adenosis is a premalignant condition especially in postmenopausal women or in premenopausal patients after prolonged use of birth control pills or after hormonal therapy for assisted fertility. There are frequent cases of adenosis that develop quickly to malignant lesions, discovered on 4–6-month follow-up US examination, with various ductal or lobular cancer forms.

The US BI-RADS classification must include these lesions in the third category, being assumed that atypical lobular hyperplasia increases by fourfold the risk for subsequent development of invasive carcinoma and lobular carcinoma in situ increases the risk by tenfold. The usual therapy of the lobular hyperplasia is either a simple expectation or follow-up exams or aggressive treatment such as chemotherapy or bilateral preventive mastectomy, considered by some authors an excessively morbid procedure.

Ductal hyperplasia represents the increasing in size and number of the epithelial cells that are lining the ductal walls; it could be either diffuse or segmental, with ductal diameters increased as compared with adjacent similar range of ducts. In the DE, ductal hyperplasias can measure between 1.5 and 3 mm thicknesses, rarely more, with the central line sign more or less visible.

Anatomically, the ductal epithelium is arranged in a single layer of cuboidal cells, with rare myoepithelial cells surrounding the ducts at the periphery.

The pathological aspect of the true ductal hyperplasia presents a multilayered epithelium, with regular arrangement of the cells of uniform shape, as in usual/simple hyperplasia, or irregular arrangements of atypical cells, without malignant markers, such as in atypical hyperplasia.

Many studies demonstrated ductal hyperplasia represents a premalignant lesion, and it is assumed hyperplasia with atypia raises eightfold the risk to develop cancer. Moreover, there is *a pathological continuum,* from simple hyperplasia to moderate hyperplasia with epithelial proliferation of more than four cells, thick and florid hyperplasia with distended and obliterated lumen, and hyperplasia with atypia, ductal carcinoma in situ, and microinvasive and invasive ductal carcinoma.

The ductal lumen is empty, so the walls are seen on DE in contact as a couple of hypoechoic lines separated by a hyperechoic central line representing the virtual lumen (*the central hyperechoic line sign*). In the physiological ductal thickening, the main ducts may present longitudinal epithelial plies/folds, more salient in young breasts, with appearance of false hyperplasia on DE because of the increased thickness up to 3.0 mm and the loss of the parallelism and continuity of the central hyperechoic line. With aging, the folds become less prominent till disappearance, the walls are thinner (main duct diameter reduced progressively up to less than 0.8 mm in climax), and the central line sign corresponding to the virtual lumen is well defined.

While simple hyperplasia does not produce the thickening of the ducts, the types of mild, moderate, or florid epithelial hyperplasia are an admixture of cell types (epithelial cells, myoepithelial cells, and metaplastic apocrine cells) with variation in the appearances of epithelial cells and their nuclei and focal abnormal imaging aspect. By contrary, the atypical ductal hyperplasia is defined as a type of a ductal hyperplasia that morphologically mimics low-grade DCIS, and the risk is increased by the presence of its uniform cell population. Most lesions of atypical ductal hyperplasia are small and focal and involve only a portion of a duct or only a few small ducts measuring <2 mm. This condition is usually suspected on mammography when the microcalcifications are present, but the sign is not specific (only in 31 % cases with microcalcifications at biopsy the atypical hyperplasia was present). Microcalcifications are not a useful sign in US, either in the classical approach or FBU, but the last technique offers the advantage to illustrate the normal and abnormal ducts, which are not visible in mammography, tomosynthesis, or breast MRI.

The risk to develop malignancy was considered increased in the next 10–15 years following the diagnosis of atypia, but usually on FBU, we can diagnose earlier a small malignancy less than 5 mm in diameter; otherwise, an invasive breast cancer could appear associated with abnormal diffuse or focal thickened ducts, with benign or malignant aspects.

In premenopausal or menopausal woman, hyperplasias are easily diagnosed, and a routine follow-up is recommended; chemoprevention on the basis of combined risk factors seems to be uncertain, while a short-time follow-up FBU at 6-month interval would be the most cost-effective noninvasive option.

In DE, the ductal hyperplasias are easy to diagnose by comparing the suspect ducts with the surrounding ductal range and relating to the clinical data (age, lactation). We can find cylindrical long thicker ducts, up to 2.5–3.5 mm diameter, with the central line sign present in the simple hyperplasia, or segmental thickening without well delineation of the lumen in suspected atypical hyperplasias. In all cases, there is no periductal abnormal vasculature visible on Doppler examination, and a good tissue elasticity is confirmed by the score 1 Ueno (green, yellow, and red) for the ducts or the score 2 Ueno if including the surrounding glandular stroma.

As a differential diagnosis, we should distinguish the ductal hyperplasia from the ductal papilloma, which will be illustrated in the next section.

Many cases present both ductal hyperplasia and ductal ectasia, with the lumen fully filled with some amount of fluid of various echogenicities: transonic for serous-type fluid and hypoechoic to isoechoic for the protein-type fluid, which may be represented by milk, pus, mucinous secretions, or bloody surge. High-resolution transducers allow the distinction between the ductal walls and the ductal content, but sonoelastography is better even in case of inspissated ducts. Moreover, the possibility of detecting small intraductal papillomas in the ductal fluid is easy to demonstrate by this radial technique of FBU.

6.5 Radial Scars and Complex Sclerosing Lesions

Radial scars and complex sclerosing lesions are not truly breast scars, but they are considered benign pseudo-infiltrative lesions of uncertain significance. They are characterized by a complex structure, centered by a fibroelastotic core with entrapped ducts, and surrounded by radiating ducts and lobules displaying variable epithelial hyperplasia, adenosis, ductal ectasia, and papillomatosis. The term "radial scar" is generally used, but it was proposed for lesions measuring less than 1 cm, whereas the term "complex sclerosing lesion" was designated for lesions measuring 1 cm or larger.

Radial scars are considered for the precursor lesions for atypical epithelial proliferations, including atypical intraductal hyperplasia, atypical lobular hyperplasia, lobular carcinoma in situ, and DCIS, but there are no evidences of the interval length between the benign and the premalignant stages of evolution.

The mammographic features of radial scars are nonspecific and may mimic carcinoma. The aspect is usually of a "black star" with long, thin spicules radiating from a radiolucent central area, while the breast cancer presents a dense central opacity surrounded by spicules. By far, the mammographic aspect has the best correspondence with the gross pathology for the radial scar/complex sclerosing scar, because the image on the film is obtained by the projection of the whole 3D lesion; the sectional imaging methods (tomosynthesis, MRI, US) usually do not describe the abnormal findings with the same term as do the mammography and the pathological report.

The role of FNA cytology in diagnosis or of the core biopsy is limited; thus, a spiculated lesion suggestive of radial scar or complex sclerosing lesion at mammography should be fully surgically excised.

MRI features are equally nonspecific in the radial scar and complex sclerosing scar; the findings were described as masses, architectural distortions, non-mass lesions, focus, and no abnormalities (occult), with or without suspicious enhancement with paramagnetic contrast, with a significant number of cases mimicking breast invasive carcinoma [12].

US in the classical technique, used for a complementary exam, has borrowed the terms from the mammography lexicon, with nonspecific sonographic aspects for the radial scar; nevertheless, US used as first intention method of examination is not able to identify such a lesion, except for the palpable lumps. The US in such cases is useful as a method for guided biopsy, but the diagnosis is not significantly improved.

FBU, as a sectional technique, is not able to illustrate a radial scar as it is represented on mammography, but it is able to identify any parenchymatous abnormality over 2–3 mm and to characterize the risk of malignancy without biopsy. DE allows the proving of the ductal connection of the lesion in any type of breast; the sclerosing process is suggested by the acoustic shadowing and the irregular contour, as in malignant lesions, but the vasculature is either unapparent or of benign type, with few poles and thin vessels with an arcuate course. The sonoelastography may present a score 2, 3, or 4 Ueno, but usually the complex/summation-BGR score is present. Sonoelastography may overestimate the diagnosis due to the sclerosing intensity. In suspect cases, a short-time follow-up of 3–6-month interval is recommended instead of the surgical biopsy (Figs. 6.29, 6.30, 6.31, 6.32, 6.33, 6.34, 6.35, 6.36, 6.37, and 6.38).

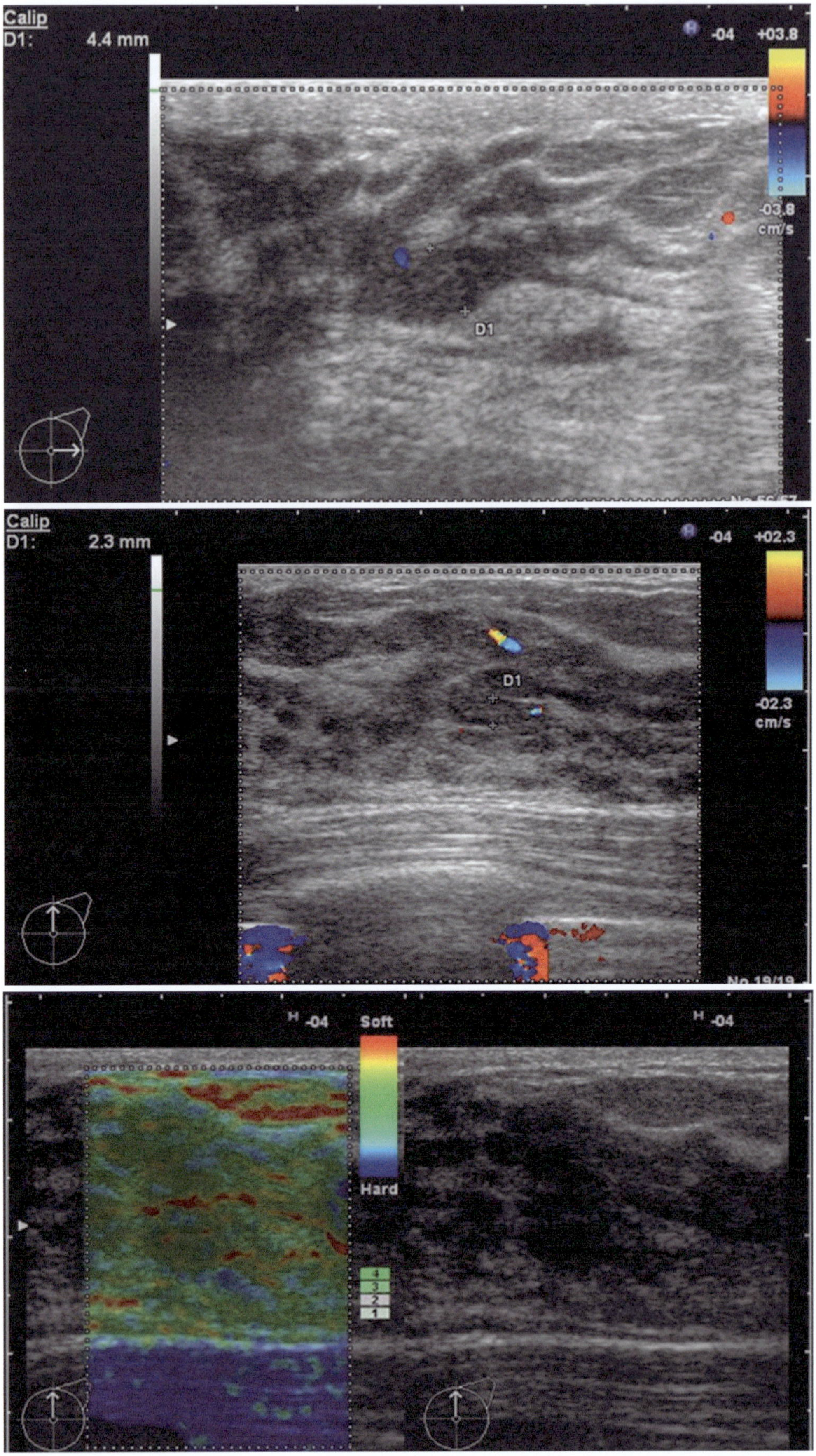

Fig. 6.29 Diffuse ductal-lobular hyperplasia with loss of the ductal central hyperechoic line and benign-type sonoelastogram

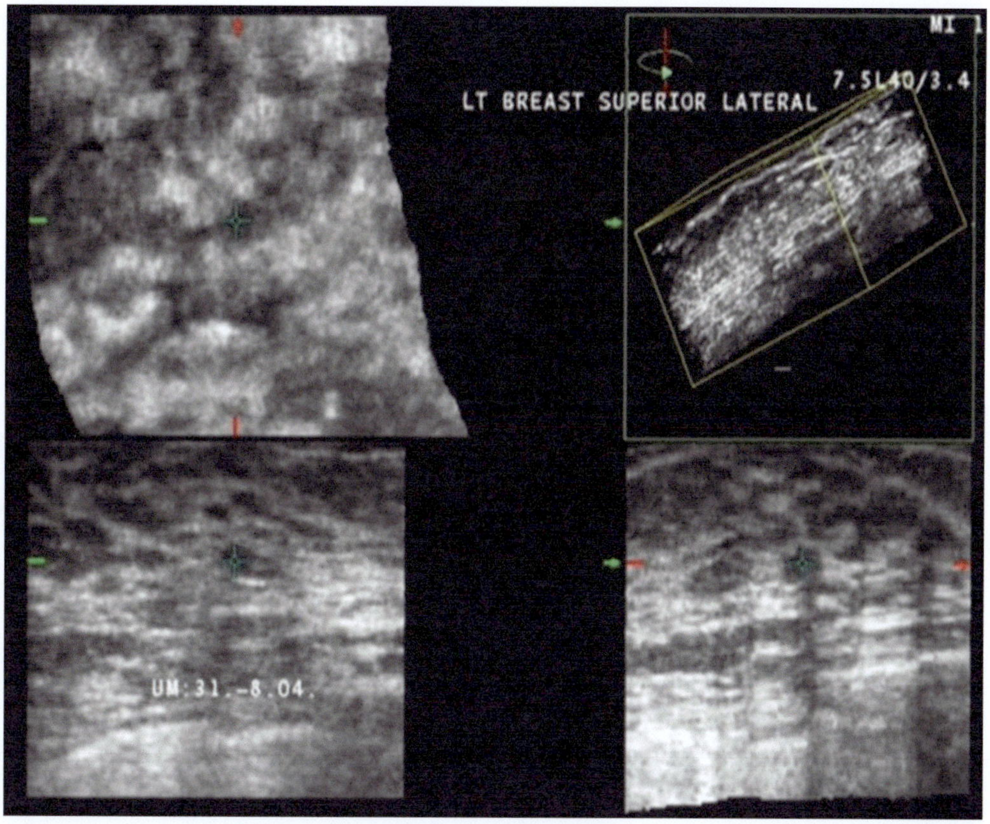

Fig. 6.30 Utility of the 3D US in the assessment of the breast parenchyma: the hypertrophied lobules in adenosis are better depicted, with their connection to the ductal trees and their irregular contour with micronodular aspect in all 3 planes (the same lobule is marked in three orthogonal planes)

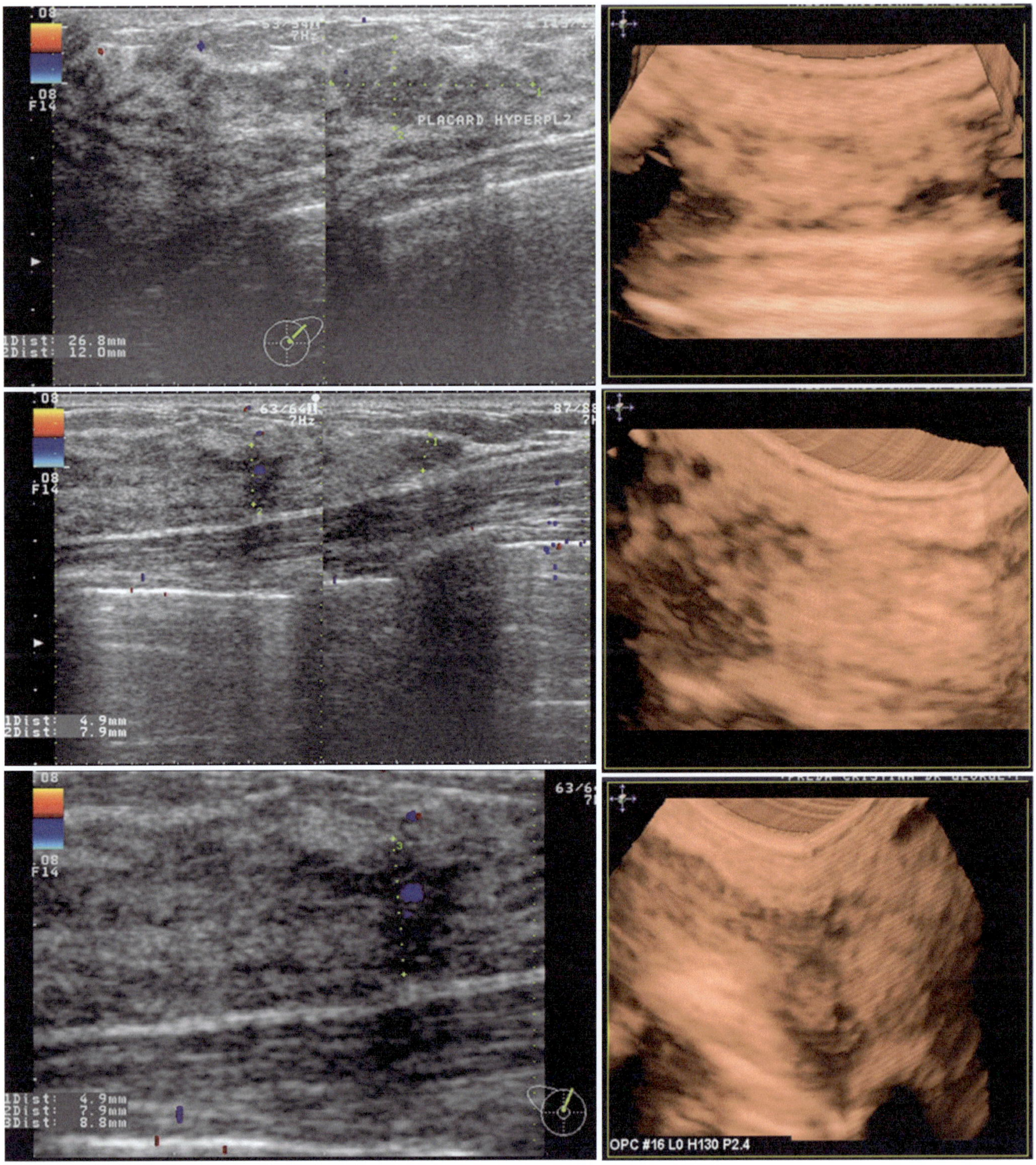

Fig. 6.31 Utility of the 4D US associated to the DE in the evaluation of the lobular hyperplasia: despite of the nonperforming yet 4D transducers and of the lack of software for the 4D acquisitions of the soft tissues, especially for breast examination, we can use the available 4D for better understanding of the breast anatomy. The volumic representations are useful especially for surgeons and in special cases for oncologists

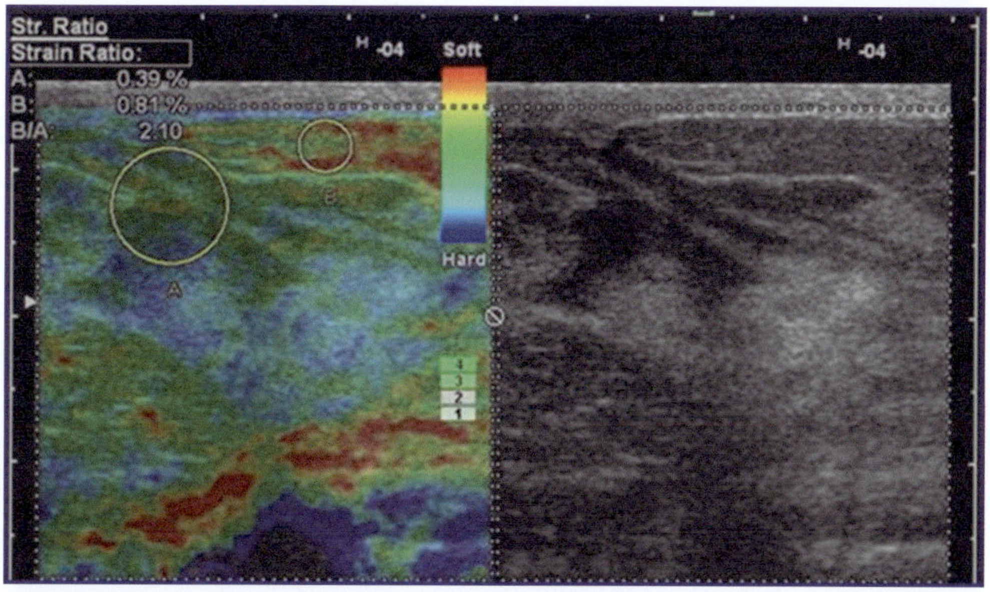

Fig. 6.32 Ductal hyperplasia—score 1 Ueno, US BI-RADS 1–2 (age related); the periareolary thickened ducts have abrupt ending and loss of the central line sign

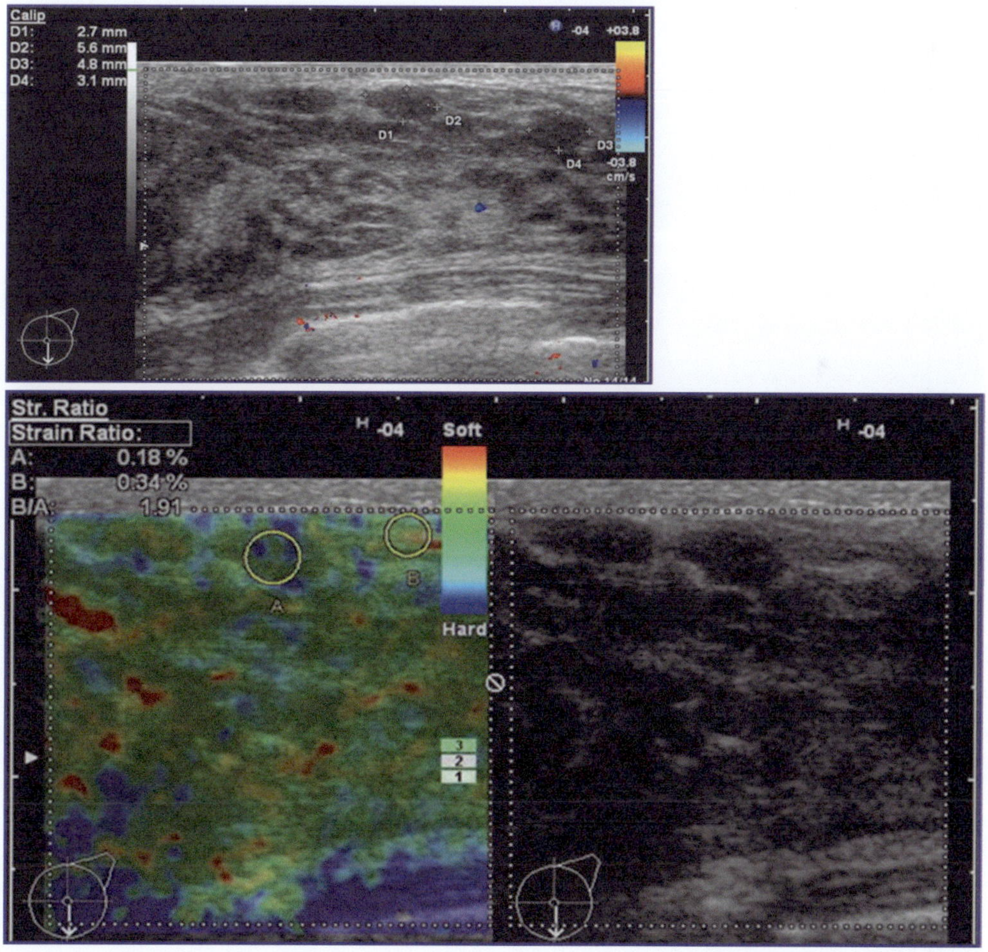

Fig. 6.33 Lobular hyperplasia—score 2 Ueno, no vascular abnormality, US BI-RADS 2 assessment

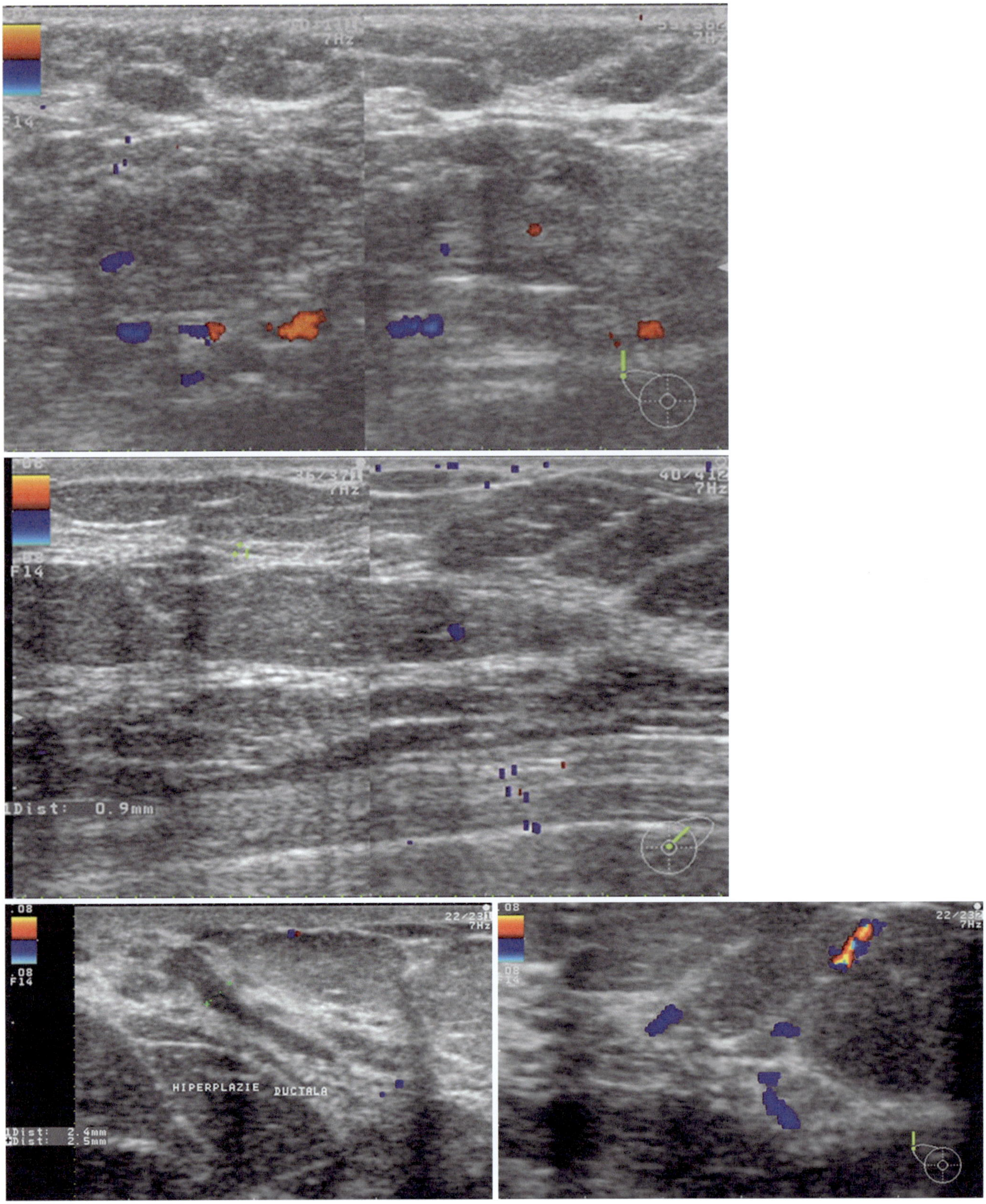

Fig. 6.34 Ductal-lobular hyperplasias in a fatty breast, with parenchymal atrophy as basic structure; the salient vasculature at Doppler is significant for developing activity and could be considered as risk factor

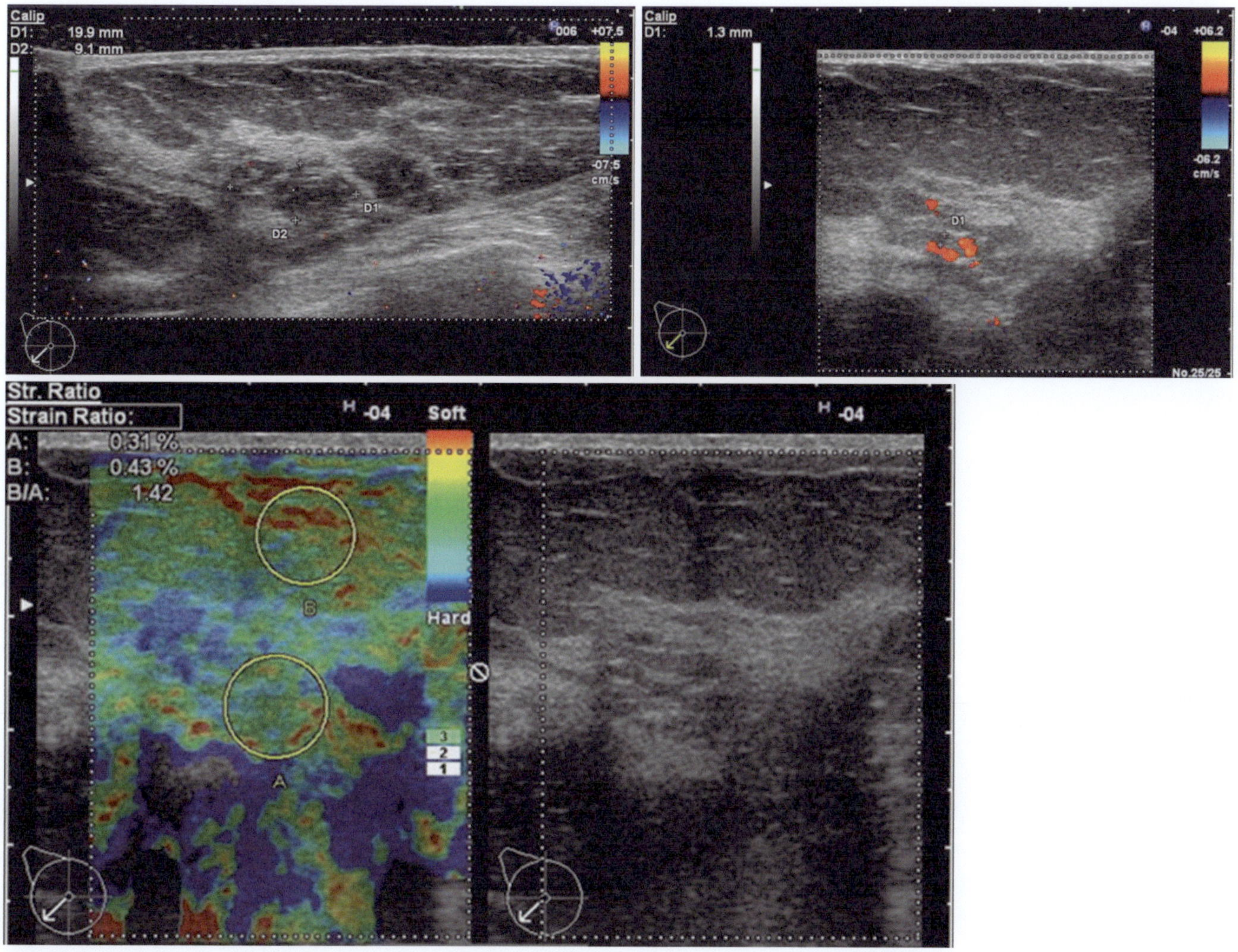

Fig. 6.35 FBU in a 51-year-old patient: focal ductal-lobular hyperplasia with salient new vasculature, score 2 Ueno, and low FLR of 1.42, assessed by US BI-RADS 3, because there is a small risk of developing breast cancer. The increased Doppler signal in the pathological area is the main descriptor, while sonoelastography is just complementary; a short-term follow-up is mandatory

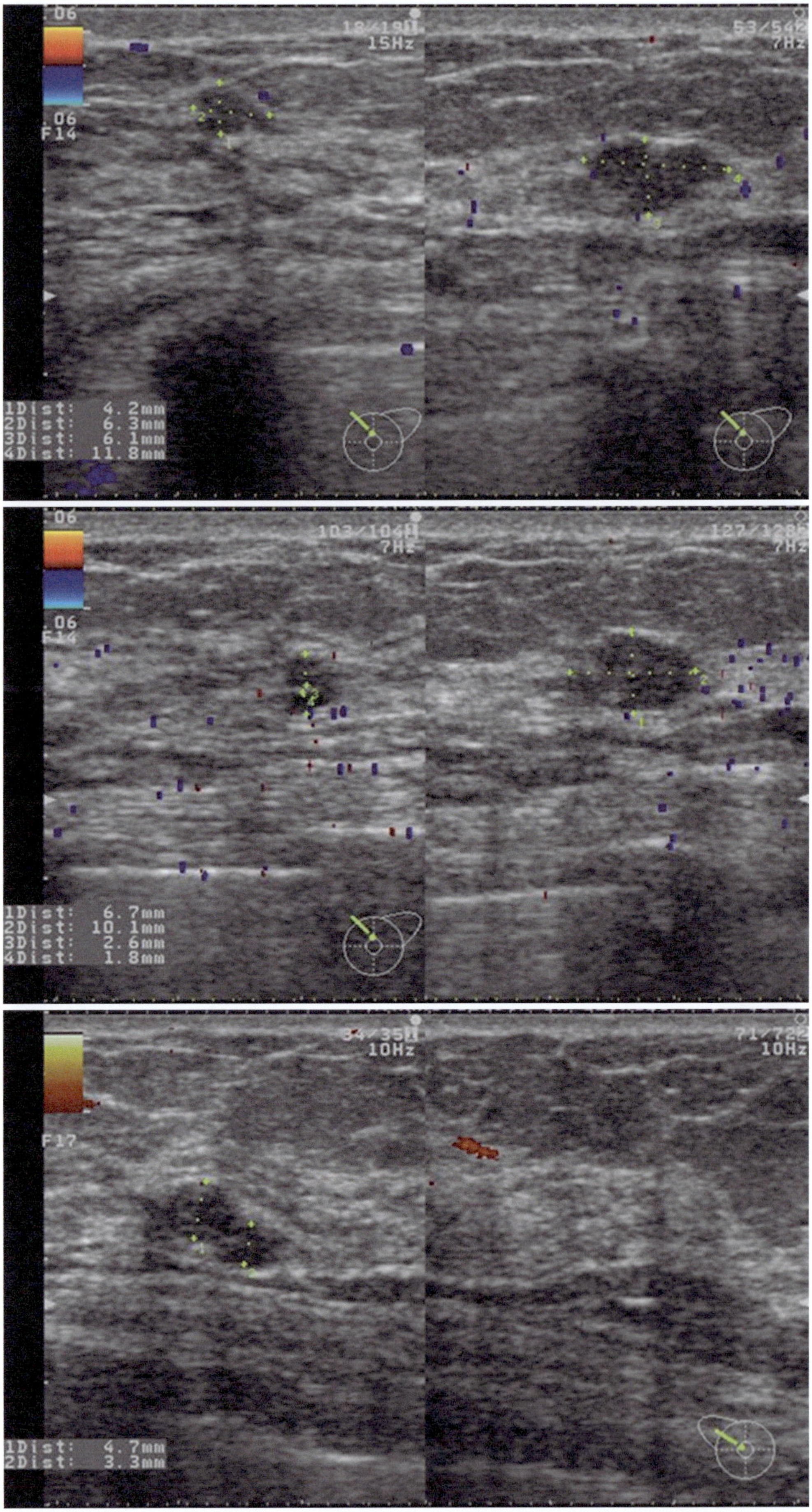

Fig. 6.36 A 49-year-old patient: bilateral nodular adenomatous hyperplasia; the peripheral new vessels are present only in the largest lumps, with benign aspect suggesting a developing fibroadenoma

Fig. 6.36 (continued)

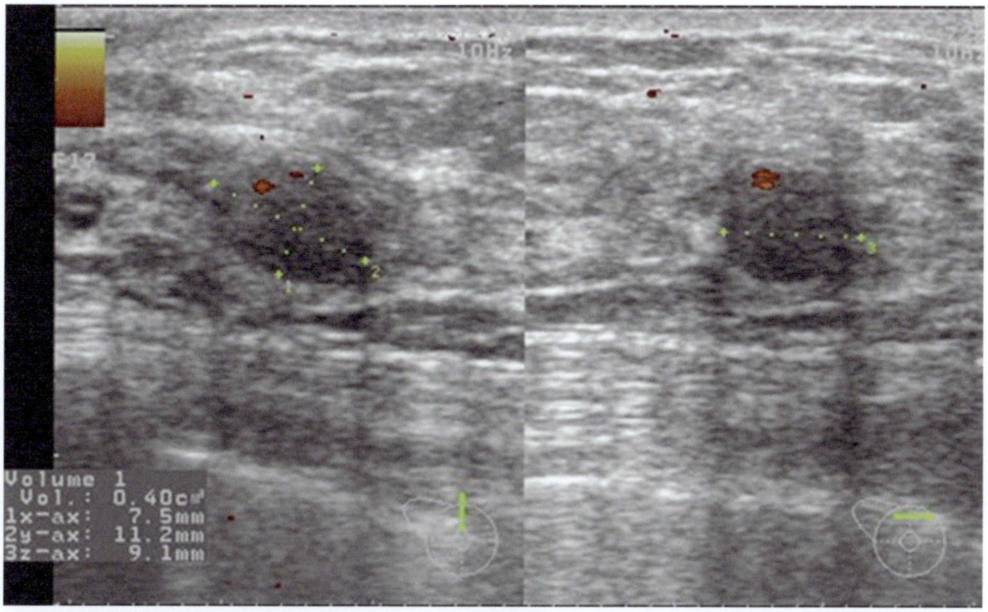

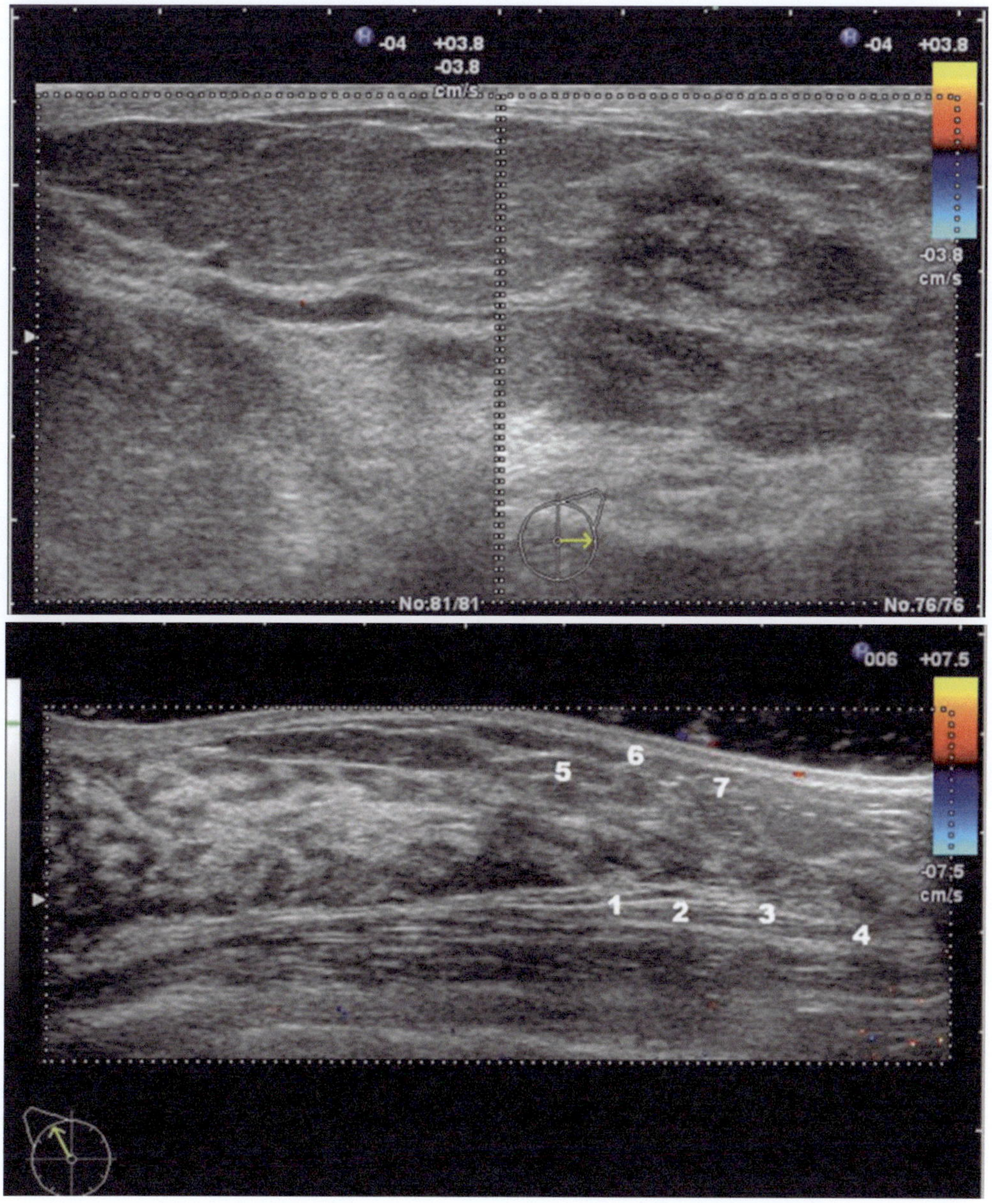

Fig. 6.37 Different aspects of ductal-lobular tree: a terminal enlarged ductal branching in ductules and ending in lobules apparently confluent without salient vasculature (*upper picture*) may be considered a normal aspect in young adult breast, but it suggests ductal-lobular benign hyperplasia in elder patients. Surrounding the ductal-lobular tree are distinct TDLUs located each side of the main duct, as the trees on both sides of a road

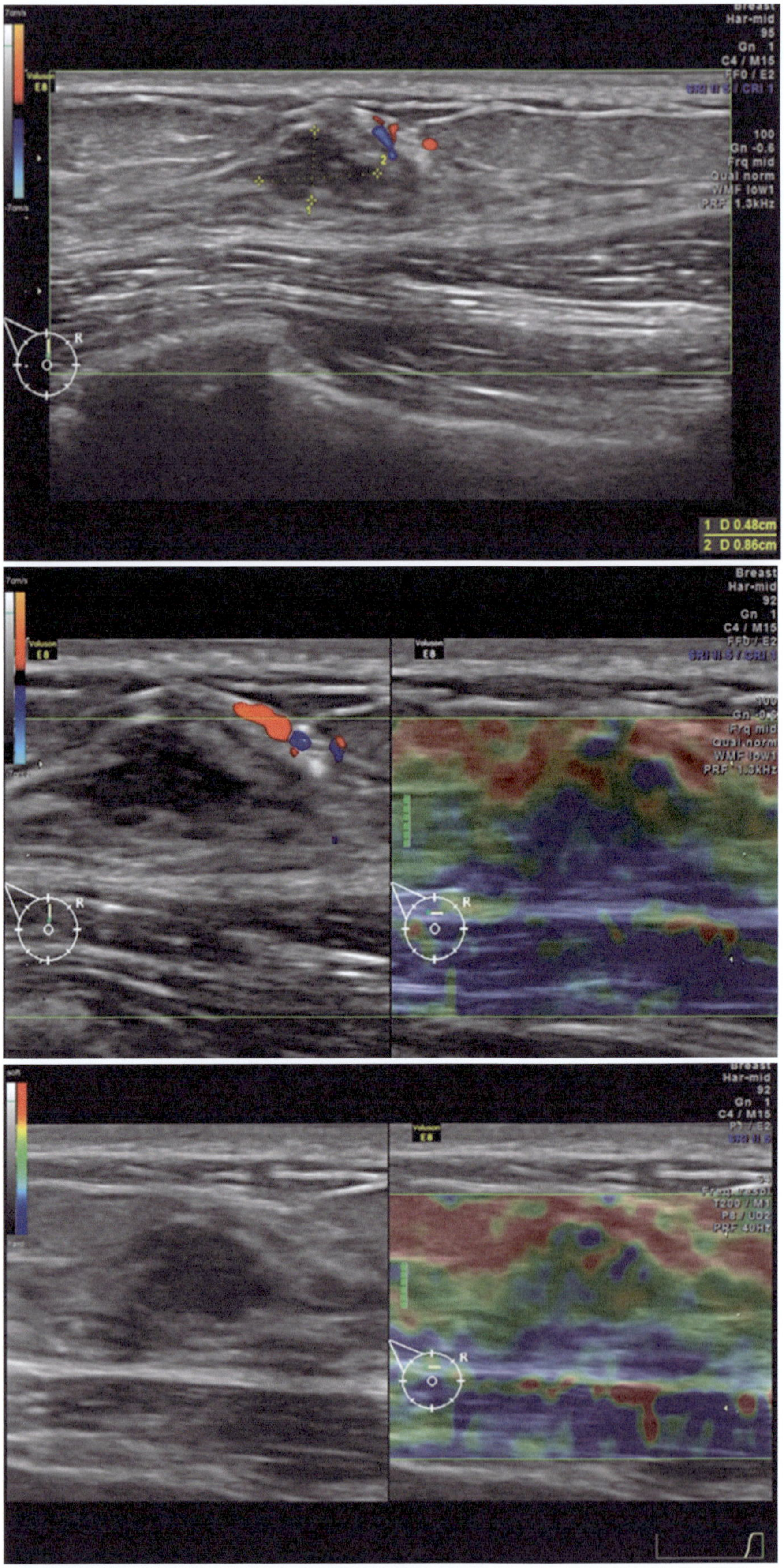

Fig. 6.38 Pseudonodular hyperplasia of mammary lobules in a TDLU, with the terminal duct oriented to the left side of the image towards the nipple; the hypoechoic aspect with irregular margins could be suspect in 2D US, but the peripheral vasculature and the score 2 Ueno with summation-BGR area are highly suggesting for adenosis with fibro-micro-cystic components

6.6 Fibroadenomas

Clinically, fibroadenomas are mobile nontender breast masses. These are the most common benign solid breast tumors, occurring most frequently in women in their reproductive years. Multiplicity and bilaterality are common features in all ages and seems to be correlated with the hyperestrogenism.

Fibroadenomas are heterogeneous tumors, composed of fibrous stroma, proliferating ducts, and acinar tissue. The epithelial and stromal components vary in amount, accounting for some variation in the ultrasound scanning. It is considered a polyclonal proliferation, thus benign; the relationship between terminal ducts and multiple blind-ending acini is well maintained in the earlier stages, which are referred as fibroadenomatous nodules or fibroadenomatous hyperplasia. A well-developed fibroadenoma is formed by coalescence of smaller fibroadenomatous nodules, explaining the expansion of this lesion by central proliferation named *concretion* and coalescence of peripheral hyperplastic lobules named *accretion* [13].

Mammography is not sensitive for small fibroadenomas, or some centimetric fibroadenomas cannot be differentiated from cysts especially in the case of dense breasts; the coarse calcifications with the characteristic radiological popcorn-like appearance are rare findings.

US scans show the classic benign features of a fibroadenoma, named by Stavros [1, 2] and completed by the US BI-RADS lexicon: a well-circumscribed isoechoic or some hypoechoic mass that may be oval, round, or lobulated (three or fewer circumscribed microlobulations). Other features of benign solid masses at US include horizontal growth greater than the vertical growth, the long axis commonly lying parallel to the skin surface, with depth-to-width index less than 0.7 for benign nodules [14]. The posterior acoustic enhancement with lateral shadowings are less intense than in the case of a cyst; these signs described by Kobayashi [15] are reinforced when increasing the pressure on the lesion with the transducer or when using THI and are suggesting benignity, but there are some mucinous cancers with similar posterior effects. Those fibroadenomas that present hyalinization or macrocalcifications can exhibit confusing shadowing on US.

The diameter commonly ranges from 2 to 3 cm or less, although some may grow considerably larger. The term "giant fibroadenoma" is reserved for fibroadenomas that are 10 cm or more in diameter, and the differential diagnosis with phyllodes tumor is mandatory.

In FBU we will find the same morphological aspects of fibroadenomas as described in the classical US, but also we can demonstrate the connection of the fibroadenomas with the ductal tree, easy to visualize and interpret using the radial scanning. These lesions appear mainly in teenagers or young women (15–30 years old), with dense breasts and usually with hyperestrogenism, presenting diffuse ductal or lobular hyperplasia. The associated dysplasia explains the multiplicity of fibroadenomas that usually are found frequently bilateral, of different sizes, and associated with adenosis or sometimes with fibrocystic mastopathy.

DE can demonstrate the lobular origin of the fibroadenoma, the depth-to-width ratio less than 0.7 being salient only for the fibroadenomas larger than 1 cm, while the smallest lesions have usually an inverse depth-to-width ratio, similar to the normal lobules that are initially perpendicularly oriented to the ductal axis and thus to the skin; they appear progressively oblique as they are growing and finally become horizontalized [16, 17]. Furthermore, FBU with high resolution offers the explanation of lobulated fibroadenomas, which are composed by 2–4 lobules grouped in a mass (*accretion*), with thin septations from the surrounding stroma and with individual connections with the galactophorous duct, proving their origin. In advanced stages, fibroadenomas become more homogeneous, but the connection with the ductal tree is well illustrated both in dense or fatty breasts. The radial and antiradial scans are standardized and offer the possibility of a volumic estimation, which is better to consider in the follow-up exams than simply 2–3 axes randomly measuring.

The complete US characterization of a fibroadenoma includes the vasculature, which presents a characteristic peripheral few branches, with curved coarse, "in basket," of regular shape and centripetal orientation. The number of the poles and the size of the new vasculature are proportional with the tumor size, and the radial scans offer the possibility to demonstrate the vascular origin from a superficial or deep part of a Cooper ligament or from the periareolary vascular ring. Contrarily to other organs, in breast spectral Doppler, the velocimetric indices RI, PI, and S/D are usually lower in the benign tumors than in the malignant ones, perhaps due to the desmoplastic reaction responsible for the increased stiffness, frequently encountered in breast ductal or lobular cancer. For fibroadenoma, RI is usually less than 0.65, but the quantitative spectral Doppler is less significant than the qualitative color or power Doppler. 3D power Doppler is very suggestive for fibroadenoma, with the characteristics described above. A significant vascular sign was proposed by a Japanese group, the incident angle of the plunging artery of breast tumors, which is absent in fibroadenoma and present in breast cancer, with a cutoff point of 30° for the sensitivity of malignancy of 86 % and the specificity of 88 % [18].

The aspect of the smallest fibroadenomas is less specific than those of centimetric tumors; only the connection with the ductal tree and the absence of a salient vasculature with probes up to 12 MHz may suggest benignity. The course benign calcifications are rare findings in fibroadenomas and are less visible in US than on mammography, but the advantage is that FBU visualizes always the tumor, while mammography can visualize only some tumors, otherwise only the (micro)calcifications. On classical US and FBU, fibroadenoma's calcifications are usually eccentric, as nonspecific hyperechoic spots with or without posterior shadowing. The recent long high-frequency probes will provide better visualization of the vasculature and of the internal echoes, and the US semiology will be adapted.

For the doubtful cases, the use of sonoelastography allows a more specific diagnosis, avoiding unnecessary biopsy. Most fibroadenomas present a score 2 Ueno, but some infracentimetric lesions may present the score 1; the score 3 Ueno was described for fibroadenomas by the promoters of the sonoelastography, but it is rarely found, while the lesions with popcorn calcifications on mammography may present a score 4 Ueno, mimicking malignancy, discordant with the vasculature of benign type. It results to FBU being the best approach for the diagnosis of the "solid" benign lesions, with fibroadenomas included. The quantitative sonoelastography may add valuable information, a low FLR with a cutoff value of 4.7 (5.0) being accepted for the benign nodule without visible internal calcifications (Figs. 6.39, 6.40, 6.41, 6.42, 6.43, 6.44, 6.45, 6.46, 6.47, and 6.48).

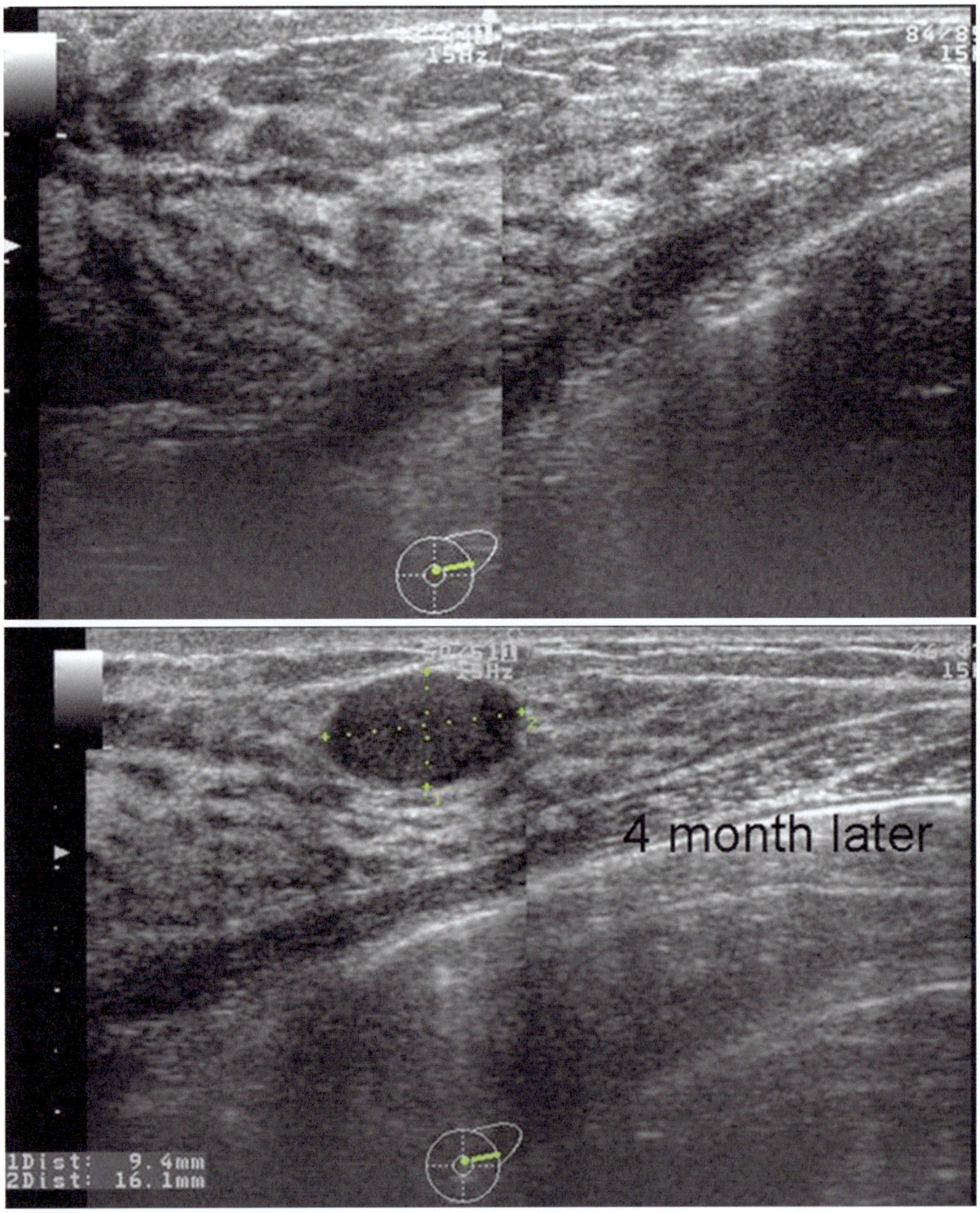

Fig. 6.39 Left breast with mastodynia in young breast and moderate lobular hyperplasia with nodular development in a 4-month interval; the benign characteristics based on Stavros are suggesting for fibroadenoma

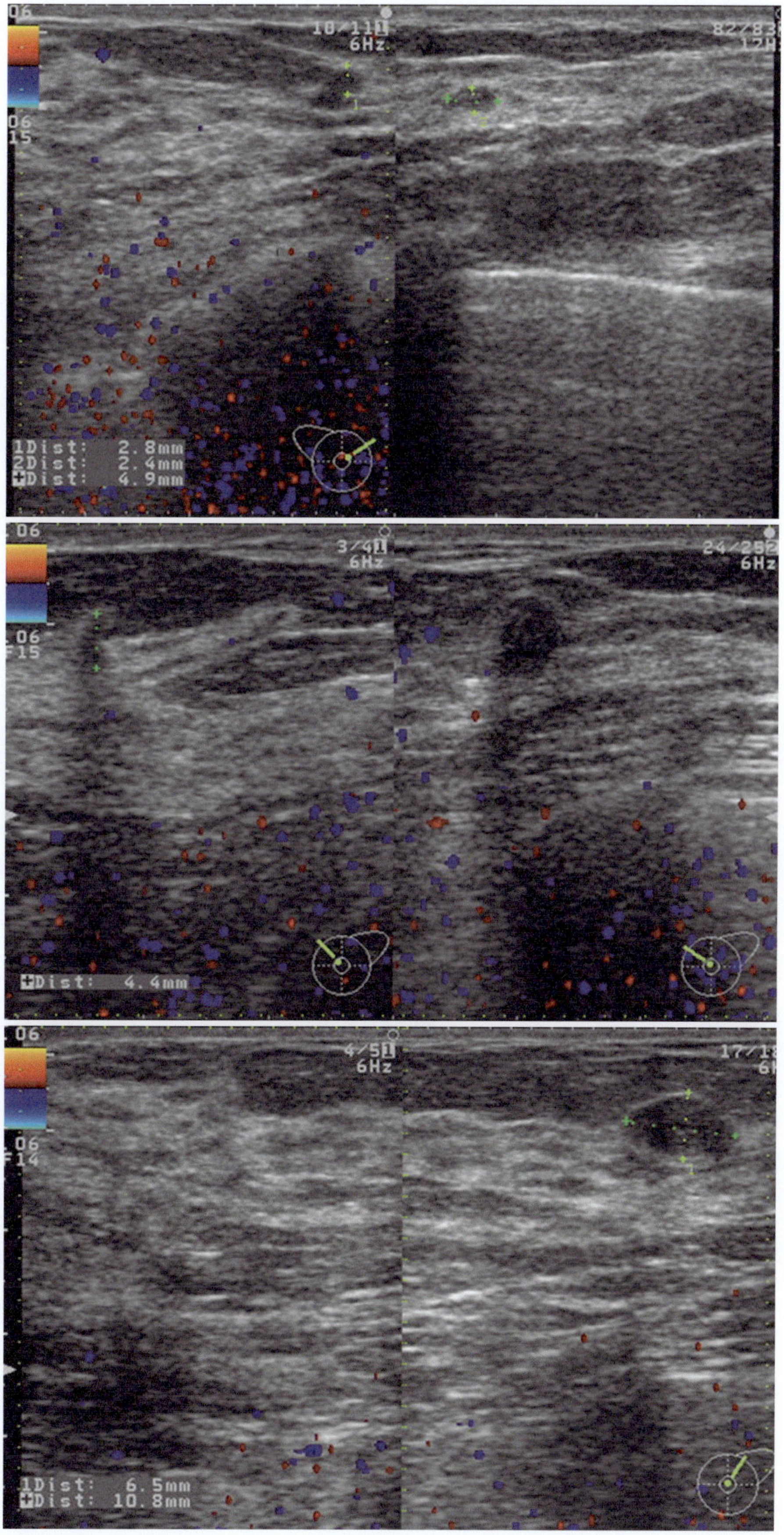

Fig. 6.40 Developing fibroadenomas: initially the deep-to-wide ratio is >1, because of the orientation of the lobule, and then the fibroadenoma enlarges and lies parallel with the skin and the deep-to-wide ratio change in subunitary

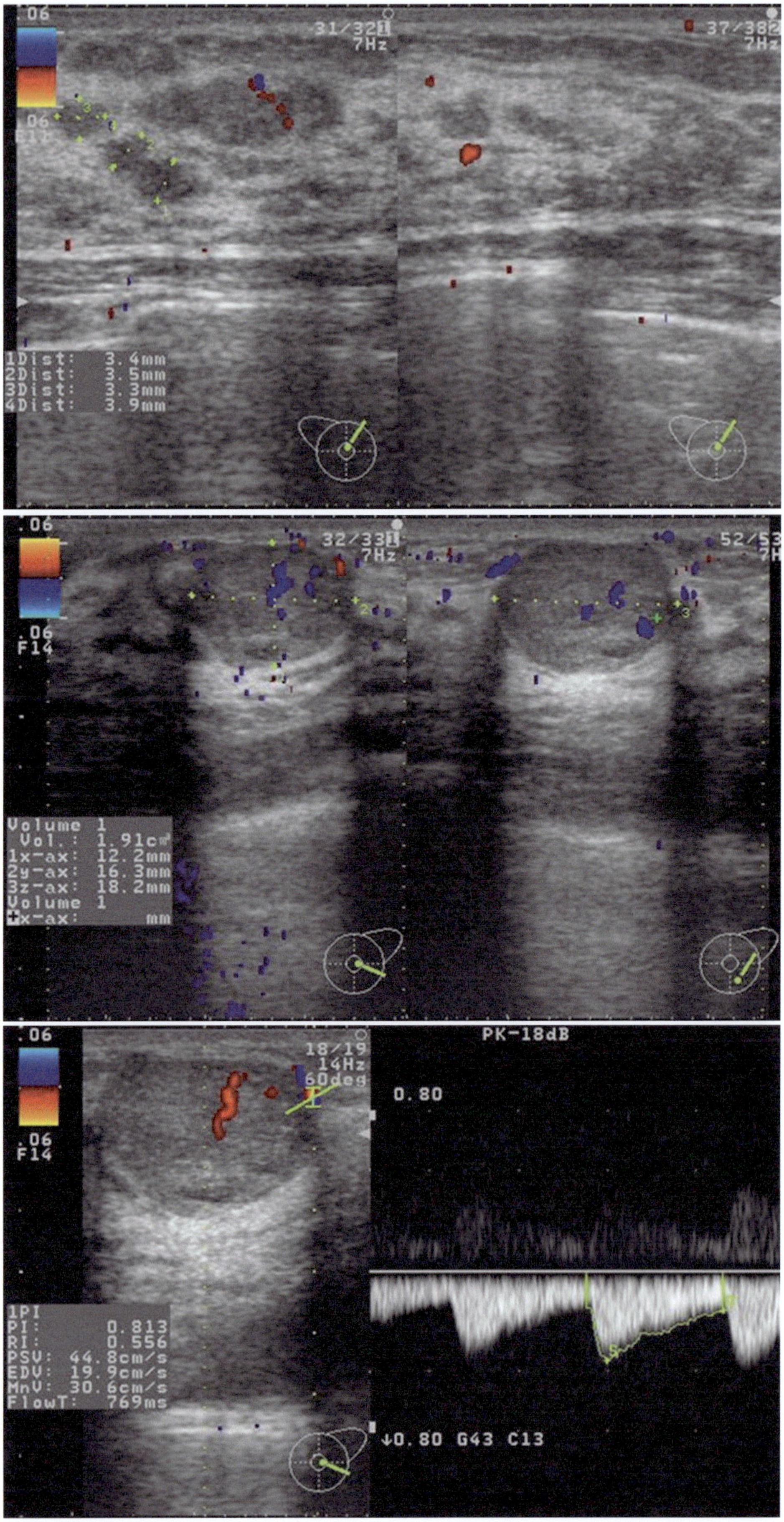

Fig. 6.41 A 20-year-old patient: developing fibroadenomas with different stages, from lobular hyperplasia to lobular accretion and final developing nodular lesion, with benign Stavros criteria and benign vasculature

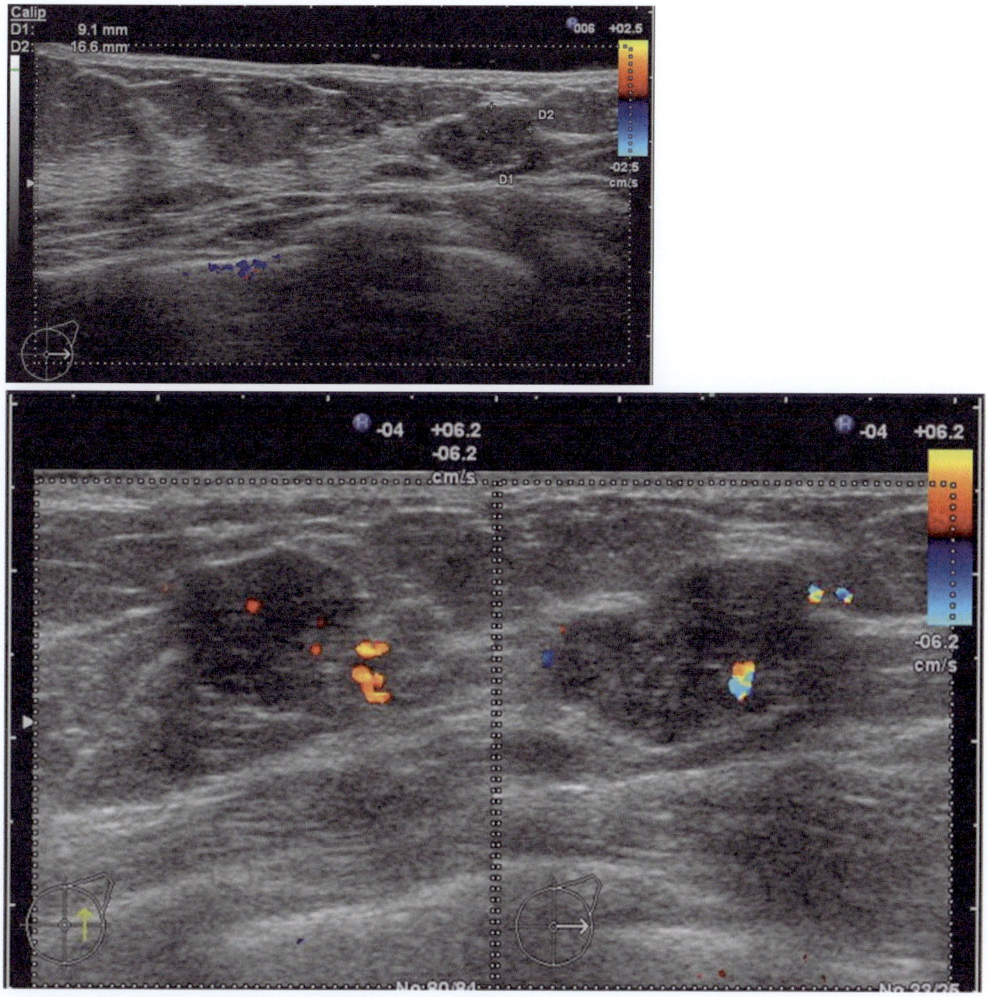

Fig. 6.42 A 28-year-old patient: L 3:00 nodular lesion, with Stavros criteria for benign lesion; the lesion is similar to the fatty tissue, but the increased vasculature of benign type in Doppler is useful for the detection and further evaluation

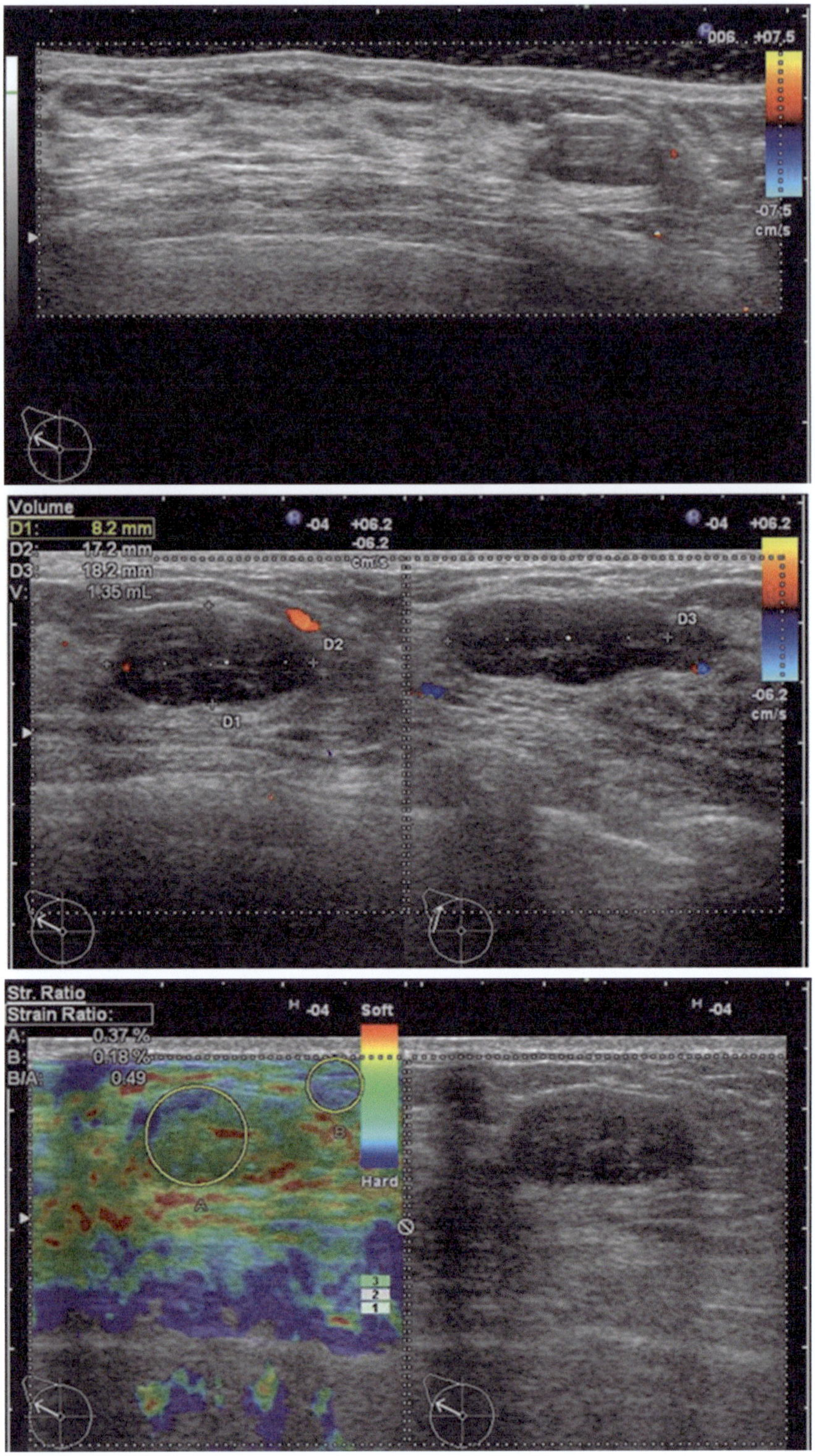

Fig. 6.43 A 34-year-old patient: typical fibroadenoma in ductal US, with few peripheral vessels and RTSE score 2 Ueno with low FLR (0.49–1.52)

Fig. 6.43 (continued)

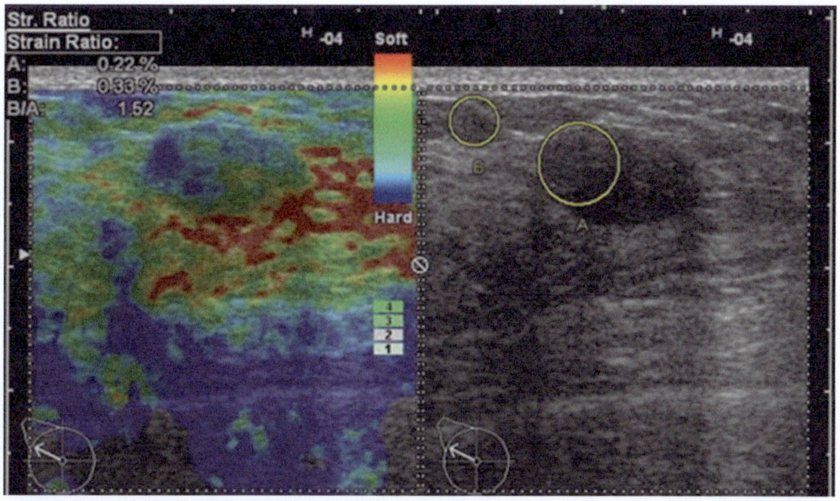

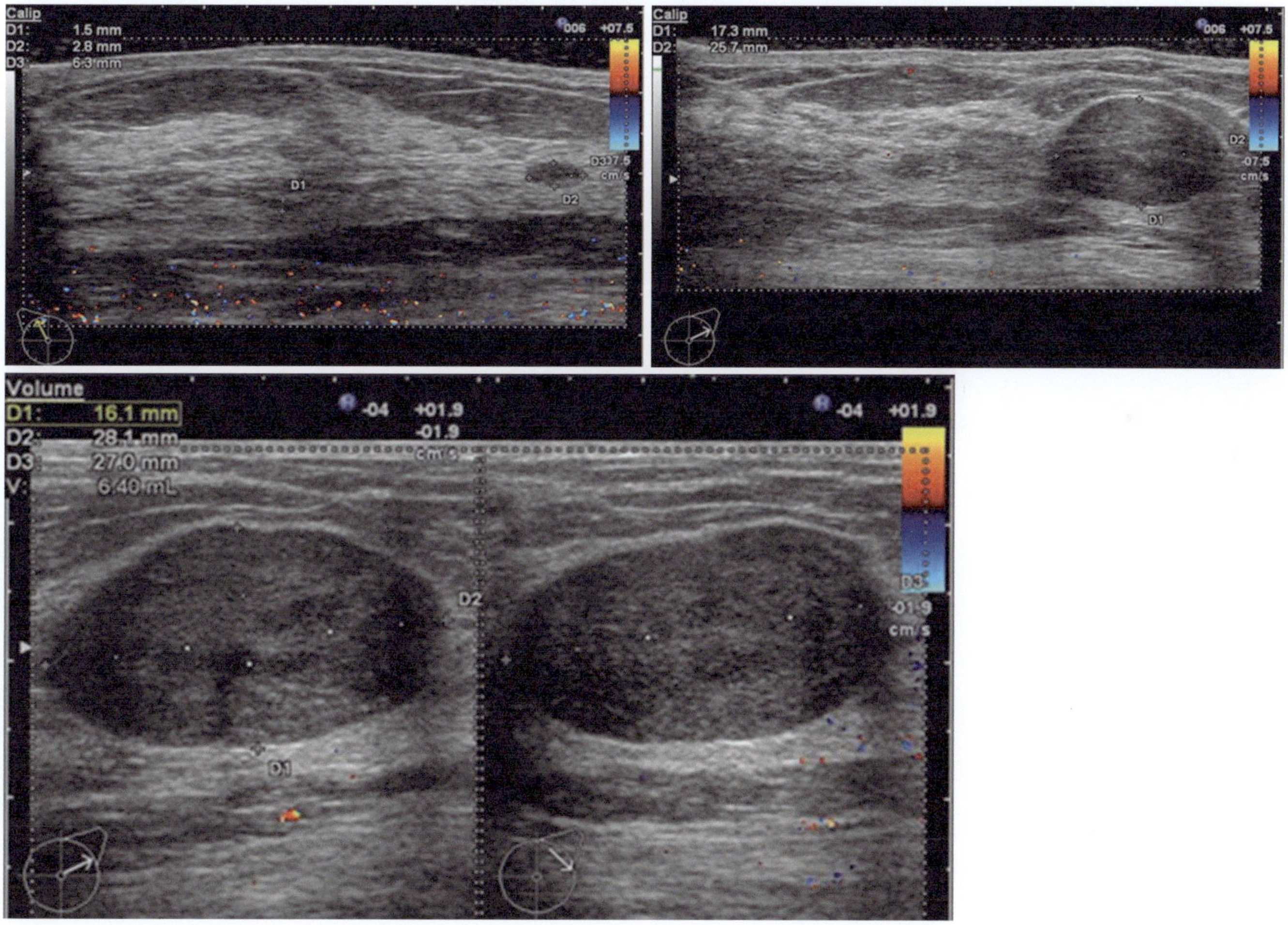

Fig. 6.44 A 52-year-old patient: R 11:00 small infracentimetric lobular hyperplasia, with benign features; L 2:00 typical fibroadenoma based on the Stavros criteria and Doppler characterization. RTSE presents a score 2 Ueno and low FLR

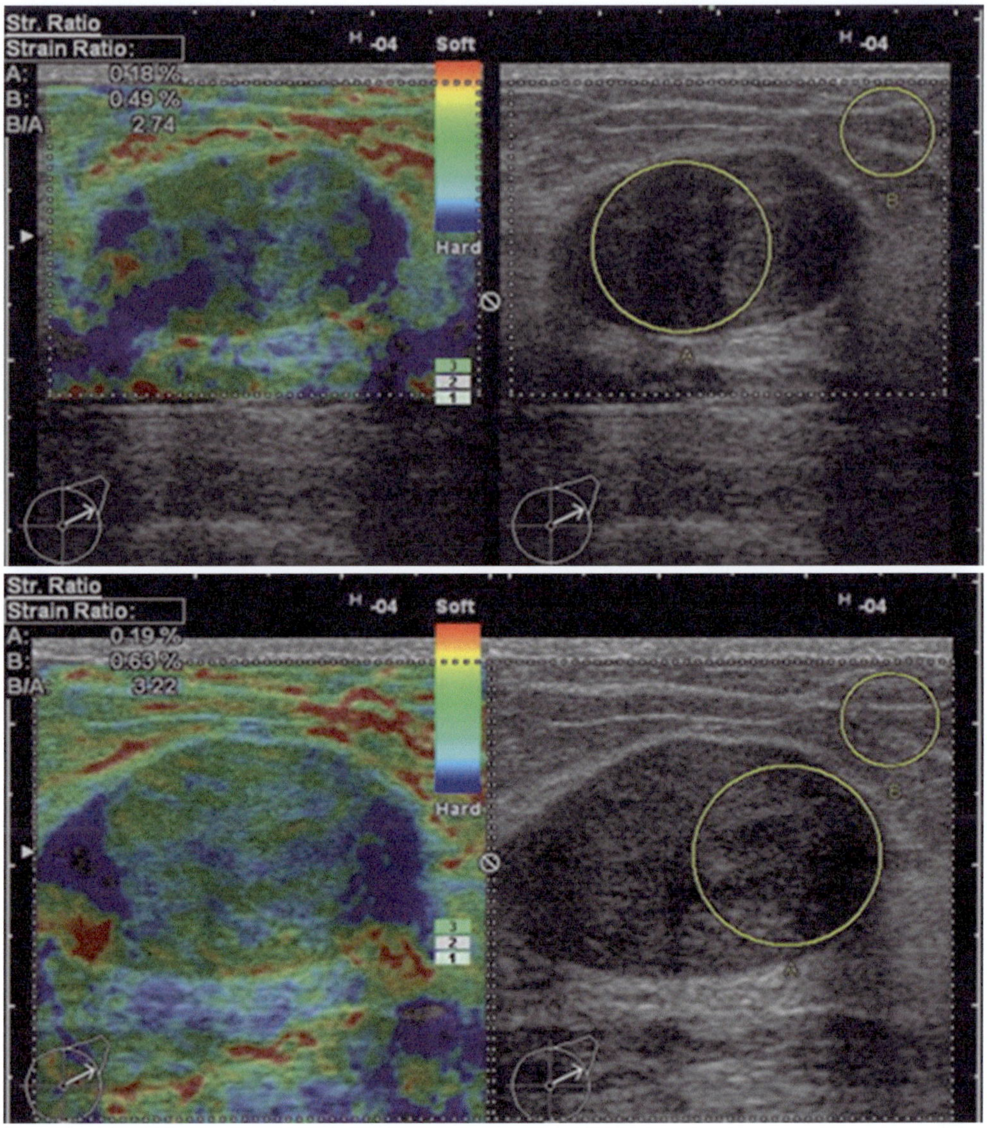

Fig. 6.44 (continued)

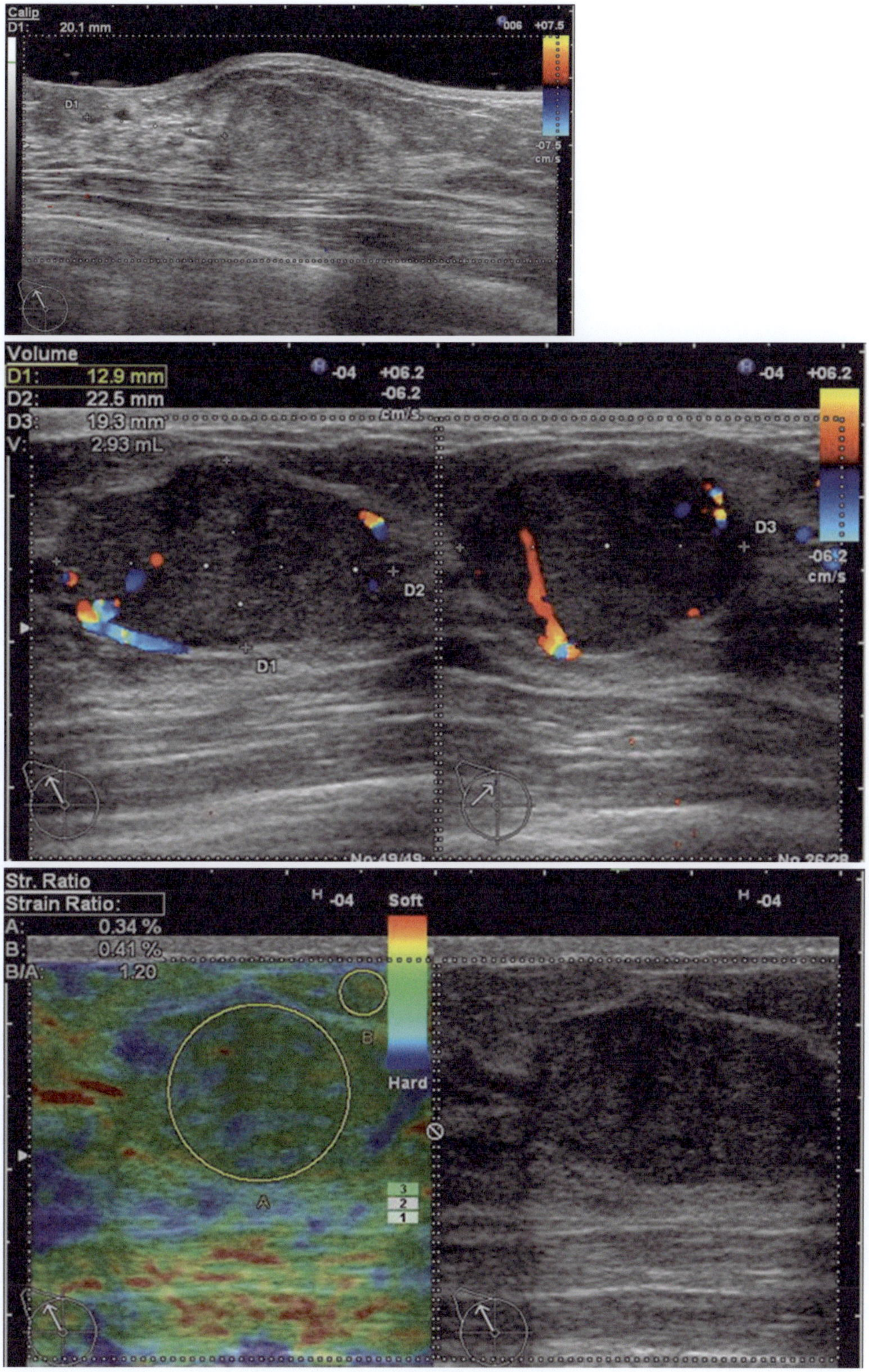

Fig. 6.45 FBU demonstrating an R 11:00 mass with benign characters based on Stavros, benign vasculature with peripheral arcuate course, and acute penetration angle; sonoelastography is concordant with a score 2 Ueno and a low FLR of 1.20, appropriated to the fat strain. DE offers a large view necessary to demonstrate the precise location of the lesion and its ductal connection, essential for the mammary etiology of this isoechoic mass; radial and antiradial scans allow the volumic characterization of the mass

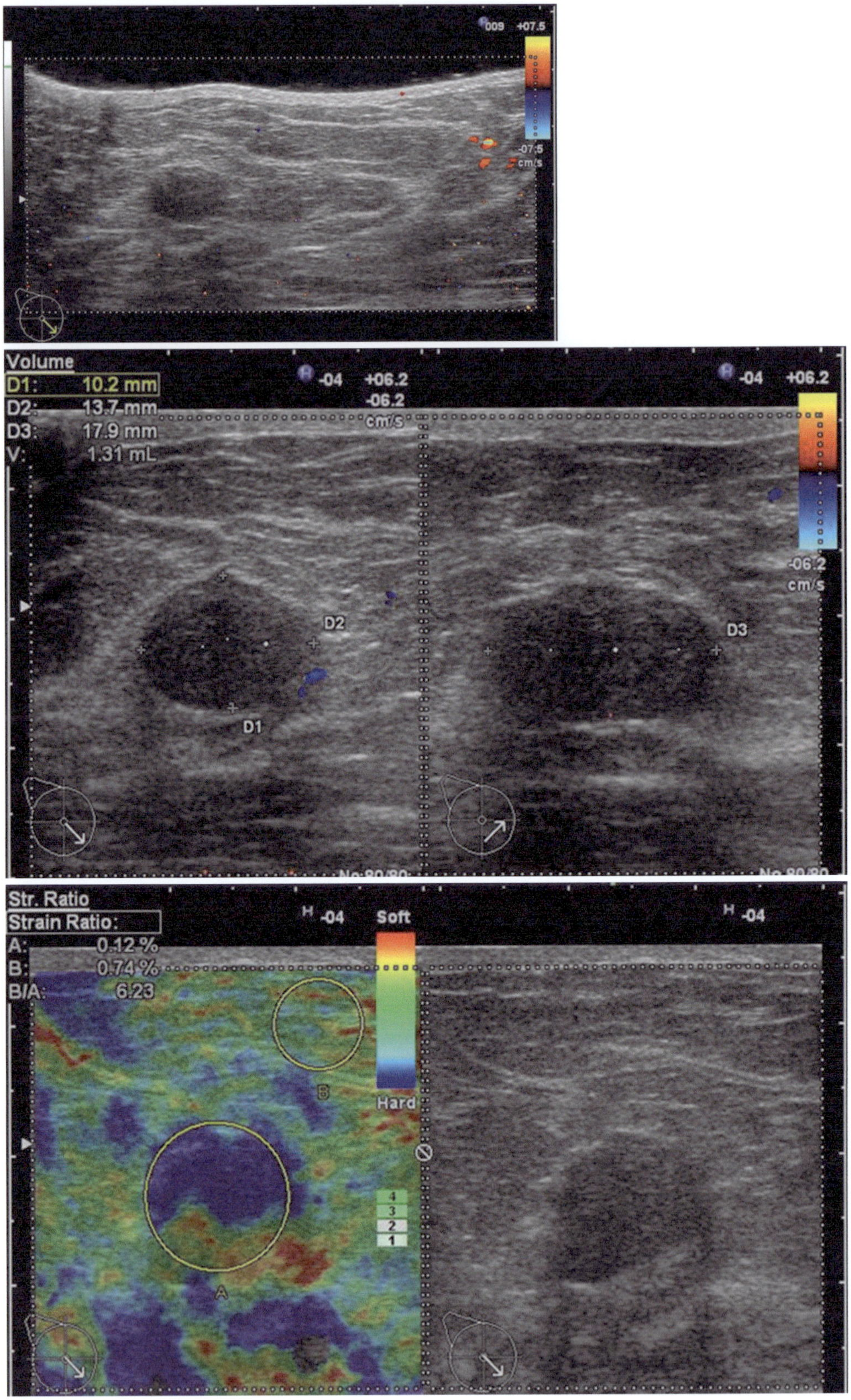

Fig. 6.46 Utility of FBU in the differential diagnosis of fibroadenoma with nodular fibro-micro-cystic dysplasia: 2D features are similar to fibroadenoma, but the Doppler signal is weak in the periphery without internal visible vasculature, and SE presents BGR score as in cystic lesions

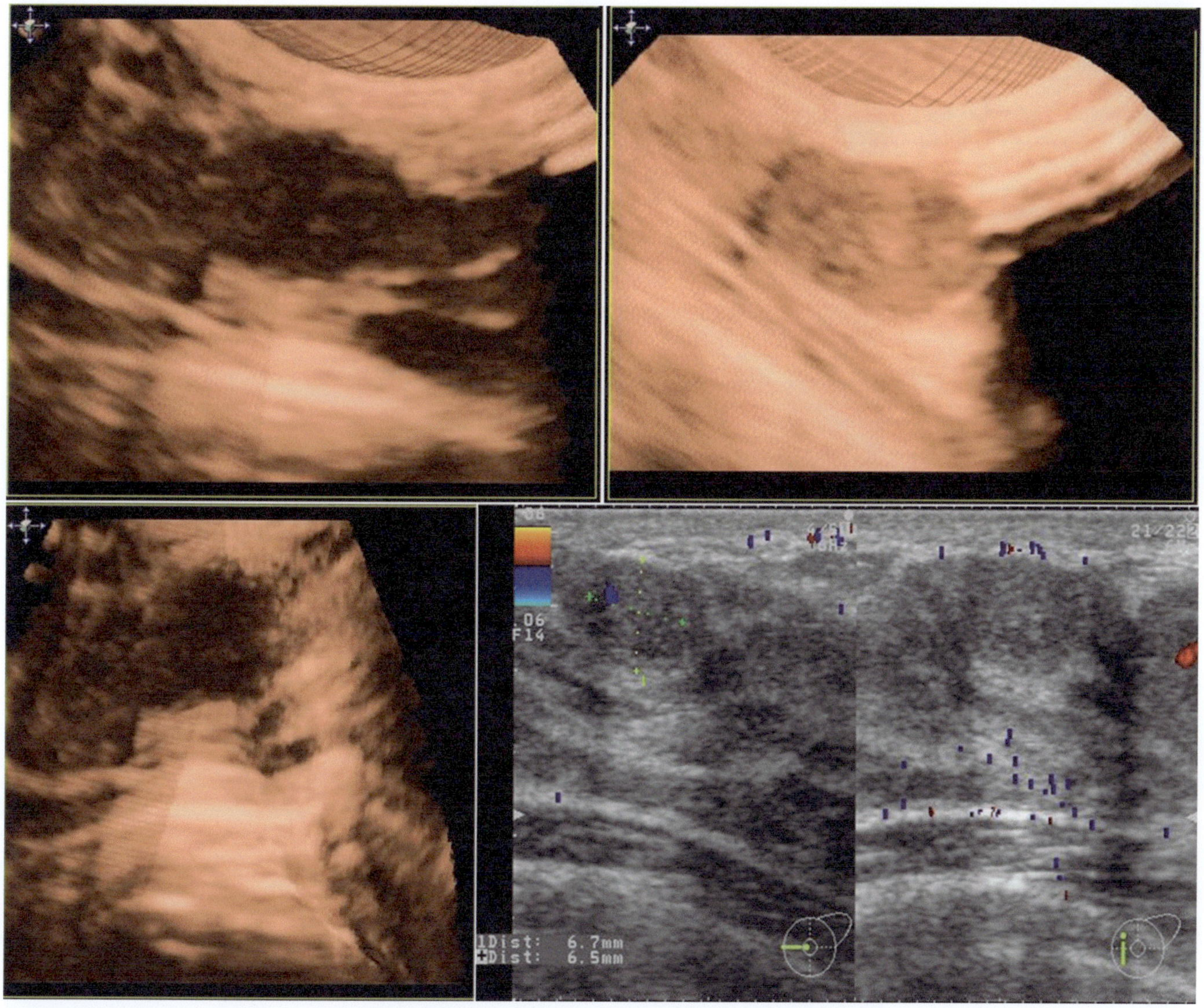

Fig. 6.47 A 19-year-old patient with L 9:00 small fibroadenoma; the mass could be characterized both in DE with radial and antiradial scans and in 3D/4D US. In this case, 4D acquisition allowed the complex data analysis, with adjustment of opacity, cutting, and rotation of the selected volume, which are useful in the increasing of contrast and better illustration of the rapports with the ductal system; volume rendering techniques are appreciated especially by the surgeons and the oncologists, but are more relevant for the patients that have to take sometimes a difficult decision

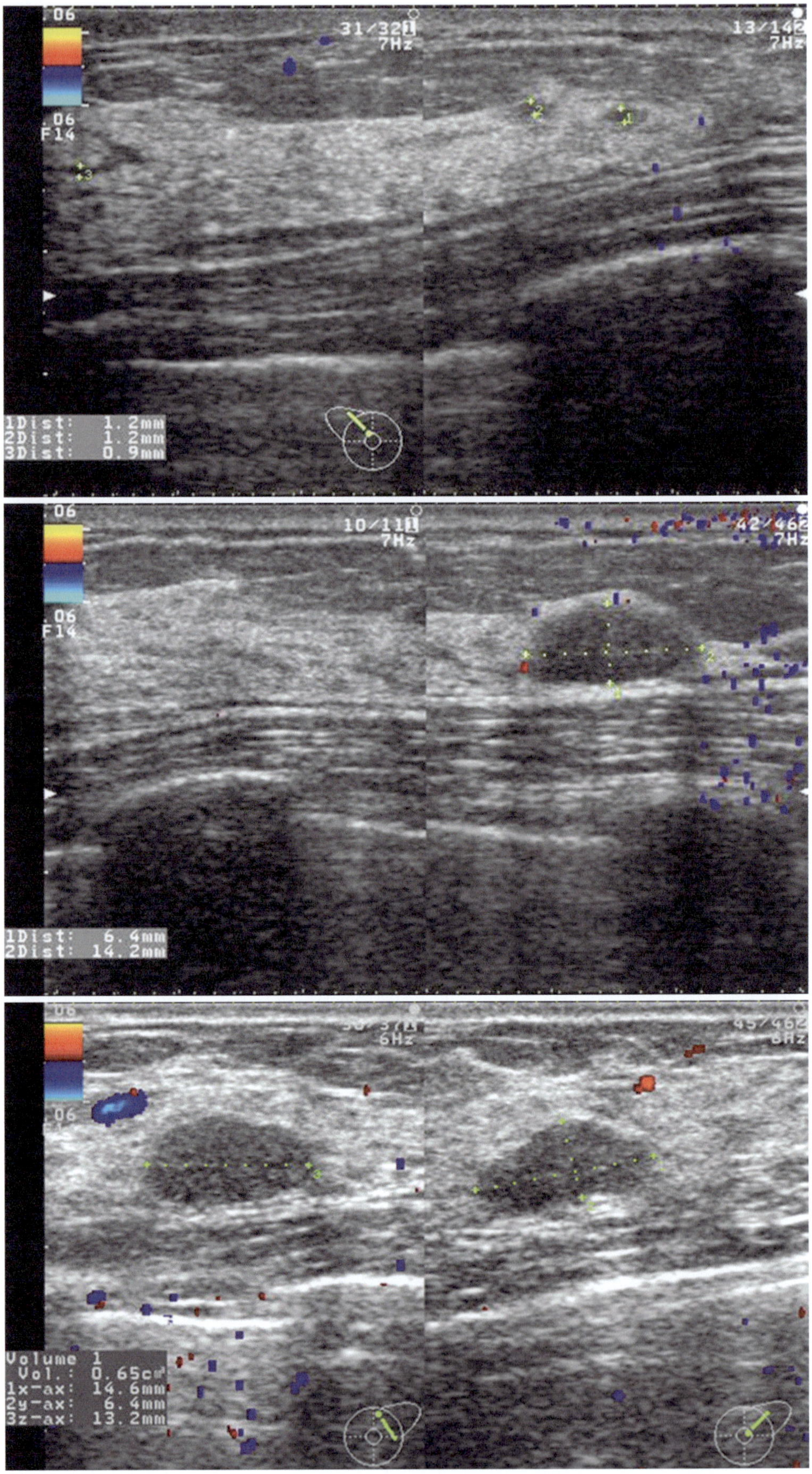

Fig. 6.48 A 49-year-old patient: ductal physiological atrophy, remnant lobules, and a fibroadenoma without changes during 6 months. The evolution is better evaluated when comparing the tumoral volume and the vasculature, in this case the reduced vasculature being a good predictor for benignity

6.7 Phyllodes Tumors

Phyllodes tumors are fibroepithelial tumors usually indistinguishable from fibroadenomas by radiological and imaging evaluation, although they tend to be larger (4 cm or greater) or exhibit rapid growth.

Phyllodes tumors account for less than 0.3–1% of all breast neoplasms. The mean age of patients is 45 years, prior to menopause, but they can occur in adolescents.

Phyllodes tumors are histologically described as resembling intracanalicular fibroadenomas with increased, heterogeneous stromal cellularity. They differ from fibroadenomas, showing cysts with intracystic epithelial proliferations with highly cellular stroma and the presence of mitotic activity. Phyllodes tumors are classified in two types: benign phyllodes tumors containing few mitoses and minimal cellular overgrowth, whereas malignant phyllodes tumors are showing marked hypercellularity and substantial mitotic activity, with potential recurrence after surgical incomplete excision without clear margins.

The mammography is not very useful in the diagnosis of the phyllodes tumors, because the presence of the tumors is always diagnosed clinically, and the radiological features are unspecific: large rounded-oval or lobulated masses, generally well circumscribed, with smooth margins. A radiolucent halo may be present, and calcifications (typically coarse and plaque-like) may be seen in a very small proportion.

In the classical US, it is not possible to differentiate the benign phyllodes tumor from the fibroadenoma, but the diagnosis is suggested by the rapid growth, huge size, and heterogeneity with cystic areas. On ultrasound, an inhomogeneous, solid-appearing mass containing single or multiple, round or cleft-like cystic spaces and demonstrating posterior acoustic enhancement strongly suggests the diagnosis of phyllodes tumor. Doppler signal is usually present in the solid components.

The malignant phyllodes tumors present the same characters such as the breast cancer: a hyper-vasculature, an increasing hypoechogenicity, and an increased stiffness on sonoelastography that have high sensibility and specificity for malignant development. Sonoelastography seems to have the best specificity for the phyllodes tumor, with better differentiation between benign and malignant lesions [19, 20]. The characteristic sign for phyllodes was described as an almost specific and constant elastic pattern with an elastic center and inelastic outer limits, referred to as the "ring sign"; by contrarily, it was found in just 5% of all fibroadenomas [19].

The advantage of using the FBU in phyllodes tumor is the possibility to explore all mammary lobes and thus the whole breast parenchyma in addition to the tumoral characterization similar to the classical US, completed with Doppler and RTSE. On the contrary, the breast outside the phyllodes tumor is not possible to be examined by classical US because of short linear transducers or by mammography, due to the high tumoral opacity that determines high electrical parameters of acquisition and thus high-level X-ray dose which overexpose the rest of the mammary tissues. Moreover, the usual large volume of the phyllodes with a higher stiffness than the rest of breast structures does not allow a good compression, and the quality of mammogram could not be assured (unequal pressure, insufficient tissues stretch).

The whole breast examination is possible using breast MRI, with the inconvenience that the method is more expansive and less available. Moreover, MRI cannot differentiate phyllodes from fibroadenomas, both of them presenting hyposignal T1 and T2 and heterogeneous contrast enhancement; when present, in 21 % cases, the significant increase of T2 signal in the surrounding breast tissue is more specific for phyllodes [21]. As a negative result, MRI overestimates the malignancy based on a suspicious signal intensity-time course both in phyllodes and fibroadenoma, with up to 30 % false-positive results. Tumor hypersignal on T1-weighted images and irregular cyst wall corresponded histopathologically to hemorrhagic infarction and necrosis, respectively [22].

The examination of the rest of tissues of a breast with phyllodes is mandatory, because behind or adjacent of a large phyllodes tumor, usually benign, we can discover a smaller malignant lesion, which is omitted by the mammography and the clinical exam.

Interval enlargement of a "fibroadenoma" represents an indication for needle biopsy, but large lesions (i.e., >4 cm) may qualify for excision out of hand because needle biopsy may not be representative of the pathology in the whole lesion due to its heterogeneity (Figs. 6.49 and 6.50)

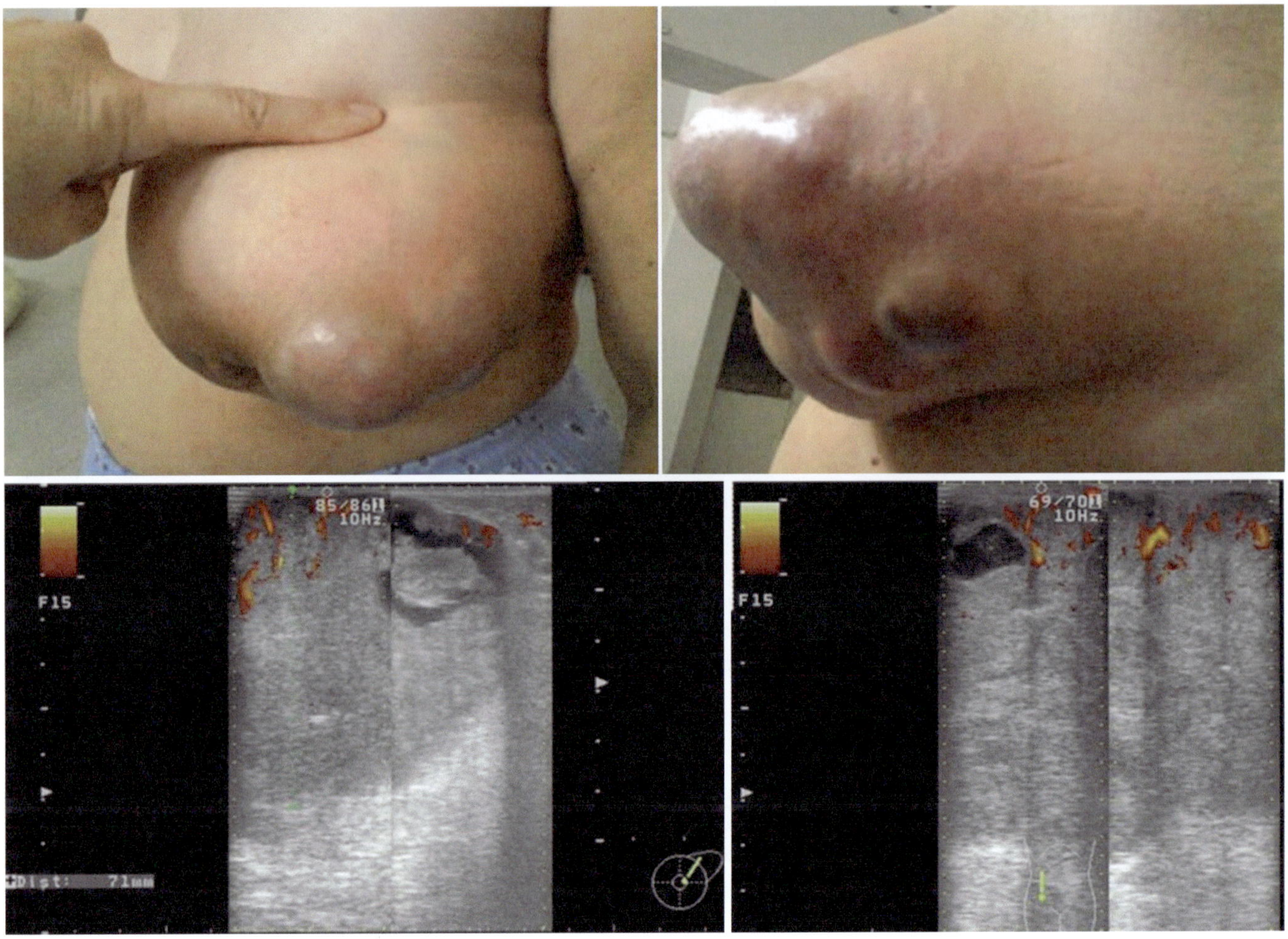

Fig. 6.49 Huge left breast tumor in a 58-year-old patient, with mixte predominant solid structure and small irregular areas of fluid content; the characters of apparent benign tumor with posterior enhancement and lateral shadowings (the Kobayashi signs) and disproportional reduced vasculature were compatible with the benign-type phyllodes tumor

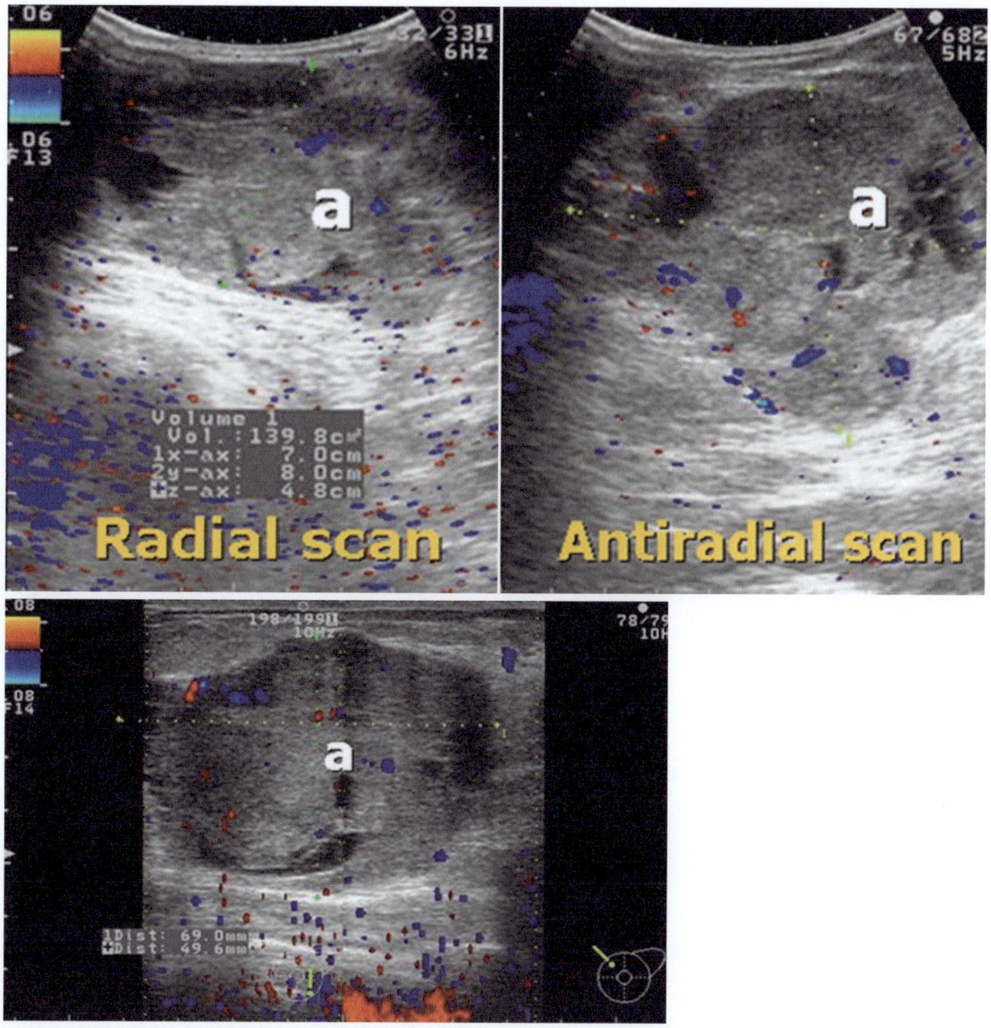

Fig. 6.50 A 39-year-old patient, with history of long use of birth control pills and a small lump in the left breast known from 3 years, when classical US diagnosed 1 cm "fibroadenoma" with negative complementary mammogram; 3-year follow-up mammography presented a huge mass, suspect phyllodes. A biopsy confirmed a benign type of phyllodes tumor. DE illustrated a tumor of up to 8 cm size, estimated to be 139.8 cm^3, heterogenic, mostly of solid structure with small cystic areas, with benign-type vasculature sustaining the diagnosis (*a*). Behind the huge tumor, there were detected multiple smaller hypoechoic lesions (*b*, *c*, *d*), with multilobulated contour, without significant posterior effects, but with malignant-type new vasculature, representing lobular multifocal invasive carcinoma. The lower figure represents a symmetric scan in the contralateral breast

Fig. 6.50 (continued)

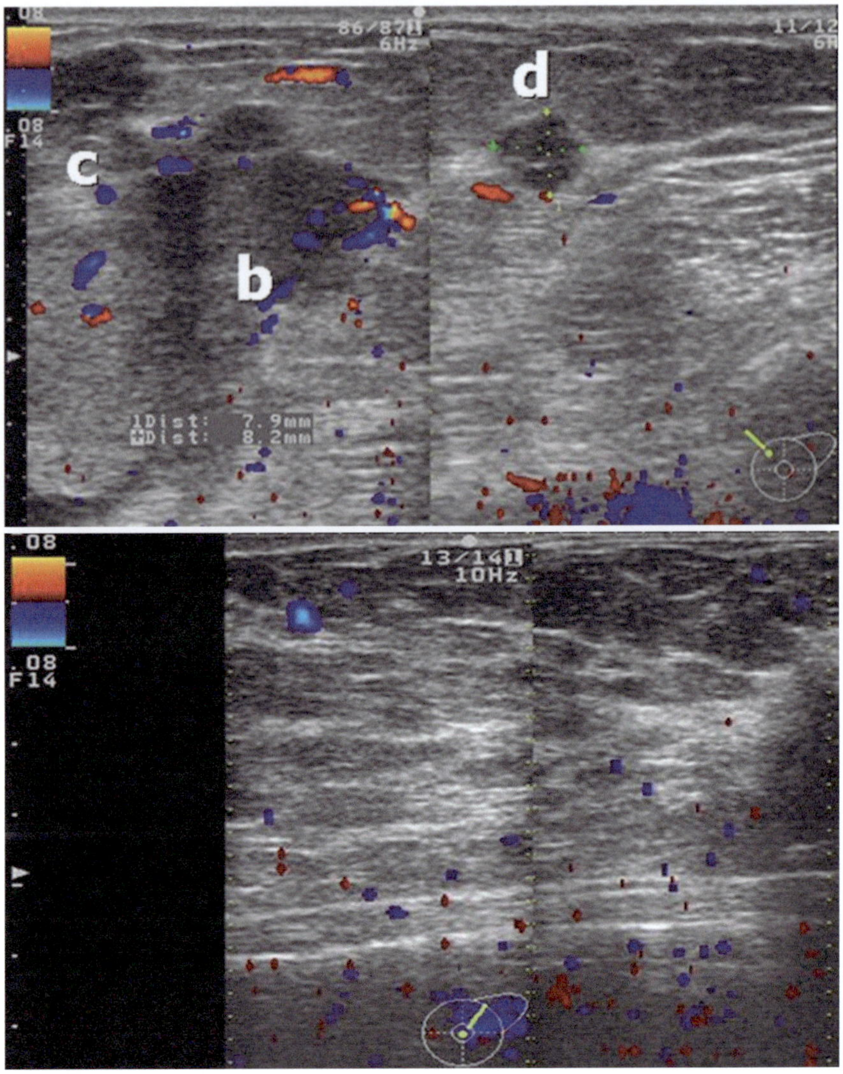

6.8 Hamartomas and Lipomas

Hamartomas and lipomas differ from fibroadenomas largely because of the presence of fat; they are more easily recognized mammographically, and there are some specific characters in US.

Hamartoma is considered a developmental error (the Greek term *hamartia* means "fault" or "defect") and can occur at a number of sites, in almost all types of tissues (organs), from the bony hamartomas to the neural lesions (the von Recklinghausen disease) and to the pulmonary, ovarian, testicular, and digestive hamartomas, Cowden syndrome, and so on. Despite the widely accepted epidemiology with the most frequent occurrence of this lesion in women older than 35 years of age, due to the fact that not all tumors are palpable and not all young women or all girls are examined for screening, it is logical that the late diagnosis does not exclude the earlier development, possible in puberty when the mammary bud is branching into mammary lobes. This point of view is concordant with the terms of "hamartoma" and "breast within a breast," with suggesting appearance in mammography.

Breast hamartoma was initially described by Arrigoni in 1971 [23] and may present clinically as a painless soft lump, sometimes with large size but slower development as compared with the phyllodes rapid growth; more often, hamartoma may also present as unilateral breast enlargement without a palpable localized mass, but with specific findings in mammography.

The pathology identifies in hamartoma a benign proliferation of fibrous, glandular-epithelial components and fatty tissue, all present in a normal breast, but without a radial architecture, and surrounded by a thin capsule of connective tissue; the structure justifies the term of fibro-adeno-lipoma.

Mammography typically demonstrates a well-circumscribed, round to oval inhomogeneous mass surrounded by thin capsule, comprising of both radiolucent areas considered as fatty tissue and radiodense components interpreted as fibroglandular tissue. The lesions may be of any size if incidental findings, but when clinical changes occur, usually the hamartomas are large and the breast size is significantly increased as compared with the opposite.

In the classical US examination, hamartoma appears as partially demarcated heterogeneous regions, containing variable amounts of hypoechoic tissue (representing fat) and echogenic "fibroglandular" elements. Because it resembles the normal breast tissue, usually it is difficult to delineate the margins and its aspect is not specific; when detected, it appears as a benign "tumor," softer than fibroadenoma. In fact, US examination is usually performed as a complementary technique, and the diagnosis is mainly based on the mammographic aspect.

Nevertheless, in DE it is easy to demonstrate the hamartoma that is not connected to the branches of the ductal-lobular system, but seems to contain some curved ducts with the central line sign without radial orientation, together with lobules, glandular stoma, and unspecific hypoechoic areas; the vasculature is often less visible or of benign aspect, and the sonoelastography is suggesting benignity with reduced scores. Moreover, FBU allows to analyze the surrounding mammary lobar structures, which are compressed, displaced, but with the normal orientation towards the nipple preserved; the largest hamartomas and the surrounding tissues are better demonstrated by using a long linear probe, eventually provided with a water-bag device, than with a short probe or even with a panoramic scanning-type SieScape, which has a less resolution and cannot allow correction of measurements in all axes.

Other lesions containing fat include fat necrosis that will be discussed in the next section and lipomas.

Lipomas have a variable appearance from homogeneous, hyperechoic, and poorly demarcated regions within fatty tissue to heterogeneous masses elsewhere in the breast. In mammography, lipomas are better illustrated in the dense breasts as a radiolucent mass with no calcification (in rare situation, there may be areas of fat necrosis presenting as calcification), sometimes delineated by a thin, peripheral fibrous capsule.

Lipomas are frequent findings in US, but they are difficult to be recognized on mammography in fatty breasts; in US they appear usually as nodular lesions, with irregular not well distinct contour, located in the mammary fatty tissue, without salient vasculature in Doppler examination, having posterior effects of benign type based on Kobayashi and benign SE of score 1 or 2 Ueno. In the breast, small lipomas appear usually as hyperechoic 1–2 cm tumors, because of the large amount of adipocytes of small size, thus having high internal echo level; these lumps are more often multiple, of different sizes, and sometimes palpable, especially when the patient has lost weight, and usually similar lesions are found in the subcutaneous fatty tissue anywhere in the body or the limbs (multiple lipomas may be congenital syndromes or acquired disease).

Large lipomas may present thin capsule, and septae, a hypoechoic aspect, are palpable and the glandular structures are dislocated. Large lipomas are rare, usually unique findings, sometimes acquiring huge volume, with rising risk of malignant degeneration towards liposarcomas, but without increasing the relative risk for developing a "true" breast cancer, we are meaning epithelial malignant proliferation in a ductal or a lobular cancer. The large, hypoechoic lipomas should be differentiated from the normal hypertrophic fatty spaces usually in the menopausal breasts, delineated by the Cooper ligaments that tend to be elongated, with arcuate course.

In conclusion, lipomas and hamartomas may compress breast parenchyma, but they have no connections with the ductal tree, and the heterogeneous internal findings have no suspect vasculature or significant reduction of the elasticity. The expectative and US follow-up examination seems the best attitude, avoiding unnecessary biopsies. When the large size of a hamartoma or breast lipoma arrives to clinical discomfort or to esthetical reasons, the surgical treatment is recommended after an accurate evaluation of the whole breast architecture, because there may be found different associated lesions.

It is recommended to correlate US with mammography and use combined diagnostic criteria to guide management of these benign lesions (Figs. 6.51, 6.52, 6.53, 6.54, 6.55, 6.56, and 6.57).

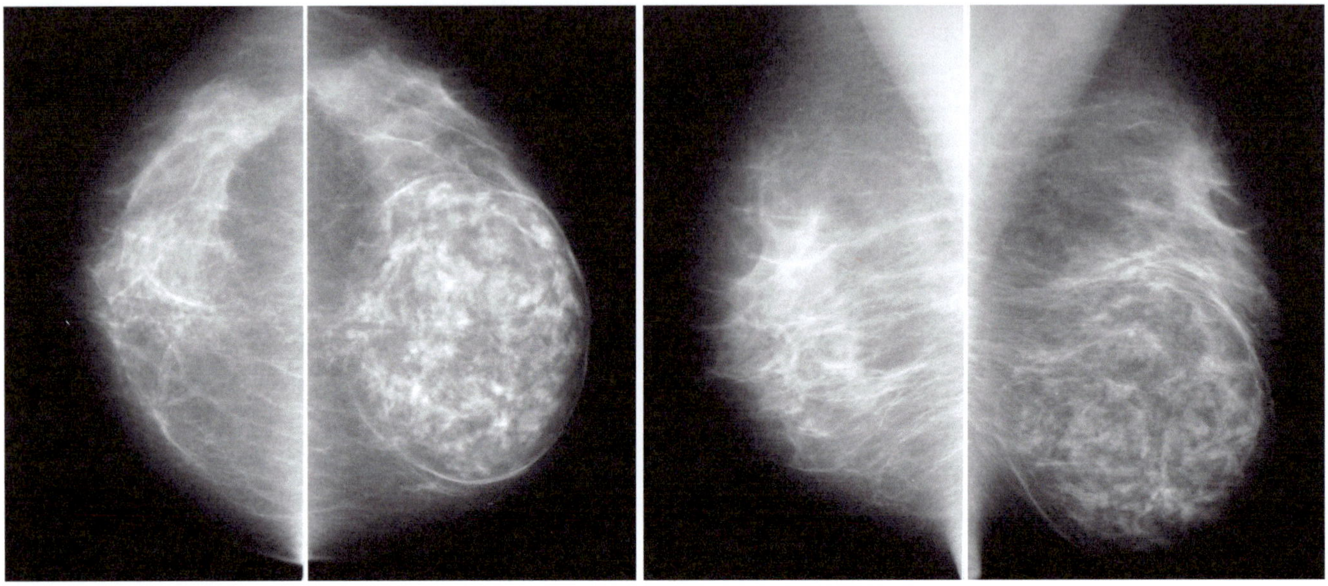

Fig. 6.51 Plain-film mammography in a 47-year-old patient with left breast hamartoma: thin fibrous capsule of a large mass that is located in the lower quadrants, with heterogeneous content

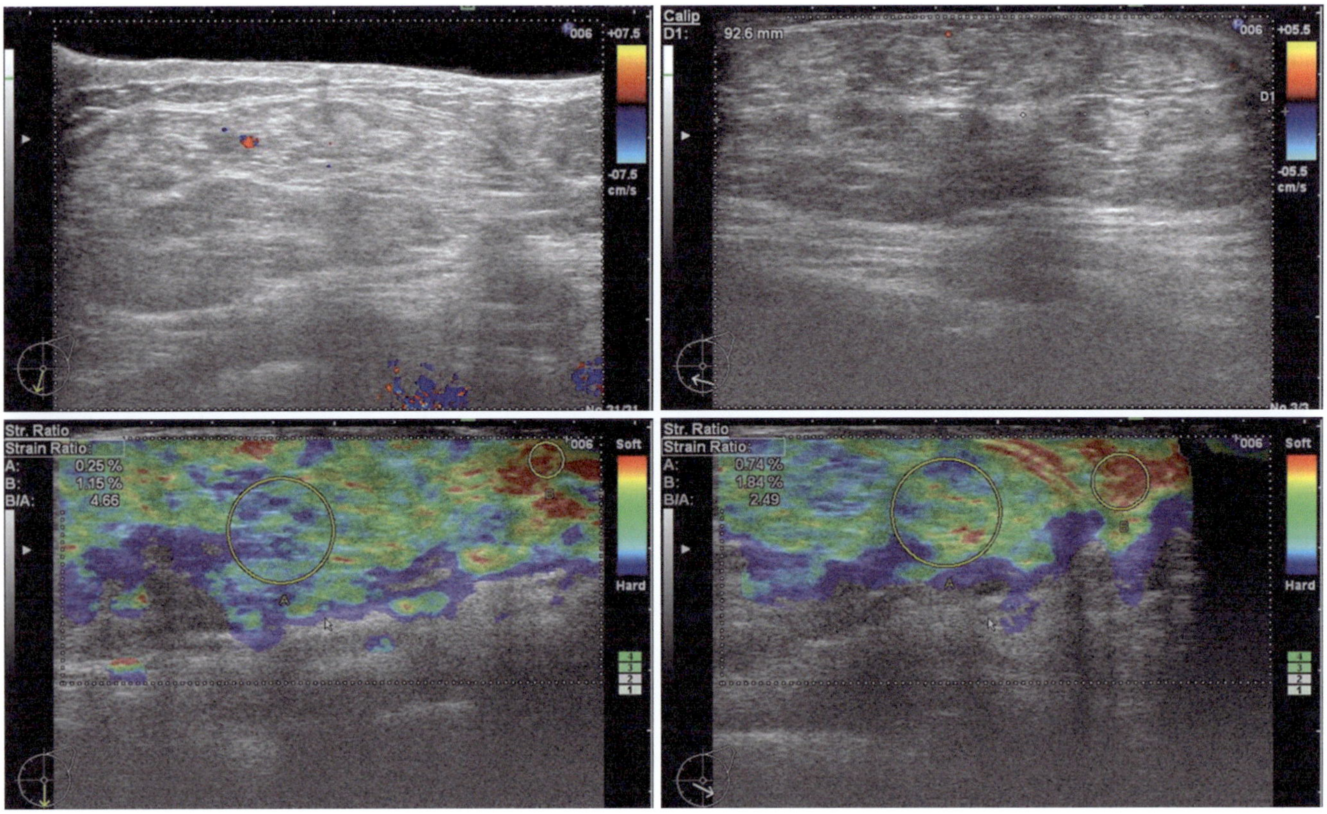

Fig. 6.52 The same case: FBU with Doppler DE and sonoelastography in radial scans (**a**, **c**) and in antiradial scans (**b**, **d**), with illustration of the capsule, of the mixte glandular and fatty content, with less vasculature and score 2 Ueno

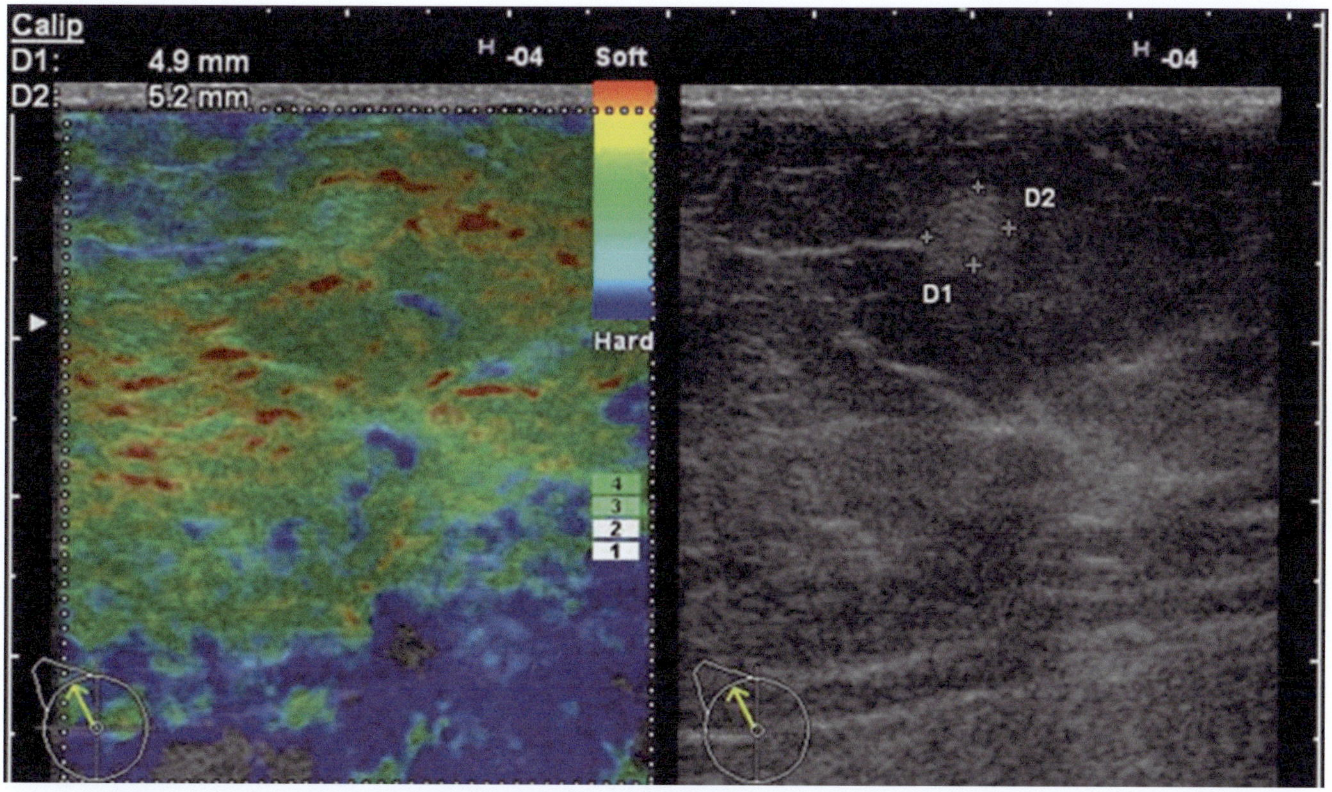

Fig. 6.53 A small hyperechoic lesion on the superficial fascia, without ductal connection, with benign features

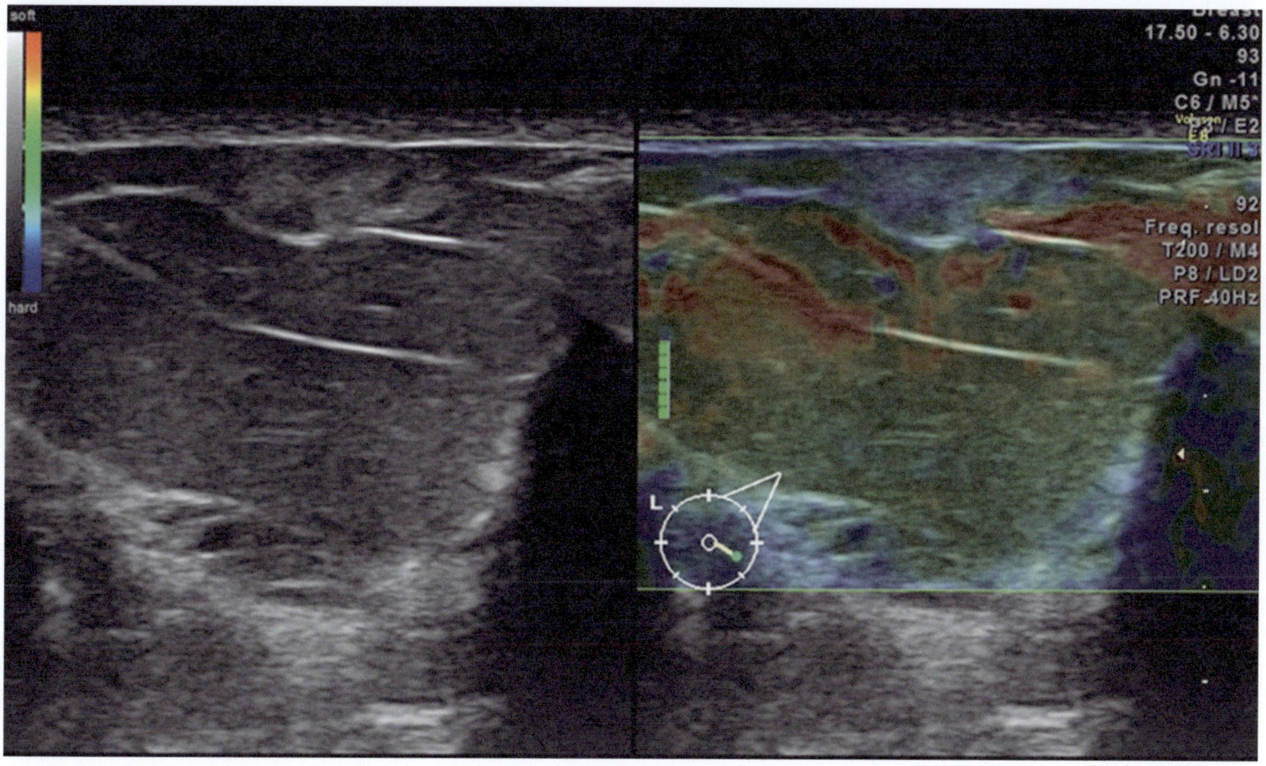

Fig. 6.54 A superficial lipoma, between the basal membrane of the derma and the fascia superficialis; the hyperechoic lesion without posterior significant effects has a reduced elasticity, being constraint by the two continuous structures

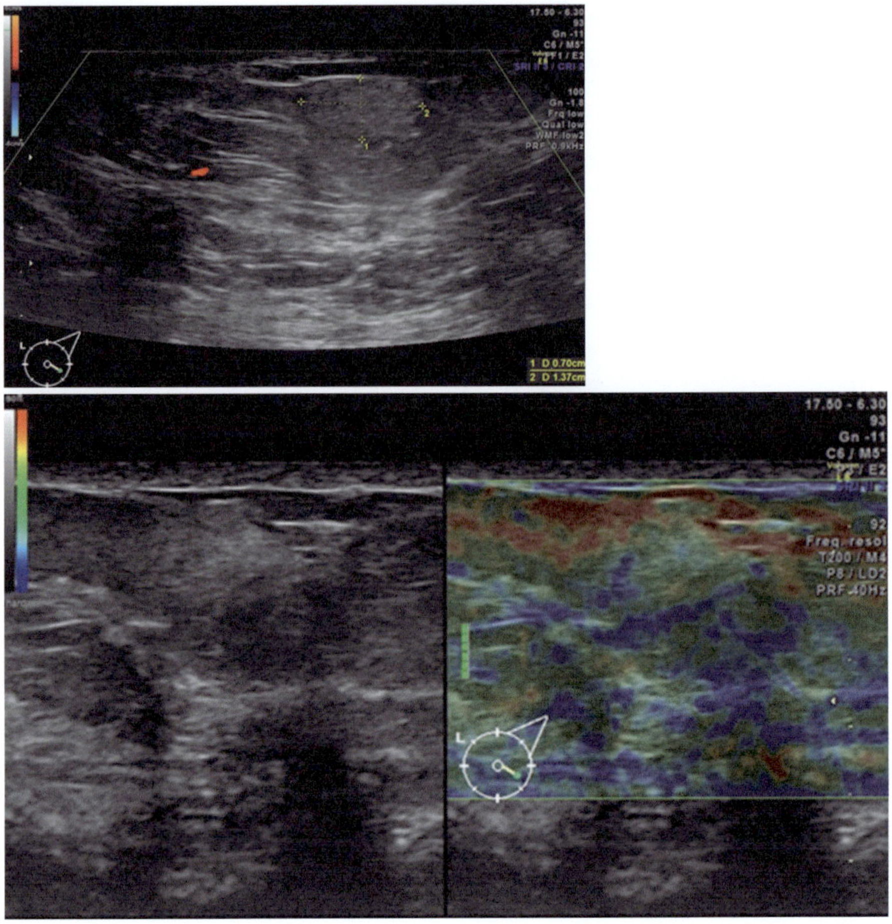

Fig. 6.55 A premammary lipoma located beneath the fascia superficialis, in the premammary fatty layer; this type of hyperechoic lesions without ductal connection, with benign descriptors based on Stavros, and with scores 1–2 Ueno, sometimes palpable and usually painless, rest unchanged for many years and are usually multiple in the breasts and elsewhere in the subcutaneous fat

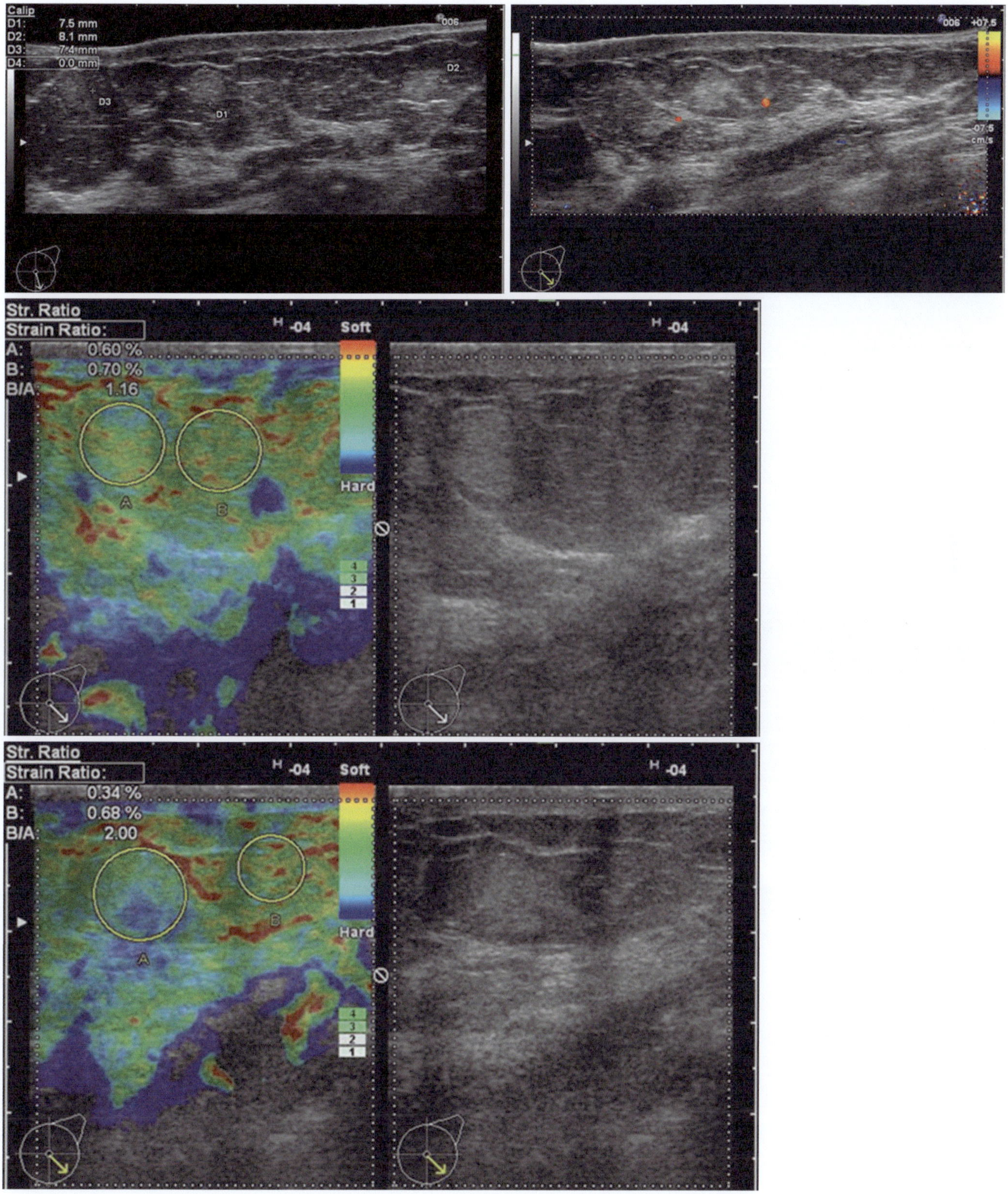

Fig. 6.56 Familial multiple lipomatosis, an autosomal dominant condition, with multiple lipomas on the trunk, included breasts, and limbs. The general aspect is similar to the glandular tissues, but the location between the Cooper ligaments inside the fatty tissue is demonstrative

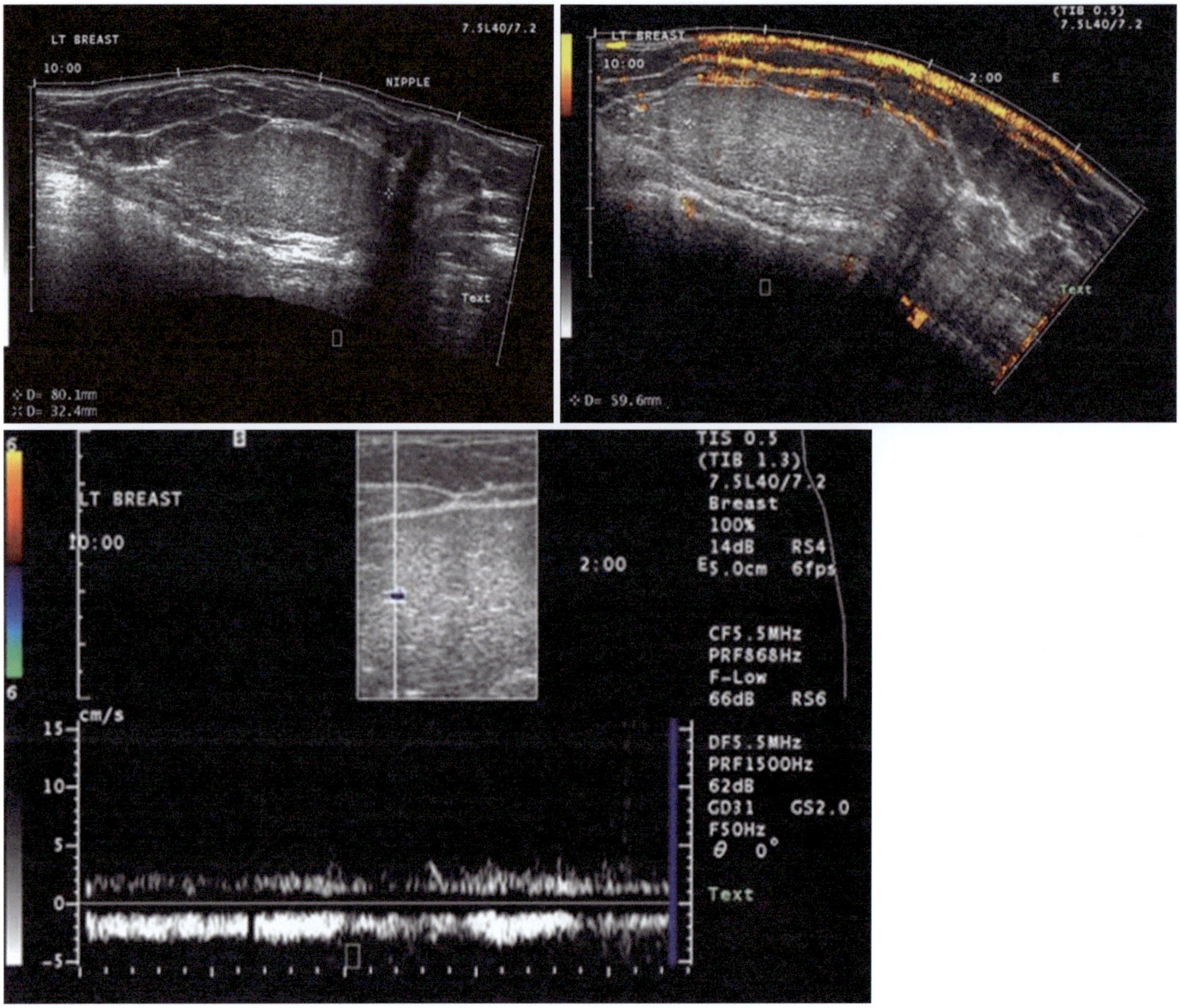

Fig. 6.57 Large breast lipoma in the premammary fat, with thin vessels and a pseudocapsule; the panoramic view (SieScape) is useful for a whole estimation of the anatomy, but the measurements in the horizontal plan are approximate

6.9 Fat Necrosis

Fat necrosis of the breast represents a benign nonsuppurative inflammatory process of the adipose tissue. It occurs usually secondary to accidental or surgical trauma, frequently after breast reconstruction because of lack of vasculature in transplanted tissues; some cases arise after animal bites, otherwise after radiotherapy. In rare cases, fat necroses may be associated with breast carcinoma or any lesion that provokes suppurative or necrotic degeneration (mammary ductal ectasia with overinfection spread in the surrounding tissues, fibrocystic disease with large cyst formation).

Clinically, fat necrosis may mimic breast cancer if it appears as an ill-defined palpable mass, associated with skin retraction, ecchymosis, erythema, and skin thickening, usually described as “orange peel skin.”

Mammography may present dense, spiculated mass and skin thickening; the classical US and breast MRI may not always distinguish fat necrosis from a malignant lesion. Even the macroscopic appearance of this benign lesion can suggest a malignant tumor. However, the histological diagnosis of fat necrosis presents no problem, as it is characterized by anucleated fat cells often surrounded by histiocytic giant cells and foamy phagocytic histiocytes. Excisional biopsy is required if carcinoma cannot be excluded.

As an alternative, FBU offers the possibility to evaluate the malignancy risk and to better locate the lesion, which has no connection with the galactophorous ductal tree, as it is the case of breast cancer; moreover, fat necroses may present diffuse contour and it is less delimited from the surrounding fatty tissue, the vasculature is not so intense as in breast cancer, and the sonoelastography demonstrates either a score 2 Ueno or a complex BGR score; in some cases, especially in fat necrosis after radiotherapy, the subcutaneous fatty tissue presents a diffuse increased strain, but the glandular tissue with the ductal tree and surrounding stroma appears with normal elasticity. Deep fat necrosis may be difficult to differentiate from the breast cancer on DE, but the clinical history, combined with Doppler, and strain assessment are useful in the differential diagnosis; a short-time follow-up FBU is recommended, and the biopsies are reserved in special cases with unclear evolution.

Fat necrosis (cytosteatonecrosis) may appear as hypoechoic small lesions, with a hyperechoic rim corresponding to the surrounding fibrous reaction or to the serohematic post-traumatic infiltration in the fatty tissue; the whole area has a reduced elasticity on palpation and usually is painful. The evolution may be either resorption after conservative treatment or fibrous organization and pseudotumoral aspect; some lesions may calcify. The satellite axillary lymph nodes usually confirm the inflammatory process, presenting a hypoechoic aspect of the central area of the hilum, consistent with benign histiocytosis (Figs. 6.58 and 6.59).

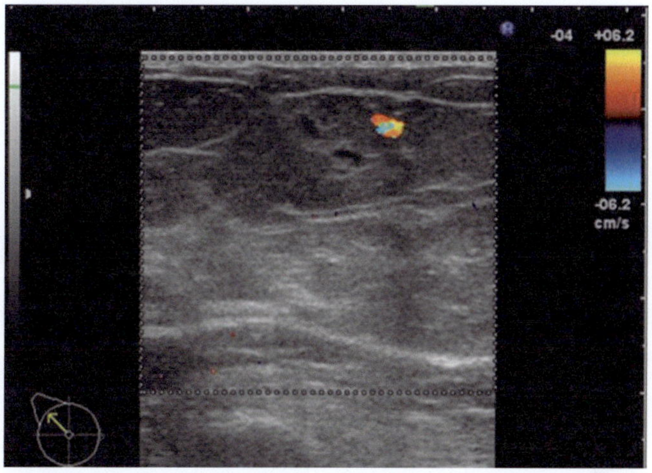

Fig. 6.58 Premammary fat necrosis with pseudocystic lesions without ductal connection in an old post-traumatic area

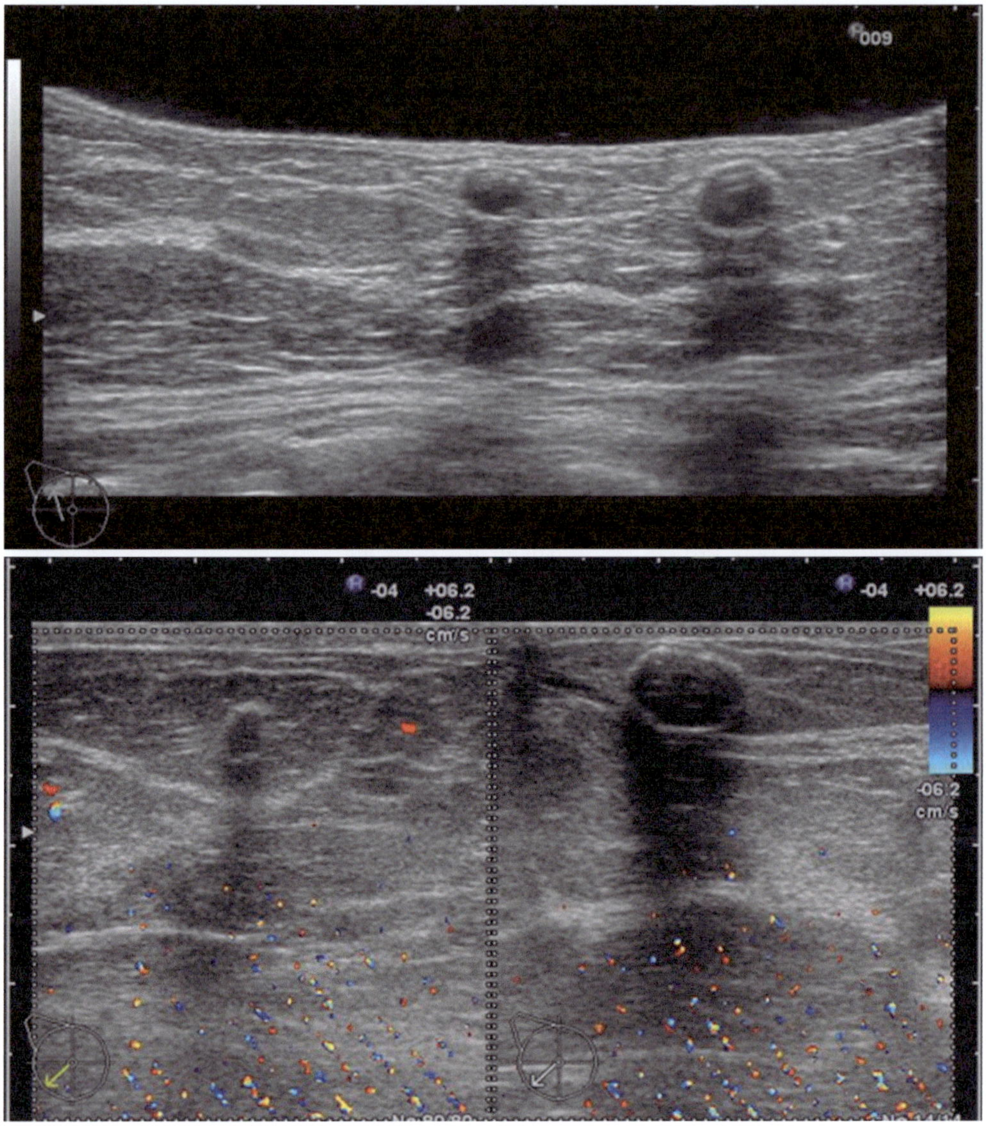

Fig. 6.59 Cystic calcifications in the premammary fatty tissue, without any connections with the remnant breast parenchyma in a postmenopausal breast; an old traumatic history could be considered for the etiologic factor

Fig. 6.59 (continued)

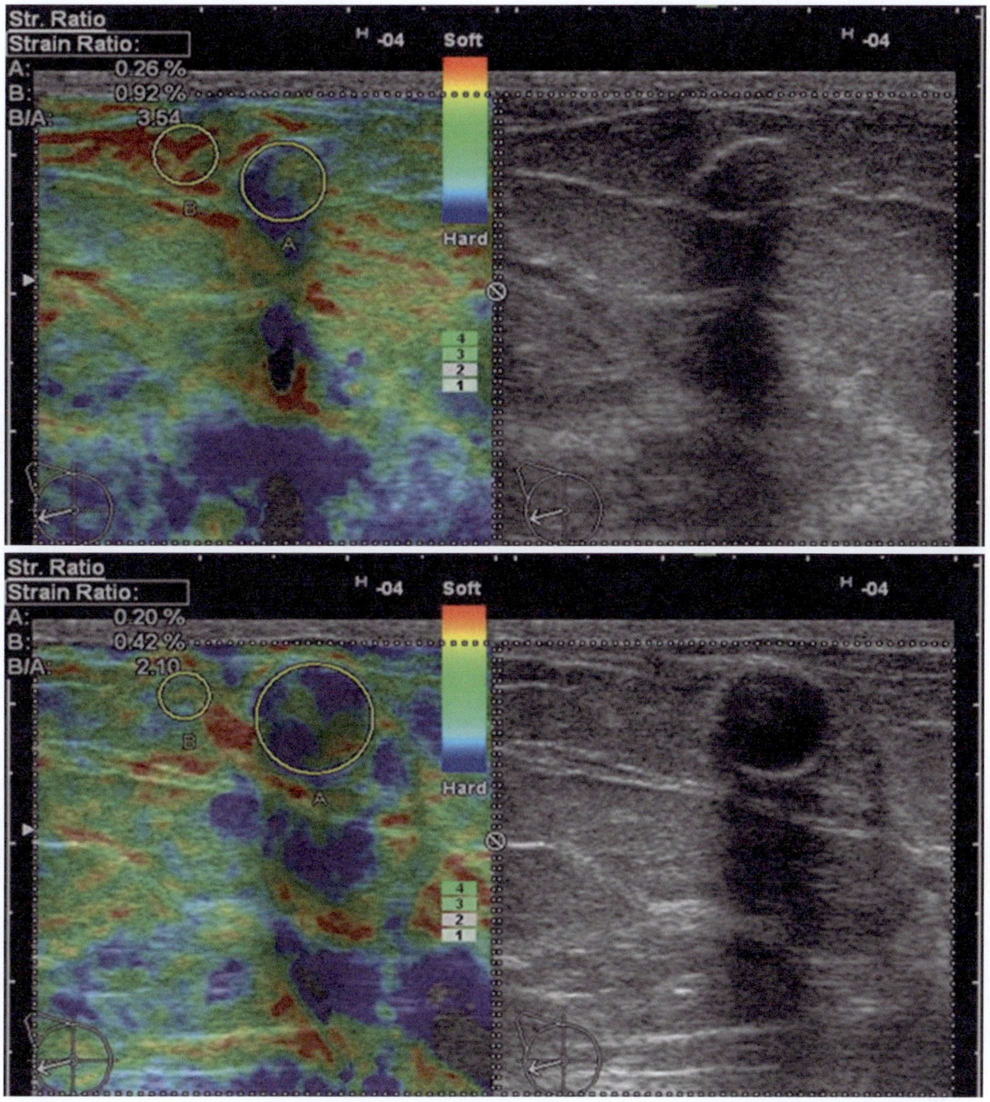

6.10 Papillomas

Breast papillomas are single formations of epithelial fronds supported by a fibrovascular stroma, a fibrovascular core covered by an epithelial layer with arborescent development. They are most frequently located in the subareolar region within major ducts but also occur peripherally, some with intracystic location. Serous or serosanguineous nipple discharge is commonly present, and the involved duct is distended and occasionally cystic. The bilateral and multicentric development suggests some systemic risk factors, such as hormonal disorders or prolonged use of contraceptive pills.

In the classical US, papillomas are described generally as hypoechoic or fibroglandular tissue, but the expression "fibroglandular tissue" is not an anatomically precise structure. Papillomas may be a discrete, well-contoured, and gently lobulated or microlobulated masses, or they may conform to the shape of a duct and can be outlined by fluid if lying within a cyst or distended duct.

In the FBU, the intraductal location is better demonstrated, usually with a central periareolary development, determining an abrupt narrowing at the limit with the peripheral normal duct. More frequently the vascular core is undetectable on Doppler, but if a lesion with a papillomatous aspect has a significant vasculature on Doppler, the differential diagnosis with an atypical hyperplasia or a DCIS is mandatory.

There are two types of papilloma, better differentiated on Doppler DE: solitary papilloma, with a central periareolary location, involving the large ducts, almost always benign, and multiple papillomas, with a lobular origin and spreading to the ducts. The precise mapping on DE of the papillomas offers a good follow-up of these lesions, and any sign of suspect evolution entails a therapeutic intervention, either a DE biopsy, or a surgical biopsy.

On sonoelastography, papillomas are soft structures, with a score 1 or 2 Ueno, while the malignant intraductal proliferations present the score 3 or 4 Ueno.

The nipple surge is usually associated with papilloma when the excretory ducts are permissive; it may be serous or viscous, citrine to dark green, or brown-bloody type, and the bacteriological tests demonstrate usually an over-infection with different types of staphylococcus or streptococcus, which may be a trigger for the proliferation of the ductal epithelium. In nipple surge, especially with bloody aspect, the clinical practice is oriented especially to the cytological research, while the chronic infections of the breast usually are ignored or underestimated (see Sect. 6.14).

Some ducts with ectasia and inspissated content could mimic ductal papillomas, but the ductal diameter decreases gradually, and the elasticity is higher, of score 1 Ueno or of BGR type.

The risk of malignant evolution of the ductal papilloma is very low, while there are many cases with large benign papillomas, sometimes remnant after surgical removal of other adjacent lesions; moreover, the papillomas occur mainly in the periareolary regions of the ducts, while malignant proliferations have for the initial site the TDLUs, usually with peripheral location (Figs. 6.60, 6.61, 6.62, 6.63, 6.64, 6.65, and 6.66).

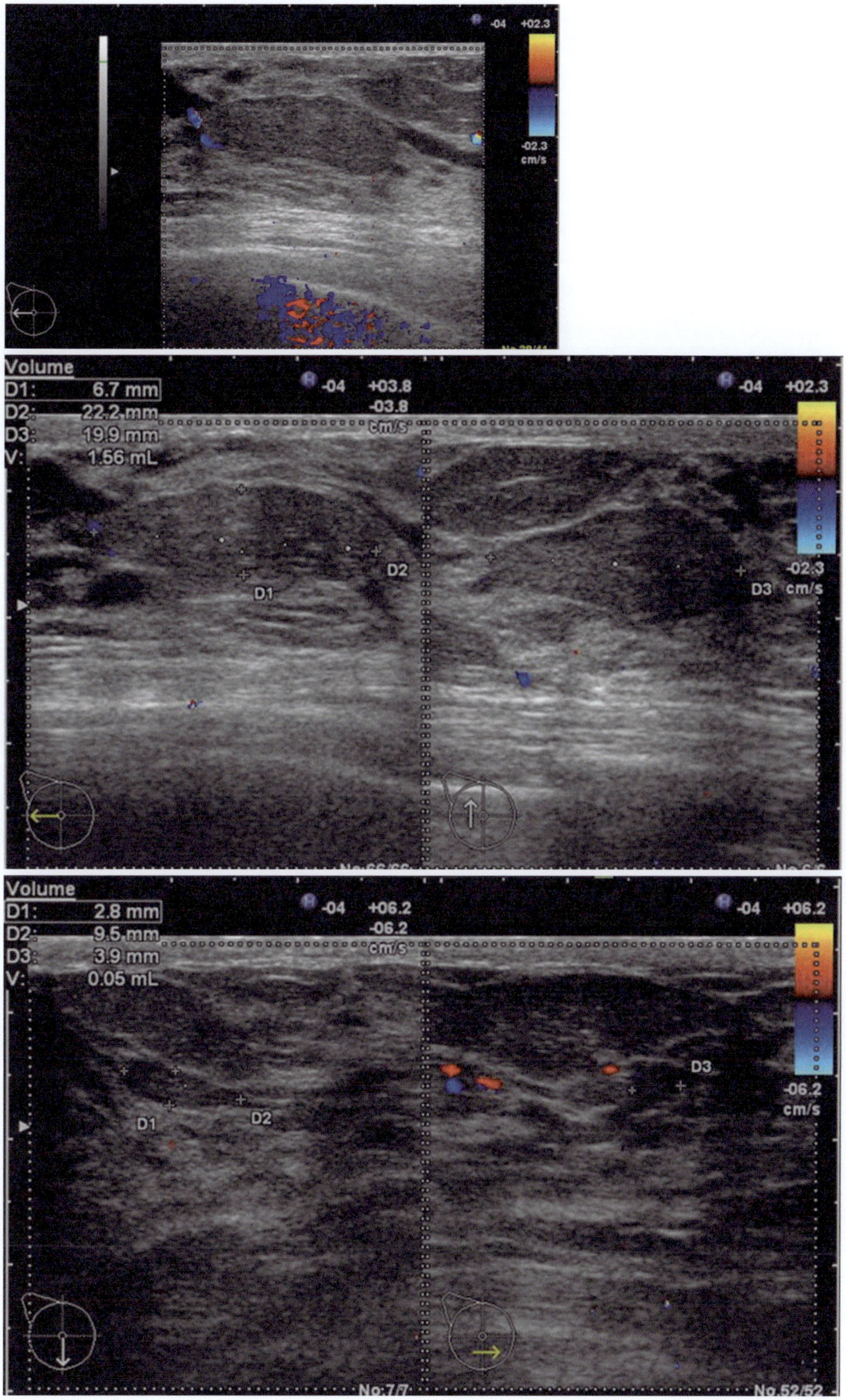

Fig. 6.60 Doppler DE: central ductal voluminous papillomas, with segmental ductal distention, an ovoidal shape with iso-/hypoechoic structure, and a vascular pole. Small ductal ectasia outside the intraductal mass and in the adjacent ducts may be responsible for the nipple surge

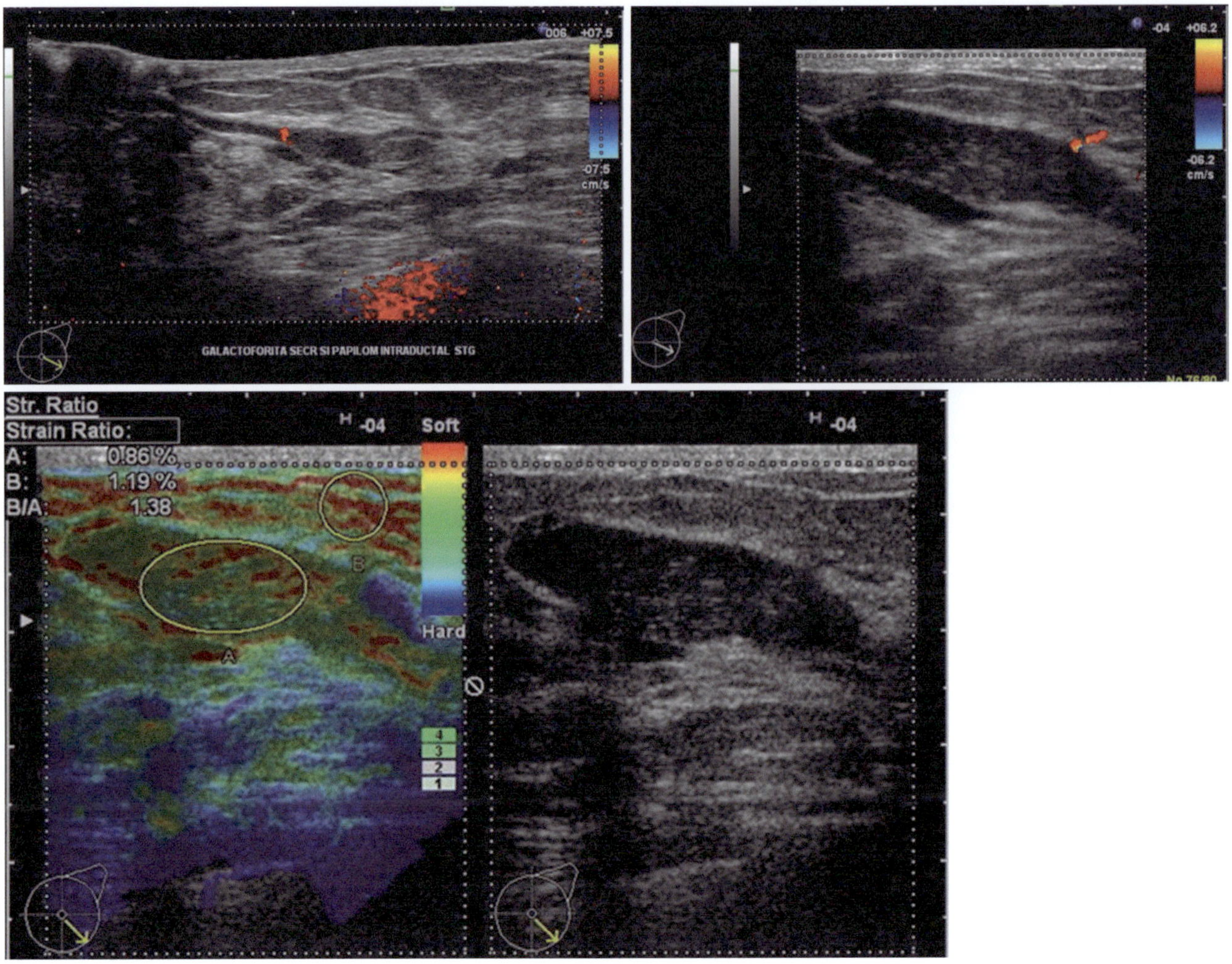

Fig. 6.61 Ductal papilloma with nourishing vessel and score 1 Ueno with low FLR

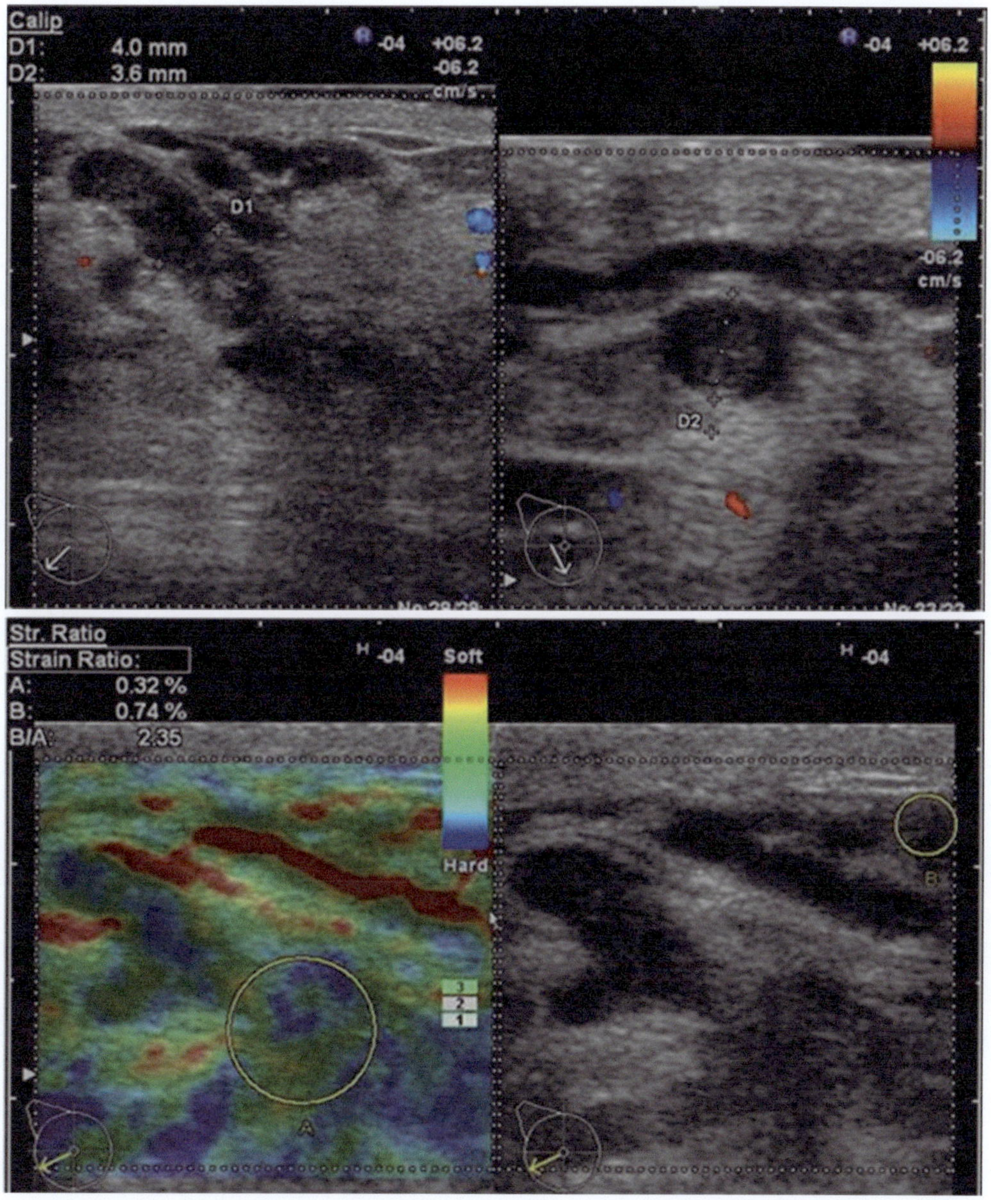

Fig. 6.62 Radial and antiradial scan in the R 8:00 demonstrates an enlarged duct fulfilled with a heterogeneous structure and low elasticity score 3 Ueno. Simple ductal ectasia with score 1 Ueno is visible in the vicinity. The differential diagnosis with DCIS is required, and cytology from the nipple surge is mandatory

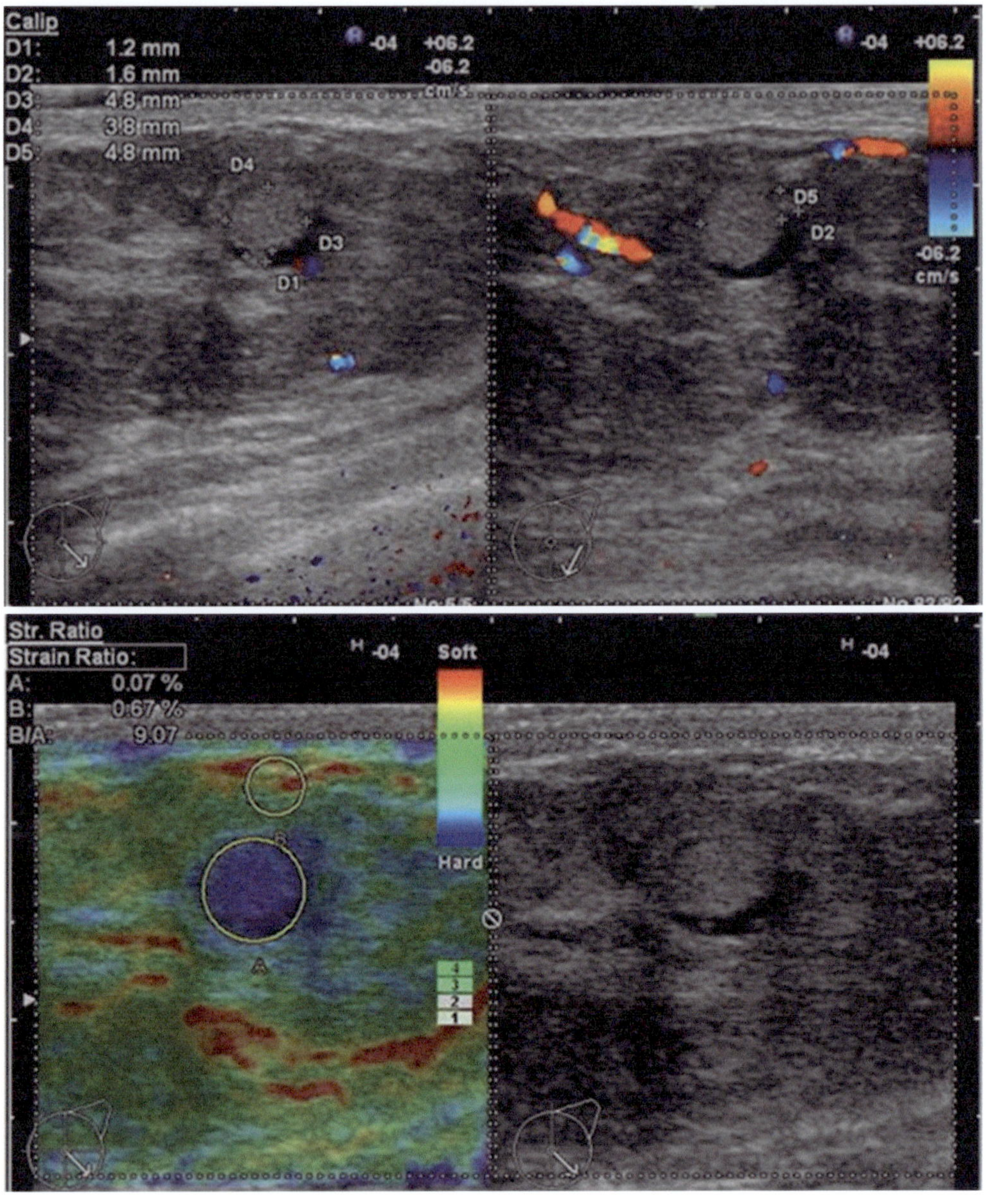

Fig. 6.63 Radial and antiradial scans at L 4:00 illustrate an intracystic papilloma; the sonoelastographic score 4 Ueno is overevaluated due to the high tension in the cystic walls; the benign-type lesion diagnosis is based on the absence of the new formation vasculature

Fig. 6.64 Papillomas

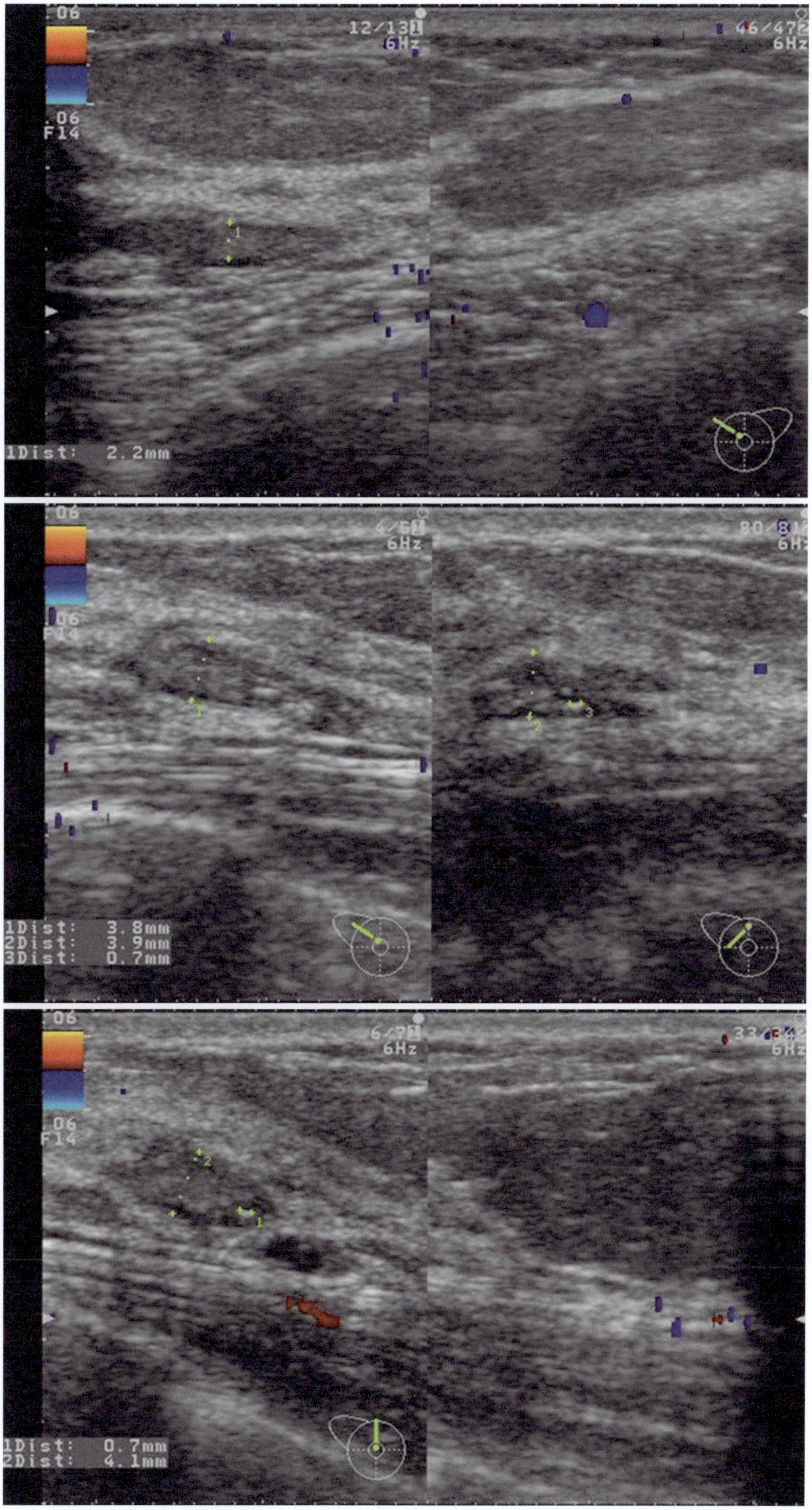

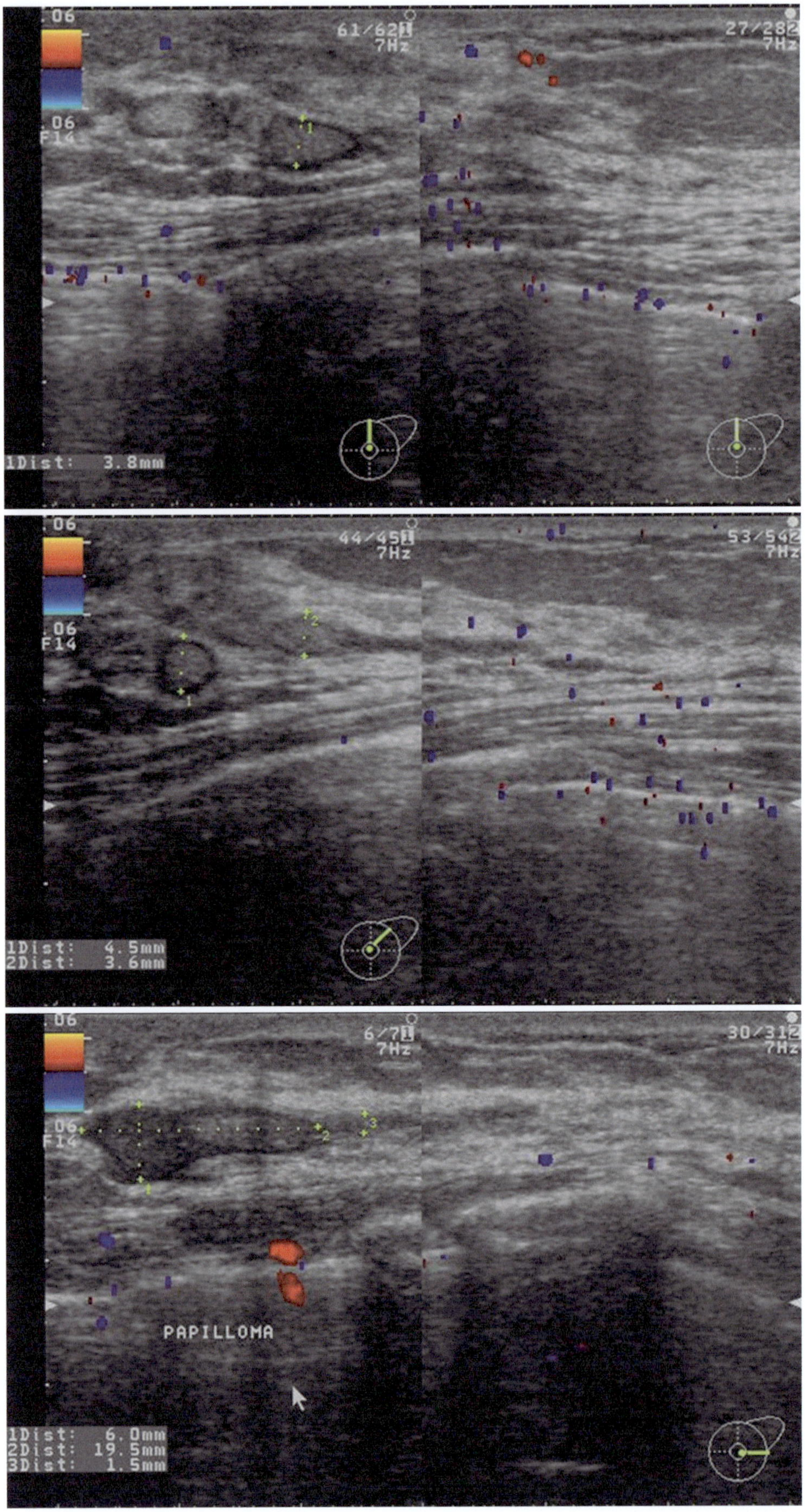

Fig. 6.65 The same case: bilateral central intraductal papillomas, with segmental thickening by intraluminal masses delineated by the ductal walls, as a hypoechoic rim

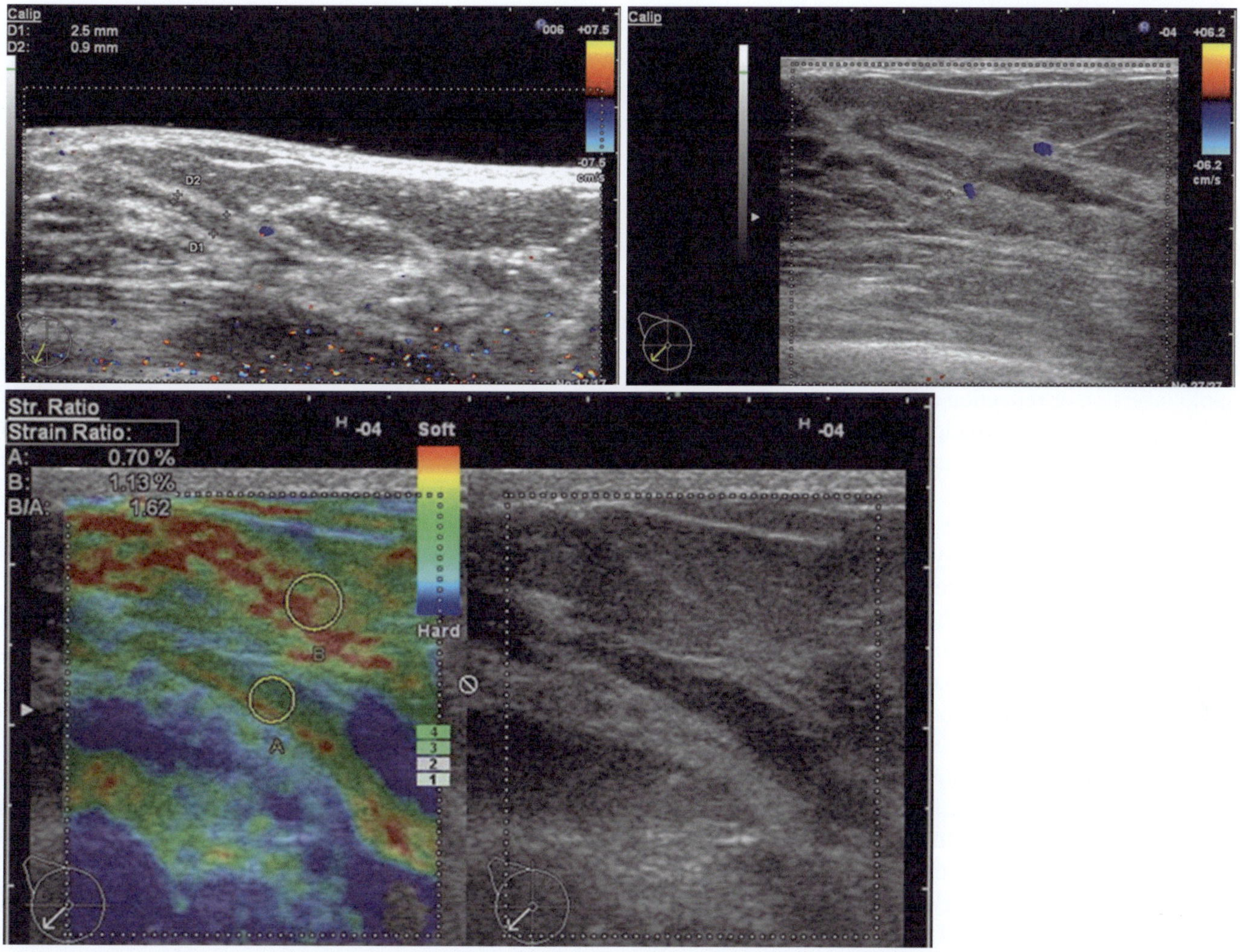

Fig. 6.66 Ductal thickening with loss of the central intraductal hyperechoic sign (long probe acquisition); the short probe with higher frequency demonstrates the ductal walls and inhomogeneous intraductal content, with hypo- and isoechoic aspect mimicking intraductal papillomas and ductal fluid. The SE aspect of score 1 Ueno in the dense segment and BGR score in the hypoechoic content are concordant with an inspissated duct

6.11 Ductal Ectasia

Ductal ectasia (periductal mastitis, plasma cell mastitis, secretory disease) is characterized by focal or segmental distention of one or multiple ducts and may be associated with inflammation and periductal fibrosis. Ductal ectasia commonly affects the subareolar ducts but may also involve the smaller peripheral ducts.

Classically, ductal ectasia is a disease of primarily middle-aged to elderly parous women, who rarely present with nipple discharge or a palpable subareolar mass, but usually with noncyclical mastalgia; in advanced stages, nipple inversion or retraction may occur. However, the disease may be present in young nulliparous woman, associated with the cystic dysplasia and even in advanced gynecomastia.

Ductal ectasia may manifest as a painful and/or palpable area, or the process may be asymptomatic and apparent only at imaging evaluation. Sometimes the patients affirm nipple surge; otherwise, the active hand expression of the nipple and of the periareolary area may demonstrate different color and consistency of the mammary secretion.

The etiologic factors are not clear; generally, fewer cases present high level of the serum concentration of prolactin, associated with mammary increased vasculature, visible at US with Doppler, from which some cases may develop microadenoma of the hypophysis confirmed by MRI. Most cases with normal prolactin present a chronic overinfection of the mammary secretion, with various bacterial factors. Food intake of hormones was incriminated in many cases, but the specific studies are missing, despite the change in food regimen which was benefic in proved cases.

The dilated ducts contain usually eosinophilic, granular secretions and foamy histiocytes both within the ductal epithelium and the lumen. The inspissated luminal secretions may undergo calcifications, rarely visualized in US, but usually proving milky secretions with or without overinfection.

The mammography may detect ductal ectasia in asymptomatic woman with fatty breasts or when there are present characteristic microcalcifications.

Classical US shows tubular anechoic structures or ducts filled with echogenic debris, and there may be associated nipple discharge. The random scans or the scans in the sagittal and transverse plans do not allow a precise location of the lesions, and thus the sensibility of the method is reduced, because most ductal ectasia may be underdiagnosed if the nipple discharge is absent or may be misinterpreted as small cysts.

FBU provides excellent visualization of distended ducts and, unlike mammography, distinguishes them clearly from the surrounding parenchyma. Typically, one or more tubular structures radiate towards the nipple, presenting thin walls and a content with low-level echoes, similar to breast-feeding type, but without significant increased vasculature. The smallest amount of secretion can be demonstrated on FBU by the presence of the *central double line sign*, usually less than 0.2 mm in diameter. Some cases may develop small papillomatous thickening of the walls, without vascular signs; others are associated with terminal cysts. The sonoelastography illustrates in small ectasias, up to 1–2 mm in diameter, a score 1 Ueno, with the content colored in red and the walls colored in green; in larger ectasias, the BGR score is more probable, as in cystic lesions. The inspissated ducts are hyper-/isoechoic but present the same strain as the fluid content, allowing the differential diagnosis with ductal papilloma, with a score 2 Ueno, or with DCIS, with a score 3 or 4 Ueno.

No indication for intervention or follow-up has been established for mild ductal widening. Irregular thickening, frond-like tissue, or masses within the duct should encourage biopsy because these may represent intraductal carcinoma or papillomatosis, which carries a high risk of malignancy; however, targeted biopsy is difficult to perform, and it can be replaced by a short-time follow-up on Doppler DE or by other noninvasive diagnoses, such as sonoelastography or breast MRI (Fig. 6.67).

Because there is no evidence in the literature indicating that mammary ductal ectasia is associated with an increased risk for breast cancer, it should be managed conservatively. However, ductal ectasia may be an indirect sign of breast cancer, located in the periphery of the ductal tree. The radial technique of acquisition is optimal for the illustration of the whole length of the pathological duct, increasing the detection rate of a ductal or lobular carcinoma. In such cases, Doppler examination completed by sonoelastography will be the noninvasive method of choice to evaluate the malignant risk because it is cheaper and more available than the breast MRI.

Some authors proposed various devices to aspirate the nipple surge for the screening of the breast cancer by studying its cytology; this is a false test of diagnosis, because not all breast cancers present ductal ectasia and aspirate and not all ductal ectasias allow nipple expression, some cases presenting very thin or obstructed excretory pores.

In the literature, there are few publications about the imaging diagnosis of the chronic galactophoritis in nonpuerperal cases.

FBU allowed a more precise location and description of the enlarged ducts in non-lactation period, and the bacteriological tests demonstrated only 3 % negative culture, while the rest presented infections with *Staphylococcus white haemolyticus*, *Staphylococcus aureus*, *Staphylococcus white*, *Staphylococcus epidermidis* (considered saprophyte but resistant to antibiotics), *Streptococcus haemolyticus*, and rarely *Pseudomonas aeruginosa*, *Escherichia coli*, *Candida albicans*, etc.

The chronic overinfection of a ductal ectasia or of breast cystic lesions (which can be associated) presents usually chronic inflammatory changes in the satellite axillary lymph nodes, described on pathology as benign histiocytosis, with a sonographic aspect characterized by normal cortical lymph node and vasculature, a benign-type sonoelastography, but a hypoechoic hilum, similar to the fatty tissue.

There were three described stages of the chronic galactophoritis:

- Simply ductal ectasia with/without nipple surge, with intraductal changes, and without stromal reaction
- The periductal stromal reaction, with infiltration demonstrated by SE with reduced elasticity outside the ducts; rarely there are Doppler changes
- The stromal fibrosis with ductal thinning with/without reduced fluid content and with nipple retraction, mimicking clinically and mammographically a breast cancer

The treatment with effective antibiotics and anti-inflammatory drugs may reduce the symptomatology in most painful breasts, and the correct diagnosis and follow-up FBU exams may reduce the unnecessary biopsies or surgical treatments.

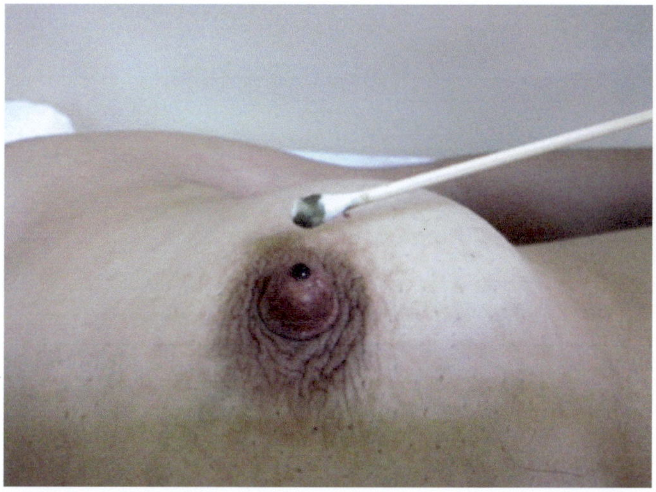

Fig. 6.67 Nipple surge with dark-green color in a ductal ectasia over-infected with *Staphylococcus white haemolyticus*. Note the absence of any clinical inflammatory signs of the skin

6.12 Galactoceles

Galactoceles, which occur during lactation or shortly after breast-feeding is stopped, are thought to be caused by an obstructed milk duct. At mammography, galactoceles may appear as an indeterminate mass, unless the classic fat-fluid level is seen. Even if the fat-fluid level is not seen, a benign finding can be determined if the fat can be identified within the mass. Classical US may show a complex mass. The diagnosis is made usually on the basis of the clinical history and aspiration, which yield a milky substance. We can also see multiple dilated tubular structures filled with echogenic material representing dilated milk-filled ducts. Given the clinical history and imaging findings, the complex mass is thought to be a galactocele.

FBU is essential in illustrating the ductal ectasia, filled with more or less hypoechoic fluid, the ductal connection with the galactocele that usually appears as a well-shaped mass; it has no internal Doppler signal but often presents peripheral increasing vasculature, which is salient in the whole breast-feeding as a characteristic sign. All clinical findings add history, pain and usually local inflammatory signs are suggestive, but Sonoelastography adds benign characterization, usually type BGR score upon Ueno.

6.13 Stromal Fibrosis

Stromal fibrosis is a frequent lesion that leads to misdiagnosis of both benign and malignant breast masses. Stromal fibrosis in the breast as a pathological entity is characterized by proliferation of stroma with obliteration of the mammary acini and ducts, which results in a localized area of fibrous tissue associated with hypoplasic mammary parenchyma. Stromal fibrosis has been named with a variety of terms including "focal fibrous disease of the breast," "fibrosis of the breast," "fibrous mastopathy," "fibrous tumor," and "focal fibrosis" of the breast.

The classical ultrasonographic appearance of the stromal fibrosis is described with different ranges from ill-defined hyperechoic tissue to a well-defined hypoechoic mass. Because there are no significant US signs, the diagnostic alternative is either short-time reexamination or diagnostic biopsy. FBU allows to differentiate the stromal abnormality from the pathologies of the ductal-lobular tree and thus to differentiate the lesion from the parenchymatous breast cancer. In addition, the benign aspect is characterized by the absence of new/hyperfocal vasculature. The posterior shadowing of the Cooper ligaments can be confusing, and SE with increasing strain indices could suggest a malignant lesion, but there is no concordance with the other signs on DE, and Doppler signal is reduced (Figs. 6.68, 6.69, 6.70, 6.71, 6.72, 6.73, 6.74, 6.75, and 6.76).

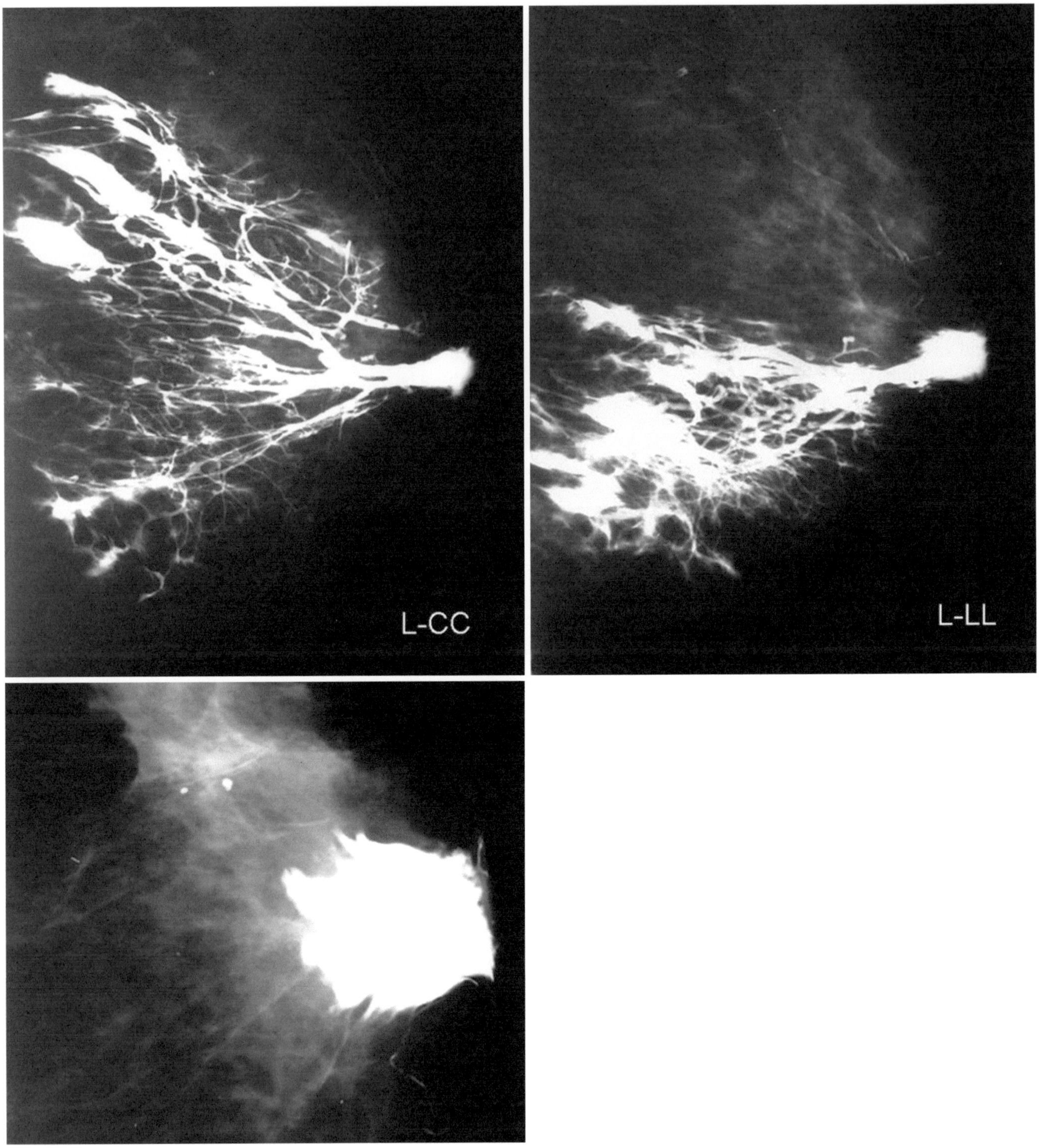

Fig. 6.68 Plain-film mammography with ductography: the duct size is artificially increased by the distention of the lumina after iodinate contrast agent injection and by the ductal flattening during mammographic compression; the ducts are superposed in a 2D projection, or may be not filled in, and thus may rest unexplored

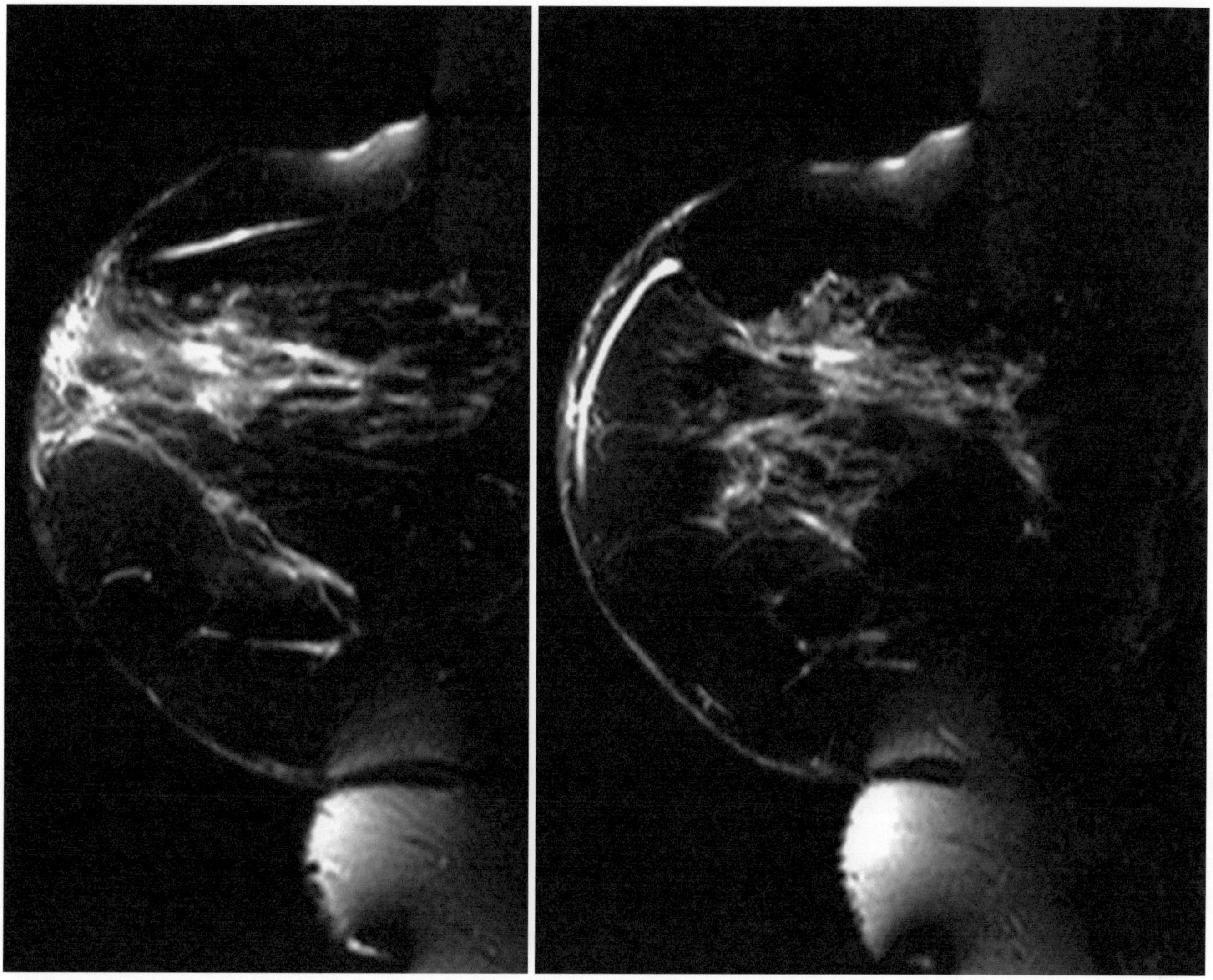

Fig. 6.69 Breast MRI with MIP reconstruction in the sagittal plan illustrates the breast' main galactophorous ducts oriented towards the nipple; they are straight because of the gravitational effect in the ventral decubitus; the technique is not usual, it is not anatomical unless for the 12:00–6:00 axe in the sagittal and 3:00–9:00 in the axial scans, but it is useful in illustrating the main ductal size

Fig. 6.70 Small ductal ectasia presenting the "double line sign," determined by the ultrasonic wave double reflection at the interfaces of the ductal walls with a few amount of fluid in the ductal lumen

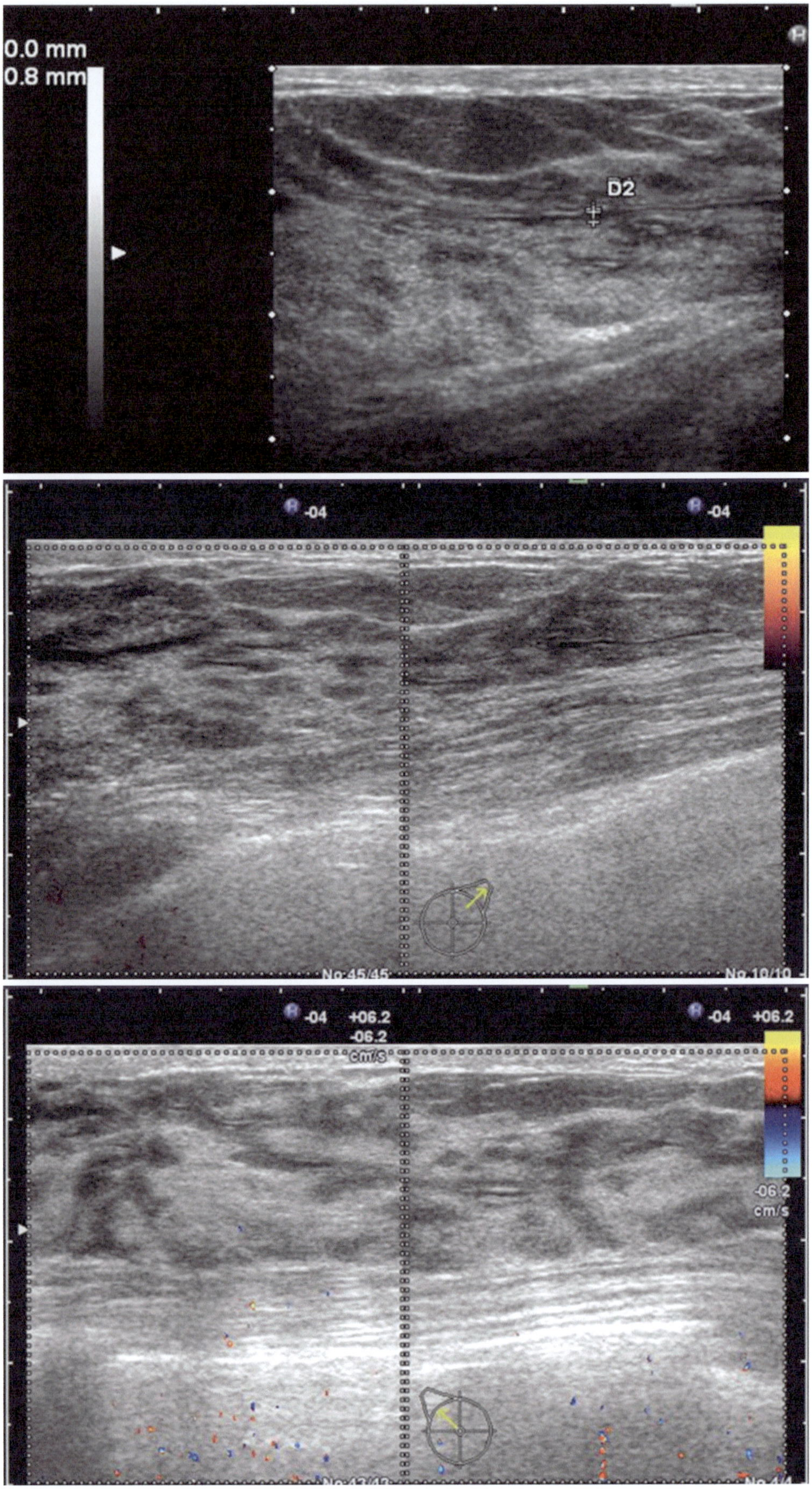

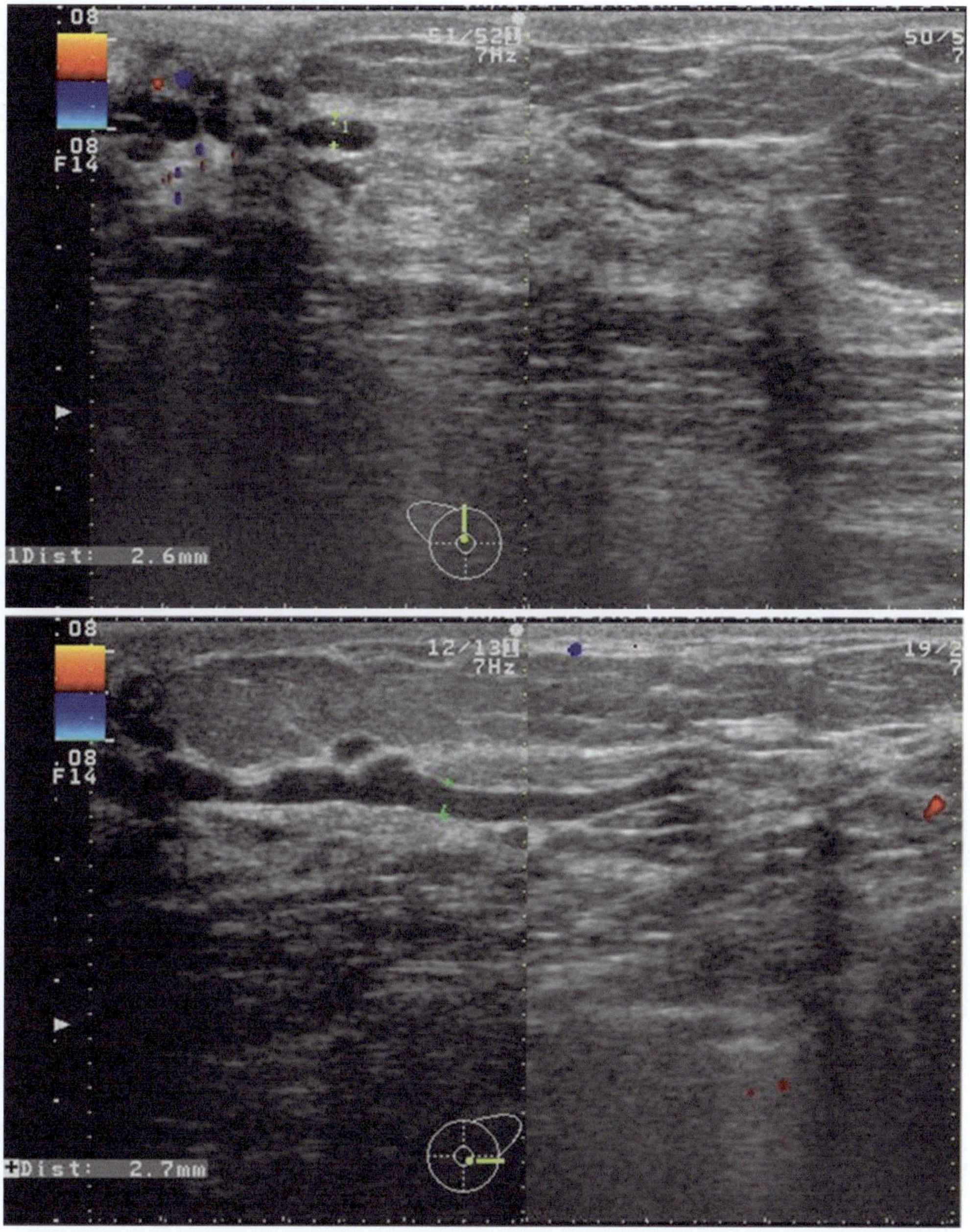

Fig. 6.71 Nipple surge with ductal-ampullary ectasia; the normal vasculature and the absence of any parenchymatous proliferations are significant for chronic secretory galactophoritis; the increasing echogenicity of the ductal fluid is correlated with high protein content and overinfection

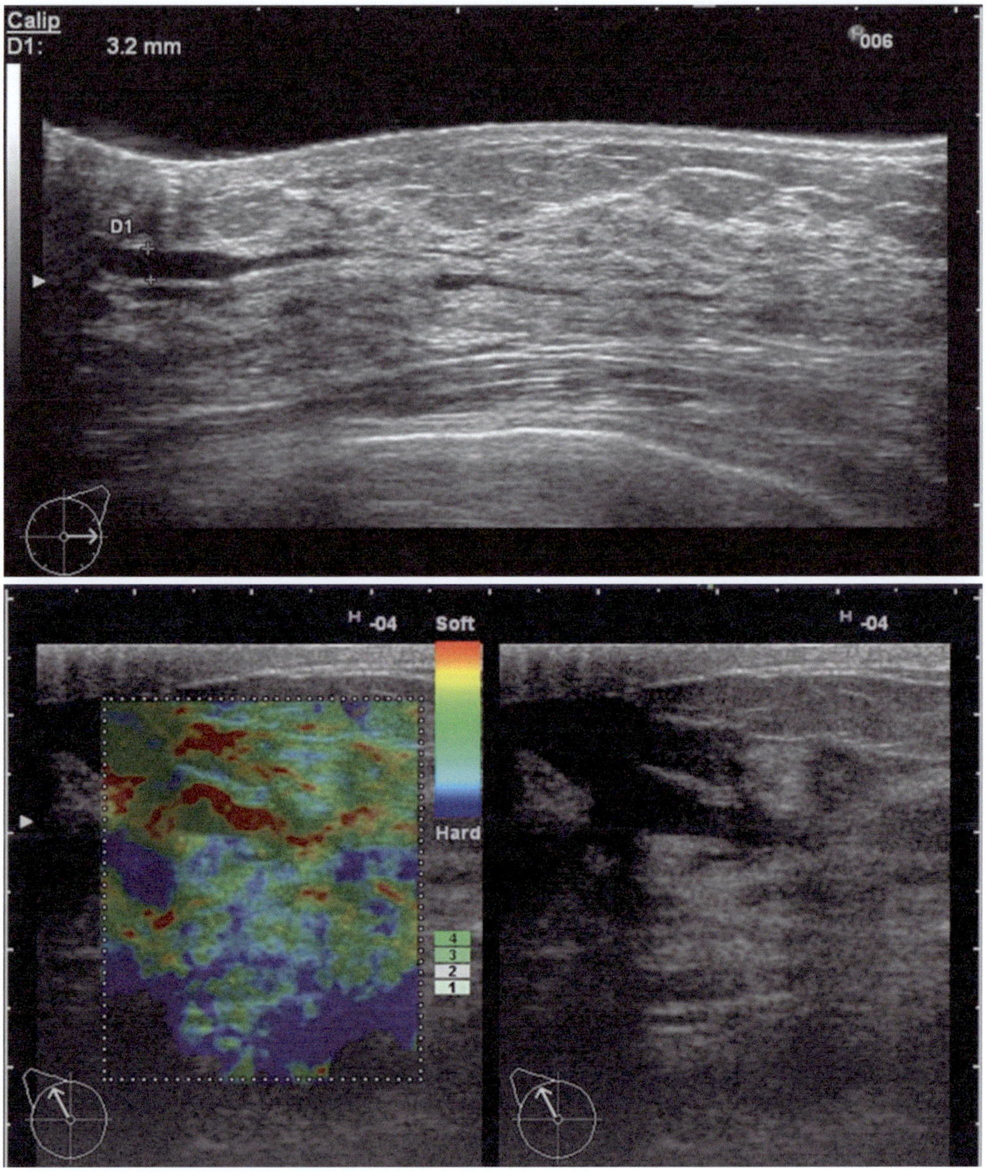

Fig. 6.72 Long probe scan in a radial plane better demonstrates the ductal ectasia; the sonoelastography presents a score 1 Ueno or BGR in significant enlargements of the ducts

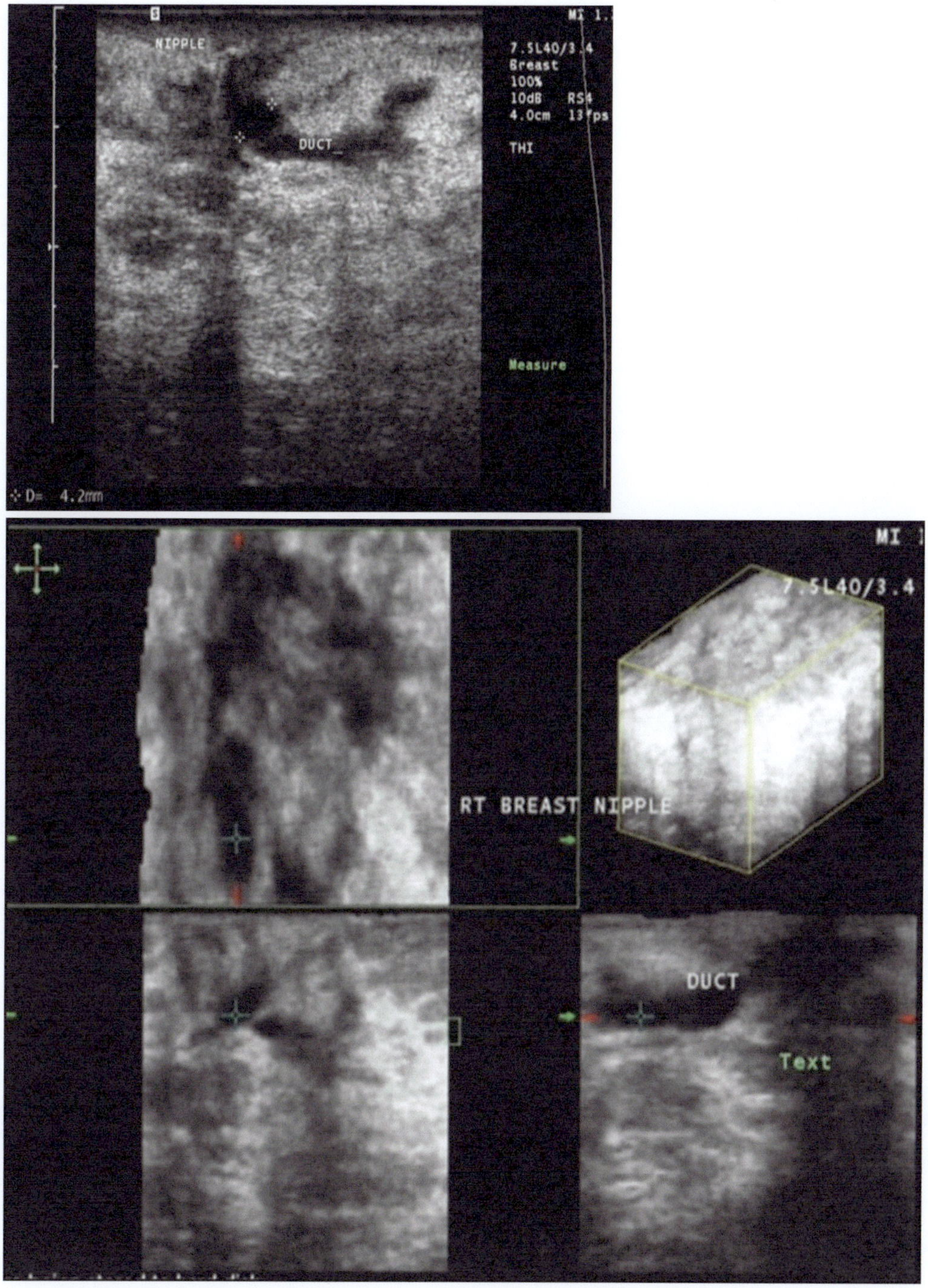

Fig. 6.73 Ductal anatomy in 3D US: the centripetal orientation towards the nipple and the cylindrical shape without Doppler signal are conclusive. The ductal ectasia was chosen for better illustration

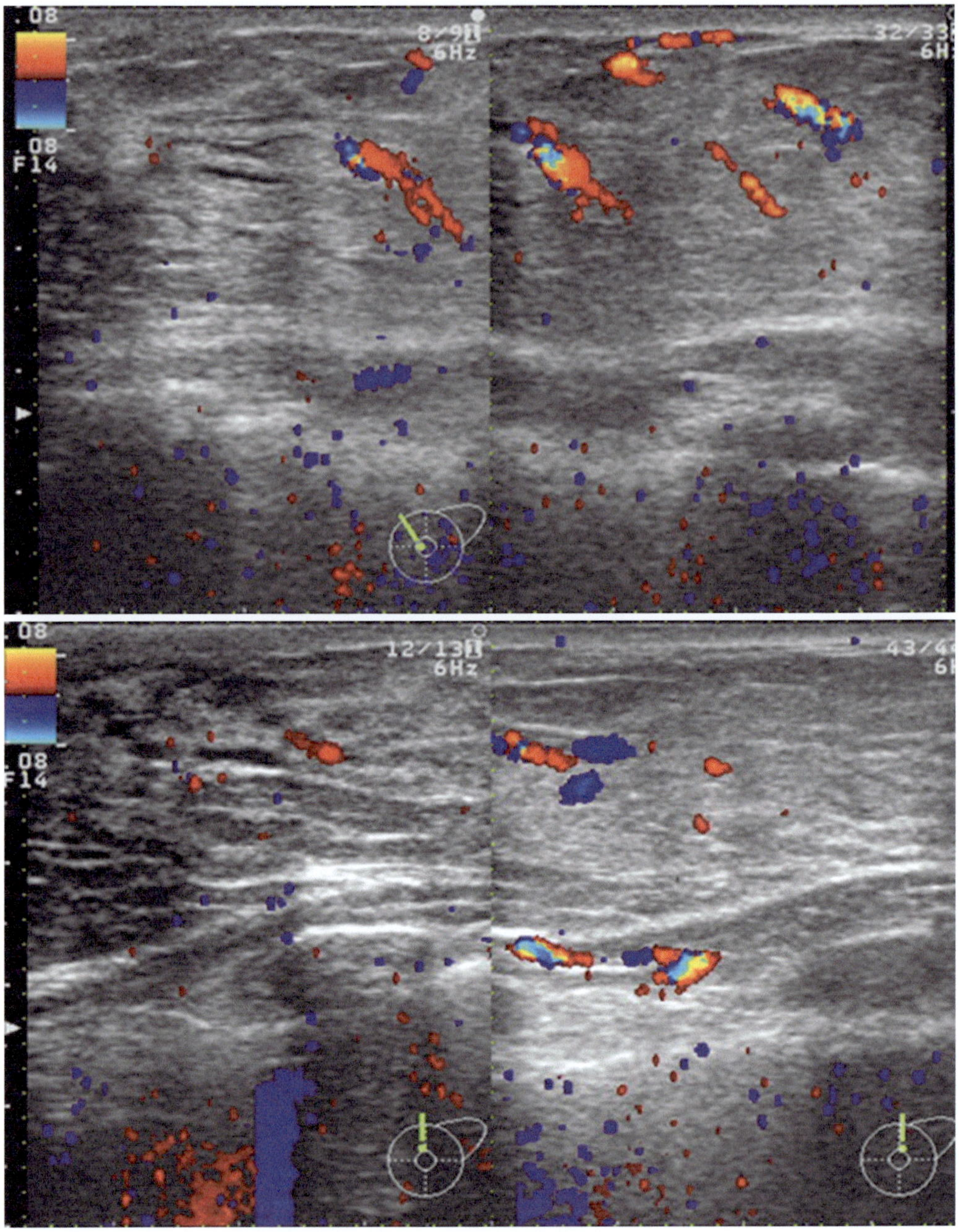

Fig. 6.74 Normal breast-feeding aspect in a 30-year-old patient presenting thin subcutaneous and retromammary fatty tissue, less echogenicity of the reduced amount of glandular stroma, small ductal ectasia, confluent glandular lobules, and a pathognomonic diffuse increased vasculature (high resolution of composed double screen radial images with a usual short probe)

Fig. 6.74 (continued)

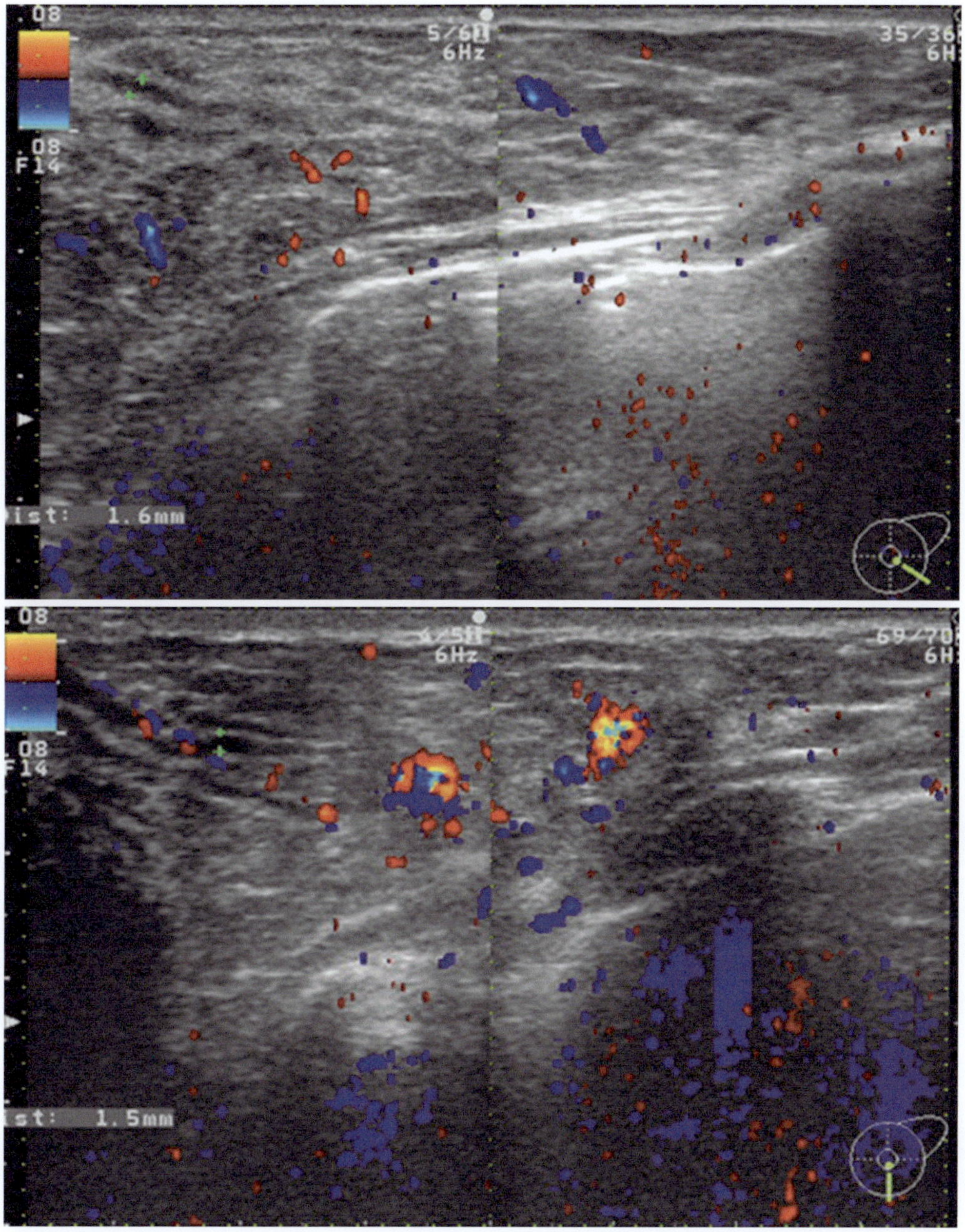

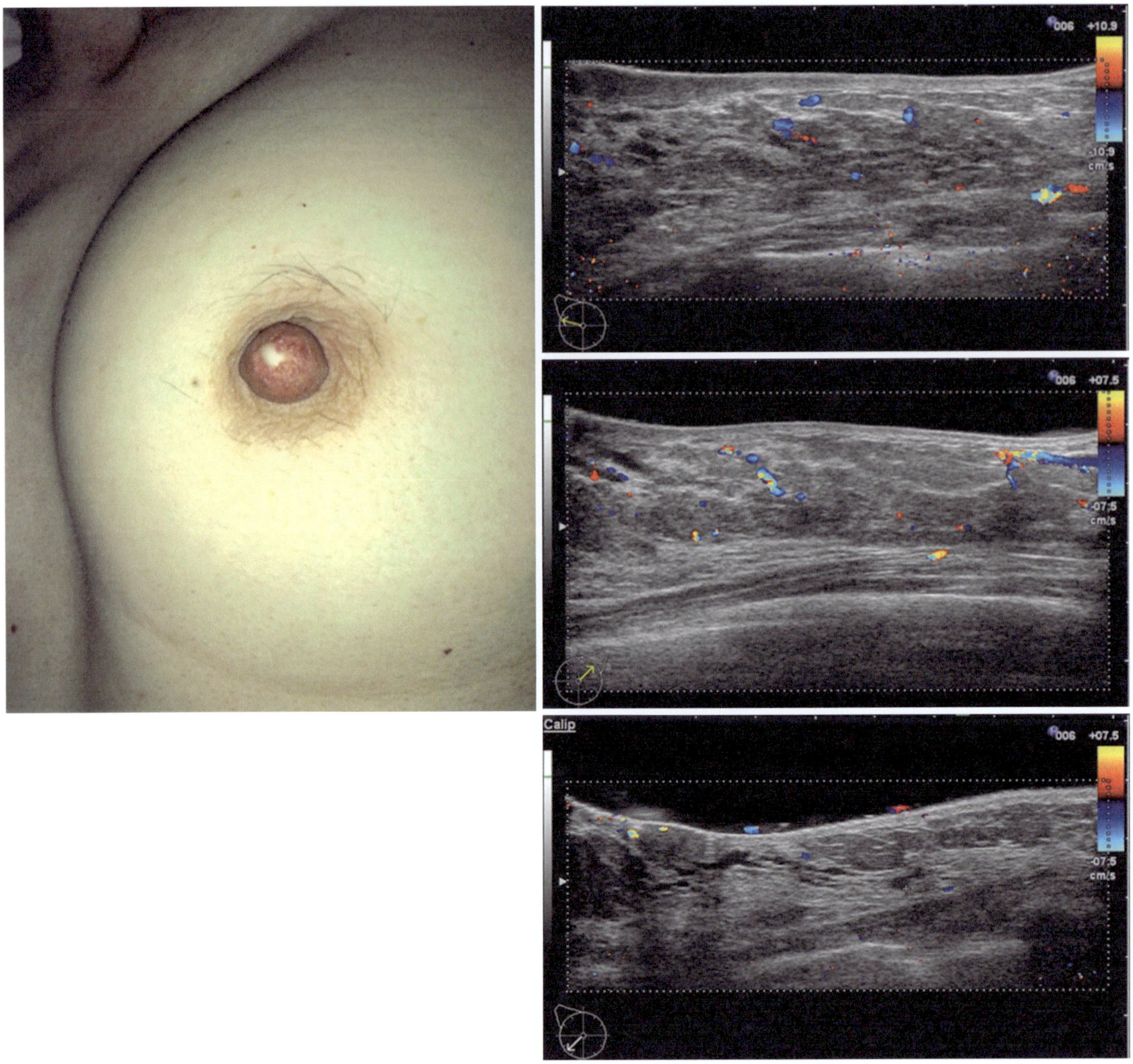

Fig. 6.75 Galactorrhea may/may not present spontaneous milky surge, or the nipple expression may be not positive, but DE illustrates diffuse ductal ectasia, lobular hypertrophy usually with confluent borders, and salient diffuse increased breast vasculature, a pathognomonic sign for physiological or pathological increase of the serum prolactin. Contrarily, the chronic overinfected galactophoritis does not present increased breast vasculature (water-bag long probe)

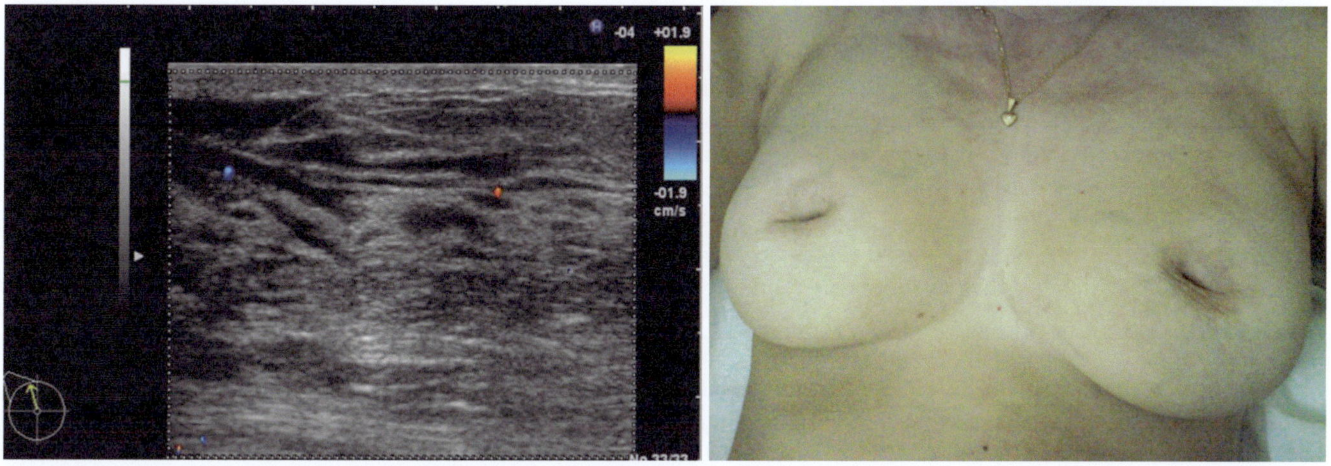

Fig. 6.76 Advanced stage of the chronic galactophoritis frequently presents nipple inversion/retraction, unilateral or bilateral, as in some breast cancer; the ductal ectasia may present various amounts of fluid, sometimes irregular ductal enlargement, or Cooper ligament increased shadowing; the diagnosis is based on the "normal" breast vasculature and absence of any suspected breast lesion

6.14 Breast Infections

Mastitis means in general opinion acute inflammation of the breast and may occur in the puerperal or nonpuerperal state and is generally rare in countries with medical assisted birth. The clinical signs respect the Celsius description: *rubor, rugor, tumor, and dolor*. The two most common types of microorganisms in acute mastitis are staphylococci and streptococci, and the imaging diagnosis is rarely requested.

Infections are believed to arise from breaks in the skin surface that allow the bacteria to enter the breast tissue, but there are many cases with *pillous folliculitis* infections or dermatitis following insects bites, without mastitis. In fact, mastitis must involve the breast lobes, with or without the surrounding fatty tissue and skin. In our experience, except penetrated trauma in the glandular mammary lobes, acute mastitis occurs from the lesions of the nipple and progresses to the periphery of the breast by the ductal tree way. Because mammary lobes may overlay but do not fusion and the lobar ductal trees do not communicate, it is possible to find mastitis isolated to a limited volume of the breast and other regions to remain uninfected.

The most frequent acute inflammation is recognized as the puerperal or lactation mastitis, which may occur in the epidemic or sporadic pattern. The epidemic pattern typically occurs in the hospital setting in nursing mothers. The small nipples, the nipple inversion, and bad hygiene during breast-feeding may initially develop nipple breaks, and then the inflammation progresses to the ducts and lobules and may extend to the lobar stroma and the surrounding tissues, including abscess formation and skin fistulae. There are few descriptions on the classical US in lactation mastitis; the main indication to perform US examination is to identify and locate an abscess that usually occurs in the subareolar location and to guide an incision and drainage associated with appropriate antibiotic therapy, which usually eradicates the infection without sequels. Doppler DE most accurately identifies the diffuse edema, the infected galactoceles which present echoic internal avascular fluid, and intense peripheral vasculature; the satellite lymphadenitis is usually present, with the preservation of the lymph node medullary hyperechogenicity at least in the periphery, but with global increased vasculature in the hilum and clinical tenderness. It is difficult to differentiate a normal breast-feeding from a diffuse mastitis, even in Doppler DE, because both of them illustrate dilated fluid-filled ducts and diffuse salient vasculature; however, mastitis is usually associated with skin thickening and subcutaneous fatty edema with hyperechogenic aspect and more homogeneous internal echoes, mainly in the lower quadrants, due to gravitational fluid migration.

The nonpuerperal subareolar infection is difficult to eradicate and may be indolent with recurrence, because it seems to be associated with breast chronic surge (secreting galactophoritis, sometimes secondary to a hormonal disturbance such as hyperprolactinemia), but the peripheral infection is not as resistant to treatment. Patients at risk for peripheral infections may have predisposing conditions such as steroid use or diabetes. We found peripheral infections of lobular cysts even in teenagers. Clinically, patients may present with a focal area of tenderness with associated erythema and pain. Classical US is performed in such patients to help identify a potential abscess collection that needs to be drained. We used FBU to precise the site and the connection of the potential infected lesion with the ductal tree, with follow-up examinations during antibiotherapy, and usually infected cysts were completely healed, while those noninfected, anechoic, and without peripheral pathological vasculature presented unchanged appearance (Fig. 6.77).

Therefore, there are much more patients with overinfected ductal ectasia, sometimes presenting yellow-green-gray nipple surge, without inflammatory periductal reaction clinically or in US, but with confirmed infection with *Staphylococcus white haemolyticus*, *Staphylococcus white*, *Staphylococcus aureus*, and others (*Streptococcus haemolyticus*, *Pseudomonas aeruginosa*, *Candida albicans*, *Escherichia coli*, etc.). We presented a retrospective analysis of 423 bacteriological tests in cases with ductal ectasia and nipple surge or aspiration from inspissated cysts, and we found in only 3 % cases of sterile probes but in 97 % cases with the presence of bacteria with significant increased resistance of antibiotics [5].

The chronic infection is sometimes confirmed by the chronic inflammation of the axillary lymph nodes, with pathological aspect of benign histiocytosis, and sonographic hypoechoic changes in the center of their hilum, without cortical or vascular abnormalities. Moreover, many pathological reports after surgical biopsies or treatments of various benign or malignant lesions affirm presence of lymphoplasmacytic interstitial breast infiltrate associated with lymph nodes histiocytosis.

As a routine, a cytological test from any colored nipple surge is recommended, but it is useful to add a bacteriological test. The main way for infection in the chronic galactophoritis has intuitively the nipple as entering point because the almost 95 % cases present a type of Staphylococcus as microbiological pathogen agent (Fig. 6.78).

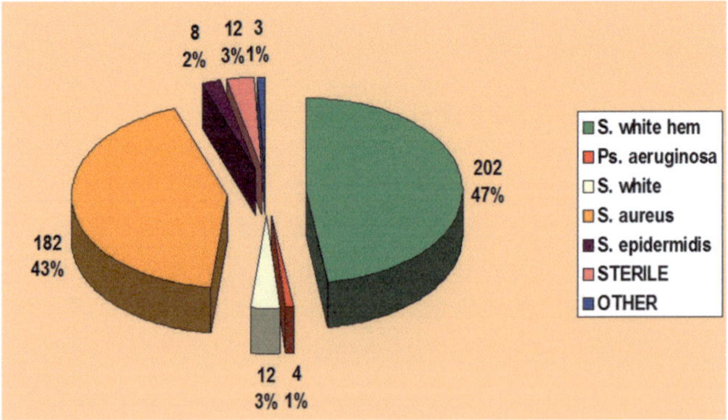

Fig. 6.77 Bacteriological test analysis of 423 samples with abnormal nipple surge: only 3 % of cases presented noninfected ductal ectasia, while the overinfected patients presented either clinical mastodynia or asymptomatic findings in screening examinations; most of chronic galactophoritis may be associated with fibrocystic dysplasia

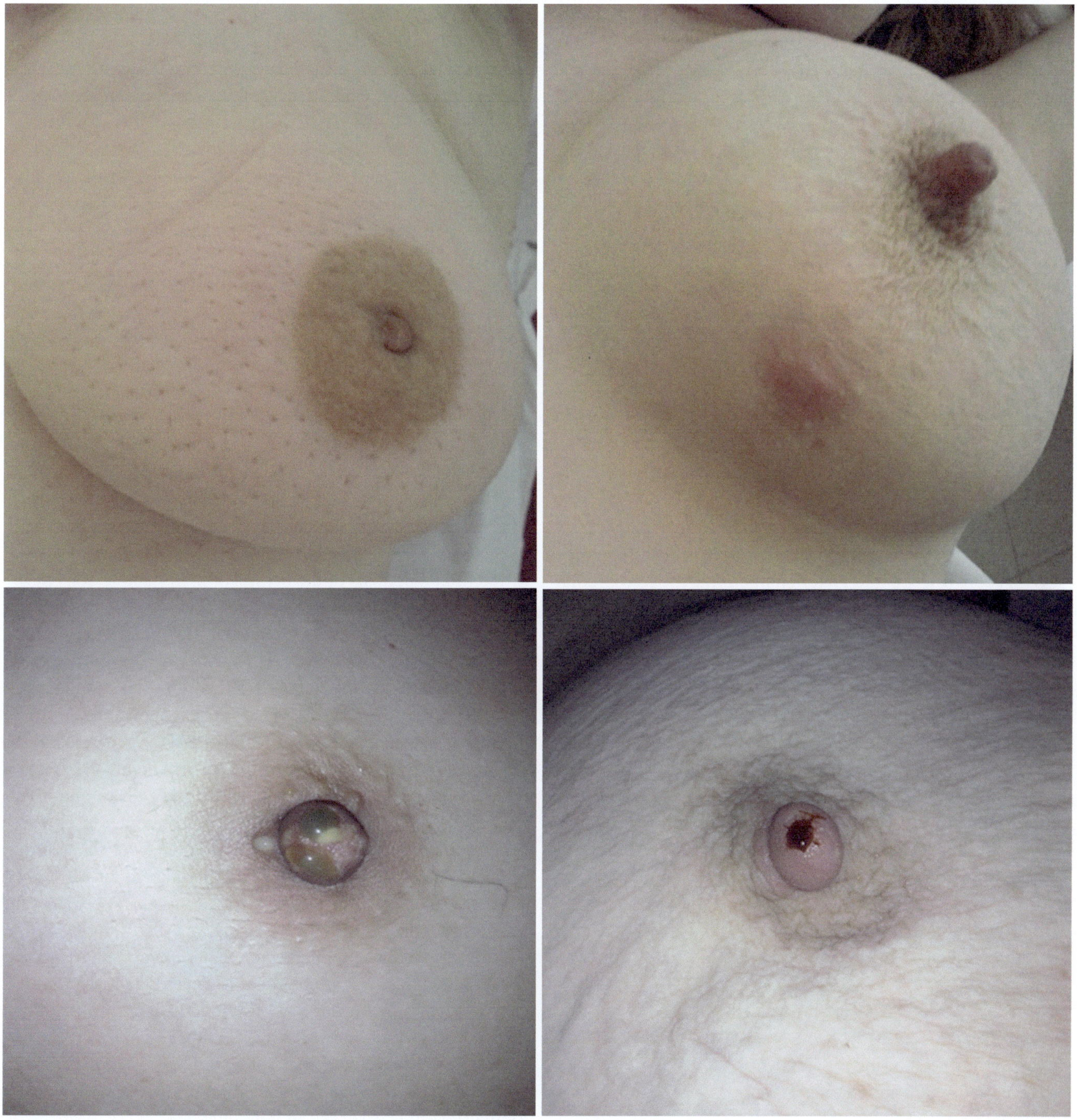

Fig. 6.78 Clinical aspect in acute mastitis (*above pictures*), the diffuse form with extended erythema, partial nipple retraction, and edema with orange peel skin; acute folliculitis has limited inflammatory area; the normal nipple is suggesting no ductal-lobular involvement. The chronic breast infection has no skin marks, but when the nipple surge may be demonstrated, we will identify abnormal color and viscosity. The bloody surge is benign in 80 % cases; the green color is usually associated with *Staphylococcus* or *Streptococcus haemolyticus* (*below pictures*)

6.15 Diseases of the Nipple-Areolar Complex

Usually, in the classical breast US, it is thought that the nipple-areolar complex is often best evaluated as a separate region of the breast [24]. We highlight that in ductal US the nipple is the starting point in any lobar acquisition and interpretation of the US scans and it is essential to establish the continuity of the retroareolar ducts, both in normal structures and ectasias, or to precise the eventually pathological mass location in relation with these structures.

For FBU examination of the nipple, we must respect some indications:

- To use much echo jelly avoiding air artifacts or better use a water bag attached to the transducer with optimal focuses and gain
- To perform at least two orthogonal scans or multiple oblique scans
- To always use Doppler facilities in the differential diagnosis
- To use sonoelastography that illustrates normal nipple with score 4 Ueno and better characterize the retroareolar structures neglecting the shadow artifact

In practice, clinical examination and screening mammography are still of central importance, but the results are unsatisfactory. Indeed, the clinical examination reveal in both benign and malignant nipple-periareolary region similar findings such as nipple discharge, thickening, and retraction; moreover, even with nonspecific mammographic views and with adjunct use of multiple imaging modalities (classical US, contrast material-enhanced magnetic resonance imaging, or both), it is often difficult to differentiate benign abnormalities from malignant ones [25].

Benign abnormalities of the nipple and of the areolar region may include:

- Mammary ductal ectasia or cyst—frequent
- Nipple calcifications
- Cutaneous horn of the nipple
- Abscess of the Montgomery gland
- Nipple adenoma

The most important malignant abnormalities of the nipple were described:

- Paget disease
- Breast carcinoma
- Primary lymphoma

Paget disease may be suspected in any persistent unilateral lesion; it is represented by DCIS, and the final diagnosis is established by nipple scrape cytology. Because there is a high risk of an underlying malignancy, present in over 80 % of cases, in most cases multifocal, frequently occult on mammograms and classical US, preoperative MRI is recommended in the selection of a conservative surgery [25]. Other authors found up to 92 % underlying carcinoma, even without any evident palpable mass (85 % cases), from which 73 % cases present multifocal evolution [26]. The differential diagnosis of Paget disease should be made with benign erosive adenomatosis of the nipple, pagetoid basal cell carcinoma, Bowen's disease, melanoma, eczema (that is bilateral), and cutaneous extension of a deep breast cancer. The mammographically findings may be isolated microcalcifications, mass associated with microcalcifications, or mass without calcifications. The widely used radiological-imaging examinations were not performing in the diagnosis of this disease, with up to 41 % negative mammograms in patients with clinically evident Paget lesions [27] and up to 64 % cases with unidentified underlying diseases in patients with no palpable mass and multifocal distribution [26].

The sonographic aspect is similar in all malignant lesions, the hypoechogenicity of the nipple and the shadowing are common findings in both benign and malignant pathology [27], but the presence of the hyper-vasculature is more suggestive for cancer.

The automatic breast scan with 3D reconstruction (the ABVS technique) intended for breast screening and offering the "plan C" for CAD diagnosis is not sufficient for the differential diagnosis of the benign or malignant lesions of the nipple-areolar complex, because of the lack of information about the vasculature and because the benign and malignant lesions intermix; moreover, the nonanatomical representations of the scans do not allow the identification of the connections between the nipple and the underlying malignancies.

Sonoelastography has some technical observations for this location. It is difficult to be performed in the nipple-areolar complex, because of accidental relief; using an increased amount of ultrasound gel for avoiding air artifacts may reduce the sensibility of the method, and the oblique scans are not correct because the strain is unequal. However, sonoelastography is useful in most cases, especially in umbilicated (inverted) nipples and areolar pathologies. Some conditions, such as nipple retraction and inversion, may have either a benign or a malignant etiology, and the history of the case completed with the FBU findings is useful in the diagnosis. The retroareolar tissues are better illustrated by sonoelastography than by US in 2D or 4D acquisitions, and the connection of the pathological nipple with distant ductal-lobular lesion is essential in the diagnosis.

There are two types of nipple inversion:

- Retractile/umbilicated nipple—reversible, the nipple can be pulled out (everted).
- Invaginated nipple—true inversion, congenital or acquired, where the nipple cannot be everted.

Congenital inversion is rare, and it is thought to result from a failure of the underlying mesenchyma to proliferate and push the nipple from its depressed position, but in fact, there is a complex pathology, with hypoplasia of the excretory ducts and pores, with further troubles in breast-feeding.

Almost 3 % of the women [28] present inverted nipple from which 73–92 % is the retractile type, with the bilateral condition occurring in almost 87 % cases [29]. The acquired cases are more frequent; some resolve themselves during pregnancy, while others are progressive, when untreated, most cases being associated with underdiagnosed chronic galactophoritis (Fig. 6.79, 6.80, 6.81, 6.82, 6.83, 6.84, 6.85, 6.86, 6.87, 6.88, 6.89, 6.90, 6.91, 6.92, 6.93, 6.94, and 6.95).

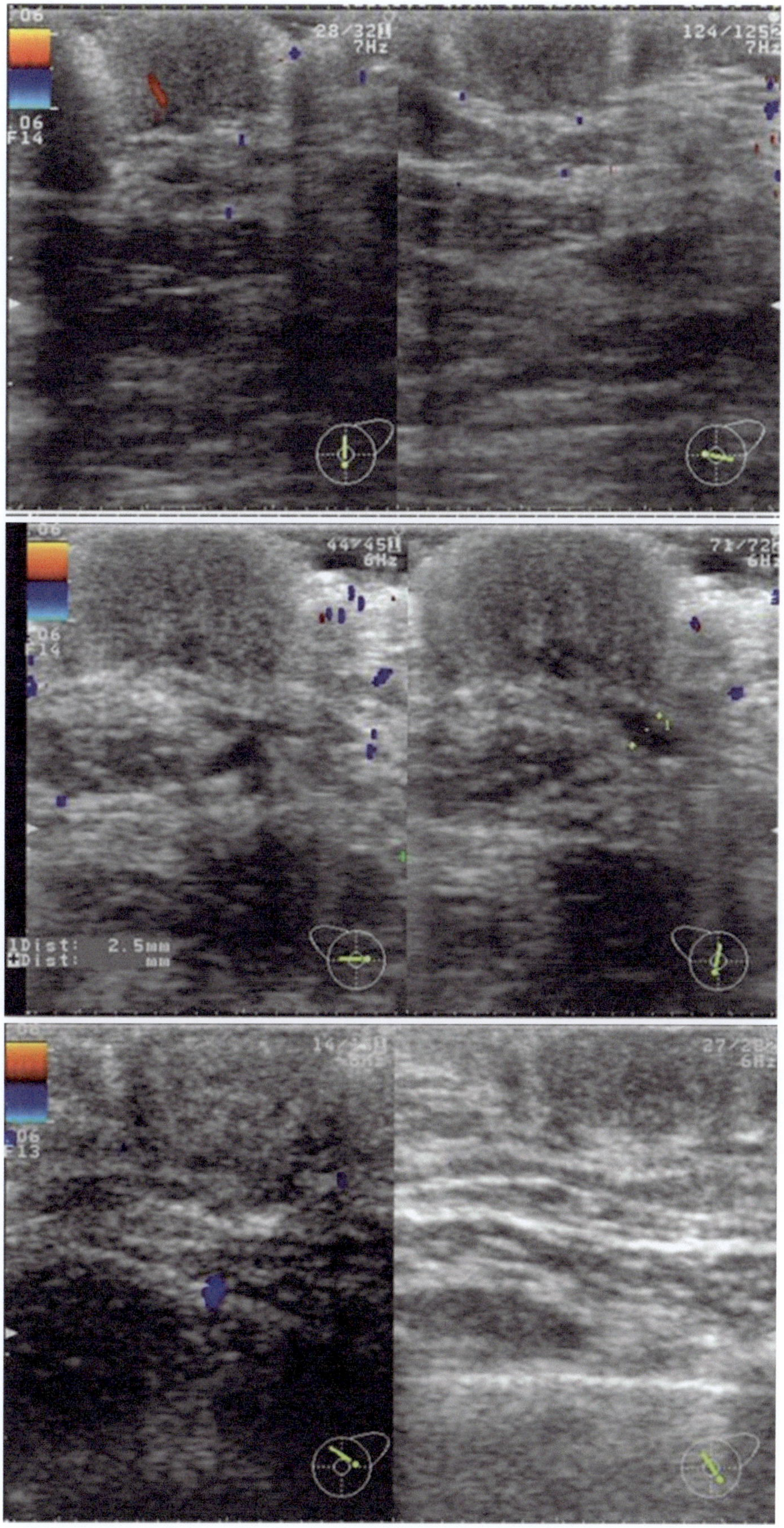

Fig. 6.79 Normal nipple with convergent ductal-ampullary parenchyma beneath it; an amount of ultrasound gel is necessary to avoid the surrounding air artifact

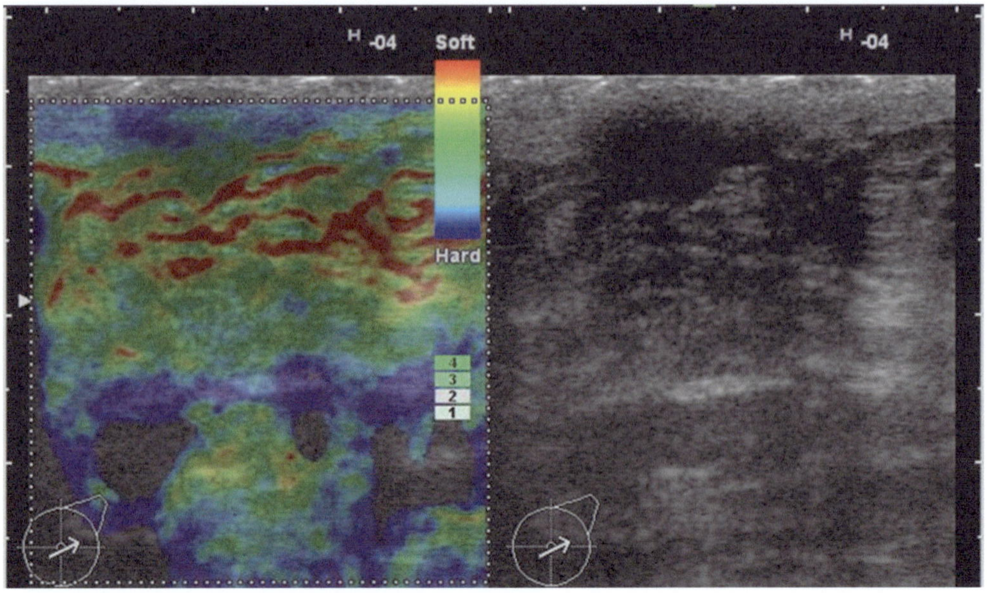

Fig. 6.80 Sonoelastography of the normal nipple presents a score 4 Ueno, with normal underlying parenchyma having a score 1 Ueno. Sonoelastography is useful even in cases with retroareolar artifacts in 2D US

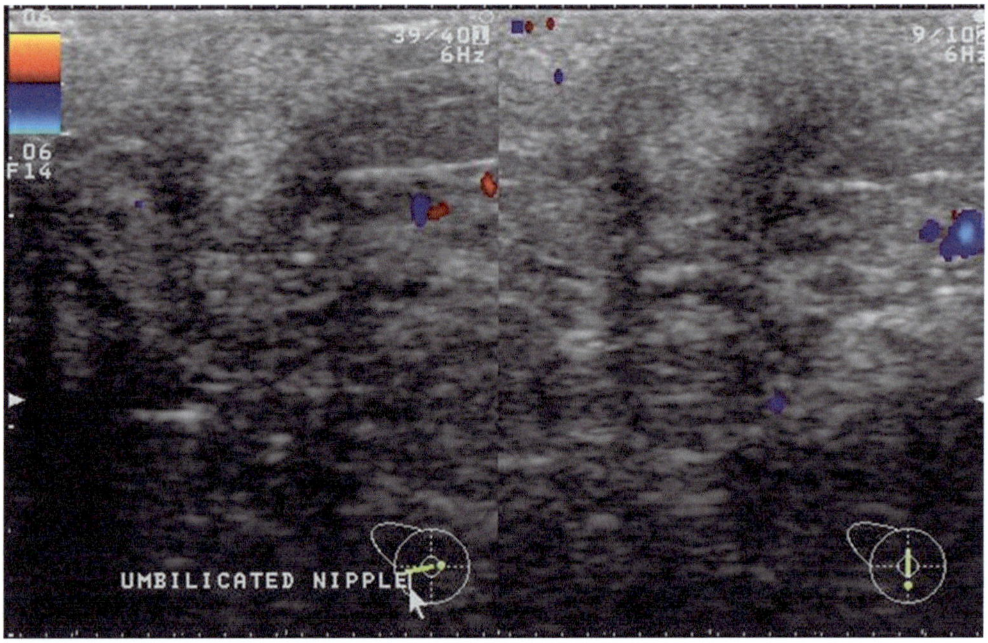

Fig. 6.81 Umbilicated nipple in a 28-year-old patient: the connection with the skin, the absence of the subcutaneous fatty tissue in the retroareolar area, the ductal-ampullary convergent structures without ectasias, and few vessels on color Doppler are the "normal" aspects

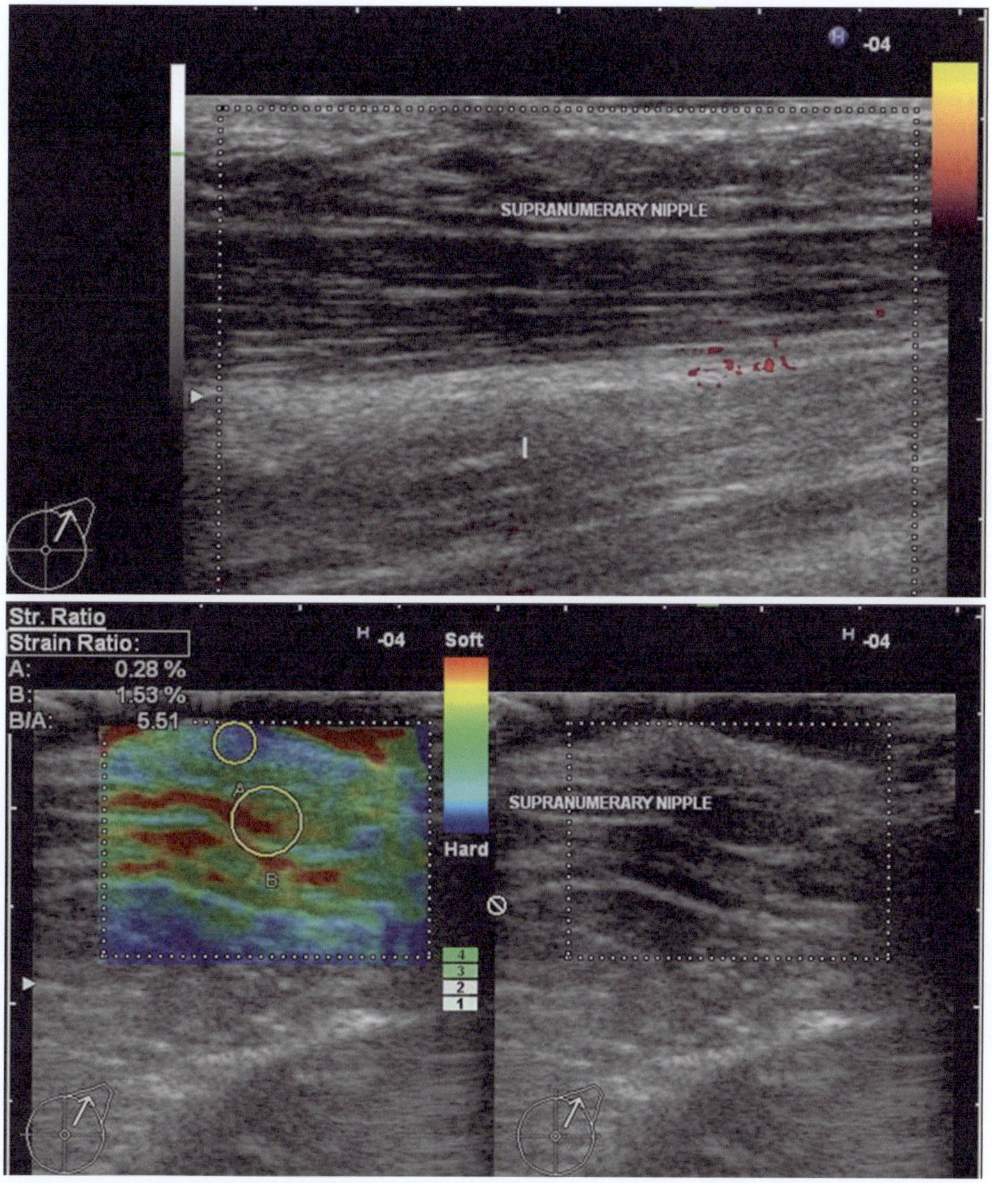

Fig. 6.82 Supernumerary nipple in a supernumerary breast in the axillary end of the mammary crest; the high strain ratio of the small nipple and of the mammary bud is similar to a normal breast

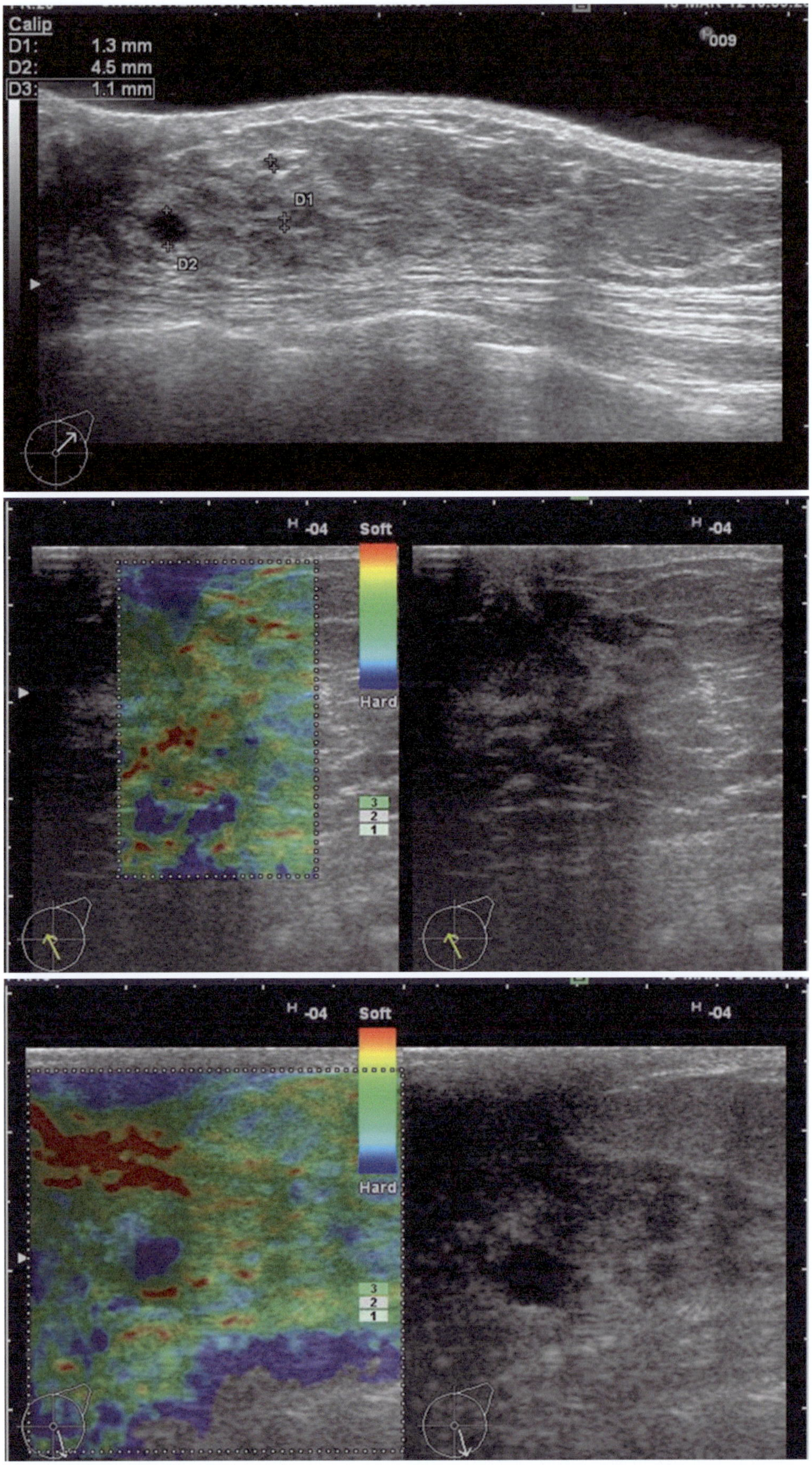

Fig. 6.83 Retroareolar ductal ectasia and cystic dysplasia, with benign aspect; sonoelastography of score 1 Ueno and BGR is "clarifying" the retroareolar shadowing artifact

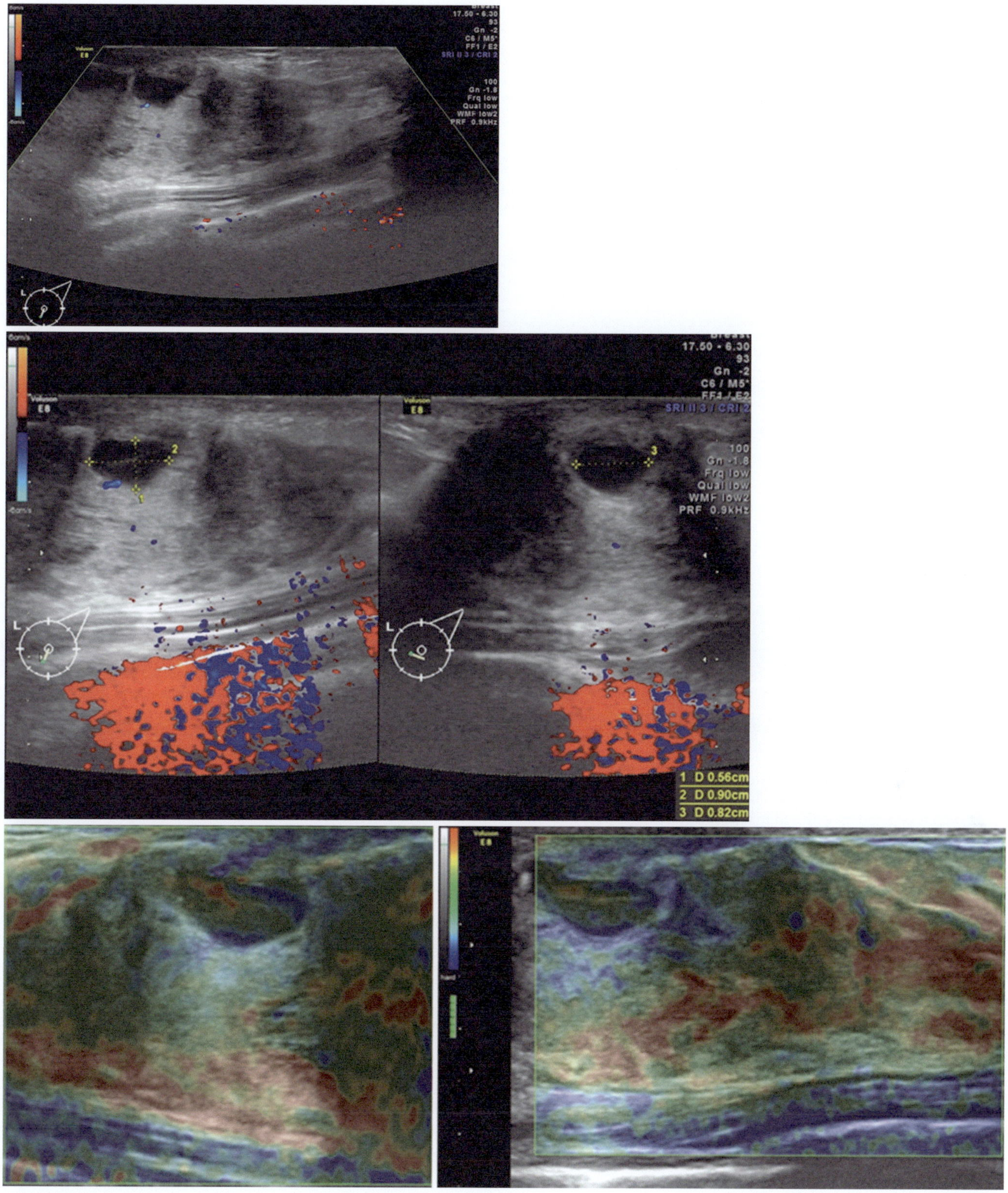

Fig. 6.84 Retroareolar cystic lesion inside the mammary branching bud in a 14-year-old patient; note the dense glandular parenchyma, with low amount of stroma characteristic to the development stage of the breast

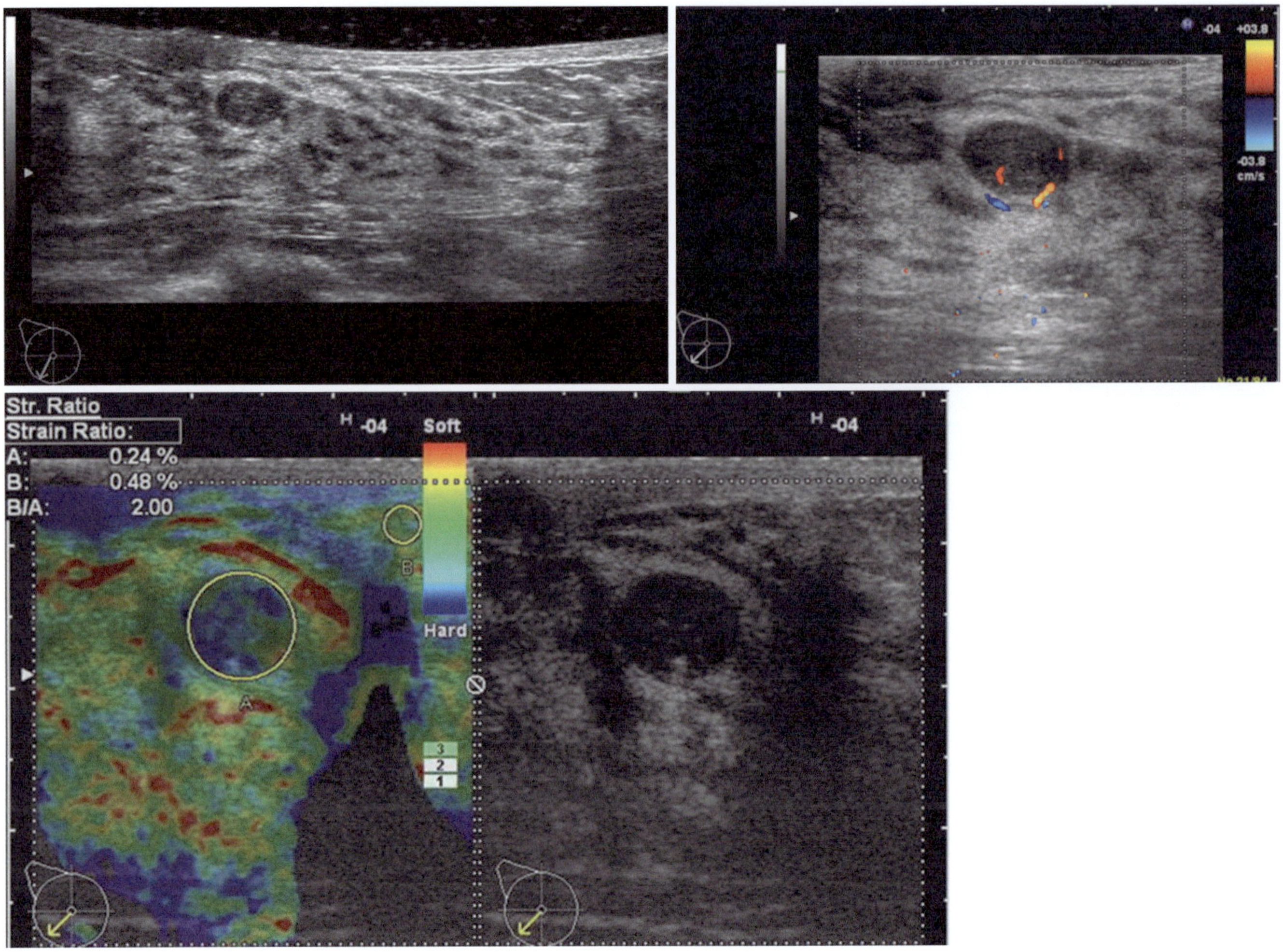

Fig. 6.85 Retroareolar solid-type lesion with benign characteristics based on Stavros, benign-type vasculature, and a score 2 Ueno with low strain ratio is concordant with a fibroadenoma; FBU is sufficient for the positive diagnosis, avoiding unnecessary biopsy, and the surgical treatment is temporized in subcentimetric lumps

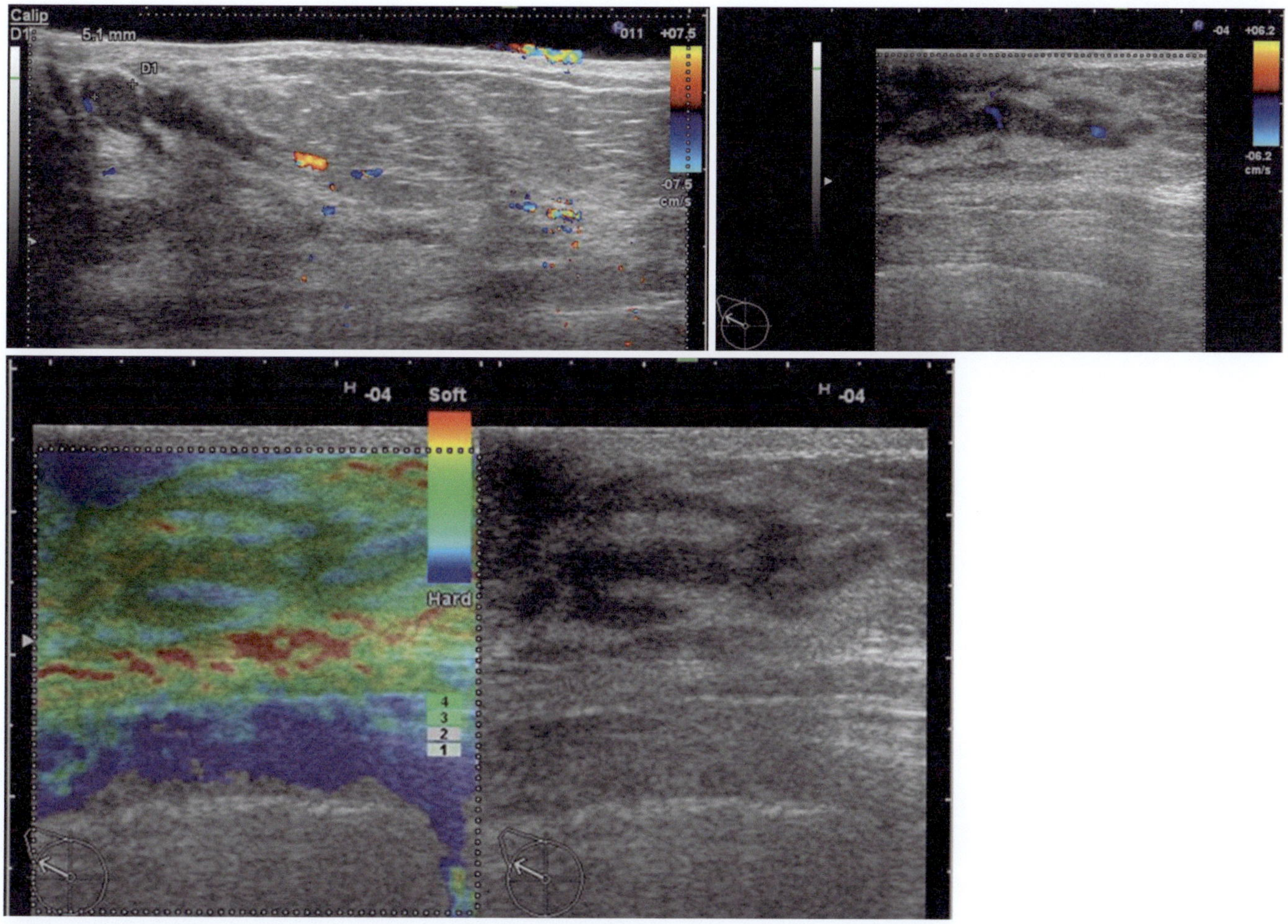

Fig. 6.86 Retroareolar ductal ectasia with small papillomas and periductal hyperemia (upper image); the differential diagnosis with ductal hyperplasia and IDCS is based on FBU evaluation, in this case the benign aspect being more probable (*middle and lower images*)

Fig. 6.87 Typically benign retroareolar complex: ductal ectasia with isoechoic content and score 1 Ueno, associated with cystic lesion of BGR score

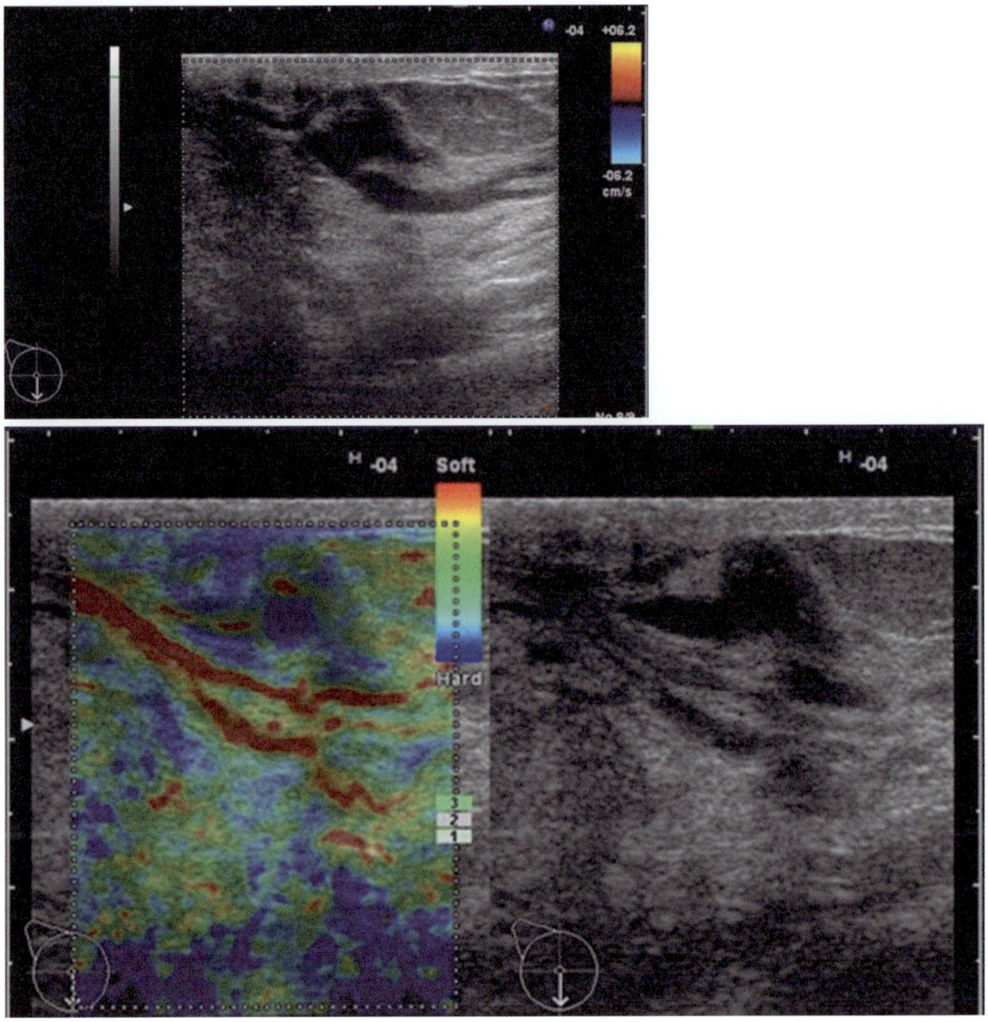

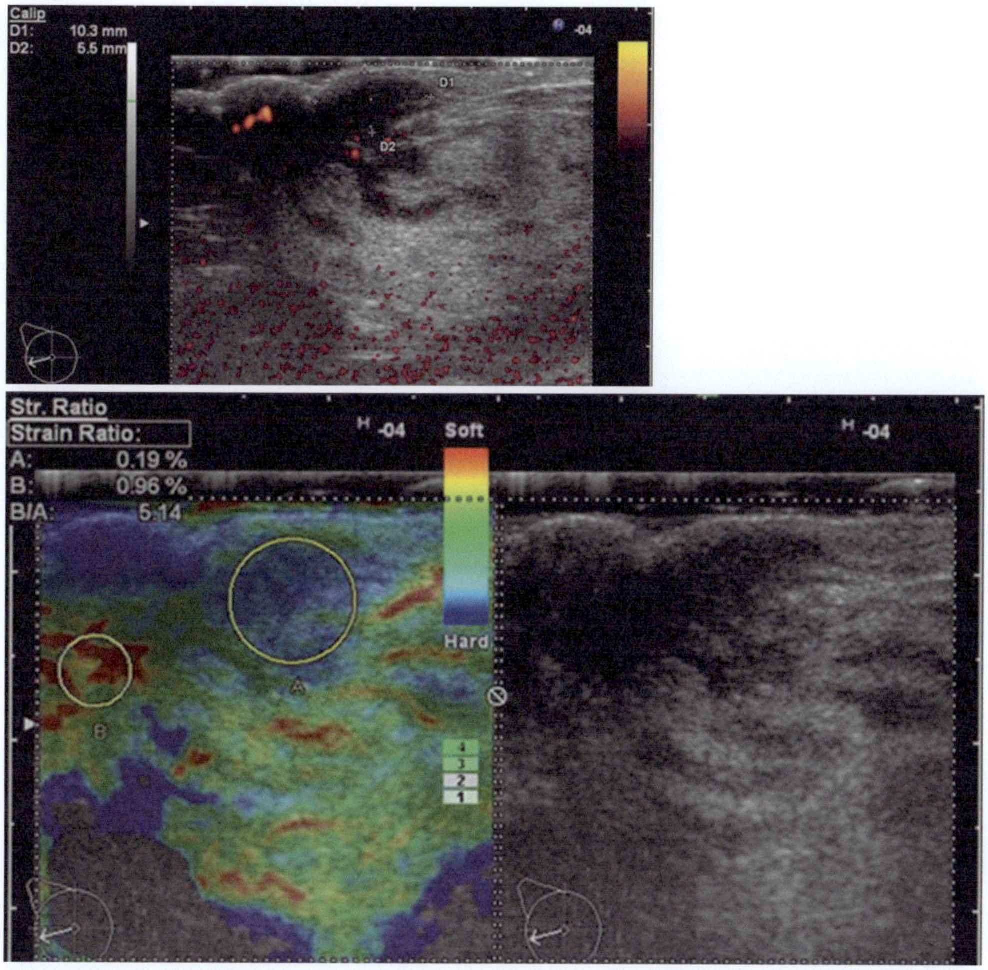

Fig. 6.88 Thickening of the nipple-areolar complex and of the emerging ducts, with new formation vasculature and high strain ratio, suggesting a suspect proliferative lesion

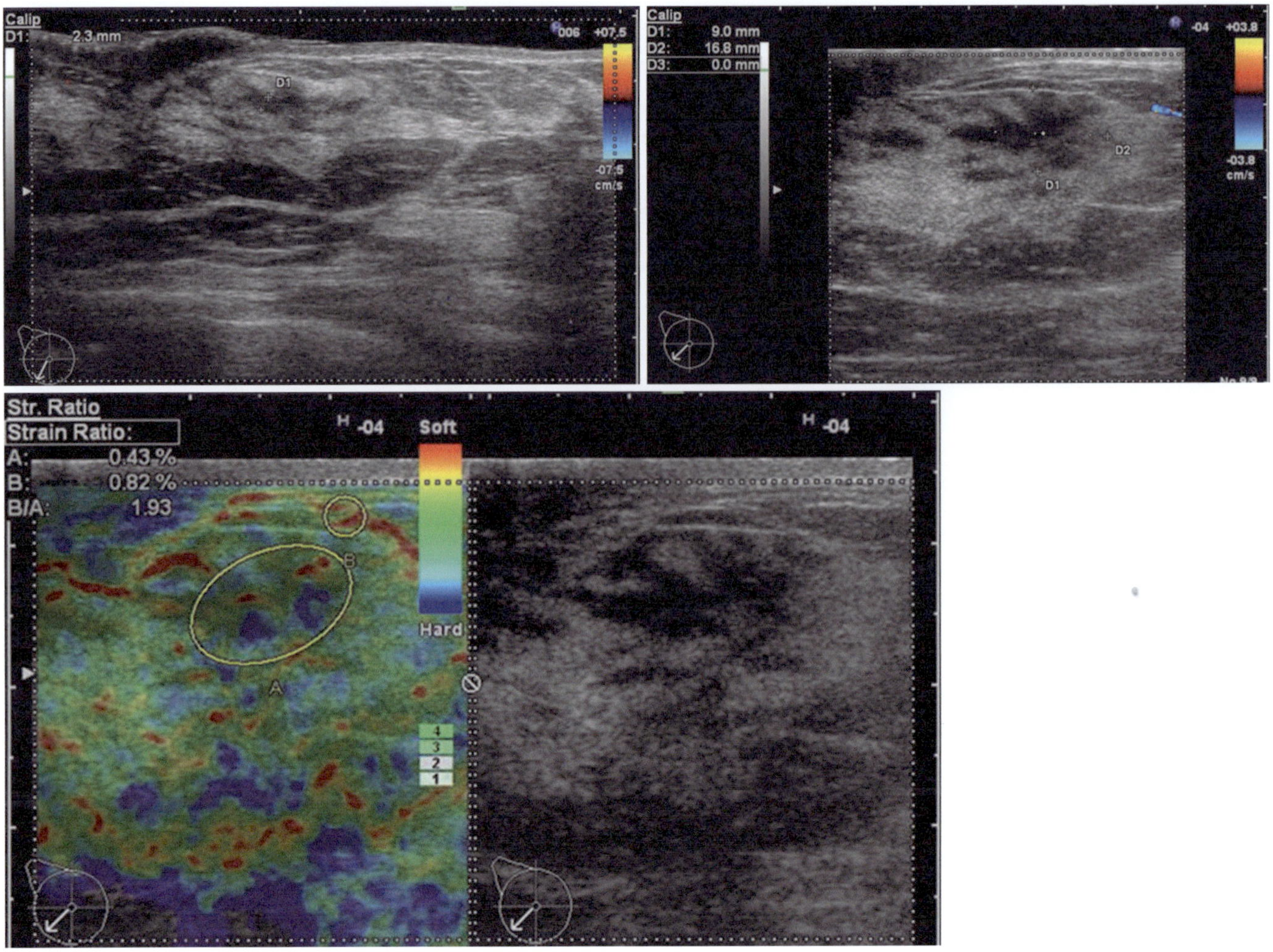

Fig. 6.89 Thickening of a radial group of retroareolar ducts, with abnormal architecture and intense hypoechoic aspect, but without posterior shadowing or new vasculature and with benign-type sonoelastogram; a BI-RADS 3 assessment with 6-month FBU follow-up examination is recommended

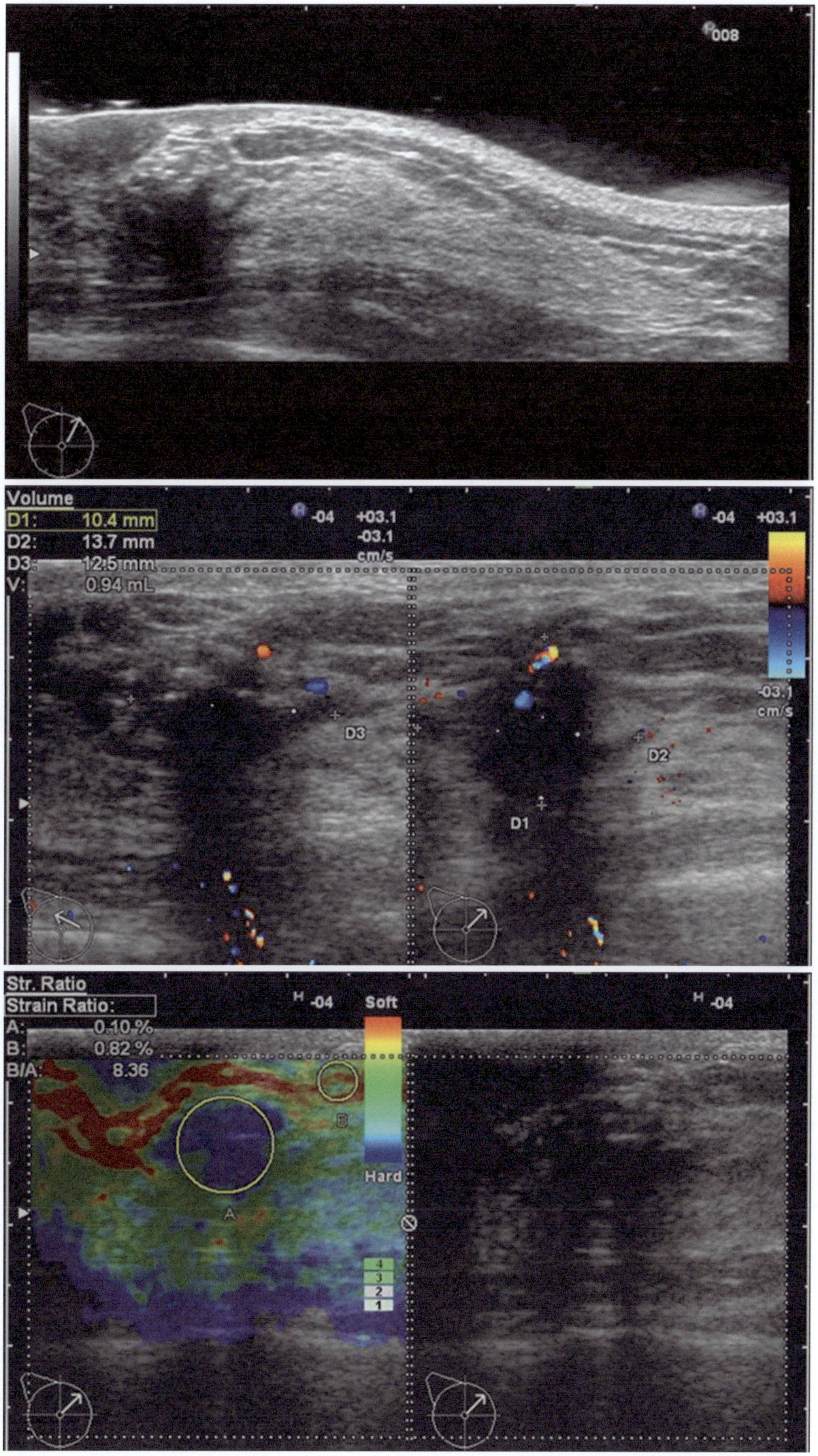

Fig. 6.90 Retroareolar deep mass with thickening of the surrounding ducts, having malignant features based on Stavros in 2D US, malignant-type vasculature with incident plugging angle and a score 4 Ueno with high FLR up to 8.36; the normal nipple is demonstrated by the sonoelastography that does not detect any hardness between the two structures

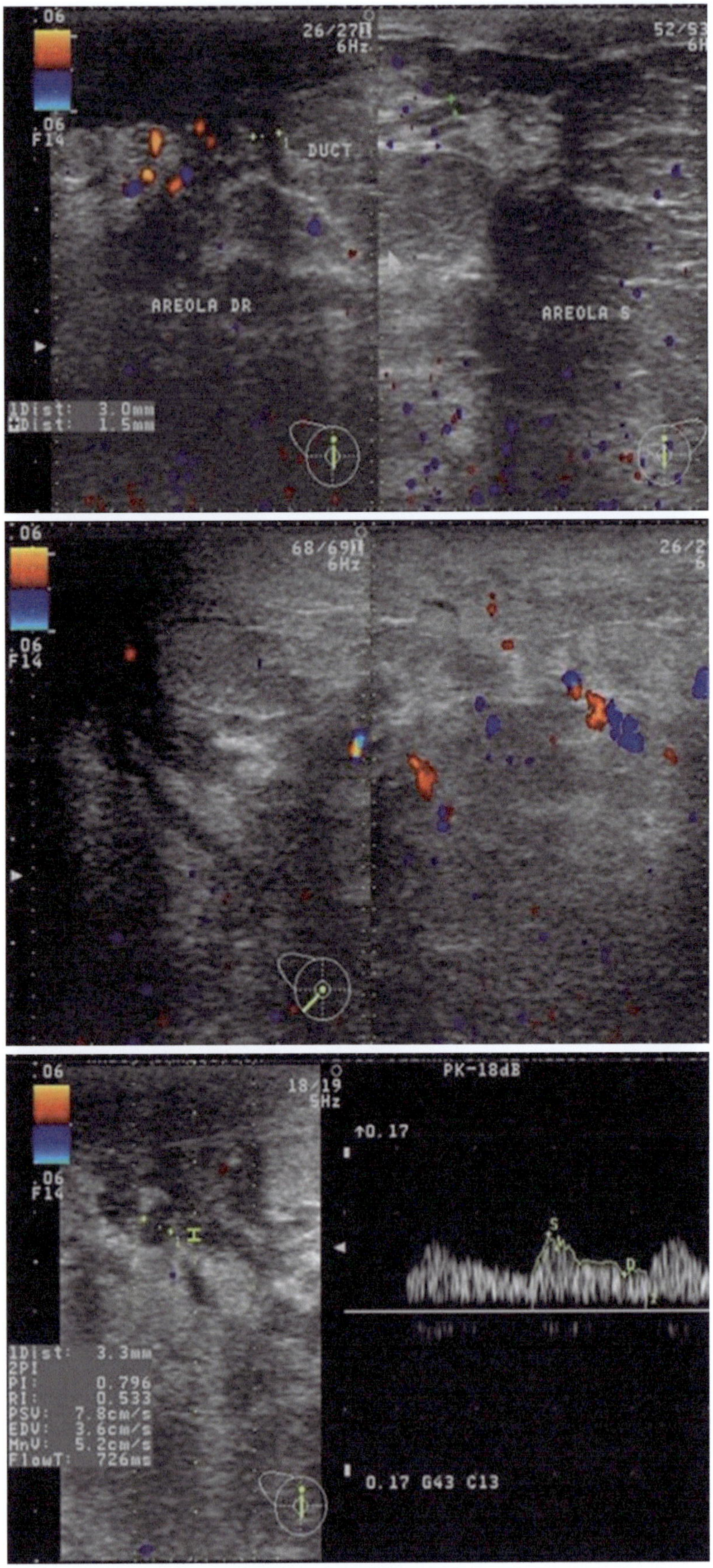

Fig. 6.91 Thickening of the nipple and areola, with extension through the emerging ducts and new formation vasculature of low velocity indices (RI, 0.53; PI, 0.79), suggesting malignant Paget disease

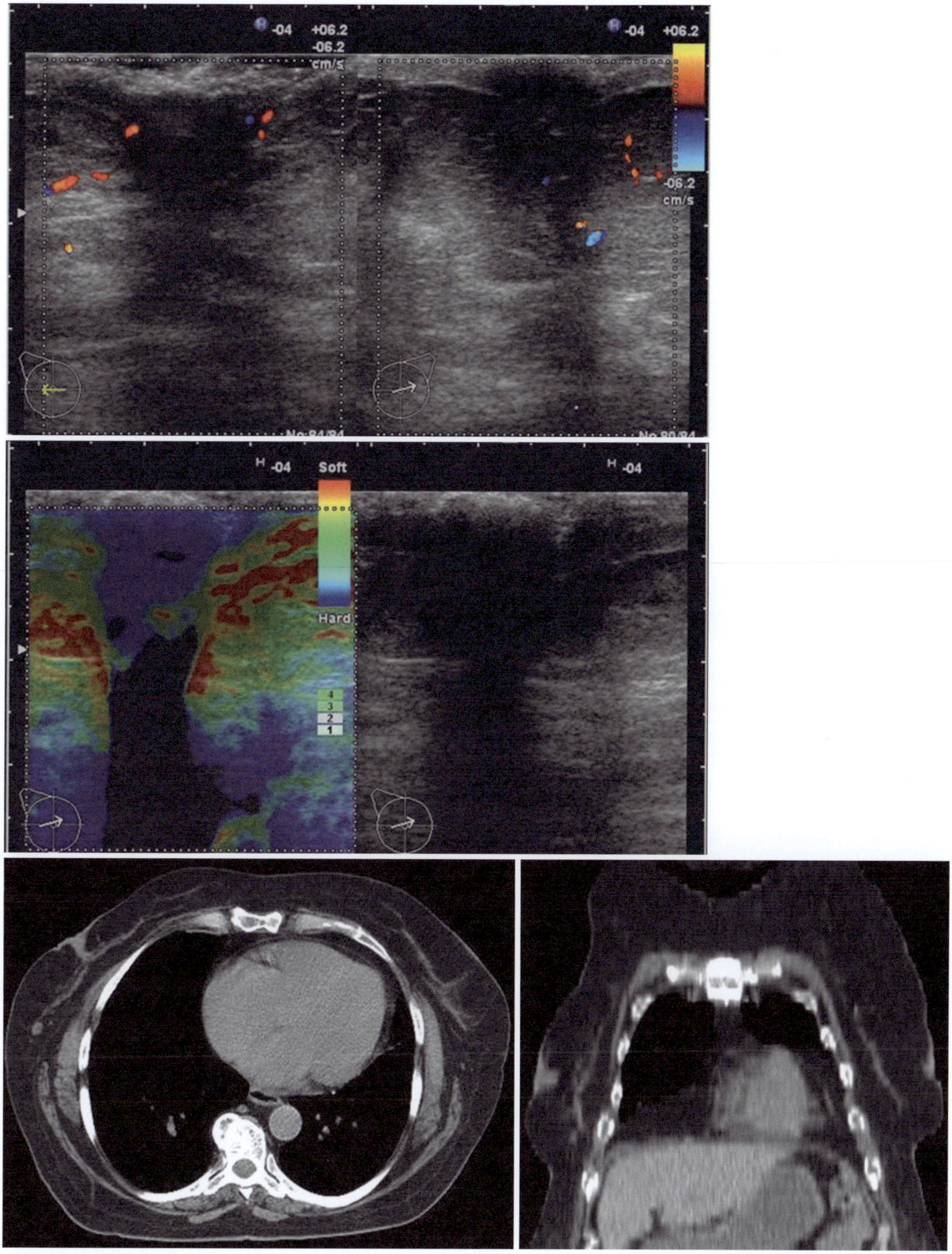

Fig. 6.92 Retroareolar malignant lesion connected to the nipple in an 84-year-old patient with Paget disease. Both FBU and CT of the same patient are illustrative for the pathological development from the deep central breast towards the nipple

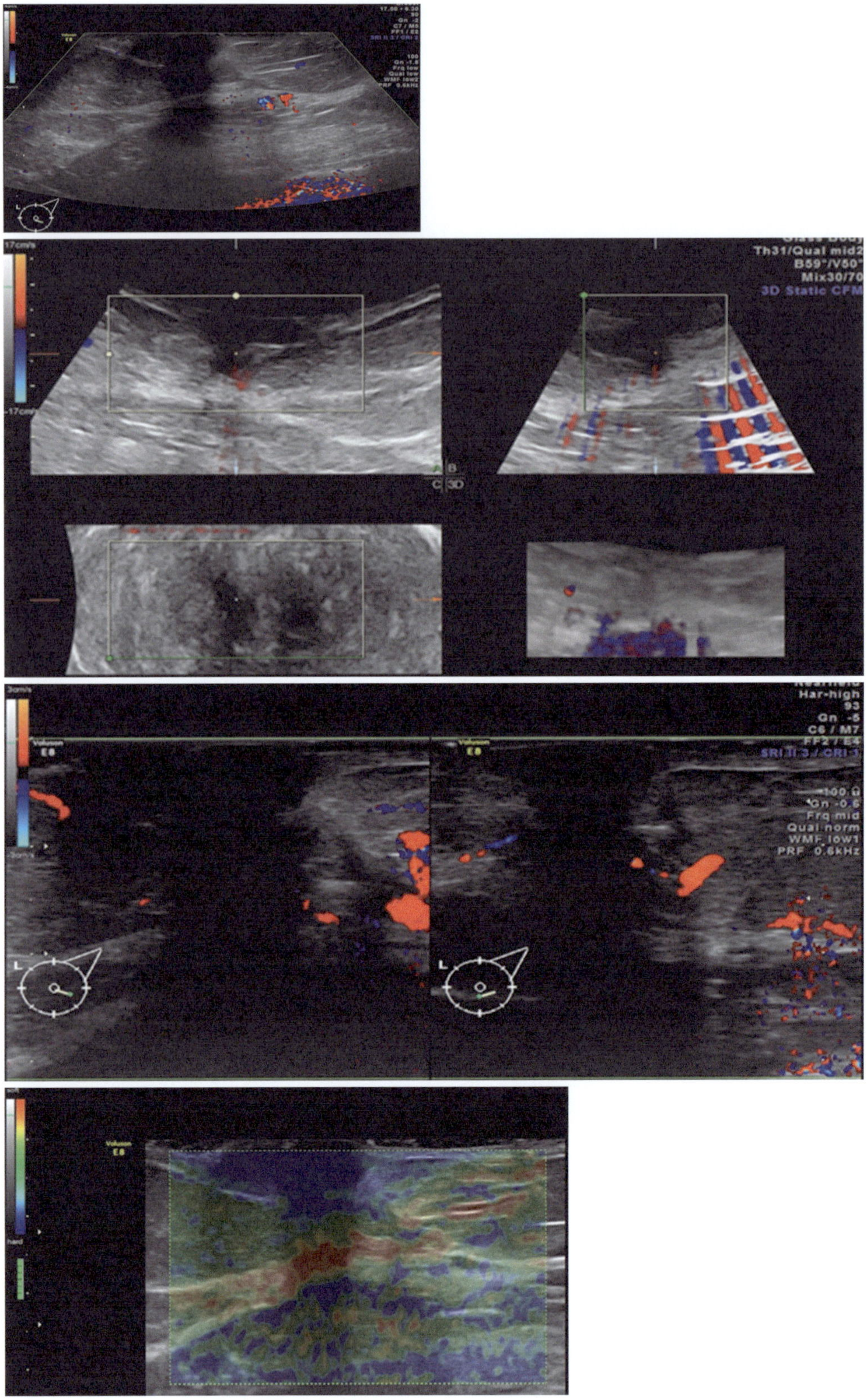

Fig. 6.93 Areolar malignant proliferation mimicking a double nipple, better demonstrated in the plan C of the 4D acquisition; the intense shadowing is similar to a typical deep lesion in malignant Paget disease, but the sonoelastography is conclusive for the unique superficial cancer (epithelioma)

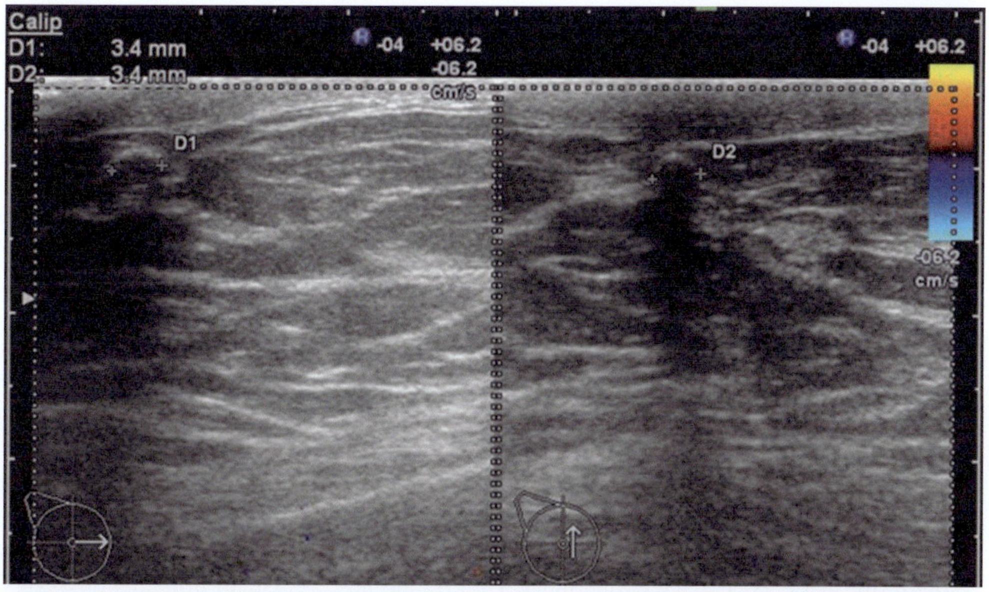

Fig. 6.94 Retroareolar calcification in eggshell without any suspect vasculature in a postmenopausal breast

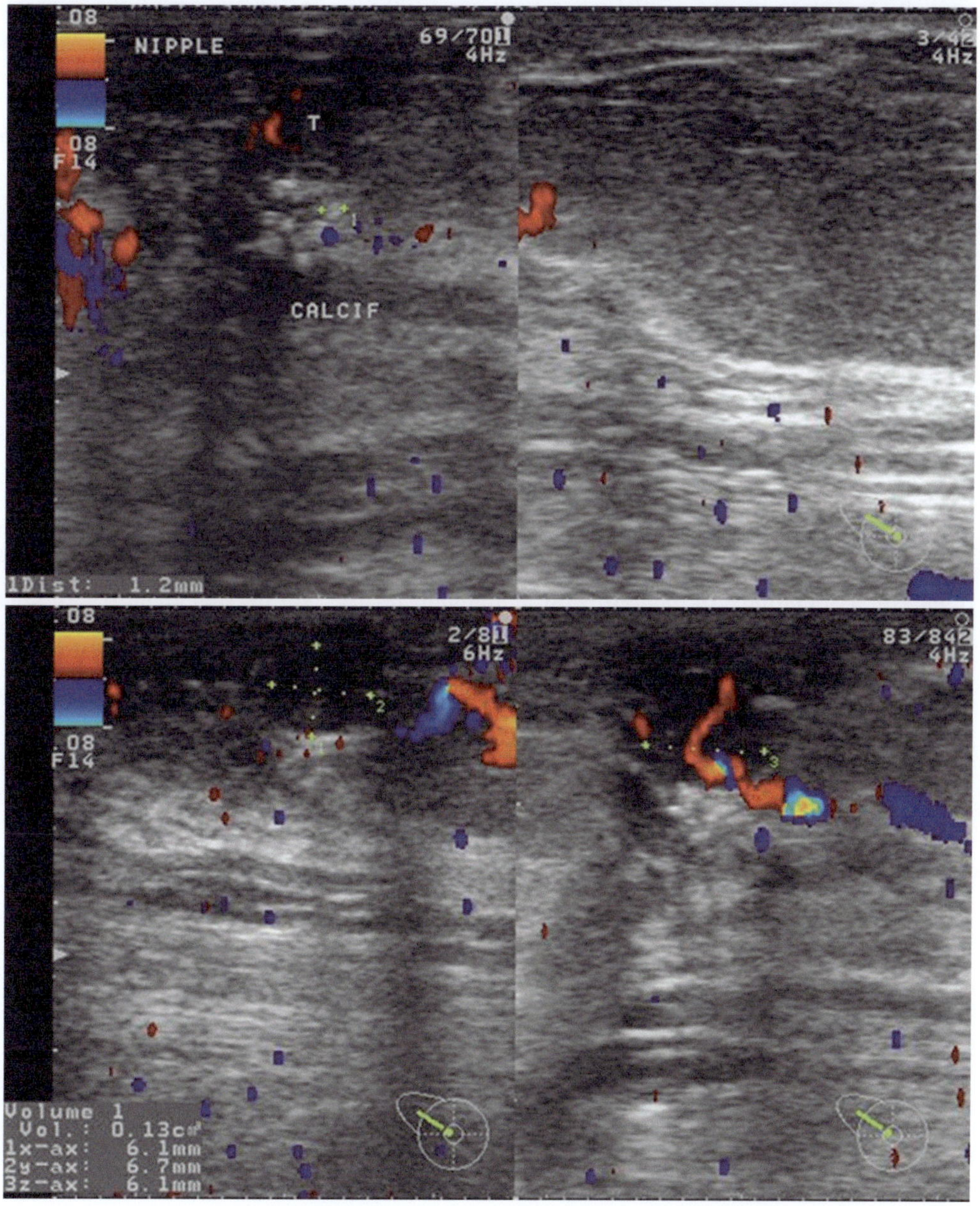

Fig. 6.95 Retroareolar malignancy with hypoechoic mass indistinct from the deepest contour of the nipple and thickened ducts with thin new vasculature

6.16 Nonpalpable Solid Breast Masses That Are Partially or Completely Obscured at Mammography

There are some pathological findings undetected on mammography and diagnosed only at US, with sonographic assessment in probably benign categories, so they can be safely managed with US follow-up. This conclusion presented by Graf and colleagues (2007) was based on a study referred to 445 breast masses that were either partially or completely obscured by dense fibroglandular tissue: 442 remained stable at follow-up (range, 2–5 years; mean, 3.3 years), two masses increased (fibroadenomas at biopsy), and one mass became palpable with cancer proved by biopsy [30].

We can resume that US is more sensitive than mammography in dense breasts, which are the most frequent type in young woman; benign masses are the most frequent in young/fertile patients; US screening and US follow-up are enough for benign findings, NPV being very good (99.8 % after Graf et al.). This study is based on classical US, which is really operator dependent and less performing than DE. It becomes irrational to recommend breast MRI associated with mammography with each 1 or 2 years as screening for risk group women younger than 40.

The key in FBU is the connection of the lesions with the ductal-lobular tree; thus, any abnormality related to the ductal thickness or content, or to the TDLUs, will be systematically identified, located, measured, and characterized by Doppler and sonoelastography; the follow-up examination is easy, and the method is quiet operator independent and safe, without limitation for the interval between examinations, which can be reduced according to the US BI-RADS classification.

The impalpable and radiologically undetectable breast lesions may be benign or malignant. Small cancers without microcalcifications are missed in almost 30 % by mammography, especially in dense breasts or in peripheral locations. In associations of benign with malignant breast lesions, both the clinical examinations and the mammography have tendency to diagnose the benign lesions and to omit the malignant, impalpable ones. Moreover, when a malignant mass is radiologically demonstrated, the multifocal or multicentric lesions may be neglected or unapparent, and the extent of the disease is underestimated, fact admitted when comparing with the results of the breast MRI.

In dense breasts, there are false-positive and false-negative mammographic results more frequent as in heterogeneous or fatty breasts; otherwise, finding breast cancer earlier does not always reduce a woman's risk to die from this disease. Because of the risk of irradiation, increased in dense breasts and in young woman with long period of screening supposed, the interval between two mammograms cannot be reduced under 2 years; in this case, the possibility of developing interval cancers will be higher.

Most benign findings that are nonpalpable and underdetected on mammography are:

- Small lesions of fibrocystic dysplasia or deeper cysts up to 1 cm in diameter
- Ductal ectasias without microcalcifications
- Small fibroadenomas or simple ductal hyperplasias
- Ductal papillomas and intracystic papillomas
- Nipple-areolar abnormalities
- Many lipomas

In some cases, there are palpable pseudomasses, with or without mammographically pathological aspect, but with normal glandular architecture on FBU; in these cases, there is usually a lack of soft, fatty tissue in the premammary layers with superficial, subcutaneous development of the mammary lobes, harder at palpation because of the glandular stroma. These pseudomasses are more sensitive, usually related to the cyclical mastodynia, due to the presence of the hormonal receptors, and the upper outer quadrant is the most frequent site of complaint due to its largest volume.

Other masses completely or partially obscured at mammography are the satellite axillary lymph nodes; when visible, usually the mammography cannot estimate the real number of the enlarged lymph nodes and has a low specificity for the malignant risk, because the small lymph nodes could be malignant, too; moreover, the micrometastases with partial involvement cannot be demonstrated radiologically. These reasons determine the almost mandatory biopsy in visible radiographic lymph nodes. Otherwise, the "benign" lymph nodes may be normal, inflammatory, or granulomatous (in sarcoidosis), with similar radiological aspect (Fig. 6.96).

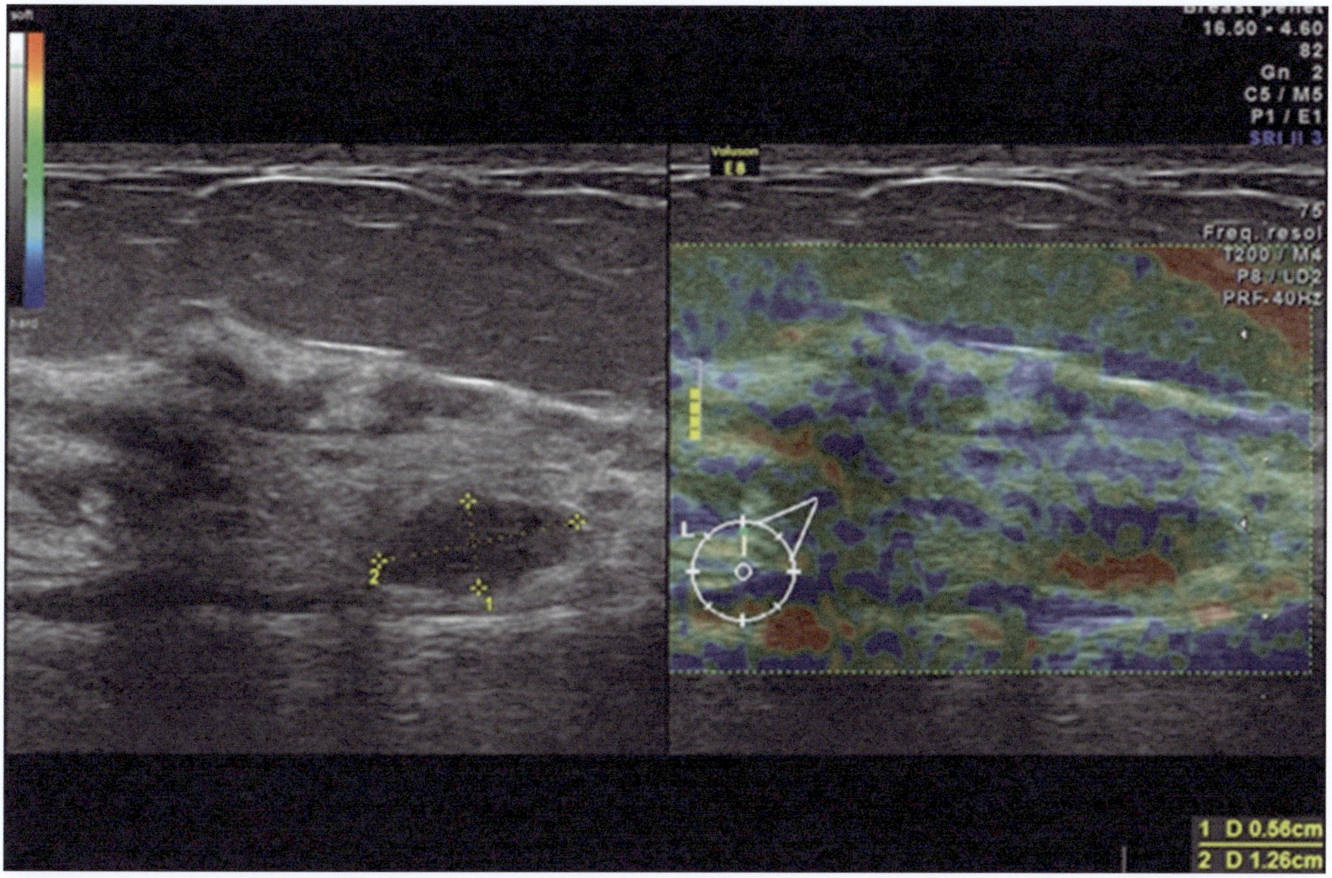

Fig. 6.96 Impalpable, deep, and inspissated cyst with isoechoic aspect and BGR score

6.17 Pseudomalignant US Lesion Appearances

In breast sonography practice, a hypoechoic mass with shadowing is worrisome for malignancy. However, occasionally benign lesions may have hypoechogenicity with shadowing mimicking malignancy such as:

- *Focal fibrosis* in the breast represents a benign entity that is characterized by abundant connective tissue (stroma) separating intervening ducts and lobules, which are often atrophic. Focal fibrosis most commonly appears as an oval mass on sonography, but not infrequently as irregular hypoechoic area with shadowing. In FBU the lesion is not connected to the ductal-lobular tree; usually, it is related to a Cooper ligament and there is no suspicious hyper-vasculature; the sonoelastography may be useful in the differential diagnosis, with a score 2 or 3 Ueno.
- *Diabetic fibrous mastopathy* is an uncommon form of lymphocytic mastitis and stromal fibrosis, which typically occurs in the long-standing type I diabetes. The FBU aspect is not specific, but the breast parenchymal pathology is usually easily excluded; in the case of suspicious lesions, short-time follow-up or biopsy is recommended.
- *Galactoceles* unrelated with recent lactation show well-defined hypoechoic masses with/without posterior shadowing, because of dense milk contents, with pseudotumoral aspect in the classical US. In FBU the positive and the differential diagnosis is easier, because there are no pathological Doppler findings and the sonoelastography demonstrates a complex BGR score. Some chronic galactoceles demonstrate fluid/"solid" level, when sedimentation of the milky contents occurs; the radial and antiradial scans are mandatory to detect the level.
- *Small cystic calcifications* usually appear on DE as 1–2 mm periductal hyperechoic lines, with or without shadowing; therefore, the best characterization of small calcifications is done by mammography, because the sensibility and specificity are unsatisfactory in US and MRI.
- *Fibroadenomas showing hypoechogenicity* with posterior shadowing are correlated with sclerosis dominant or calcifications (*coarse* or *popcorn calcifications*) at pathological examination, but they have benign-type vascularization on Doppler, and the sonoelastography presents a score 2 or 3 Ueno based on the classification.
- *Sarcoidosis* may be associated with breast cancer and may precede or follow breast cancer [31]; breast involvement in sarcoidosis is rare, less than 1 % of patients [32].

  The mammographic and physical findings could not distinguish between these lesions, and biopsy is usually recommended. The diagnosis of sarcoidosis does not exclude malignancy, because breast cancer is more frequent and the association may present. Moreover, multifocal and multicentric sarcoid granuloma may be present in both breasts and sometimes visible on mammography and sonography with irregular shape, angular margins, hypoechoic aspect, and malignant-type shadowing. MRI demonstrates patchy areas of non-mass enhancement corresponding to the same lesions, indistinguishable from the breast cancer [33]. However, the FBU may be useful to better characterize malignant lesions, demonstrating the breast parenchymal connection, either with the surrounding main ducts or with the location in a TDLU; in proven cases of sarcoidosis, the breast involvement has no significant interval changes, and a short-interval follow-up examination is suitable to repeated negative biopsies, being known that those who survive the known cases of sarcoidosis may extend to two to three decades.

  An important aspect in sarcoidosis represents the involvement of the axillary lymph nodes, which can present various aspects, from normal type to acute or chronic inflammatory form or malignant aspect. The lymph nodes with sarcoidosis may present nonspecific lymphatic adenomegalies: global enlargement, especially due to the thickening of the cortex, hypoechoic aspect by reducing of the hilum, normal vasculature, normal elastogram, or increased strain due to lymph node calcification, frequently found in sarcoidosis.
- *Fibro-micro-cystic dysplasia*, in the extended form or in the nodular form, may mimic malignancy in 2D US based on the Stavros criteria; therefore, the vasculature is in normal limits and the sonoelastography demonstrates either a BGR or a complex BGR score or a score 2 Ueno, according to the proportion of fibrosis and cystic fluid. The association of a fibro-micro-cystic dysplasia with breast cancer is not rare; sometimes, a couple of lesions is closely located, thus clinical examination, mammogram, 2D US, and MRI could overdiagnose the size and the extent of the malignancies; in such cases, Doppler associated with sonoelastography is able to distinguish their boundaries (Figs. 6.97, 6.98, 6.99, and 6.100).

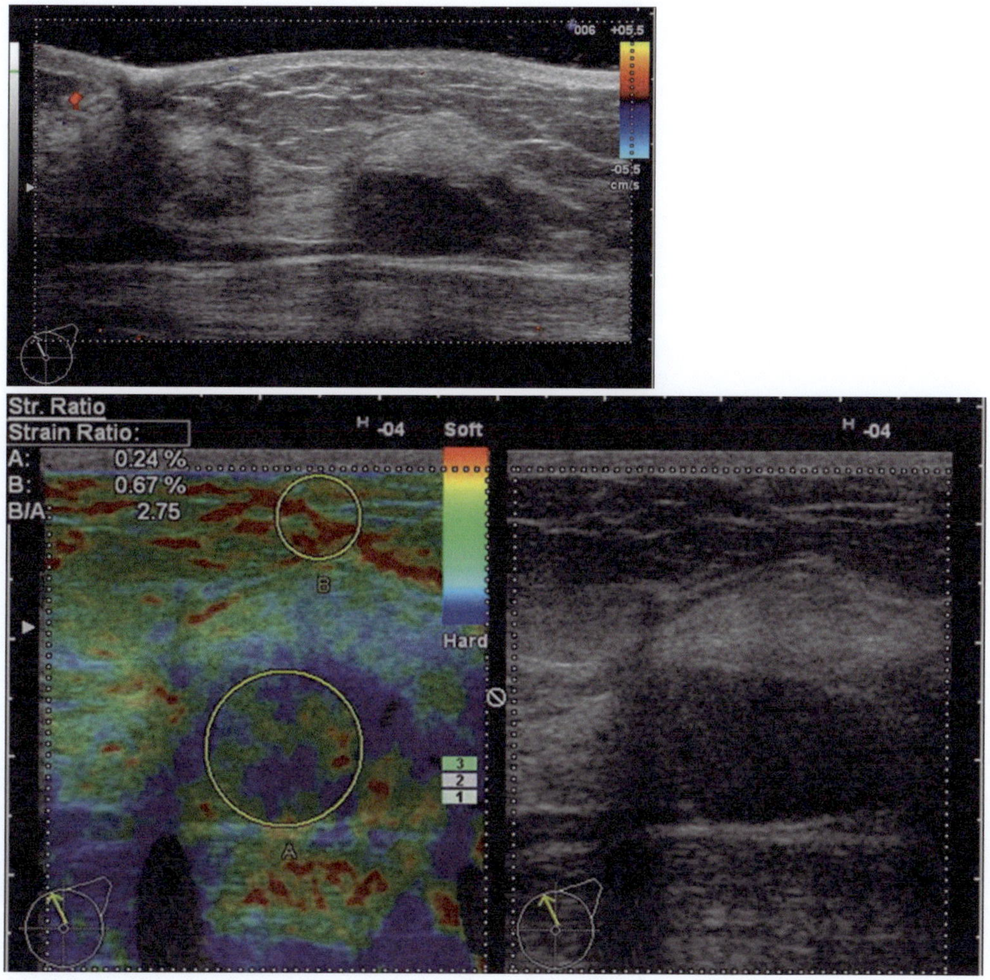

Fig. 6.97 Pseudotumoral lesion represented by nodular fibrocystic dysplasia with complex BGR score

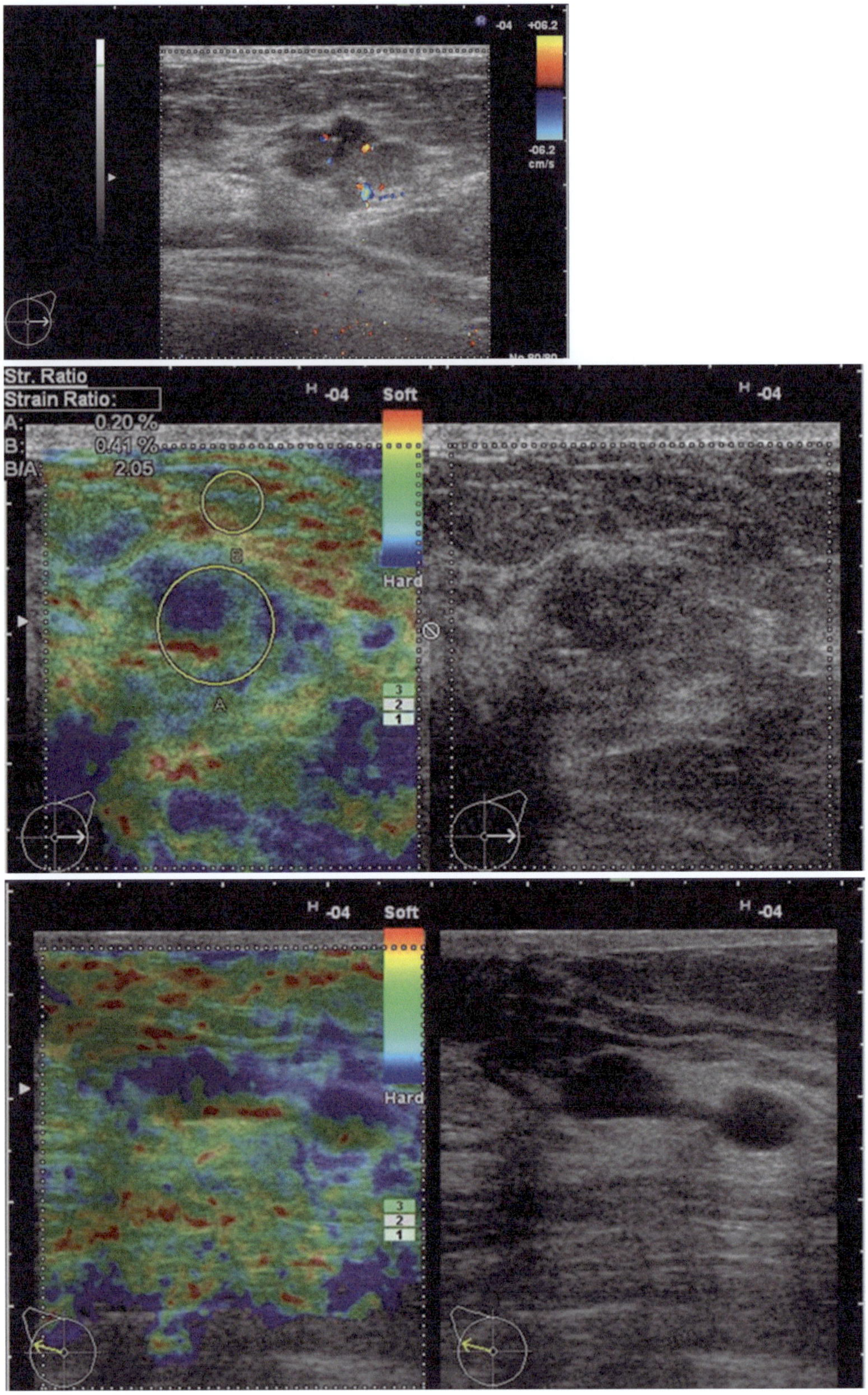

Fig. 6.98 Pseudomalignant mass in L 3:00 with multilobular contour with halo, new formation vasculature but complex strain with areas of BGR and areas of score 2 Ueno, with low strain ratio; the opposite area in the right breast illustrates ductal ectasias and cystic formation

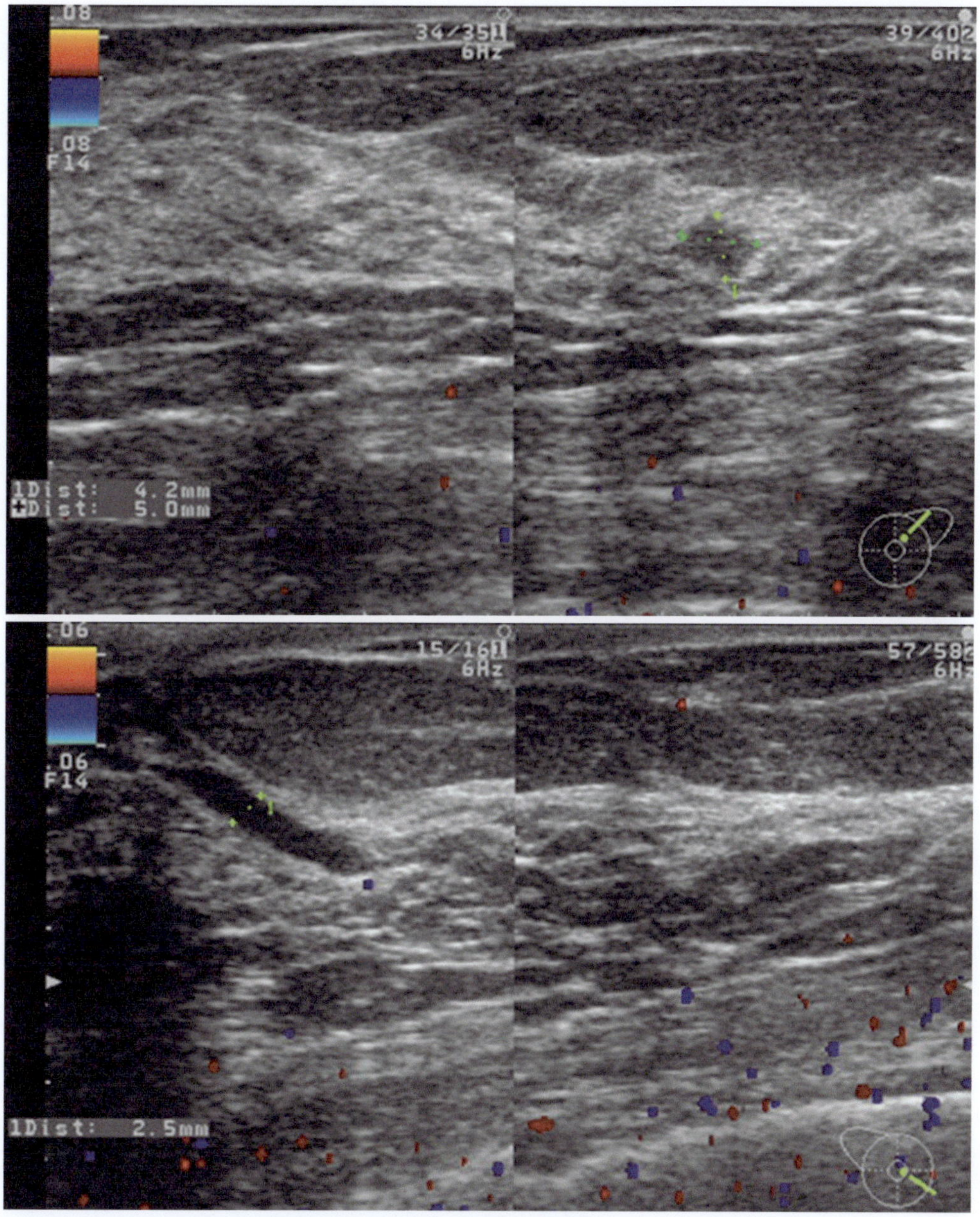

Fig. 6.99 Systemic sarcoidosis with evolution from 27 years with complex features in the breasts in a 63-year-old patient: small nodular masses, diffuse ductal hyperplasias, and central ectasias; right axillary lymph node enlargement with cortical thickening and hyper-vasculature and right supraclavicular adenomegalies with cortical thickening; left axillary lymph nodes with benign features in Doppler US

Fig. 6.99 (continued)

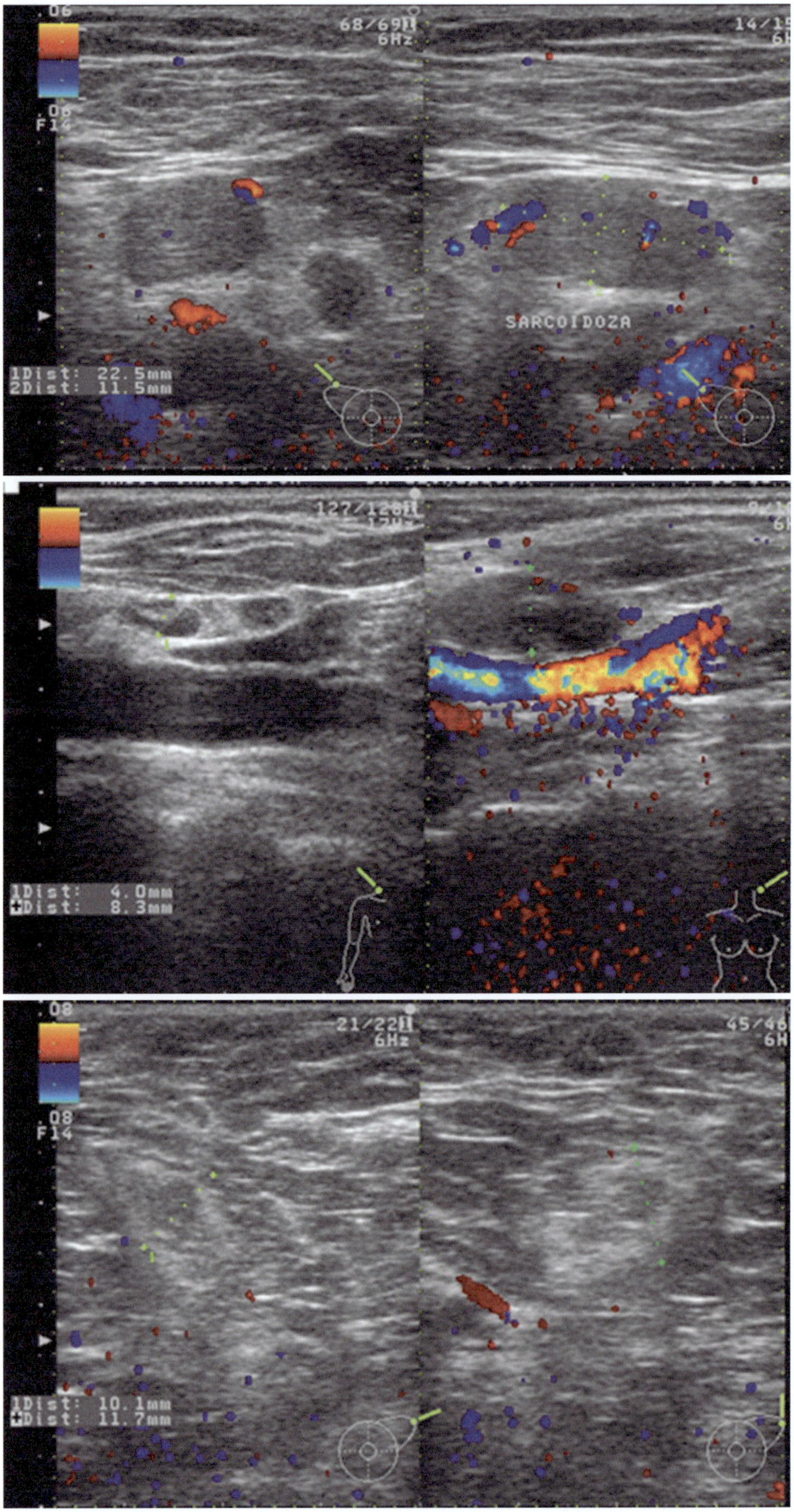

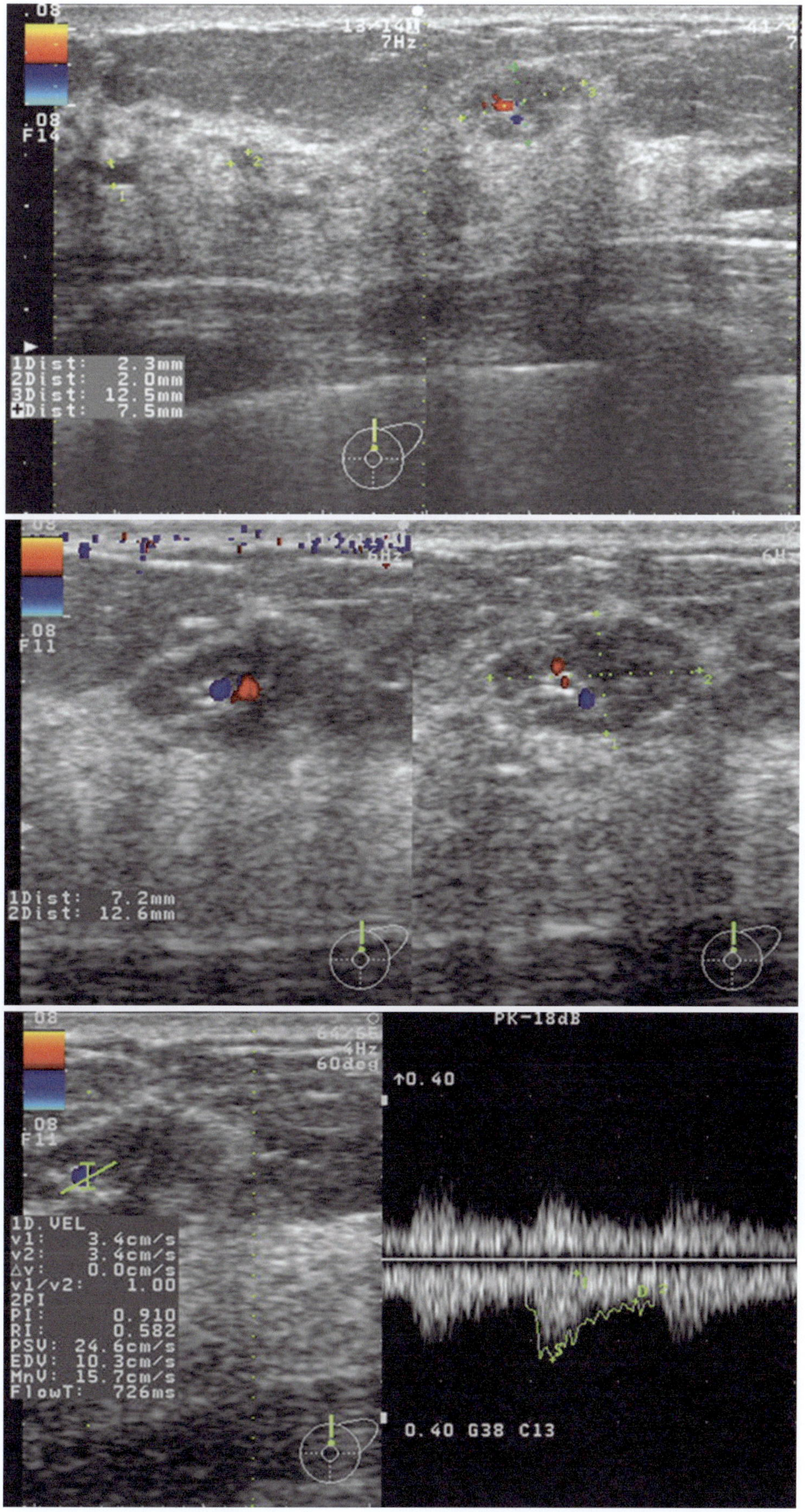

Fig. 6.100 A 41-year-old patient with history of left breast lumpectomy for fibroadenoma: at L 12:00 presents a lump in a TDLU position, less taller than wide, ovoidal shaped, with posterior acoustic enhancement and marginal shadowing effects (Kobayashi signs); the internal architecture and the vasculature in the sinus are concordant with an intramammary lymph node

References

1. Stavros AT, Thickman D, Rapp CL, Dennis MA, Parker SH, Sisney GA (1995) Solid breast nodules: use of sonography to distinguish between benign and malignant lesions. Radiology 196:123–134
2. Stavros AT, Rapp LC, Parker HS (2004) Breast ultrasound. Lippincott Williams & Wilkins, Philadelphia
3. Taylor KJ, Merritt C, Piccoli C, Schmidt R et al (2002) Ultrasound as a complement to mammography and breast examination to characterize breast masses. Ultrasound Med Biol 28(1):19–26
4. Kobayashi T (1975) Ultrasonic diagnosis of breast cancer. Ultrasound Med Biol 1(4):383–391
5. Aristida G, Ernestina A, Viorela E, Simona B (2013) New horizons in breast Doppler ductal echography: the positive and differential diagnosis of ductal ectasia, with etiopathological correlations. ECR Viena. EPOS ™. doi:10.1594/ecr2013/C-0667
6. Tot T (2007) The theory of the sick breast lobe and the possible consequences. Int J Surg Pathol 1:68–71
7. Georgescu A, Bondari S, Manda A, Andrei E-M (2012) The differential diagnosis between breast cancer and fibro-micro-cystic dysplasia by full breast ultrasonography – a new approach. ECR Viena. EPOS ™. doi:10.1594/ecr2012/C-0167, Control Nr #4281
8. Visscher DW, Nassar A, Degnim AC et al (2014) Sclerosing adenosis and risk of breast cancer. Breast Cancer Res Treat 144(1):205–212. Published online Feb 8. doi:10.1007/s10549-014-2862-5
9. Jensen RA, Page DL, Dupont WD et al (1989) Invasive breast cancer risk in women with sclerosing adenosis. Cancer 64(10):1977–1983, Pubmed citation
10. Günhan-Bilgen I, Memiş A, Ustün EE et al (2002) Sclerosing adenosis: mammographic and ultrasonographic findings with clinical and histopathological correlation. Eur J Radiol 44(3):232–238, Eur J Radiol (link) – Pubmed citation
11. Taskin F, Koseoglu K, Unsal A et al (2011) Sclerosing adenosis of the breast: radiologic appearance and efficiency of core needle biopsy. Diagn Interv Radiol 17:311–316. doi:10.4261/1305-3825.DIR.3785-10.2, Pubmed citation
12. Linda A, Zuiani C, Londero V, Cedolini C et al (2012) Magnetic resonance imaging of radial sclerosing lesions (radial scars) of the breast. Eur J Radiol 81(11):3201–3207. doi:10.1016/j.ejrad.2012.01.038
13. Ichihara S, Moritani S, Ohitake T, Ohuchi N (2005) Ductal carcinoma in situ of the breast: the pathological reason for the diversity of its clinical imaging. In: Research and development in breast ultrasound. Springer, Tokyo, pp 104–113
14. Tsunoda-Shimizu H, Kato Y, Ueno E, Endo T et al (2005) Usefulness of depth to width ratio in differentiation of regular invasive ductal carcinoma from fibroadenoma. In: Research and development in breast ultrasound. Springer, Tokyo, pp 57–61
15. Kobayashi T (1977) Gray scale echography for breast cancer. Radiology 122:207–214
16. Teboul M (2003) Practical ductal echography: guide to intelligent and intelligible Ultrasound imaging of the breast. Saned Editors, Madrid
17. Amy D (2010) Lobar ultrasound of the breast. In: Tot T (ed), breast cancer. Springer, London Limited. doi:10.1007/978-1-84996-314-5_8
18. Kujiraoka Y, Ueno E, Yohno E, Morishima I, Tsunoda-Shimizu H (2005) Incident angle of the plunging artery of breast tumors. In: Research and development in breast ultrasound. Springer, Tokyo, pp 72–75
19. Adamietz BR, Kahmann L, Fasching PA, Schulz-Wendtland R, Uder M et al (2011) Differentiation between phyllodes tumor and fibroadenoma using real-time Elastography. Ultraschall Med Suppl 2:E75–E79. doi:10.1055/s-0031-1282024
20. Li L-J, Zeng H, Ou B, Luo B-M, Xiao X-Y et al (2014) Ultrasonic elastography features of phyllodes tumors of the breast: a clinical research. PLoS One 9(1), e85257. doi:10.1371/journal.pone.0085257
21. Wurdinger S, Herzog AB, Fischer DR et al (2005) Differentiation of phyllodes breast tumors from fibroadenomas on MRI. AJR Am J Roentgenol 185(5):1317–1321
22. Yabuuchi H, Soeda H, Matsuo Y et al (2006) Phyllodes tumor of the breast: correlation between MR findings and histologic grade. Radiology 241:702–709, http://dx.doi.org/10.1148/radiol.2413051470
23. Arrigoni MG, Dockerty MB, Judd ES (1971) The identification and treatment of mammary hamartoma. Surg Gynecol Obstet 133(4):577–582, Pubmed citation
24. Da Costa D, Taddese A, Cure ML, Gerson D, Poppiti R, Esserman LE (2007) Common and unusual diseases of the nipple-areolar complex. RadioGraphics 27:S65–S77, © RSNA, 2007
25. Geffroy D, Doutriaux-Doumulins I, Labbe-Devilliers C et al (2011) Paget's disease of the nipple and differential diagnosis. J Radiol 92(10):889–898. doi:10.1016/j.jradio.2011.07.010, Epub 2011 Sep7
26. Yim JH, Wick MR, Philpott GW, Norton JA, Doherty GM (1997) Underlying pathology in mammary Paget's disease. Ann Surg Oncol 4(4):287–292
27. Günhan-Bilgen I, Oktay A (2006) Paget's disease of the breast: clinical, mammographic, sonographic and pathologic findings in 52 cases. Eur J Radiol 60(2):256–263, Epub 2006 Aug 2
28. Riordan J, Wambach K (2010) Breast related problems. In: Riordan J, Wambach K (eds) Breastfeeding and human lactation. Jones & Bartlett, Boston, pp 291–324
29. Park HS, Yoon CH, Kim HJ (1999) The prevalence of congenital inverted nipple. Aesthetic Plast Surg 20:144
30. Graf O, Helbich TH, Hopf G, Graf C, Sickles EA (2007) Probably benign breast masses at US: is follow-up an acceptable alternative to biopsy? Radiology 244:87–93, © RSNA 2007
31. Lower EE, Hawkins HH, Baughman RP (2001) Breast disease in sarcoidosis. Sarcoidosis Vasc Diffuse Lung Dis 18(3):301–306
32. Hermann G, Nagi C, Mester J, Tierstein A (2008) Unusual presentation of sarcoidosis of the breast. Br J Radiol 81:e231–e233 [PUBMED]
33. Isley ML, Cluver RC, Leddy JR, Baker KM (2012) Primary sarcoid of the breast with incidental malignancy. J Clin Imaging Sci 2:46

7 Breast Calcifications in Full Breast Ultrasonography

7.1 Breast Calcifications in US: Technical Aspects

Because the mammography still represents the main imaging method to visualize the breast (micro-)calcifications and the US BI-RADS assessment was created upon the first radiological one, the extension of the terms and the intention to interpret the sonographic images using the same descriptors added disillusion for the overall classical US accuracy. Results of both mammography and classical US have limitations that reduce their clinical usefulness, and alternative breast imaging modalities are being sought.

Indeed, the main important findings in detecting breast cancer by mammography are microcalcifications, architectural distortions, and asymmetric breast densities eventually with peripheral spiculations. Contrarily, FBU can visualize the main normal breast tissues, represented by breast parenchyma (mammary ductal tree ended by lobules) and the glandular stroma, surrounded by the pre-, retro-, or interlobar fatty tissue, delimited by the fibrous tissue represented by the network of Cooper ligaments; in addition, there are identified the main vessels and the satellite lymph nodes, and thus any abnormal benign or malignant structures issued in the breast become salient.

The typical size of breast microcalcifications ranges from 50 to 500 μm, but the size measurable using usual high-frequency transducers of up to 14 MHz is over 400 μm, usually in the domain of benign calcifications. Current ultrasound scanners do not reliably detect microcalcifications in the size range of clinical interest for breast cancer diagnosis. However, some theoretic, simulation, and experimental studies focused on the improvement of the ultrasonic visualization of microcalcifications were presented [1]. But the results are still unsatisfactory, because the use of the US as an adjuvant or complementary method for mammography (which has low sensibility in dense breasts) is wrong and confusing; otherwise, US has other descriptors, more accurate and more specific than mammography, especially when combining the results of all the developments in US, achieving the concept of FBU.

The research of the tissues' elasticity was based on clinical experience, but the best imaging method was not easy to define. Many methods have been proposed to measure the mechanical response of the tissues to the impact of a force. The method named *vibro-acoustography* uses the ultrasound radiation force to harmonically vibrate tissue and measure the resulting acoustic emission field with a nearby hydrophone. Another method, *vibrometry*, uses the ultrasound radiation force accompanied with a measurement of the resulting velocity or displacement of the vibrating tissue or object. An extension of the vibro-acoustography method using a multifrequency stress field to vibrate an object was described [2]. Resulting images of the vibro-acoustography show soft tissue structures and calcifications within breast with high contrast, high resolution, and no speckles [3]. These methods are not popular, and there are few manufacturers that implemented them in their ultrasonographic machines. Contrarily, sonoelastography was more successful, and its technique and applications were standardized and implemented by many manufacturers, becoming a technique as available and useful as is the Doppler in the US practice; however, sonoelastography can diagnose the malignancy without correlation with the presence of the microcalcifications; even admitting the strain is influenced by the presence of undetectable malignant microcalcifications.

The best characterization of the microcalcifications is realized of course by mammography. The radiologist can visualize all the microcalcifications and their shape, size, and distribution. A classification of the calcifications in benign (not cancerous), probably benign, indeterminate (not sure), and suspicious (might be cancer) was adopted. Benign calcifications tend to be round or oval, uniform in density, and scattered in the breast tissue. Suspicious microcalcifications, on the other hand, vary in shape, size, form, and density and are usually clustered in a linear or segmental pattern.

Mammography cannot diagnose small breast invasive cancer or DCIS that do not present microcalcifications; nevertheless, it is useful in detecting DCIS because 90 % of cases present microcalcifications with suggesting distribution

A. Colan-Georges, *Atlas of Full Breast Ultrasonography*, DOI 10.1007/978-3-319-31418-1_7

(branching calcifications in DCIS) [4]. Any areas of microcalcifications should be evaluated with magnification views to accurately define their morphological features as well as their number and distribution. However, there are limitations of the mammography that are due to the image blur on magnification views that may compromise image quality. Digital mammography was finally accepted as screening method, and some advantages such as good magnification without repeated exposure made quickly its success. In addition, tomosynthesis is proposed as a better technique of detection of breast cancer, microcalcifications included, but it is far the era of using it for breast cancer screening.

It is assumed microcalcifications often cannot be localized with US; however, some authors consider microcalcifications in malignant lesions that are reliably recognized by US (100 %), but they are difficult to detect in fibrocystic breast changes because of their spreading without correlation with a sonographic mass [5].

The classical US used especially as a complementary examination may be helpful in:

- The determination of the presence of a solid mass that corresponds to an area of distortion.
- Further evaluation of a palpable mass in any patient with dense breast parenchyma and negative mammographic findings.
- The evaluation of asymmetric densities seen at mammography because US can precise the differential diagnosis of the density as either a breast tissue or a true mass. Soo et al. [6] and Skaane [7] found the NPV of US with mammography for a palpable lesion to be 99.8 % and 100 %, respectively. Moy et al. [8] affirm a negative mammographic and US finding of a palpable abnormality does not exclude breast cancer, but the likelihood of breast cancer is low, approximately 2.6–2.7 %. However, the classical practice considers a palpable mass that appears solid at US which warrants further evaluation with biopsy, in the absence of the full analysis by Doppler and sonoelastography.
- The detection of the thickened ducts that are associated with malignancy: a unilateral solitary dilated duct [9] and dilated ducts associated with microcalcifications or in a non-subareolar location.

Limitations of breast US that are recognized in the classical examination (as a complementary method, with the main scans in the transversal and sagittal planes) include:

- The inability to visualize some solid masses owing to small size (particularly intraductal carcinomas) or to izoechogenicity.
- Overlap in ultrasonographic appearance of some benign and malignant lesions.
- Difficulty in identifying intraductal microcalcifications that are readily depicted on mammography in the absence of a mass. However, the noncalcified DCIS that is commonly occult or shows subtle findings of malignancy on mammography may be visible on US as a variable figured mass or nonspecific ductal changes sometimes with suspicious findings [10].

In US, microcalcifications of malignant type could not be positively identified because of the limiting factor of the low frequency of the transducers. However, microcalcifications larger than 0.5 mm could be differentiated as strong echogenic foci in hypoechoic masses. The main value of the US was the ability to demonstrate masses in the area of mammographic microcalcifications, which were associated with invasive carcinoma. Reports in literature affirm the introduction of higher-frequency 7.5 MHz transducers with automatic scanners that improved visualization of microcalcifications up to 57 % of cases but only when associated with masses; they appear as echogenic foci in hypoechoic areas and do not attenuate. Using 7.5–10 MHz real-time ultrasound equipment, ultrasound abnormalities corresponding to clustered microcalcifications were identified in 59.6–76 % cases with specificity for malignancy of 82–93 %. There is, however, lower accuracy in the positive identification of benign microcalcifications, and not all malignant microcalcifications could be positively identified on ultrasound. There is no clear distinction in whether the malignant lesions identified sonographically were invasive carcinomas, which were usually associated with a sonographic mass or pure in situ disease. Other investigators using similar equipment to localize impalpable lesions presenting solely as microcalcifications have not been able to achieve this level of detection. The use of higher-frequency ultrasound probes with operating frequencies above 7.5 MHz and claimed axial and lateral resolution of 0.1–0.5 mm improved the ability of detecting microcalcifications greater than 0.6 mm in size. Moreover, the detection of microcalcifications of 0.15 mm in size is possible using a 13 MHz transducer with an axial resolution of 0.118 mm. However, the results are mixed with sensitivities ranging from 52 to 88 % patients in the literature, but almost all authors used US as a complementary method [11].

In conclusion, the ability to visualize microcalcifications is likely to be multifactorial, depending not only on the presence of any associated sonographic abnormalities but also on operator experience.

Nevertheless, the definitive identification of benign microcalcification is comparatively lower from that of malignant disease and ranges from 33.5 to 85.7 % in prospective studies where histological correlation is available, the main size being larger than of the malignant type of up to 2–4 mm. Malignant lesions are usually more readily identified even in the absence of a mammographic detectable mass, because the breast cancerous cells are not dense and do not form a mammographic opacity in the absence of the desmoplastic reaction, while the proliferative lesion is always salient in US.

Classical US describes morphological features in DCIS with vague relationship with the breast anatomy; the presence of dilated ducts that contain flecks of microcalcifications, which may be associated to sonographic parenchymal changes or hypoechoic lesions, is included. Adjacent strongly echogenic foci representing microcalcifications are also described, but without specific location related to the breast anatomy. Masses or irregular attenuating areas may also be present particularly with high-grade or comedo DCIS, which have the appearances of the typical spiculated or irregular borders. Where invasive carcinoma is present, the positive identification of a sonographic abnormality approaches that of 100 %; the ability to visualize a sonographic abnormality is particularly high where the mammogram shows a suspicious appearance or where there is clustering of more than 10 mm in extent. In fact, the increased detection rate of malignant calcifications using ultrasound was due to the use as a complementary method, but it was not proved US can visualize with good accuracy any calcification as the first technique of diagnosis; moreover, US was exploited by investigators as a means of performing guided needle biopsy or preoperatory localizations of the mammographic abnormalities.

The mammographic classification of the breast calcifications was correlated with the risk of malignancy; this classification cannot be superposed on the sonographic findings, because the resolution is less performing and the geometrical aspect is different; indeed, if the microcalcifications are too small, under 200 μm, they may be not visualized as distinct sonographic foci, and if they are larger, usually in the benign lesions over 500 μm, they may present acoustic shadowing and their shape cannot be precise. This is the reason the usefulness in US diagnosis of the microcalcifications is poor, because the main characters used in mammography are not interpretable: the morphology, the distribution, and the change over time.

Therefore, the US examination must be correlated with the mammographic findings, and the radiological classification of the breast calcifications must be considered as the gold standard.

Breast calcifications in mammography may be:

Benign Calcifications

- Skin calcifications—tattoo sign
- Vascular calcifications
- Coarse or "popcorn-like"
- Large rodlike, plasma cell mastitis
- Round and punctate calcifications
- Lucent centered
- Eggshell or rim calcifications
- Milk of calcium
- Suture calcifications
- Dystrophic calcifications

Suspicious Calcifications

- Amorphous calcifications
- Coarse heterogeneous

High Probability of Malignancy

- Fine pleomorphic
- Fine linear or fine linear branching

ACR BI-RADS 2013 had reunified the suspicious and high probability of malignancy calcifications, because of biopsy recommended in both cases.

The lobular calcifications fill the acini, which are often dilated. This results in mammography to uniform, homogeneous, and sharply outlined calcifications, which are often punctate or round, sometimes visible accidently in US; when the acini become very large, as in cystic dysplasia, "milk of calcium" may fill these cavities, and fluid/fluid level can be demonstrated in US. However, when there is more fibrosis, as in sclerosing adenosis, the calcifications are usually smaller and less uniform, usually unapparent in US, but the pseudotumoral aspect with increasing acoustic shadowing may be demonstrated. In these cases, it can be difficult to differentiate them from intraductal calcifications in the classical US. Lobular calcifications usually have a diffuse or scattered distribution and are almost always benign.

The intraductal calcifications represent calcified cellular debris or secretions within the intraductal lumen; the uneven calcification of the cellular debris explains the fragmentation and irregular contours of the calcifications in mammography. These calcifications are extremely variable in size, density, and form, from pleomorphic to a complete cast of the ductal lumen. This explains the fine linear or branching form and distribution, specific in the radiological examination, but rarely detected by US as the first technique of examination, because different ducts are scanned in the transverse, variant-oblique, and longitudinal short plans in the same time, without anatomical relationship. Intraductal calcifications are suspicious of malignancy and are classified as BI-RADS 4 or 5.

The differential diagnosis in US is more important and more difficult as in the radiological examination. There are no sufficient studies about the sensibility and specificity of the US microcalcifications when using as the first method of diagnosis, but the overall accuracy is less 30 %, insufficient for the validating of the method. In fact, the most cases present *false-negative diagnosis* for microcalcifications, especially for the malignant ones, which are too small and are masked in the acoustic shadowing of the mass; moreover, there are microcalcifications in the glandular stroma that is hyperechoic and has no sufficient contrast toward the tinny foci. Small benign calcifications of the glandular acini are isolated and usually are underdiagnosed in US, already being without clinical significance.

The most cases of *false-positive diagnosis* are microcysts, in the nodular form of the fibro-micro-cystic dysplasia, or ductal micropapillomas associated with ectasias. In other cases, the vascular calcifications may appear as ductal or lobular lesions if the non-anatomical/random scans are performed. The Cooper ligaments are easily differentiated, but abnormal fibrous changes may be confused with breast calcifications presenting hyperechoic foci. Because of their small size, the malignant microcalcifications have no acoustic shadowing, which is more conclusive for US; thus, we cannot make the differential diagnosis of the hyperechoic foci, resulting to false-positive diagnosis.

7.2 Breast Calcifications in FBU: Improvements and Limits in Detection and Interpreting

FBU has the same limits as the classical US in the detection of the tinny microcalcifications, due to the limits of the US length wave and to their unspecific aspect: small hyperechoic foci without acoustic shadowing. As consequence, microcalcifications are not essential findings in the FBU diagnosis. However, when visible, they must be interpreted and integrated in the diagnosis.

The localization of the visible microcalcifications is more precise in FBU than in the classical US or mammography: intraductal, in the surrounding stroma, and intratumoral; the site is specified according to the clockwise notation, useful in the follow-up examination. Moreover, the salient pathological vasculature and the increased FLR are high suggestive for malignancy in the site with mammographic microcalcifications that are not visible in US.

The benign calcifications are usually larger than 1 mm, well identified as hyperechoic lesions sometimes with an eggshell aspect and with acoustic shadowing effect; the new vasculature is either absent, or the Doppler signal may present the twinkling artifact, while the FLR may be increased, mimicking malignant lesions.

FBU is useful in the managing of cases after surgical conservative therapy of the DCIS, usually diagnosed by mammography based on the suggestive microcalcifications, with/without preoperatory biopsy; recidivate in the local area after lumpectomy or segmentectomy can be demonstrated in FBU by segmental thickening of the ductal tree with loss of the central line sign; the eventual remnant axillary lymph nodes are observed during adjuvant therapy. In rare cases, in DCIS with extended microcalcifications, they are visualized by the DE of Teboul, using transducers with high resolution.

The IDC or ILC may develop in the same or in the contralateral breast after breast-conserving surgery, and 6-month interval follow-up FBU for the next 5 years should be preferred in the asymptomatic cases, instead of mammographic follow-up or of unrepeatable biopsy as the clinical practice still recommends [12, 13]. In fact, the clinical practice uses the FNAB in verifying a malignancy and the core-needle biopsy in establishing definitive preoperatory diagnosis; despite the preoperative diagnostic algorithm in case of round/oval densities, stellate lesions, or microcalcifications found on the mammogram which are usually based on the guided biopsies [14], there is no consensus about the interval between negative biopsies or histologically proved benign/premalignant breast proliferation [15].

As a conclusion, FBU and US in general are not useful in detecting and characterizing the *microcalcifications as indirect signs* of breast malignancy, as does the mammography, which is still missing up to 30 % of breast cancers because of various types of pitfalls [16]; however, FBU can detect any *proliferative abnormality of the ductal tree*, from the ductal/lobular hyperplasia to the DCIS or IDC/ILC, based on the *direct* anatomical findings (Figs. 7.1, 7.2, 7.3, 7.4, 7.5, 7.6, 7.7, 7.8, 7.9, 7.10, 7.11, 7.12, 7.13, 7.14, 7.15, 7.16, 7.17, and 7.18).

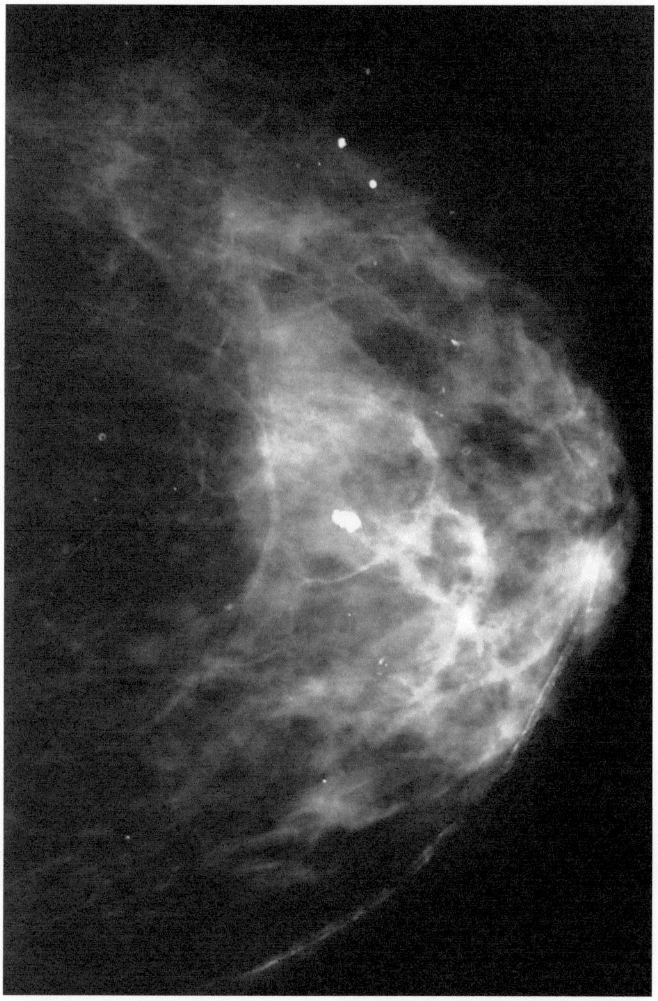

Fig. 7.1 Analogue mammography (zoomed plain-film mammography) illustrating benign calcifications

Fig. 7.2 IDC with mammographic tinny microcalcifications in the R-UOQ, visible with electronic magnification in this case; the focal surrounding increased breast density is difficult to delimitate from the rest of glandular structures and represents the stromal reaction, the tumor itself being invisible radiologically

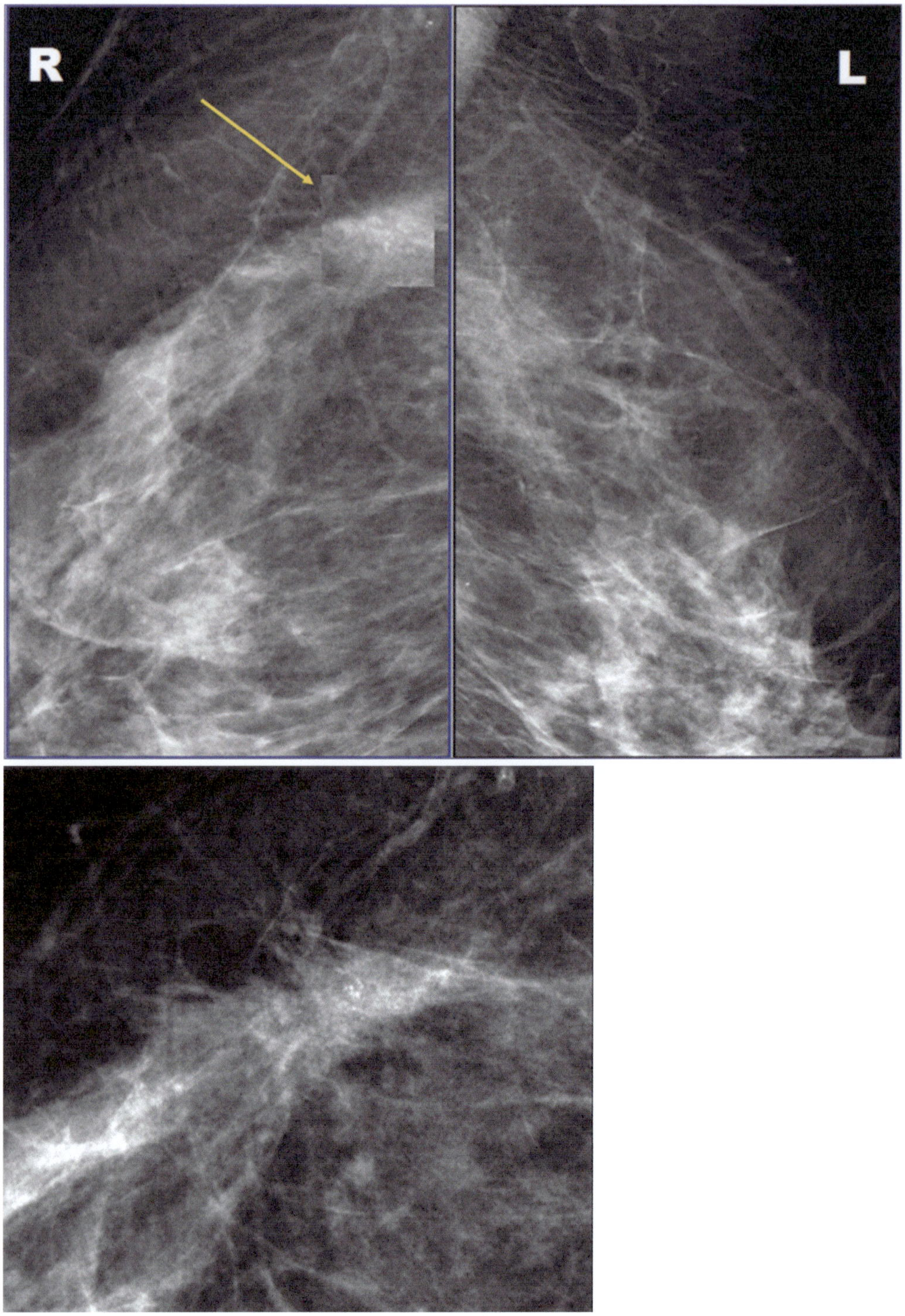

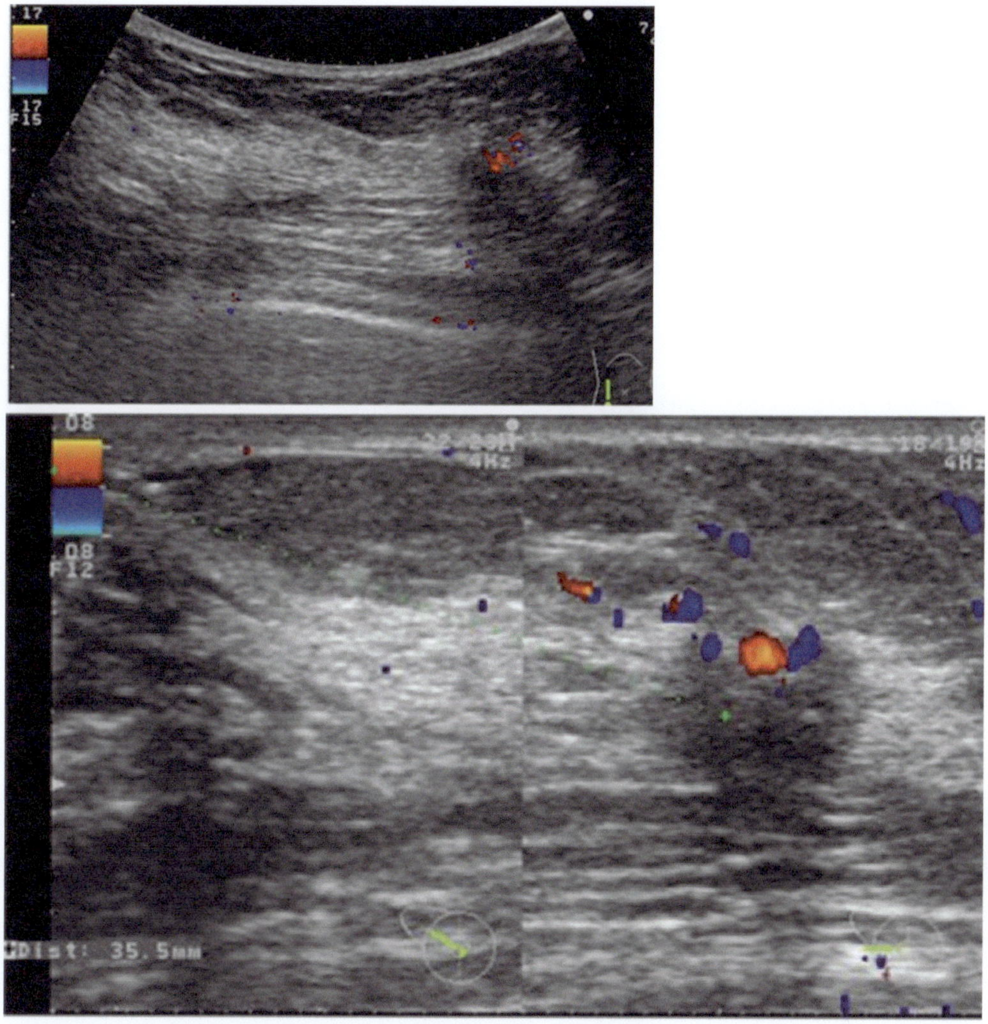

Fig. 7.3 The same case: R: 10:00 peripheral mass less 12 mm size, with ductal connection, malignant characters upon Stavros and salient new vasculature with incident plunging angle, tortuous and enlarged vessels with high velocity determining aliasing; the hyperechoic foci cannot be interpreted as microcalcifications without previous radiological information

Fig. 7.3 (continued)

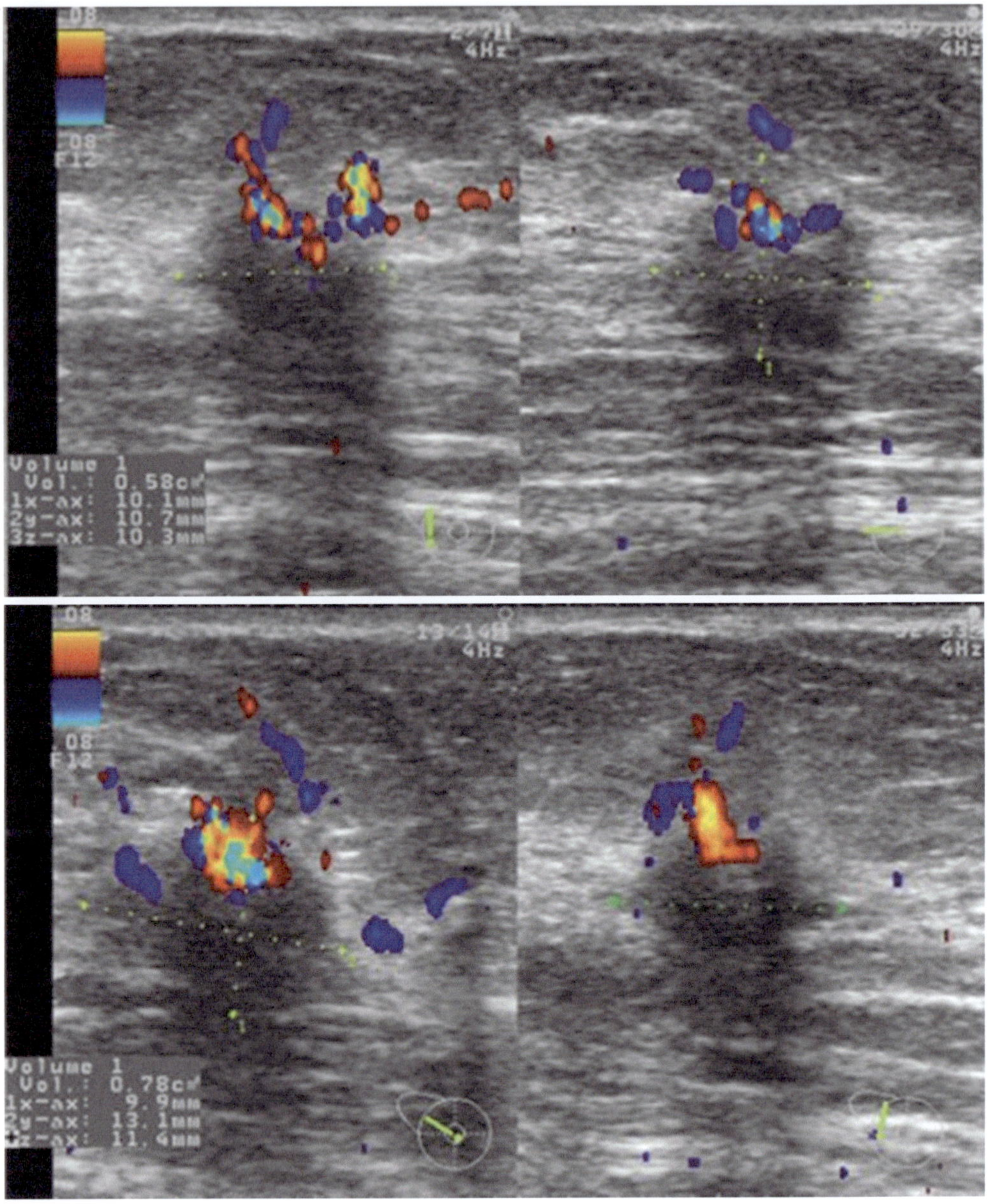

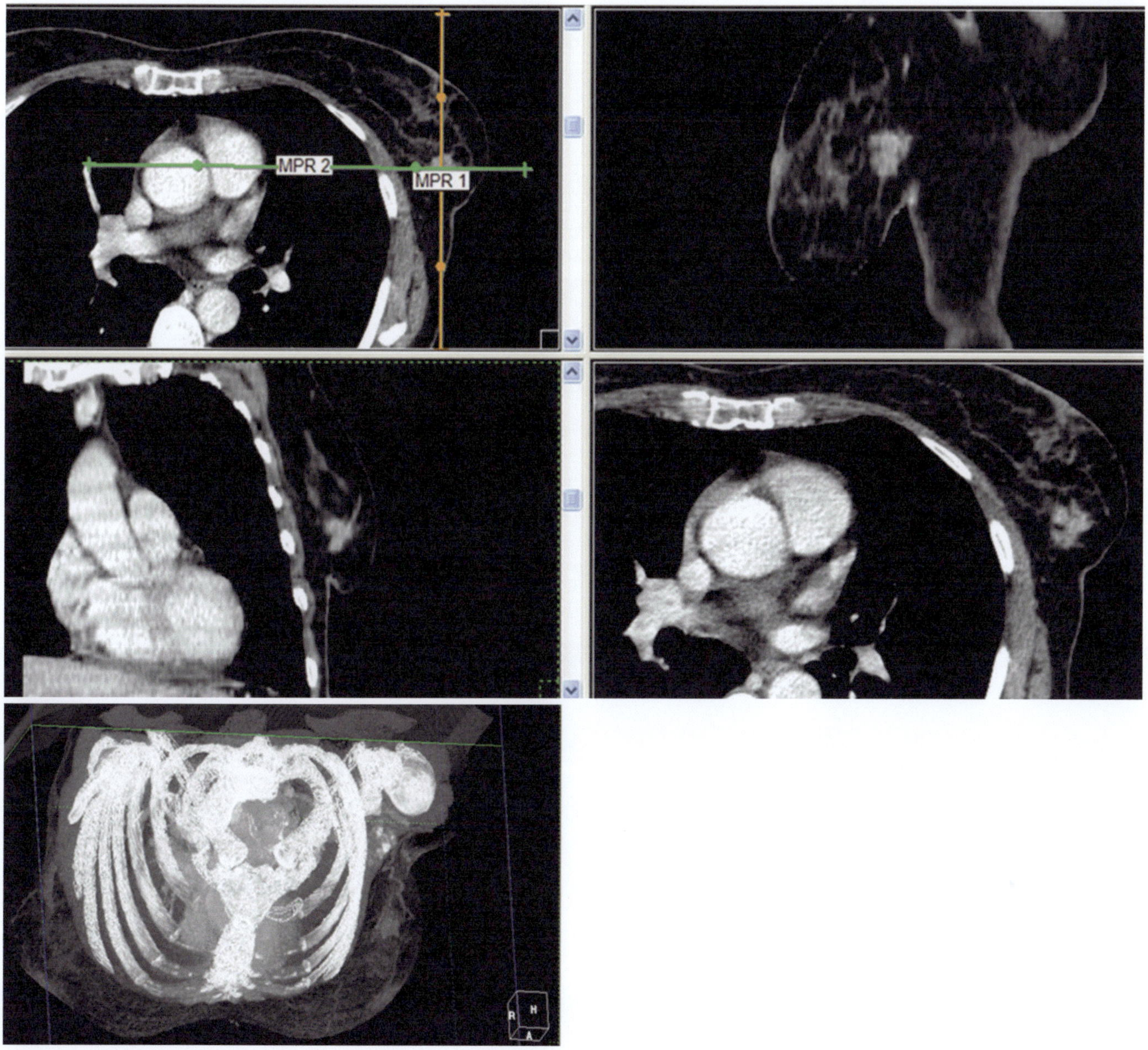

Fig. 7.4 Breast cancer with axillary lymph nodes metastasis: the multidetector CT examination with multiplanar reconstructions illustrates the breast tumor, with microcalcifications detectable at mammography, confirmed as IDC; the tumor connection with the armpit is demonstrated by the nourishing vessel and the axillary lymph nodes that present calcifications detectable by 3D reforming with bony density

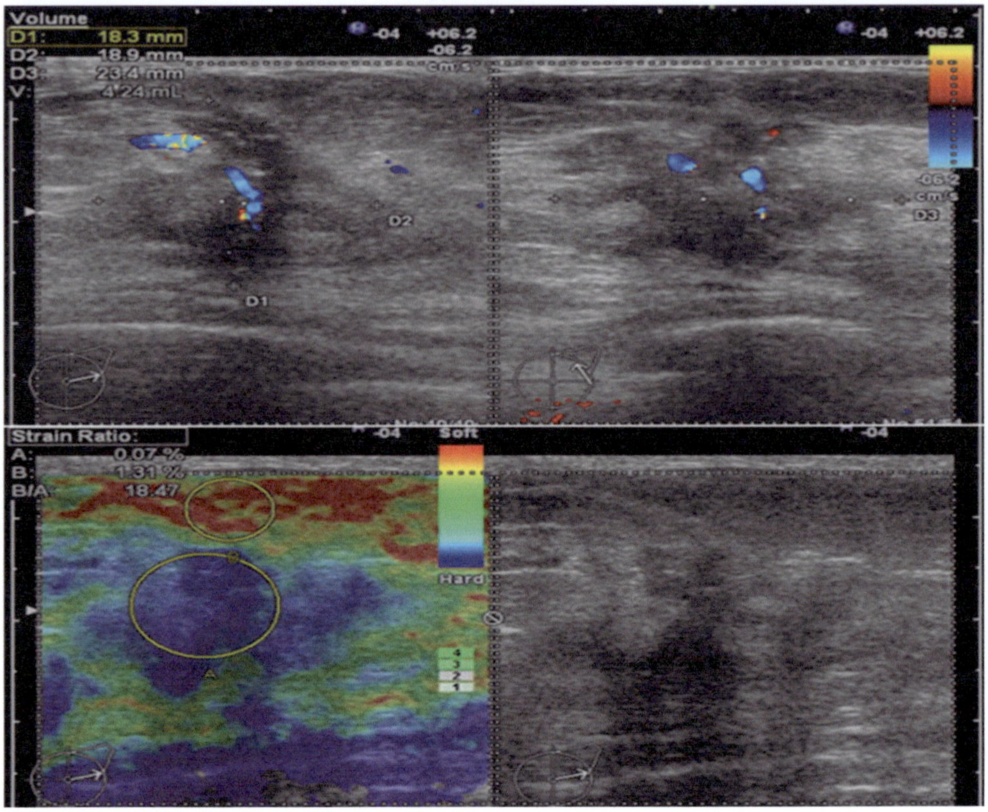

Fig. 7.5 The same case: IDC with FBU characteristic findings in L: 2:00 with irregular shape, acoustic shadowing, new vasculature with incident plunging angle, and score 5 Ueno with high FLR of 18.47. The presence of many hyperechoic foci inside the pathological mass may suggest microcalcifications in association with the other findings, but the sensibility of the method does not exceed 60 %, while other illustrated descriptors for malignity acquire an overall accuracy superior to 95 %

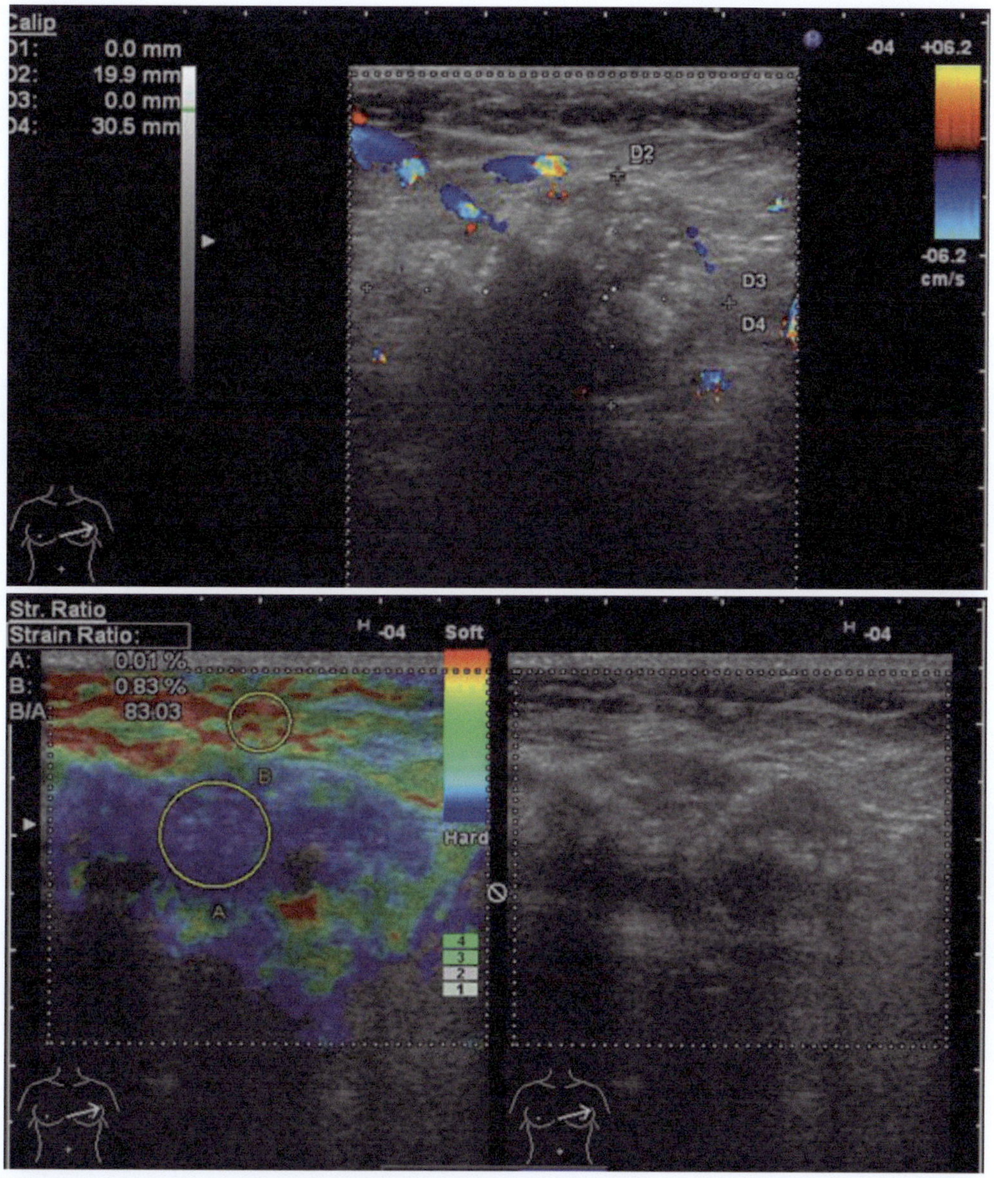

Fig. 7.6 The same case, with peripheral new vasculature of the axillary lymph nodes, small hyperechoic foci and macrocalcifications with irregular shape, hypoechoic aspect, and acoustic shadowing; the high strain is confirmed by sonoelastography with score 4 Ueno and FLR over 80.00

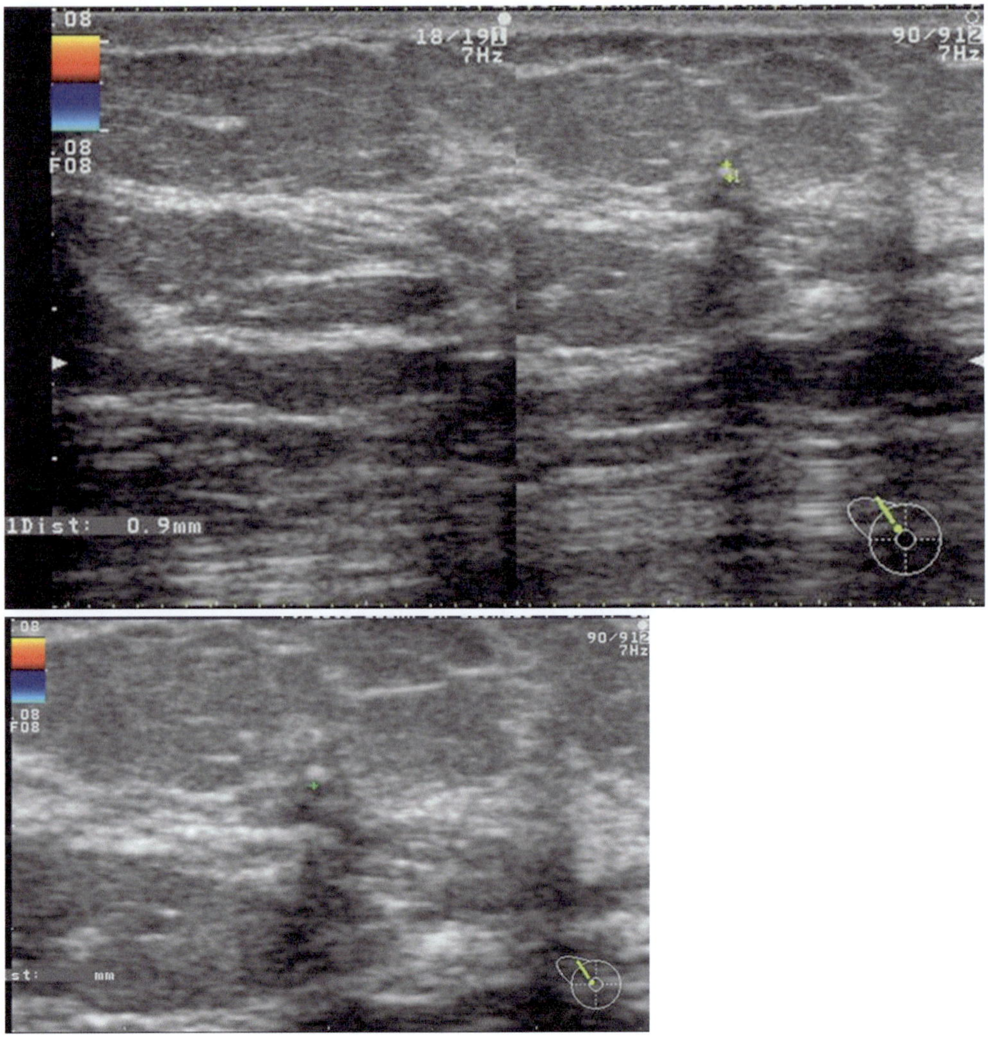

Fig. 7.7 Benign calcification of 0.9 mm, in a TDLU location, typically for a calcified lactiferous cyst; Doppler DE confirms beside the dimension, shape, location, and the absence of the new formation vessels, conclusive for the benign lesions; the acoustic shadowing is due to the Cooper ligament, these calcifications being too small for producing posterior effects

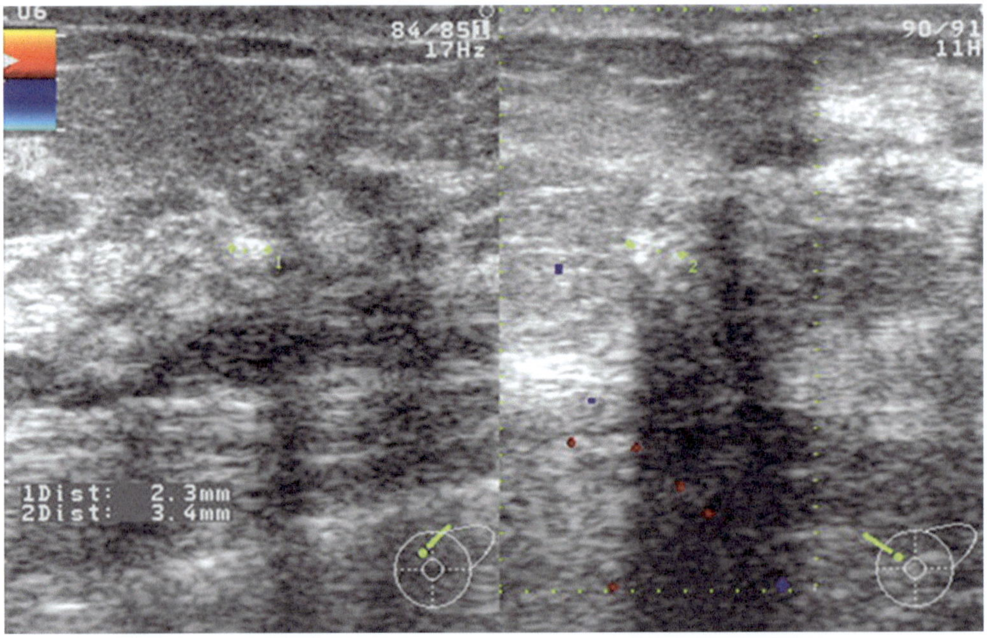

Fig. 7.8 Microcalcifications visualized on US with a size over 1 mm diameter present the characteristic posterior acoustic shadowing; these dimensions correspond to the benign mammographic microcalcifications. The finest malignant ones mammographic detectable are either not visualized or have not specific aspect on US, which has low PPV and NPV

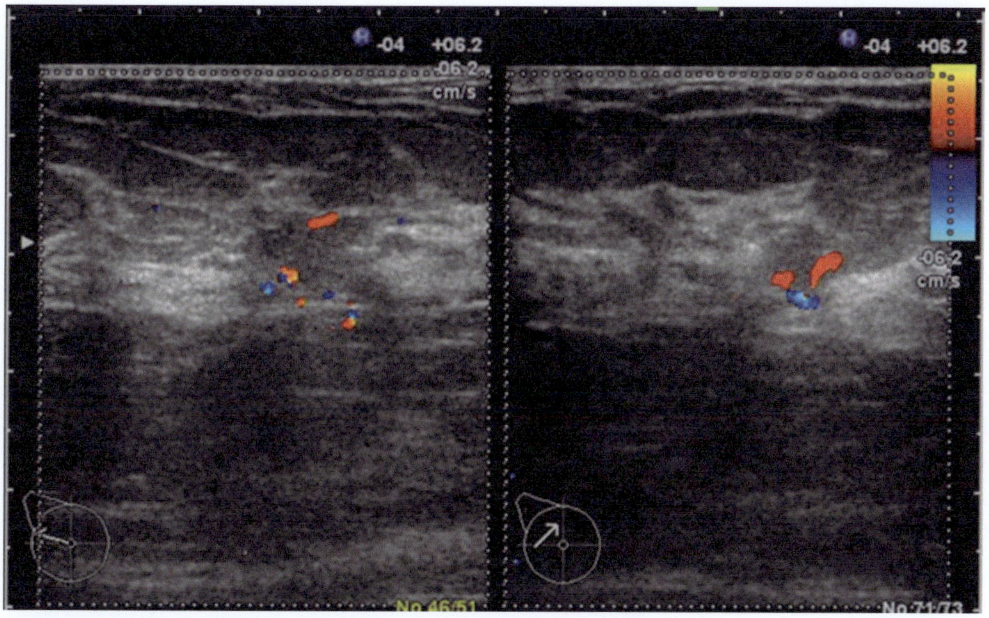

Fig. 7.9 DCIS with segmental thickening of the ducts and new formation vasculature with incident plunging angle artery; no microcalcifications detectable by US, but mammographically, they were visible as cluster of amorphous less than 0.3 mm in diameter that assessed suspect microcalcifications

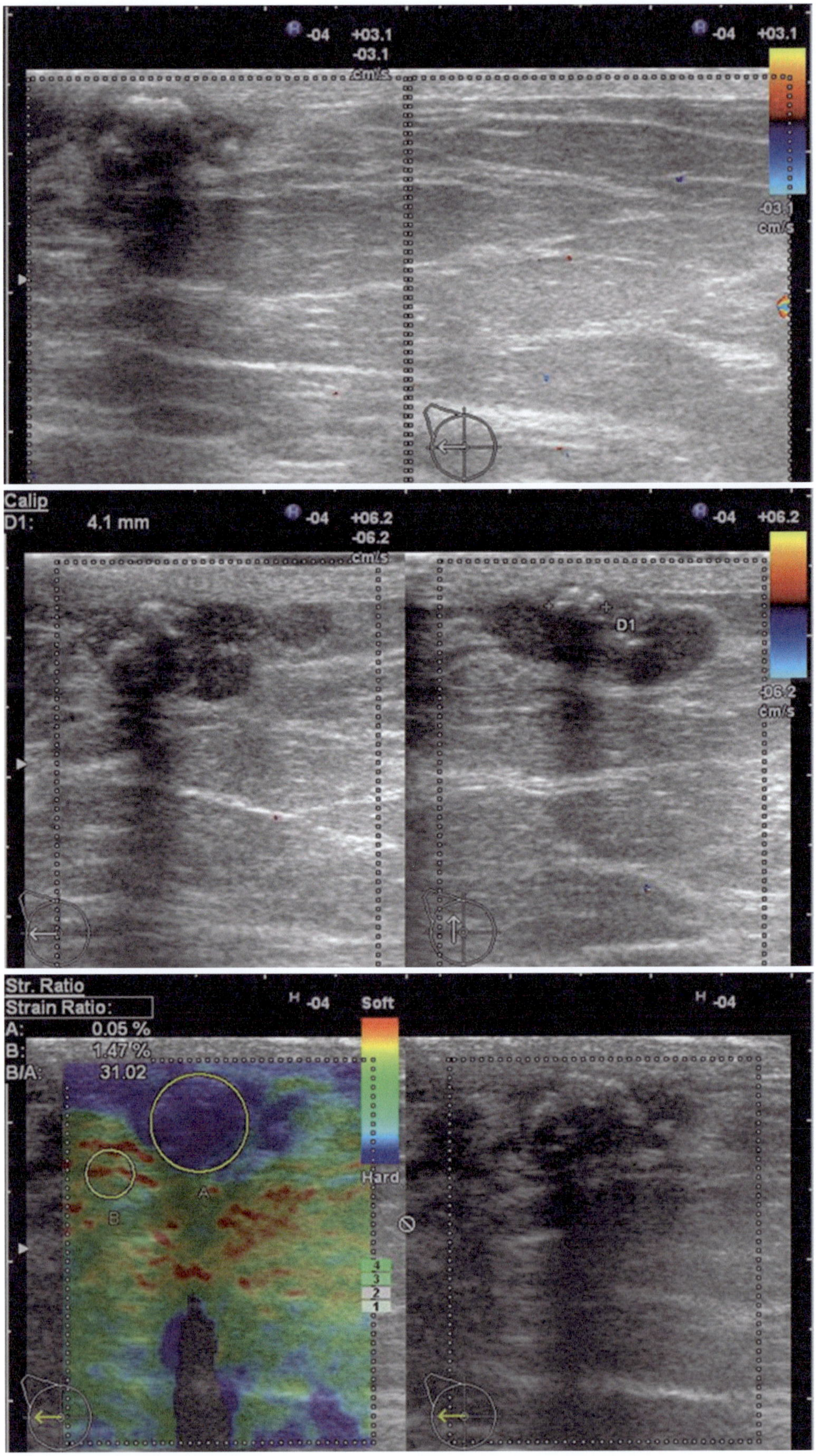

Fig. 7.10 Superficial periareolary lump in a fatty breast, with polycyclic contour, heterogeneous structure with hypoechoic aspect, and macrocalcifications in popcorn, scored 4 upon Ueno classification and with high FLR; therefore, the absence of Doppler signal argues the FBU diagnosis of benign lesion, assessed US BI-RADS 2 category, while the sonoelastographic score for this case is just estimative

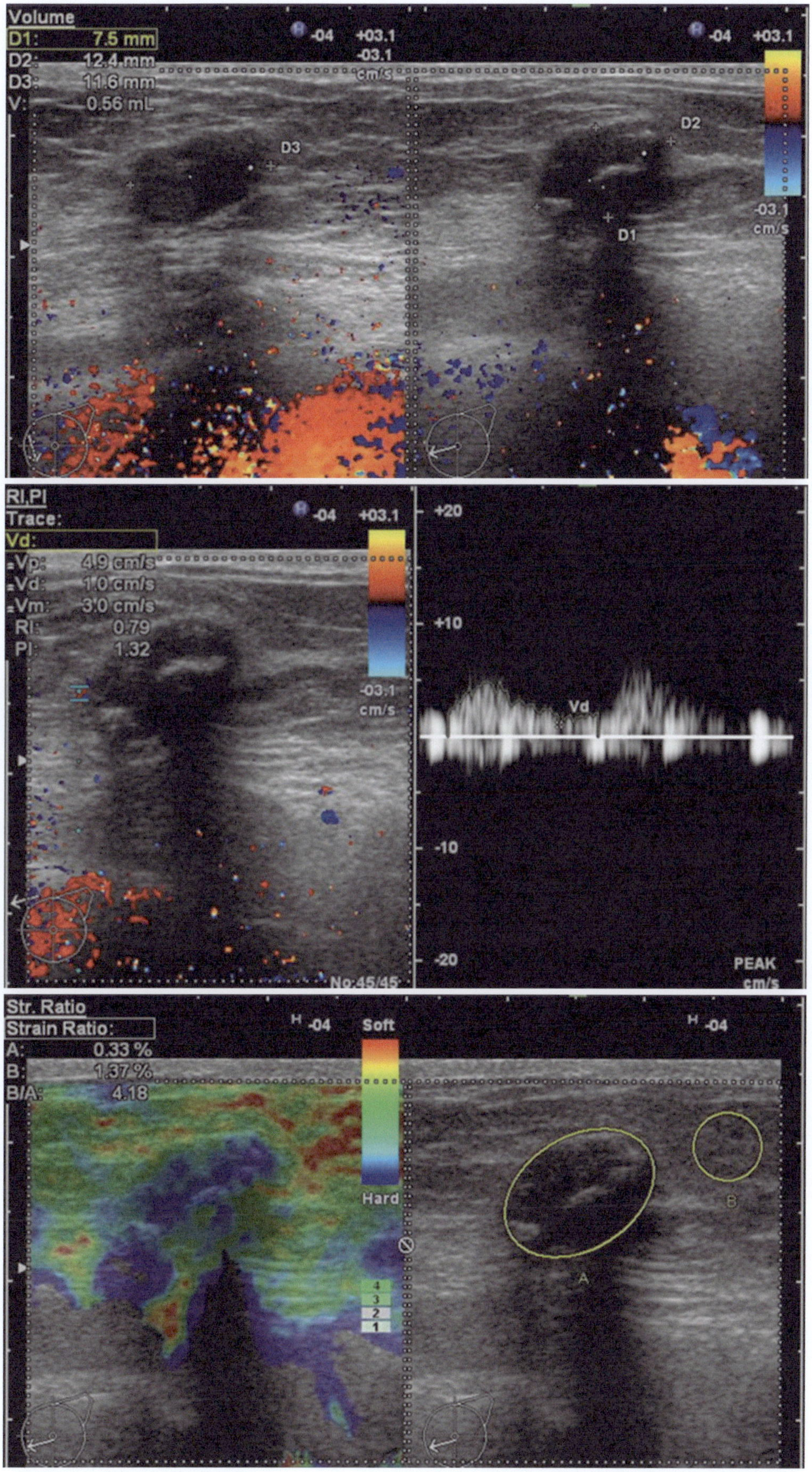

Fig. 7.11 Macrocalcifications in a cystic lesion, with peripheral vasculature and score 3 Ueno; despite the well-delineated contour, the complex aspect and the correlation between Doppler and sonoelastography can be assessed as US BI-RADS 3 category

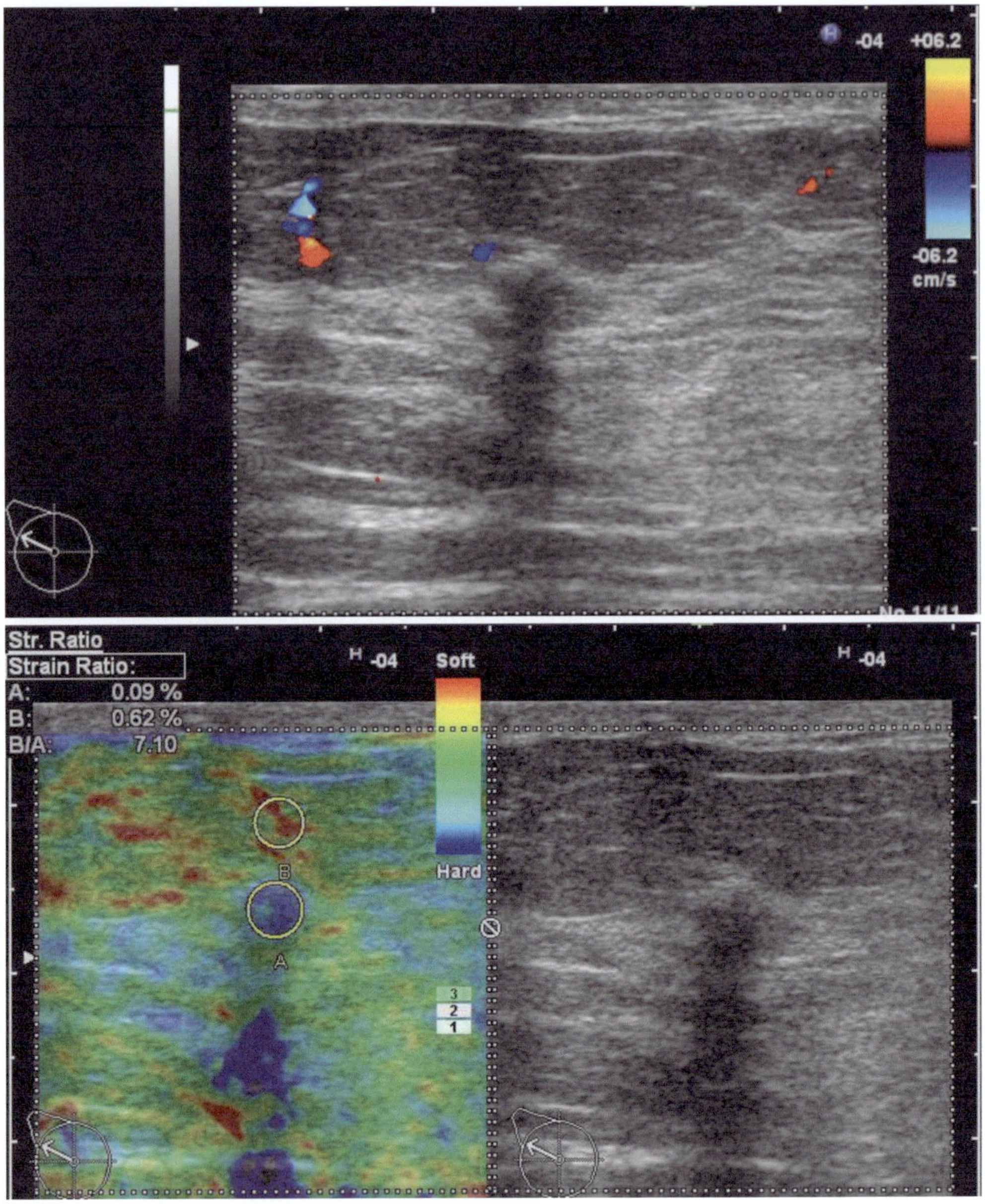

Fig. 7.12 Macrocalcifications grouped in TDLUs, with overall benign characters, despite the score 4 Ueno with high FLR (7.10); the calcifications have over 1 mm size, hyperechoic round-oval shape, and salient acoustic shadowing reinforced by the adjacent Cooper ligament's own shadow

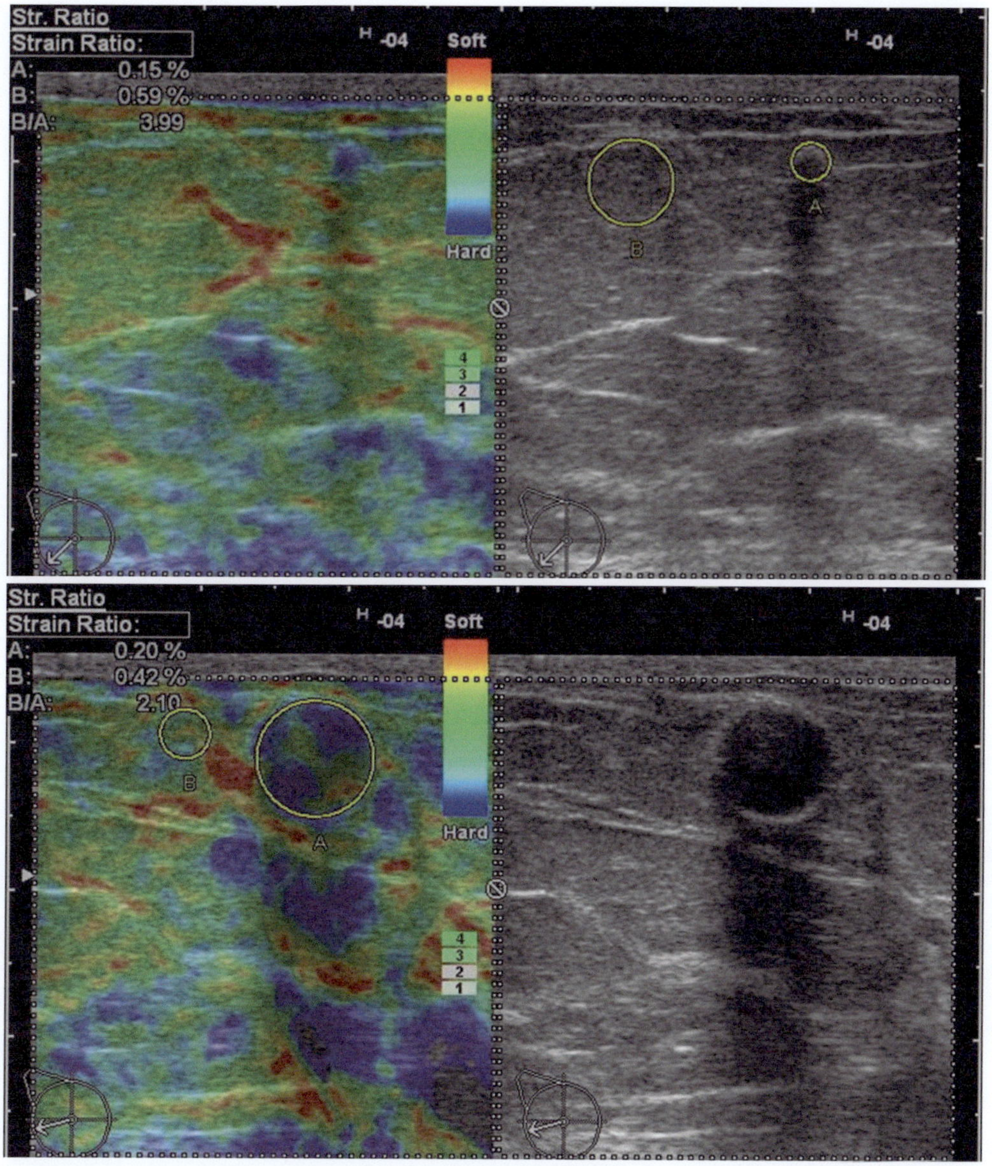

Fig. 7.13 Macrocystic calcifications presenting the eggshell sign, the absence of Doppler signal, and BGR complex score; in this case, the calcified cysts are located in the premammary fatty tissue, without connection with the remnant ductal tree, usually secondary findings after cytosteatonecrosis

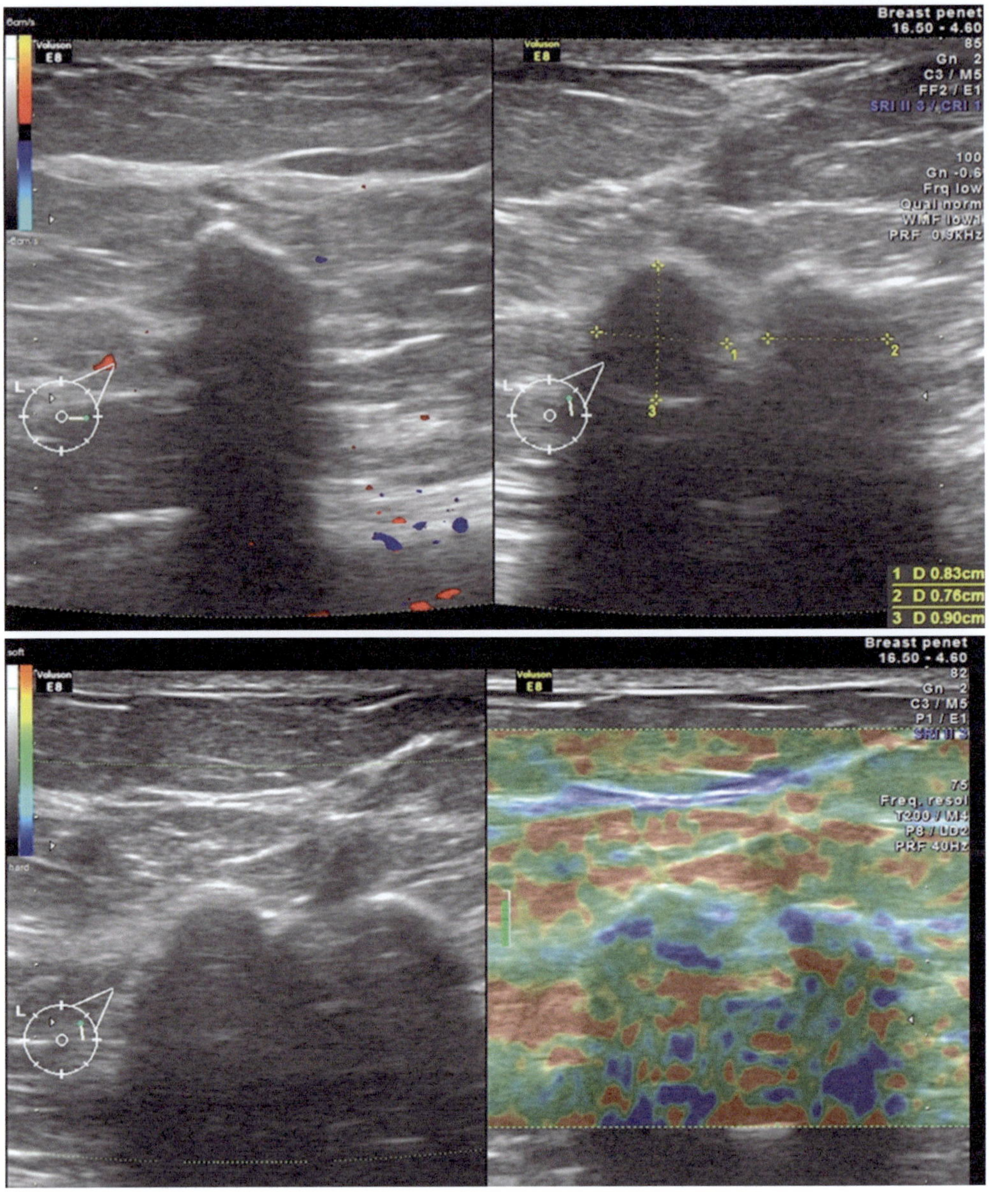

Fig. 7.14 Macrocystic calcifications in a fatty breast presenting the eggshell sign, increased acoustic shadowing, the absence of Doppler signal, and BGR complex score-type reverberation; the cysts have connection with the ductal tree, representing a form of the fibrocystic dysplasia

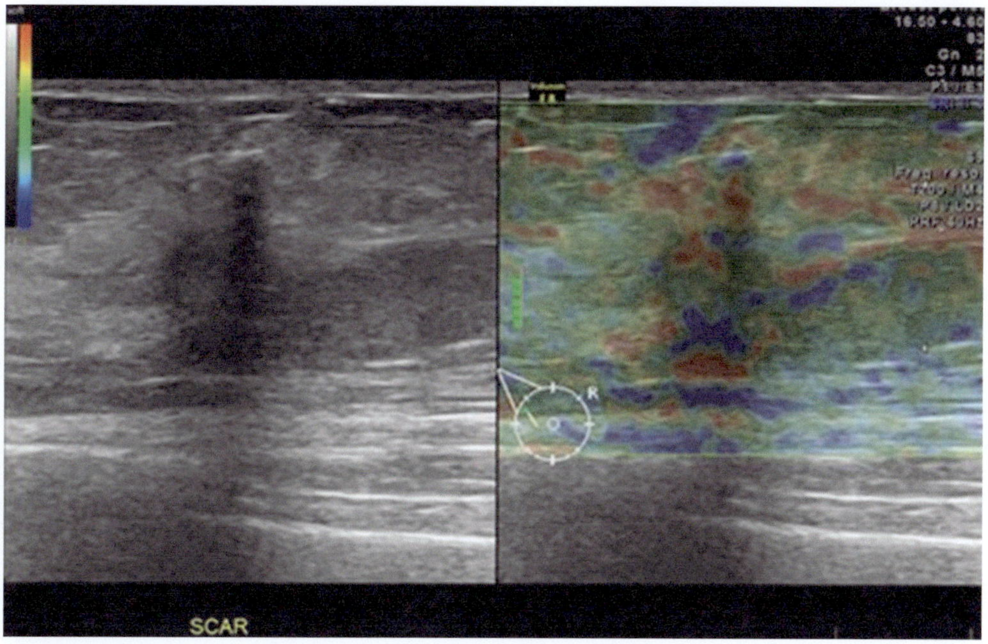

Fig. 7.15 Suture granuloma mimicking breast calcification

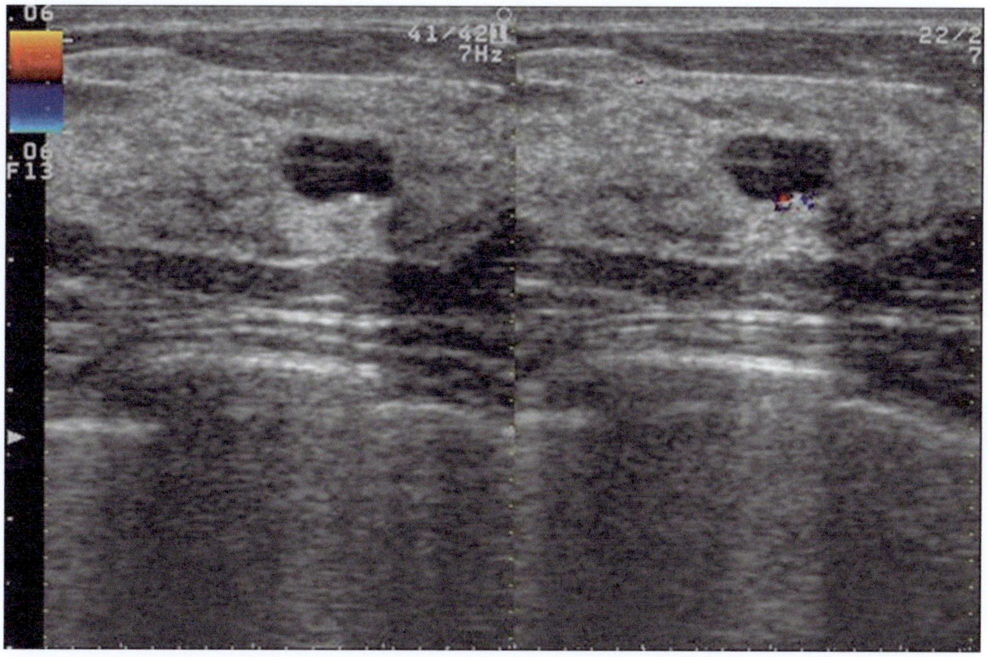

Fig. 7.16 Cystic sedimentary calcifications with hyperechoic debris presenting small Doppler twinkling artifact

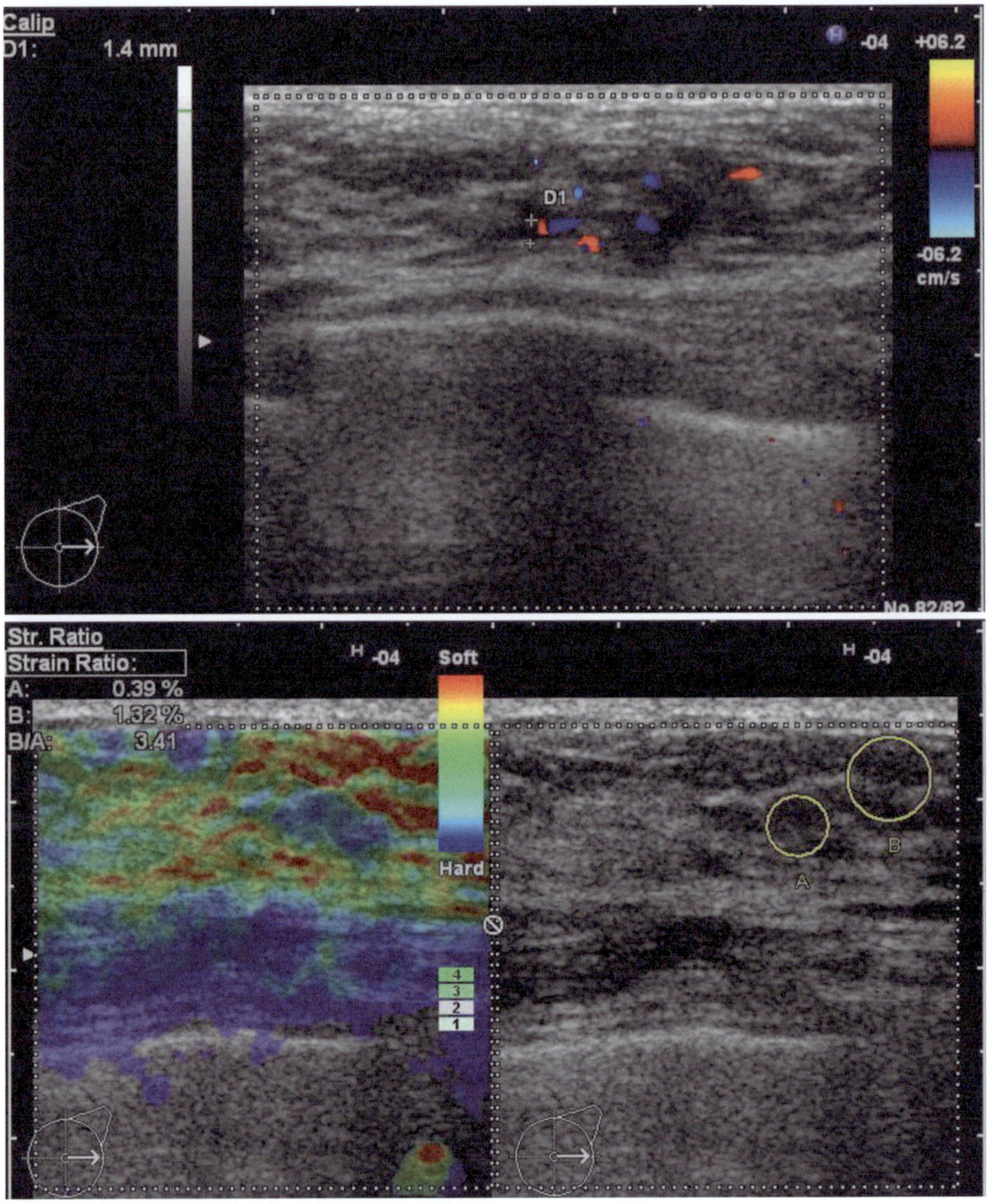

Fig. 7.17 DCIS with mammographic branching microcalcifications, unapparent in 2D US, but with suspect hyperplasias in FBU

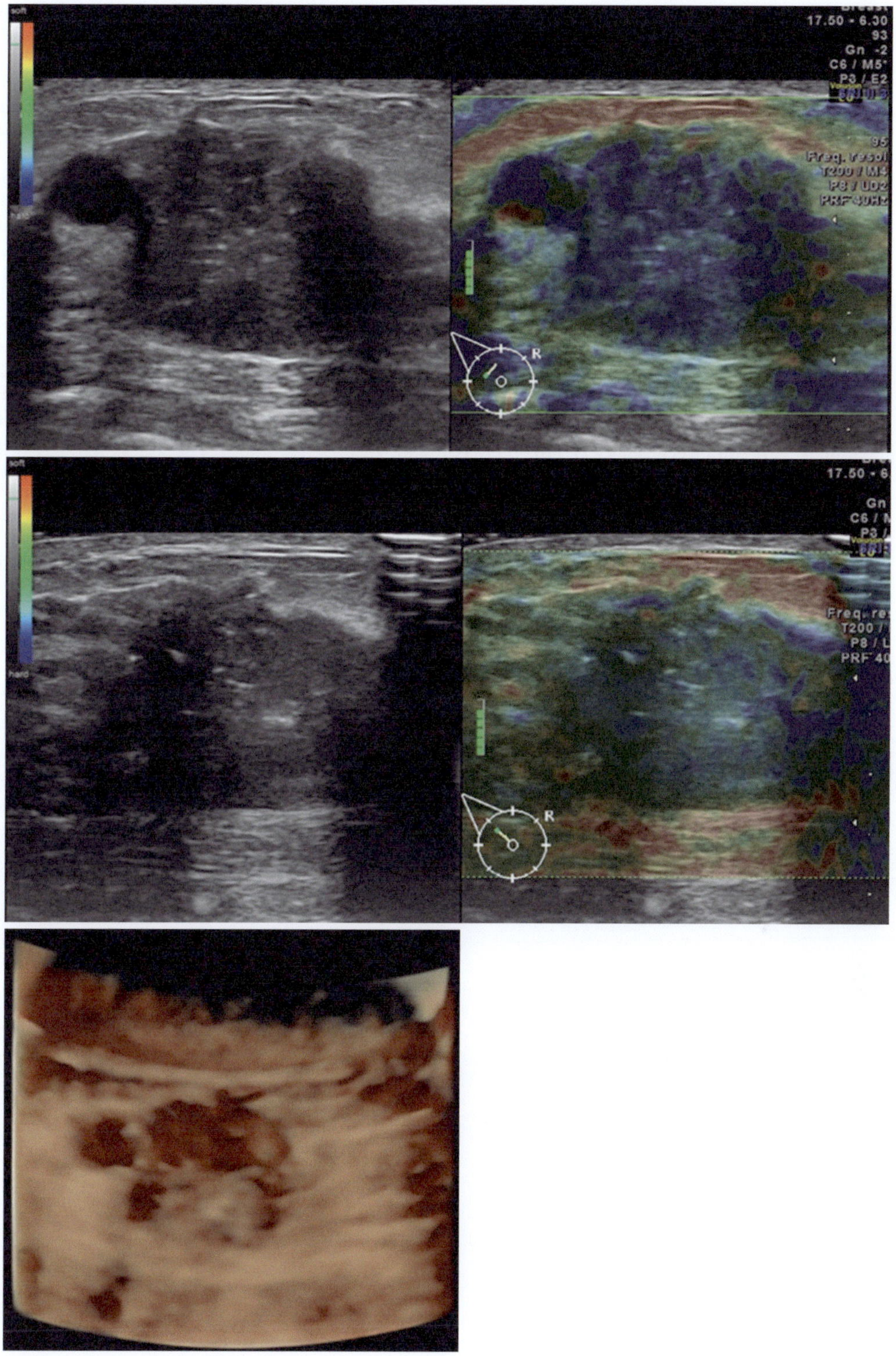

Fig. 7.18 Fibro-micro-cystic nodular dysplasia: there are tinny lesions inside the nodular dysplasia, mimicking microcalcifications with hyperechoic foci representing the posterior acoustic effect behind the almost equal hypoechoic/transonic findings, which represent the microcystic lesions. In the nodular fibro-micro-cystic lesions, usually there is a peripheral larger cyst, and the overall elasticity is of benign score; the 4D US, despite the actual insufficient developed technique, is high suggesting for dysplasia

References

1. Anderson ME, Soo MS, Bentley RC, Trahey GE (1997) The detection of breast microcalcifications with medical ultrasound. J Acoust Soc Am 101(1):29–39
2. Urban MW, Silva GT, Fatemi M, Greenleaf JF (2006) Multifrequency vibro-acoustography. IEEE Trans Med Imaging 25(10):1284–1295
3. Alizad A, Whaley DH, Greenleaf JF, Fatemi M (2006) Critical issues in breast imaging by vibro-acoustography. Ultrasonics 44(Suppl 1):e217–e220, Epub 2006 Jun 30
4. Rosen PP et al (2009) Rosen's breast pathology. Lippincott Williams & Wilkins, Philadelphia, pp 39–166
5. Gufler H, Buitrago-Téllez CH, Madjar H, Allmann KH, Uhl M, Rohr-Reyes A (2000) Ultrasound demonstration of mammographically detected microcalcifications. Acta Radiol 41(3):217–221
6. Soo MS, Rosen EL, Baker JA et al (2001) Negative predictive value of sonography with mammography in patients with palpable breast lesions. AJR Am J Roentgenol 177:1167–1170 [CrossRef]
7. Skaane P (1999) Ultrasonography as adjunct to mammography in the evaluation of breast tumors. Acta Radiol 420(suppl):1–47
8. Moy L, Slanetz P, Moore R et al (2002) Specificity of mammography and ultrasound in the evaluation of a palpable abnormality: retrospective review. Radiology 225:176–181 [Abstract]
9. Sickles EA (1986) Mammographic features of 300 consecutive nonpalpable breast cancers. AJR Am J Roentgenol 146:661–663 [CrossRef]
10. Whang KW, Cho KR, Seo BK et al (2003) Non-calcified ductal carcinoma in situ: radiologic and histopathological findings. Radiographics 23:881–895, © RSNA
11. Teh WL (2002) Chapter 10: High-frequency ultrasound in breast calcification. In: Evans A, Ellis I, Pinder S, Wilson R (eds) A diagnostic manual. Greenwich Medical Media, London, pp 139–148
12. Intra M, Veronesi P, Mazzarol G et al (2003) Axillary sentinel lymph node biopsy in patients with pure ductal carcinoma in situ of the breast. Arch Surg 138:309–313
13. Ansari B, Ogston SA, Purdie CA, Adamson DJ, Brown DC, Thompson AM (2008) Meta-analysis of sentinel node biopsy in ductal carcinoma in situ of the breast. Br J Surg 95:547–554
14. Tot T, Tabár L, Dean PB (2002) Practical breast pathology. Thieme D, New York. ISBN ISBN#: 1588900916
15. Soo MS, Baker JA, Rosen EL (2003) Sonographic detection and sonographically guided biopsy of breast microcalcifications. Roentgenol 180(4):941–948. [Medline]. Available: http://www.ajronline.org/cgi/content/full/180/4/941
16. Majid SA, Shaw de Paredes E, Doherty DR, Sharma NR, Salvador X (2003) Missed breast carcinoma: pitfalls and pearls. RadioGraphics 23(4):881–895. doi:10.1148/rg.234025083

8 Full Breast Ultrasonography of Malignant Lesions

8.1 Major Risk Factors for Breast Cancer and Breast Cancer Prevention

8.1.1 Major Risk Factors for Breast Cancer

The major risk factors for development of breast cancer in women are as follows:

- Positive family history of breast cancer in a first-degree relative
- History of benign breast disease
- Age over 40 years
- Late-age birth of first child or nulliparous
- Use of long-term estrogen replacement therapy or oral contraceptive pills
- Radiation exposure
- Alcoholic beverage consumption
- Smoking (increases the risk of metastases in lungs)

Today, it is widely acknowledged that breast cancer is found three to five times more often in women with benign lesions of the breast and 30–40 times more often in women with a nodular form of mastopathy with signs of epithelial proliferation. About 10–15 % of breast cancers are thought to be hereditary. Normal cells become cancerous as a result of certain mutagenic genes: BRCA1 in about 45 % cases and BRCA2 in about 35 % cases (*BReast CAncer Gene 1* and *BReast CAncer Gene 2*).

8.1.2 Control of the Risk Factors of Breast Cancer: Dishormonal Changes

Because benign conditions and breast cancers have many similar etiologic factors and pathologic processes, they have common risk factors, most related to dishormonal changes. The hypothalamus–hypophysis system plays an important role in the development of dishormonal hyperplasias of the breast. Some authors consider a risk factor to be the activation of the proliferative process in the hormone-dependant organs, including the tissues of breast, which are target areas for the steroid hormones of the ovaries, prolactin, placental hormones, and, implicitly, other endocrine hormones.

Estrogens have major impacts on the proliferation of the epithelial acini, lobules, and interlobular ducts. Their role is, therefore, overestimated, and the use of progesterone-based creams as an "antidote" treatment is illogical because a breast cancer may be both estrogen-receptor (ER) and progesterone-receptor (PR) positive. Therefore, the level of estrogens is correlated in ductal echography (DE) with breast parenchyma, especially with ductal diameter and the size of the lobules. In ovarian precocious insufficiency, bradimenorrhea, primary or secondary amenorrhea, or after ovariectomy, postmenopausal-type changes of the breast occur. With hormonal substitution therapy, assisted fertility treatment, or other cases of hyperestrogenism and "true" gynecomastia, the breast parenchyma presents more or less as ductal-lobular thickening.

Fibrocystic changes, considered dishormonal hyperplasias of mammas, represent one of the most common benign conditions, affecting more than 50 % of women with palpably irregular breasts, cyclic pain, and tenderness. Some findings are considered as congenital pathology, the most severe being Reclus' disease. The "sick lobe theory" of Tot considers the whole lobar unit damage present at birth [1], but the branching of the mammary bud begins at puberty, and many women develop mammary dysplasia later in adulthood or in the postmenopausal stage as result of complex dishormonal changes.

High levels of prolactin may cause breast-feeding changes similar to, but less intense than, normal pregnancies: diffuse breast hypervasculature, lobular hypertrophy, and duct ectasia with milky secretions. In chronic disorders, such as prolactinoma, chronic overinfection may be present. However, not all cases of duct ectasia present hyper-prolactin levels, and not all cases of high prolactin are associated with a pituitary lesion, found on the magnetic resonance imaging (MRI) examination. Elevated prolactin level seems to be correlated in Doppler DE with diffuse increase in the number and size of breast vessels, but no vascular changes were found in chronic secreting galactophoritis [2]. Androgens have more impact on the fibrotic process [3].

A. Colan-Georges, *Atlas of Full Breast Ultrasonography*, DOI 10.1007/978-3-319-31418-1_8

Mastodynia/cyclic mastalgia usually occurs premenstrually and may not demonstrate any changes in the breast anatomy in DE, neither ducts nor lobules being influenced in size or aspect. In the premenstrual breast, increased tenderness and reduced elasticity seem to be determined by the stromal reaction, as is frequently demonstrated by Sonoelastography (SE), which can better delineate the differences in the strain of the stroma (harder) and parenchyma (softer, score type 1 Ueno).

Breast cancer has a significant correlation with thyroidal lesions [4, 5]. Not only is the nodular goiter usually associated with breast diseases but also the diffuse goiter. In many cases, the autoimmune thyroiditis, Hashimoto's disease, is present. Thus results the recommendation to explore the thyroid by ultrasonography, in all cases, with breast screening or breast symptomatic examination.

Food hormones are associated with precocious thelarche, "true" gynecomastia, and duct ectasia. Although this correlation is accepted worldwide, there are few studies employing systematic observation in large populations of food-induced breast pathology. More evident are the effects of therapeutic hormonal intake on breast morphology. Birth control pills may aggravate or ameliorate breast dysplasia, and substitution hormonal therapy increases breast density in postmenopausal woman, increasing the risk of breast cancer. More frequent reports present breast cancer following repeated treatments for assisted fertility.

In cases of adrenal or gonadic hormonal-secreting tumors, breast changes are present in male and female patients. In children with precocious thelarche or pathological gynecomastia (at different ages than physiological breast development), in addition to food-intake of steroids and hormone-secreting tumors as causes, genetic disorders correlated with neuroendocrine imbalance, such as neurofibromatosis (von Recklinghausen disease) [6], hydrocephaly, and brain tumors may be found.

8.1.3 Prevention of Breast Cancer

Despite pathological reports of various types of ductal or lobular hyperplasias, preoperatory noninvasive diagnosis was unable to detect these changes until the advent of DE. Prevention of breast cancer was not considered before the last decade, and it is still a subject of discussion because premalignant lesions are usually not diagnosed by "classical" methods of radiological-imaging diagnosis. Mammography cannot detect any premalignant lesion, except some cases of ductal carcinoma in situ (DCIS) that are suspected because of their suggestive branching or extensive microcalcifications. The sectional methods in use do not respect the branching architecture of the ductal tree or the relationship of the lesions inside the same lobe and with the nipple. Thus, abnormal small proliferative lesions are difficult to detect and characterize. However, there are many possibilities for prevention of breast cancer, and this new vision offers better chances for patients both with and without risk factors.

8.1.3.1 Prevention by Therapy: Immunotherapy

An antitumor vaccine would be ideal for prevention, at least in high-risk patients. RESAN is one such novel drug that has been proposed to be administered in combination with surgical and oncological methods. The aim of the so-called vaccine is to destroy small metastases and prevent relapses after surgical treatment of breast cancers, which may result in absolute cures. The immune action of the drug is a result of the glycoproteins that are analogous to fragments of tumor-associated antigens of breast cancer [7]. These glycoproteins, included in the composition of the vaccine, imitate 6–50 different peptide fragments (each with 7–30 amino-acids) of each of the cancer antigens listed below:

1. Ovarian carcinoma antigen CA125 (1A1-3B) (KIAA0049)
2. Mucin 1 (tumor-associated mucin)
3. Breast carcinoma-associated antigen Df3
4. Cancer associated surface antigen
5. Adenocarcinoma antigen ART 1
6. Serologically defined breast cancer antigen NY-BR-15
7. Serologically defined breast cancer antigen NY-BR-16
8. CA 19-9

Tumor markers such as CEA, CA 125, CA 19-9, CA 15-3, and tumor-associated mucin can be used to monitor the treatment of breast cancer. The risk of recidivism could be reduced by using such a vaccine in patients with dishormonal mastopathy or benign tumors such as fibroadenomas. It could prevent malignant tumors in healthy people and those with positive heritable anamnesis or tumor markers that are higher than in normal. Moreover, it has been proposed as a complementary treatment in preventing and curing endometriosis [8].

Another vaccine that is currently in stage 3 of trials is NewVax (Nelipepimut-S), which is the immunodominant nine amino-acid peptide derived from the extracellular domain of the oncogene HER2, present in 85 % of breast cancer cells. The vaccine binds to antigen-presenting cells (APCs) that migrate in the lymph nodes and, after binding the cytotoxic t lymphocytes (CTLs), which rapidly replicate and migrate in the whole body "attracted" by the antigen HER2, recognize, neutralize, and destroy the HER2-expressing cells. Long-term protection against tumor recurrence is promising. Nevertheless, there is much more research aimed at the true prevention of primitive breast cancer. The results are far from satisfactory because the etiology of the disease is multifactorial and some causes are still unknown.

8.1.3.2 Prevention of Breast Cancer by Diagnosis of Premalignant Lesions

A true screening method must diagnose both premalignant and malignant breast lesions. Unfortunately, except for DE, no current method of radiological or imaging diagnosis is able to detect normal ducts and lobules, essential in depicting small abnormal changes. The methods in use for screening are intended for early diagnosis of breast cancer that is already developed but clinically unapparent. Thus, the real incidence of the breast cancer will not decrease with the use of these techniques, but at least the survival rate should increase.

Techniques used worldwide for the early detection of the breast cancer are, in decreasing order of their accuracy, as follows:

- Breast MRI
- Breast tomosynthesis
- Digital mammography and computed aided diagnosis
- Analogue mammography
- Classical ultrasonography

Ductal ultrasonography, which the authors refer to as DE, being the only anatomical imaging method, has an intrinsic high sensibility in detecting the breast's normal ductal-lobular tree and its physiological and pathological changes, with a resolution up to 0.4 mm for the actual transducers. The use of Doppler increases the specificity, without any supplementary contrast agent, and the sonoelastography is a complementary tool in differential diagnosis, resulting in higher overall accuracy.

8.2 Histologic Aspects of Breast Cancer and Correlation with Mammography and Ductal Echography

There are histological characteristics of breast cancer that determine some specific features of the radiological and ultrasonographic images and are not adequately understood by radiologists and, consequently, by clinicians. Therefore, understanding the anatomical basis of the image's formation is important in diagnosis and therapeutic decision making.

8.2.1 The Large-Format Section in Surgical Pathology: The Best Pathological-Imaging Correlation of Breast Carcinoma

The large-format section (LS) of breast pathology has, for more than a century, been a research tool to better understand breast microanatomy and the relationship between radiological images and pathological features [9]. Beginning in 1906, Cheatle used LS in cases of breast cancer to better understand the relation between a neoplastic mass and the surrounding normal tissue and the possible existence of premalignant changes [10, 11]. Furthermore, many researchers have used this method to study the early phases of breast cancer development, proving the importance of analysis with large sections of the branching ducts. Thus, in 1973, Wellings and Jensen concluded that most breast carcinomas arise in the terminal duct lobular unit (TDLU), the main site of the different morphological malignant features [12]. The precise location of the lesion in a TDLU can be visualized only by full breast ultrasonography (FBU) in all cases, because the radial scan allows the detection of all TDLUs at the intersection of the main ductal axis with Cooper's ligament, and Doppler can illustrate the nourishing vessels arising from the superior or inferior segments of that Cooper's ligament. The mammogram, being a volumetric projection to a surface, can visualize only the peripheral TDLUs located to the radius 9:00 and 3:00 for the cranial-caudal view, or to the radius corresponding to the medial-oblique-lateral view (e.g., between 7:00–8:00 and 1:00–2:00, for the left breast). Similarly, MRI examination can visualize the TDLUs located only to the radius 12:00, 3:00, 6:00, and 9:00, the rest of the scans being oblique to the main ductal axes.

More recently, many authors have highlighted the value of LS in the diagnosis of breast malignancy, especially in the precise determination of tumor size, multifocality and cancer extension, vascular invasion, and extension of the DCIS and lobular carcinoma in-situ (LCIS) [13], with good cost/benefit evaluation [14]. However, most authors performed randomly large sections, omitting the radial distribution of the breast ductal tree, and the relationship between their findings and breast anatomy was incomplete.

The best application of LS in the analysis of breast pathology is represented by the *theory of the sick lobe* of Tibor Tot [1, 15]. Indeed, the breast lobes are individual units, without peripheral delimitations by septae or other structures, but with unitary function and pathology (either benign or malignant).

The use of large-format histological sections redefined the terms *multifocality* and *multicentricity* of breast cancer. Their better understanding allowed better evaluation of prognosis and treatment [16]. In classical ultrasonography, used as a complementary tool with mammography, the distinction between multicentric and multifocal cancer is arbitrarily defined, according to the breast quadrants, the unique radiological feasible segmentation of the breasts, which is easily to realize by combining the acquisitions of the cranial-caudal and medial-lateral views. The lesions located in the same quadrant are "multifocal," whereas the lesions located in different quadrants are "multicentric." These arbitrary definitions are dangerous in therapeutic decision making because the lobes with individual ductal trees may overlap in the same quadrant. As a consequence, there can be present in the same quadrant different cancers in different lobes, with different cellular-types and evolution, representing true multicentric cancers. In addition, a mammary lobe may extend to a few adjacent quadrants, and thus the same tumor may disseminate intraductally in two adjacent quadrants, determining multiple monoclonal lesions, or true multifocal cancers.

Tot's classification of breast cancers, based on the sick lobe theory, is logical and offers a better basis for decision making about therapy [17]:

1. *Unifocal cancer* – better prognosis
2. *Multifocal cancer* – in the same lobe (lobar cancer), with worse prognosis, usually with axillary lymph node involvement (in 75 % of cases)
3. *Multicentric cancers* – in different lobes, in the same breast or bilateral
4. *Diffuse cancer* – (5 % of cases) extension is present in many lobes and quadrants, with greater aggressiveness

The number of the lesions was found to be higher in the cases of examinations of large sections than in small, conventional blocks. It is logical that the use of large, anatomical radial scanning in ultrasonography is better than small scans used as a complementary examination of the lesion and of its proximity. The large pathological section is obtained after surgery, but the large scan, with dedicated, long, linear transducers, allows better diagnosis in vivo, with the possibility of measuring the size of the lesion and the extent of disease by locating the multifocal and multicentric breast cancers. Nevertheless, the accuracy of the available ultrasound devices is lower than that of microscopic analysis, but it allows a significant improvement in the preoperatory diagnosis.

Large sections were used in the last century for understanding, diagnosis, and management of pathological lesions of the breast and organs such as lung, brain, kidney, ovary, and colon [9]. The limitations of their availability are related to the manufacturing of the adapted cryothome.

8.2.2 The Main Pathological and Imaging Classifications of Breast Carcinoma

Because the radiological imaging methods of diagnosis of breast cancer have a logical and physical similarity to gross appearance on pathological examination, we have chosen the classification of Martin, which has been well known since 1882 [18]:

Pathological Classification of Breast Cancer Based on Martin (1882)

A. Usual Breast Carcinoma
   - In situ carcinoma (ductal, lobular)
   - Mass-forming carcinoma (invasive)
   - – Knobby carcinoma
   - – Stellate carcinoma
   - – Circumscribed masses (pseudo-benign appearances):
     1. Medullary carcinoma
     2. Mucinous carcinoma
     3. Poorly/undifferentiated carcinoma
     4. Cystosarcoma phyllodes
     5. Mixed carcinomas (usually intraductal and medullary or mucinous)
   - – Invasive lobular carcinoma
B. Unusual Malignant Breast Lesions
   - Carcinomas: inflammatory, tubular, metaplastic and anaplastic, apocrine, adenocytic, fibroadenoma and carcinoma, invasive colloid, recurrent
   - Carcinosarcoma
   - Sarcomas: cystosarcoma, liposarcoma, angiosarcoma
   - Metastatic malignant lesions: metastatic carcinomas, melanoma, carcinoid, hypernephroma, angiosarcoma, neuroectodermal tumor, lymphoma
   - Paget's disease
   - Breast carcinoma in children
   - Breast carcinoma in pregnancy

"Knobby" carcinoma is a term proposed by Gallager and Martin [19, 20] to describe the type of invasive breast carcinoma made up of innumerable, tiny, circumscribed masses as small as 1 mm, which coalesce but do not fuse into groupings, each knob remaining separate from the others. As a consequence, when analyzing the whole tumor, we see the knobs protruding from the edges. The edges of the knobby carcinoma become indistinct, with unsharp borders in mammography and and a multilobular/multi-cyclic appearance in ultrasonography. This form of breast was found by the authors to be the most common, comprising up to 47.7 % of all invasive cancers, and its major extensions are in the mammary ducts, usually proximally toward the mammary areola, following the line of minimal resistance. That corresponds to the demonstrations of Teboul, which proved by DE the intraductal dissemination of multistep evolution, the metastases decreasing in size proportionally with the distance from the main tumor. The centripetal or centrifugal dissemination is explained by the minimal resistance of the ductal content. This manner of malignant spreading is confirmed by Tot and colleagues in the sick lobe theory [1]. Gallager and Martin, in 1969, used serial whole organ sections with gross and microscopic viewing, which were easily compared with mammograms. Tot and coworkers, in 2007, used large-format histologic sections, from the nipple to the periphery, similar to radial scanning of the DE, to demonstrate the lobar architecture and the intraductal dissemination of BC.

Stellate carcinoma usually arises in older women, has a distinctive shape with peripheral spicules, and represents the best-known type of breast cancer. However, stellate cancer, with its peripheral stromal reaction determining the spicules, has a better prognosis than knobby cancer, with an absolute survival rate of 70.8 % versus 57.6 % cases based on Martin [18].

Circumscribed masses are mostly represented by medullary and mucinous cancers, which account for less than 5 % of cases. Medullary cancer may develop in young or older women and tends to be located at the periphery of the breast, mimicking a benign lesion on the mammogram. It can be connected to a dilated duct with centripetal orientation toward the nipple.

The mucinous carcinoma tends to lie superficially, has a low density on a mammogram, and the centripetal ducts may be distended by mucin and tumoral cells. The skin may be infiltrated, up to exophytic lesions, but the axillary lymph nodes are rarely involved. Survival rate is higher than in the knobby and stellate forms. However, survival depends on the precise preoperatory diagnosis of the extent of disease, because the whole organ pathological reports may present associated dilated tumor-filled ducts, dilated lymphatic vessels, and other satellite small cancers, unapparent on mammography. Mucinous cancers may present both multifocal and multicentric lesions, and before the use of DE, no preoperatory method could demonstrate the real extent of the disease. Breast MRI may demonstrate the multiple lesions, but the arbitrary scanning planes do not allow the illustration of their connections.

8.2.3 Multifocal and Multicentric Breast Carcinoma

According to Tot, the real local extent of disease can be classified in three major types of breast cancer that can be found by pathologic examination using large sections, which are related to the ductal tree:

- Unifocal lesion, usually located in a TDLU, with various sizes and local extension
- Lobar cancer, with secondary dissemination intraductally, following minimal resistance
- Diffuse cancer

A study by Tot et al. (2011), performed on 574 consecutive cases diagnosed using large sections, found that invasive carcinomas were multifocal in 24 % and diffuse in 5 % of cases, percentages that are largely superior to those published in paper based on conventional blocking [17]. Simultaneously, Teboul recommends following the anatomic criteria and observing the epithelial structures in vivo using DE, which allows for assessment of cancers, and presuming localization in vivo and the type of malignancy (2010). According to his classification, there are three main types of breast cancer [21]:

- Lobular carcinoma (10 % of cases)
- Diffuse carcinoma with involvement of a duct, its branches ,and terminal lobules (25 % of cases); this corresponds to lobar cancer in Tot's classification
- Ductal-lobular and ductal focal cancers (65 % of cases), corresponding to unifocal lesion in Tot's classification

Multifocality has a great impact on survival, as the risk of death from breast cancer is higher in patients with multifocal and/or diffuse carcinomas when compared with those with unifocal carcinomas. Multifocality can be useful in the evaluation of the risk of axillary involvement by breast cancer metastases. According to Baldovini [22], 71.42 % of patients with multifocal tumors exhibited axillary lymph node metastases, whereas 40.54 % of those with unifocal tumors showed axillary nodal involvement.

Radiological differential diagnosis of multifocal and multicentric cancer was established arbitrarily, by necessity, to standardize localization of a mass on orthogonal projections: cranial-caudal and medial-lateral (oblique) views. As a consequence, the mammographic distinction is established by the location in a quadrant: inside the quadrant there are "multifocal" cancers, and in different (even adjacent) quadrants there are "multicentric" cancers. This classification does not reflect the breast anatomy and, therefore, is not concordant with pathologic reports. Nevertheless, this classification is still in use and is important in the surgical treatment of breast cancers, accompanied by the risk of missing foci and recurrence of the disease.

Because of the intralobar dissemination of breast cancer, and the unapparent connection between two lobar branching trees, it is logical for multifocal cancer to spread initially in the same lobe, with similar types of malignant cells (monoclonal). Cancers present in different breast lobes may have more probable different malignant-type cellularity, being multiclonal lesions. Because the lobes may overlap, it is possible using ultrasonograpy to visualize different lobar structures in the same quadrant, even on the same radius, with the potential to develop multicentric cancers. The arbitrary division of a breast in quadrants, while useful for reporting lesions, is not correlated with the lobar distribution. As a consequence, it is possible for a mammary lobe to lie at the border of two quadrants, extending to both sides, as has been proved by Cooper's models [23], with presence of some multifocal cancers simultaneously in different quadrants.

Mammography (analogue or digital) is not suitable for the detection of multiple cancers. Even breast tomosynthesis and breast MRI, which are used more frequently to detect multiple lesions, are not accurate in the differential diagnosis of multifocal and multicentric malignancies. DE, being an anatomical *in vivo* examination, changes the arbitrary delimitation and is able to detect lobar multiple lesions, the multifocal cancers connected to the same ductal tree, whatever the quadrant. Diffuse cancer is easily recognized by MRI examination, but DE findings may be suspect, especially when adding Doppler and sonoelastography, with further evaluation by biopsy or MRI evaluation.

8.2.4 Size and Extent of Breast Cancer

Determining the size of the lesion is important for the characterization of T value of the TNM (tumor, nodes, metastasis) staging of the breast cancer. When the lesion is unique, with well-shaped borders, such as knobby cancer and pseudo-benign rare types, the largest diameter is considered the lesion's size. For the most accurate measurement, the volumetric measurement is more conclusive, especially when preoperatory treatment is intended.

The size of the stellate form of breast cancer is difficult to measure. Some authors recommended measuring the size of the central mass, ignoring the surrounding spicules and the halo as they are determined by the stromal reaction. Others believe that the spicules are the way tumoral cells spread, and the real extent calls for measurement of the whole visible lesion.

To measure the local extent of the disease, multifocal cancer requires evaluation of all distinguishable lesions (determining each lesion's size) and calculation of the global volume of these masses. The best methods for evaluation are breast MRI and FBU with the ductal tree analysis. According to Teboul, the DE technique indisputably shows that malignancies often demonstrate a greater spatial extent than has been suspected by other techniques. Indeed, this method allows direct perception of a malignant diffusion by sprinkling or distinct fragmentation of the main detected malignant masses. The fragmentation into several malignant tiny nodules or malignant clusters is found close to the main malignant lesion or at a distance along the affected duct, as demonstrated by the theory of the sick lobe [21].

8.3 Breast Cancer and Ultrasound Diagnosis Applying Old and New Criteria

Breast cancer staging using the Union for International Cancer Control (UICC) TNM classification was issued in 1960 (joined since 1987 with the staging system of the American Joint Committee on Cancer, or AJCC) and includes five stages [24]:

- *Stage 0*: The cancer has not spread farther than the ducts, DCIS, the lobules, LCIS.
- *Stage I*: The tumor measures 2 cm or less and has not spread to the lymph nodes or other tissues.
- *Stage II*: The tumor is between 2 and 5 cm in size, and/or the cancer has spread to one to three auxiliary lymph nodes on the same side; tumors of 5 cm without any metastases to lymph nodes are also included.
- *Stage III*: Tumors less than 5 cm in size with metastases to four to nine auxiliary lymph nodes; tumors bigger than 5 cm with metastases to one to nine auxiliary lymph nodes; tumors that have spread locally (close to the breast) and usually involve the skin, chest wall, or nine or fewer auxiliary lymph nodes.
- *Stage IV*: A cancer of any size that has spread to the other parts of the body, most often the bones, lungs, liver, brain, or distant lymph nodes.

The most common breast malignancies are of ductal epithelial origin (almost 80 %) and are either confined to the duct (in situ or intraductal) or infiltrative (invasive). Lobular cancer represents 10–15 % of cases, usually as multifocal disease; stromal cancers and rare forms, including atypical cancers and metastases, are less common (5–10 % of cases).

It is widely accepted that, although mammography is the primary imaging modality for the early detection of breast cancer, classical ultrasonography (for the majority, the only known ultrasound technique), used in conjunction with mammography, can further increase the cancer detection rate.

There are different pathologic characteristics that account for some variability in ultrasound appearance. Most invasive ductal carcinomas exhibit irregular or ill-defined margins related to infiltrative and reactive fibrotic desmoplastic components. Carcinomas of uniform cell type or types that do not invade aggressively may appear as well-circumscribed masses, such as mucinous or papillary carcinomas; intracystic carcinomas are rare but usually noninvasive with well-defined margins, mimicking benign lesions on mammography.

Because early diagnosis is desirable in the fight against breast carcinoma (allowing faster treatment that is more effective, less aggressive, and has a great probability of cure), it is essential to have at our disposal a technique making possible to detect with certainty all the variations, abnormalities, or lesions of the breast at an infracentimetric stage. Moreover, it would be ideal to detect premalignant lesions, the most important factor in reducing the incidence of a malignancy. For example, by using the Papanicolaou test to detect and treat cervical dysplasias, cervical cancer incidence was reduced [25], and prostate cancer incidence was reduced after the introduction of PSA (prostate-specific antigen) screening [26]. This will be possible using DE as a technique of examination and guidelines for the diagnosis of breast diseases, combined with Doppler and sonoelastography for the full characterization of the lesions. This is the concept of full breast ultrasonography, as introduced by Amy [27].

In a study by Amy that included 5,010 cases, all patients were investigated systematically by mammography and DE. The study concluded that DE score detection is higher than that of radiological examination [28]. Moreover, contrary to other published studies, the author claims to have never encountered mammographic-visible lesions that were not detected by DE. In addition, we consider that lesions visible only in one mammographic projection, cranial-caudal or oblique, usually called "opacities" (to differentiate them from "masses," visible on two to three projections), are better characterized by DE because of the anatomical scanning. Moreover, Amy's report highlights the significant number of multifocal cancers diagnosed with DE, which consequently involve surgical and chemotherapeutic treatment changes.

DE diagnosis applies to anatomical scans the same Stavros criteria of breast lesions that are used in classical ultrasonography, which are the basis for the ultrasound Breast Imaging Reporting and Data System (BI-RADS) assessment [29, 30]. Stavros reported a 98.4 % sensitivity for diagnosis of malignant masses using classical ultrasonographic criteria for malignancy, including spiculation, nonparallel orientation, angular margins, marked hypoechogeneicity (relative to fat), shadowing, calcification, duct extension and branching pattern, and microlobulations. These results reflect the high resolution of state-of-the-art equipment and expanding skills of radiologists, but classical ultrasonography should be assumed as a complementary examination of a precise area with suspect clinical or mammographic findings.

In classical ultrasonography, suspicious masses identified on ultrasound should always be correlated with mammography, or more recently with MRI, which can depict the lesion and eventually the multicentric/multifocal malignancy.

The halo sign, proposed by Takehara in 1976 and reaffirmed by the Japan Society of Ultrasound in Medicine in 2005 [31], represents the hyperechoic marginal zone that is the expression of a scirrhous carcinoma that invades and spreads into the surrounding tissues. In recent years, the Japan Association of Breast and Thyroid Sonology refined the description and defined a peritumoral "boundary zone," existing on a "border" between the "tumoral margin" at the inside part and the "periphery" at the outside [32].

The complete characterization of a malignant breast lesion is presented in the previous Chap. 5, Sects. 5.2 Ultrasound Diagnostic Criteria and 5.3 Lexicon for Breast Lesions in the fundamentals of ultrasound breast BI–RADS classification. However, the criteria for the differentiating benign from malignant breast lesions are not specific and, even when they are used in combination, the specificity of the method is modest, less 70 % according to most authors.

The use of three-dimensional/four-dimensional (3D/4D) acquisitions as a second step in ultrasound examination may be useful. It is proven that spiculations are more easily seen in the coronal view than in other variant orthogonal views. Moreover, 16 % of benign cases and 90 % of malignant cases are detected with spiculations [33]. Siemens presented a technique of automatic breast volume scanning (ABVS), which offers the coronal plan with accuracy. However, in this technique the sagittal and transverse plan are not useful in screening and detecting premalignant changes because there is no anatomical relationship with the nipple and the ductal tree.

The characterization of the vasculature represents one of the most important criteria of diagnosis, more important than shape, orientation, posterior effects, and so on. Although FBU demonstration of a normal or an abnormal duct or lobule is not difficult with state-of-the-art ultrasound instruments, the demonstration of the intraductal or periductal vasculature cannot be always successful with conventional color Doppler or power Doppler acquisitions. However, the absence of detectable vessels in a solid-type lesion is a negative predictor for malignancy. When visible, the vasculature of the benign masses has less three poles, with a peripheral arcuate course and oblique plunging angle, described by some authors as "basket-type new vasculature." On the other hand, malignant lesions show new vasculature with the number of poles depending on the lesion's size. In the case of small malignancies, new vessels are visible beginning when the tumor reaches 3–4 mm diameter, with the poles increasing progressively. Malignant lesions usually present larger vessels than the surrounding glandular tissues, with higher velocity compared with the normal vasculature in the surrounding regions and sometimes demonstrating an aliasing effect. In addition, the most important sign of malignant new vasculature is the incidence angle of the plunging vessels, which is almost pathognomonic [34].

Three-dimensional Doppler ultrasound may better demonstrate the differences between benign and malignant vascular patterns [35]. The technical evolution of ultrasound machines, including software development, will allow rapid and reproducible volumetric acquisitions, available even for examination of small parts. Actually, the 3D/4D transducers have only small resolution for Doppler reconstruction in breast tumors.

In some cases, there are cysts with echoic content that may mimic a solid benign lesion. Otherwise, a small cancer, usually a second or a third intraductal dissemination of the main tumor, may have undetectable vasculature, but they conserve the irregular shape and the posterior acoustic shadowing of the main tumor and are connected with the same ductal tree. In such cases, the evaluation of periductal angiogenesis using contrast-enhanced ultrasound is recommended. A study by Chou [36] of the efficacy of contrast-enhanced ultrasound (CEUS) in the identification of ductal pathology in women with abnormal nipple discharge found that CEUS has 100 % sensitivity. For intraductal papillomas or carcinomas, ultrasound detected 12 pathologies out of 13 patients, and CEUS showed positive results (i.e., either intra- or periductal contrast flow signal) in all patients (13/13), whereas the specificity was 71.4 % (positive CEUS in periductal mastopathy and occasionally fibrocystic changes).

The use of CEUS was found to be correlated with MRI wash in–wash out curves and with a CEUS specificity of 87.5 % (similar to ultrasound alone) and a sensitivity of 100 % [37]. However, there were some lesions with a false-positive diagnosis: two hypervascular fibroadenomas in young women and a phyllodes tumor. This study demonstrates that evaluation of the vasculature as a single descriptor is not sufficient in positive and differential diagnosis, which is an argument for using FBU as a complete examination utilizing the assets of US. In addition, the use of CEUS has some limitations, the most important being its invasiveness (there are proved side-effects), costs, and lack of an observer agreement regarding vascularization patterns [38].

The use of Doppler techniques has proved useful as a follow-up exam in treated breast cancer, with reduction of vasculature as response of chemotherapy [39–41] or reduced vascular pattern in post-radiotherapy mastitis. Contrarily, an increased number and diameter of vessels are present in developing breast cancer. Most authors agree with Kumar et al. [42], who proved that Doppler scoring correlates well and can be accurately used to objectively predict the pathological response to chemotherapy in patients with locally advanced breast cancer.

8.4 Particular Clinical–Imaging Aspects of Breast Carcinoma

There are some particular clinical and imaging aspects of breast carcinoma that have incomplete descriptions in the typical model of malignancies, but there are some specific findings that are presented in the following.

8.4.1 Inflammatory Breast Carcinoma

Inflammatory breast carcinoma is also called carcinomatous mastitis. Clinically it has an acute appearance, with painful tenderness, orange peel-like skin thickening, hyperthermia redness involving more than a third of the breast, increase in size and heaviness, and lymph node enlargement, mimicking inflammation. These signs are not determined by infection or injury as in real mastitis. Sometimes an inverted nipple occurs. More often, no mass can be felt. This form of breast cancer is caused by malignant cells blocking lymph vessels in the skin and premammary fatty tissue.

Carcinomatous mastitis accounts for about 1 % of all breast cancers in United States, but the diagnosis and reporting seems to be an underestimation. This cancer occurs usually in young women after birth control treatment abuse or in the older women, in whom it is easier to eliminate a nonmalignant mastitis. It is more common among African-American women and in overweight and obese women.

The prognosis is the worst, as it is more aggressive than the common types of cancer. In fact, there is never an early stage with this breast cancer, being diagnosed at least in stage IIIB (locally advanced) or even stage IV, with distant metastases. However, some cases have no findings on the mammogram, or the edema may be present but unspecific. The affected breast may be larger and denser than the contralateral breast, similar to the clinical findings. Moreover, tenderness and swelling can make it difficult to perform a mammogram. The clinical presentation being in the advanced stage, the screening mammogram is not useful.

Characteristic classical ultrasound findings with inflammatory breast carcinoma are diffuse, irregular thickening of the skin and subcutaneous layer. Sometimes it is possible to identify a tumoral mass with irregular margins and internal hypoechoic necrosis in the parenchymal layer. The subcutaneous fatty tissue becomes more echogenic, and the distinction with the hyperechoic glandular stoma is less defined.

Dilated branching pattern of lymphatics in subcutis fatty tissue could be more distinctively evaluated on ultrasound than on MRI. Most authors believe that the association between a tumor with lymphatic dilatation on ultrasound and enhancement of thickened skin and parenchyma on MRI could be useful for the diagnosis of the inflammatory breast cancer [43, 44]. However, the description is vague and nonspecific, and, in the absence of the clinical examination and patient's history, differential diagnosis with infectious mastitis or inflammatory changes after radiotherapy is difficult to make by radiological and classical sonographic examination. MRI can detect abnormal regions not visible on mammogram and it is used to guide the biopsy.

In DE, the aspect is less specific. The thickening of the skin and fatty tissue, which has a hyperechoic aspect with the dilated hypoechoic branching pattern of lymphatics, make it difficult to examine the ductal-lobular structures, which may present ectasias (in benign mastitis the enlarged ducts are better delineated). Cooper's ligaments are thickened with increased posterior acoustic shadowing. The hyperemia is diffuse, as in inflammatory benign mastitis, whereas in post-radiotherapy mastitis the vasculature is reduced. The differential diagnosis between benign-type mastitis and inflammatory breast cancer may be possible by adding sonoelastography. There are few observations about its application for carcinomatous mastitis, but in our experience the benign type presents an inversion of the strain ratio. The skin and subcutaneous fatty tissue present increased strain compared with the glandular lobar structures that are "softer." The malignant type has less strain of the thickened skin and subcutis layer, with increased diffused hardness of the glandular lobes, such as in diffuse lobar cancer. An additional observation about the malignant type is that the axillary lymph nodes are almost always involved with malignant characters. If the breast biopsy is not accurate in such cases, an axillary lymph node biopsy is easier to perform and offers a quick diagnosis.

Staging of the inflammatory breast cancer needs further investigations, by with multi-detector computed tomography or PET-CT. According to the American Cancer Society, after the TNM staging, all inflammatory breast cancer is classified T4. If the collarbone (supraclavicular or infraclavicular) lymph nodes or the internal mammary lymph nodes are involved, without distant metastases, then it is the stage IIIC. If no more than the axillary lymph nodes are involved, it is the stage IIIB. The presence of distant spreading of the disease is stage IV.

8.4.2 DCIS and LCIS

Despite the pathological examinations that make differences between ductal and lobular carcinoma in situ, in the literature there are some disagreements concerning the start zone of these cancers and the imagistic findings. It is widely accepted that DCIS arises in the hormone-sensitive epithelial cells of the peripheral ducts, in the area of TDLUs, so in the proximity of the lobule. There are also locations in the peripheral segments of the main ducts, which allow easier intraductal centripetal/centrifugal dissemination. DCIS may be associated with the ductal papilloma centrally located in a large duct, but the evolution and pathogeneses are different, the papilloma being a benign lesion without risk of malignancy, whereas DCIS may develop in invasive carcinoma [45]. There are some papillomas with apocrine, squamous, mucinous, clear cell, and sebaceous metaplasia with benign prognoses. They are usually not detected by mammography because microcalcifications are usually absent. Sclerosing papillomas may mimic a pseudoinvasive pattern [46] and in sonoelastography may present increasing strain ratio, but there is not a pathological new formation vasculature. Some papillomas may display focal proliferations of a mildly atypical, monotonous cell population identical to grade 1 DCIS or atypical hyperplasia, rarely grades 2 and 3. These lesions were designated as *atypical papillomas*, with excellent prognosis, estimated at nearly 100 % survival at 10 years [47].

Papillomatosis, or peripheral/multiple papillomas, is represented by papillary proliferations within multiple TDLUs or in the ductules. Usually it is an incidental microscopic finding, because mammography cannot distinguish them from the other breast opacities, except in cases with microcalcifications or nodular masses [48]. Even in DE, differential diagnosis with adenosis or small LCIS is difficult, except in cases with nipple discharge, when associated duct ectasia is visualized and cytological tests are performed from the nipple surge.

In DCIS and LCIS, neoplastic growing cells fill and distend the duct without disrupting it. DCIS is an incidental discovery in an asymptomatic woman or in a woman with a painful breast. Rarely it is discovered in nipple discharge cases or after suspect microcalcifications in mammography. The clinical incidence is only 1–3 %, whereas the mammographic incidence is 8–25 %, and practically it could be more because not all DCIS present microcalcifications. With nipple discharge, DCIS was found in 26.8 % of cases with bloody discharge, 13 % of cases with serous discharge, and in no cases with discharge of other types, according to Hou et al., as quoted by Svane [49].

A study by Takebe and Izumory from 1997 to 2003 confirmed a DCIS that was nonpalpable and without discharge or mammographic calcification, which they named "3 non-DCIS." They found well-defined 3–10 mm masses connected to the ducts, without posterior attenuation or other malignant well-known findings [50]. This aspect can be detected with best accuracy only by following the normal anatomy, ductal size, and distribution, as done in DE, and not randomly checking an eventual clinical or mammographic negative abnormality, as in classical ultrasound.

DCIS may involve a unique segment of a duct, but sometimes it extends to multiple ducts by the unfolding process or develops in many sites simultaneously. DE can demonstrate the ductal connection between the lesions, which appear as thickened ducts, with loss of the central hyperechoic line sign, sometimes with inhomogeneous ductal content. The new periductal vasculature is rarely found with the actual transducers, but the elasticity of the whole area and of the ductal tree inside the pathological region may be reduced compared with the healthy lobes. Without treatment, this lesion may develop in few years into an invasive ductal carcinoma (IDC). The problem is hunting it out. DCIS is asymptomatic and painless in this stage and not all cases have an invasive evolution. The high-grade DCIS has the most risk.

Morphological aspects of DCIS are classified as follows:

- Comedocarcinoma
- Papillary carcinoma
- Cribriform carcinoma
- Solid carcinoma

Doppler DE can at least suspect a DCIS when demonstrating a segment with abrupt margins, well-shaped thickening of a duct, with or without shadowing, but with a local periductal detectable vasculature or/and an increased stiffness. Positive diagnosis becomes difficult when the lesion is associated with ductal hyperplasia, as is usually presented in the pathological reports, but a short-interval follow-up (2–3 months) is more useful without any more risk than an ultrasound-guided biopsy. With ultrasound equipment it is not possible to differentiate the atypical ductal hyperplasia from the DCIS. The value of Doppler DE has yet to be demonstrated because there are few encouraging reports regarding the actual state-of-the-art.

High-grade DCIS may present characteristic microcalcifications at pathology as well as mammographically. However, with ultrasound there are few visible microcalcifications with the usual high-frequency probes (7–12 MHz). Hyperechoic spots without shadowing (less than 0.4 mm in diameter) are nonspecific findings. When transducers of 18 MHz or more will become available, they will improve the vascular pattern detection. In ultrasound this is more useful than blind identification of microcalcifications (the manufacturer technical development will allow to the US to become the examination of first-intention). Mammographically, the microcalcifications appear in DCIS as numerous, with segmental distribution and irregularities in size, density, and shape (linear or branching shape, suggesting ductal spreading of the malignant cells and the calcification of the necrotic material).

Although DCIS is considered noninvasive, neoplastic cells have been observed in the sentinel nodes, so the systematic examination of all axillary, subclavicular, and internal mammary lymph nodes must always be performed.

There is not a control interval guideline in suspected DCIS on ultrasound, but, in our experience, performing a follow-up control in 3 months is useful, with increasing intervals if stationary or regressing lesions classified as ultrasound BI-RADS category 3 are found. If the developing evolution of the suspect DCIS is proved, a change of the assessment to ultrasound BI-RADS category 4 is justified and can be supported by the possibility of developing a well-known "interval cancer" encountered in the screening mammography. As a consequence, there are some recommendations for complementary examinations (mammography, breast MRI, serological tumor markers determination, or guided biopsy).

A particular form of DCIS arises with sclerosing adenosis. In classical ultrasound, sclerosing adenosis is usually difficult to detect because of the neglect of the normal anatomy with the connection of the pathological findings to the ductal-lobular tree. However, ultrasound still seems to be useful in the diagnosis of DCIS, which appears as an irregularly shaped hypoechoic lesion, usually as a non-mass-forming lesion (nonpalpable), whereas mammography misinterprets sclerosing adenosis with DCIS as an invasive carcinoma (emphasized diagnosis) [51]. Doppler DE is able to provide more diagnostic accuracy because sclerosing adenosis is easy to visualize in postmenopausal women with normal atrophied parenchyma associated with segmental ductal-lobular hyperplasias. Any supplementary abnormal structure connected to the ductal-lobular tree, with suspect features such as irregular shape, shadowing, abnormal increasing vasculature, or increasing size on short follow-up interval, require further investigation and is referred to as ultrasound BI-RADS category 4. Further research is needed on sonoelastography of sclerosing adenosis associated with malignant lesions because of the risk of emphasized diagnosis, but if it is correlated with the other sonographic descriptors, the diagnostic could be more appropriate. Quantitative sonoelastography seems to be more accurate than the qualitative modality, and the FLR (fat-to-lesion ratio) with the cut-off level 4.70 (5.00) as results from the Amy's reports and from our researches proved more specific. The greater the ranges of the FLR, the greater risk of malignancy. FBU might be able to solve one of the most important causes of false-positive ultrasound diagnosis.

LCIS is the other noninvasive breast cancer. It is limited to the lobule area without breaking the basement membrane, but it can develop into an invasive form. As with DCIS, there have been observed involvements of the sentinel lymph nodes [52]. Usually there are multiple simultaneous lobular involvements in young women, which may be misdiagnosed in FBU as adenosis because of their small sizes and lack of malignant characteristics. In the accentuated forms of adenosis, a 3-month-interval follow-up ultrasound is recommended, associated with dynamic evaluation of tumoral markers. It would be erroneous to consider FBU as a method of differential diagnosis of the pathological type of lesions, but the intention of the method must be limited to finding lesions as early as possible, determining their precise location, and classifying them in a risk category.

Invasive lobular cancers (ILC) are characterized by the multiplicity of their foci. Because of their small size, usually less than 1 cm, they are more easily recognized in FBU. Because there is no evidence of important secondary features on the skin and superficial fascia, ligaments or fatty signs, or architectural disorders, lobular cancers may be missed on mammography, especially in dense breasts. After Teboul, lobular carcinomas appear in DE preferentially located in TDLUs, as a few hypoechogenic lobular enlargements on the skin side of the duct, growing perpendicularly to the duct, isolated from each other and measuring about 5 mm in longitudinal diameter. If Doppler examination is added, the regional vasculature may be increased according to the size and extension of the lesions. The sonoelastographic aspect is not typical, but the overall elasticity is reduced compared with the rest of the breast areas.

8.4.3 Diffuse Breast Carcinomas

Diffuse breast malignancies are difficult to recognize in mammography in the absence of microcalcifications. MRI examination is more sensitive, but it is not a first intention examination. Classical ultrasound has low sensitivity and specificity.

The pathological examination demonstrates a lack of focal arrangement and evidence of spreading of the malignancy in and along ductal-lobular structures. DE illustrates the normal and abnormal ductal tree and thus is able to display two types of patterns of diffuse cancers at initial stages [21]:

1. Anatomical, showing a thick and long linear spreading of malignancy in ductal-lobular structures (slow-growing cancers).
2. Brambles, showing a rather more restricted diffusion, displayed as a thin and irregular tree network developing into some local terminal ductal branches or the close interstitial space and fatty tissue (acute diffuse malignancies and recurrences in scars).

In the intermediate stages of the diffuse malignancy, the lobules enlarge with diameter up to 15 mm, in small number as dominant foci upon Teboul, with small enlargement of adjacent lobules as new foci; their orientation initially perpendicular to the main duct and skin, as in normal lobules, progressively becomes oblique. In advanced stages, these diffuse malignancies appear as extended, hypoechogenic areas, with acoustic shadowing, developed in the whole lobe with almost no remaining recognizable organized ductal-lobular structures. Sonoelastography may add valuable information with diffuse increasing of the lobar strain in a large volume of the breast.

8.4.4 Carcinomas with Pseudo-Benign Appearance

The best-known circumscribed masses with pseudo-benign appearance are presented in the above classification. However, there are multiple malignancies with false appearance on ultrasound. There are a few (less 5 % of all of carcinomas) with pseudo-benign appearance on two-dimensional (2D) ultrasound, both in classical ultrasound and in DE. This means that they can have an oval width-to-depth shape, with more or less regular but clear borders, without malignant shadowing or even with posterior echo enhancement and small lateral shadowings, such as benign posterior findings described by Kobayashi. The most important lesions with these ultrasound findings are mucinous and medullary carcinomas, which have regular internal architecture with low attenuation, and breast lymphomas and leukemic infiltrations, usually in acute leukemia, which may appear as a solid-type infiltration or as a diffuse mixed echo-texture. The pseudo-benign, well-delimited masses may become suspect in FBU by their new formation of rich vasculature demonstrated by Doppler evaluation. Furthermore, the diagnosis can be reinforced by sonoelastography, which is highly sensitive. These lesions, classified with the score 4 Ueno, appear in blue without a peripheral light blue boundary zone (because of the lack of desmoplastic reaction, as in infiltrating carcinomas). It results that FBU can address one of the most important causes of false-negative ultrasound diagnosis in breast cancer management.

8.4.5 Nipple and Retroareolar Carcinomas

The nipple and the retroareolar volume must be distinctly explored by ultrasound, in multiplanary acquisitions, with water-bag probe or adequate echo jelly, which is used to fill the skin irregularities and to offer an image without relief deformation. There are many types of malignancies related to this initial developing root and final functional station of the lobar trees.

The most important lesion involving the nipple is Paget's disease, with a long benign evolution and sometimes malignant changes. The mammographic findings are nonspecific in Paget's disease, because the nipple and areola rarely have nonspecific changes, and the examination is limited to an evaluation of the extent of a primary carcinoma, which may be obscured in dense breasts [52]. The sonographic findings in Paget's disease are more various and correlated with the clinical signs. A study by Choi et al. detailed the most important clinical manifestations compared with the ultrasound findings, with remarkable results considering the technology of 2001:

- Nipple retraction
- Bloody nipple discharge
- Nipple eczema
- Subareolar mass

Ultrasound was better than clinical examination in detecting the mass as a hypoechoic lesion with irregular borders. The second important finding was the irregularly dilated major lactiferous ducts associated with a mass, specific to ultrasound examination and never demonstrated by mammography [54]. Other findings such as calcifications and parenchymal distortion were rarely described and seem to be imitations in interpretation borrowed from the mammographic lexicon. Otherwise, the most frequent mammographic findings were increased subareolar density, parenchymal distortion, microcalcifications (branching and granular shapes), and the presence of a mass. Mass detection was superior on ultrasound, which detected 12 of 13 masses, compared with mammography, which detected 4 of 12 masses.

A study of nipple malignancies explored using 3D sonogram multiplanar images and volume-rendering transparent minimum projection mode in 184 histologically proven breast cancers and reported that 41 breast cancers were suggestive of Paget's disease ($n=3$) and pagetoid extension of breast cancers ($n=38$) [55]. The following were found: nipple duct dilatations (41/41), nipple parenchymal stromal distortion (40/41) (sic), calcifications in nipple duct or lactiferous sinus (20/40), disrupted high echoic nipple skin (40/41), and mass in the nipple and subareolar area (12/41). False-positive lesions were breast cancers with duct ectasia ($n=5$), breast cancer with chronic perivascular inflammation ($n=1$), and focal post-inflammatory dermal fibrosis ($n=1$). This study is important because it describes the most frequent findings in Paget's disease, but some findings are unclear (nipple parenchymal stromal distortion) or useless because of clinically evident signs (disrupted high echoic nipple skin). Otherwise, it is important to note that other cancers with a nipple-areolar location may present the same aspect. Ultrasound is useful, especially in the differential diagnosis of a malignant lesion from an inflammatory one, such as infected cysts or ductal-ampullary systems, and also for a summary examination of the whole breast.

For the differential diagnosis of retroareolar lesions, especially for the assumption of malignancy or benign-type mass or dilated ducts, FBU is recommended as the most-performed, noninvasive, and available technique. Because the normal nipple has a high strain, appearing in blue, sonoelastography is useful in detecting retroareolar and periareolary abnormal stiffness, allowing better guidance for biopsy in suspect cases.

8.4.6 Breast Cancer with Nephrotic Syndrome

Paraneoplastic nephropathy/membranous glomerulopathy refers to glomerular disease without specific etiology that develops in parallel with cancer evolution phases (improvement, remission, recurrence) [56]. The most common neoplasias associated with paraneoplastic glomerular disease are Hodgkin's lymphomas and lung and gastrointestinal tract carcinomas. A few cases of nephrotic syndrome and breast cancer have been reported.

Membranous glomerulopathy is caused by immune complexes that build up in the kidney, resulting in a thickening of the vessel walls within the kidney filters. Despite the small number of cases with this association reported in the literature, it is possible that some cases are underdiagnosed or neglected. The ethyological-pathological diagnosis is important because the surgical and chemotherapeutical treatment of breast cancer can resolve the nephrotic syndrome, and, inversely, the resolution of proteinuria with hypoproteinemia might be a measure of cancer control [56]. An important aspect of the reported cases with paraneoplastic membranous nephropathy associated with breast cancer was the advanced local stage, with most cases presenting invasive ductal cancer, with or without any lymph node involvement [56].

The nephrotic syndrome is considered a rare complication of breast carcinoma, but the incidence may be underestimated because of either a missing diagnosis, misinterpretation as different etiologies, or even because of the metachronous association of proteinuria and hypoproteinemia with advanced breast cancer. In a report of Valcamonico et al. [57], the nephrotic syndrome appeared 5 years after the diagnosis of breast cancer. Despite the absence of a widely accepted experimental model of the association of glomerulopathy and cancer, the remission of proteinuria after complete healing of the neoplasia represents clinical proof of etiological correlation.

The differential diagnosis must include the irreversible renal injuries induced by the oncological treatment, such as pamidronate treatment in advanced breast cancer [58]. In these cases, the glomerulopathy associated with tubular-interstitial damage determines irreversible renal failure that does not improve after discontinuation of the treatment.

8.5 Satellite Lymph Node Metastases in Breast Cancer

8.5.1 Diagnosis of the Satellite Lymph Node Metastases by Classical Methods and FBU

Physical examination and plain ultrasound of axillary lymph nodes offer an evaluation that is not always precise. The metastasis in the sentinel lymph node can be detected in some cases only by Doppler imaging [59]. Contrast-enhanced interstitial ultrasound lymphography, with subcutaneous injection, was successfully tested in 2003 as an alternative to the sentinel node biopsy, with 85–94 % sensitivity [60].

Not all axillary findings are lymph nodes and not all lymph nodes detectable with ultrasound or mammography are malignant. Usually, there are more than 15 axillary lymph nodes, but not all normal axillary lymph nodes are detectable because of their small size and because their features are similar to the lobules of the fatty tissue. As a consequence, if some lymph nodes are salient, they must be characterized as well as possible. Those that are undetectable are assumed as benign/normal [61].

A study by a Korean group, presented in 2003, included 114 patients with axillary abnormalities and found 35 cases with benign lymphadenopathy: 21 nodal hyperplasias, 8 tuberculosis, and 6 histiocytic necrotizing lymphadenitis. The malignant lymph nodes ($n=20$) were represented by nine nodal metastases from breast carcinoma and one lymphoma. Other non-lymphadenopathy structures included accessory breast and its related abnormalities in 28 cases, 17 cases of benign skin lesions, a cystic lymphangioma, and a lipomatous tumor [62].

Before the widespread use of the sonoelastography, Doppler imaging was the first technique added to classical ultrasound that proved to be useful for determining whether sentinel lymph node biopsy is indicated [59].

The risk of false-negative results in axillary lymph node biopsy is proportional with the stage of the breast cancer and the location in the upper outer quadrants [63]. In a study of 512 women with breast cancer, axillary lymph node metastases were present in 6.1 % of T1a-b cases, 25.1 % of T1c, 28.7 % of T2, and 35 % of T3. The probability of nodal involvement in negative lymph node biopsy (false negative) was calculated between 1.3 % for T1a-b, up to 6.3 % in T1c, up to 7.5 % for T2, and 9.7 % for T3. The authors concluded the patient may be better informed about the axillary lymph node dissection decision based on the calculated risk of metastases, but the evaluation is only statistical, not case related.

The evaluation of the satellite lymph nodes is important before therapeutic decision making. Mammographic detection has a low sensitivity and poor specificity. MRI has a high sensitivity but low specificity, which increases the biopsy rate. Ultrasound detection of the lymph nodes has a variable accuracy according to different authors, because the technique and the criteria for diagnosis are different. It is important to discriminate between "benign-type" and sentinel lymph nodes in patients with breast cancer. The node seen as the most malignant looking or located closest to the tumor was defined as a sentinel node on ultrasound. Sentinel node biopsy will be a standard technique in breast cancer treatment. Therefore, preoperative examination of axillary lymph nodes needs reevaluation.

In gray-scale ultrasonography it is often difficult to judge lymph node metastasis only by the morphologic assessment, the general sensitivity being less 45 % and the specificity less than 70 %. A classical ultrasound description of a lymph node with a round shape rather than an oval shape, a ratio of the wide to the long axis greater than 0.5, or a wide axis larger than 1 cm is suggestive of a malignant lymph node, in addition to hypoechoic internal structure, with loss of hyperechogenicity of the node's sinus.

Better results are obtained using ultrasonography with Doppler and sonoelastography. Salient new vasculatures, especially in the cortical regions, combined with low elasticity are the most important findings with high accuracy for malignancy. Often, the sentinel node appears as a focal thickening of the cortical region, with asymmetrical shape and local cortical hyper vasculature, the aspect is more specific than the lymph node diameters. These observations related to partial lymph node involvement are confirmed by a study by Britton et al. that presented the results of core biopsies in different ultrasound types of axillary lymph nodes:

- No visible nodes had normal histology after surgical biopsy.
- Normal ultrasound lymph nodes presented micrometastases in 3 of 70 cases.
- Uni-lobulated cortex lymph nodes were malignant in 7 of 17 cases.
- Multilobulated cortex lymph nodes were malignant in 17 of 31 cases.
- Absent hilum with smooth cortex were malignant in 7 of 9 cases; those with absent hilum with lobulated cortex were positive in 5 of 6 cases [61].

When the characterization of axillary lymph nodes was based on 2D assessment of their size, shape, vasculature with Doppler exam, and internal echoes using THI (Tissue Harmonic Imaging), the accuracy was good, up to 95.8 %, with sensitivity 90.8 % and specificity 97.6 %, according to Kusama et al. [64]. The value of Doppler ultrasound was proved in cases with axillary metastases in no palpable lymph nodes, with high accuracy (the sensitivity, specificity, positive and negative predictive values, and accuracy of ultrasonography were 86.49 %, 93.62 %, 91.43 %, 89.8 %, and 90.48 %, respectively, according to Esen and colleagues [66]).

Because of the lack of standardization, the correlation between the ultrasound size and the histopathologic size of the lymph nodes has low value, but Doppler examination is useful in determining response after chemotherapy, with a significant increase in the resistance index and pulsatility index values, according to Rashmi et al. [67].

The normal aspect of the axillary lymph nodes is described in Chap. 3.

8.5.2 Differential Diagnosis of Armpit Lumps

A. *Benign* Armpit Lumps

Some axillary lymphadenomegalies with transverse diameter greater than 10 mm, which may be benign findings, are wrongly designated on mammography as adenopathies because of their increased size. The main differential diagnosis must refer to the following:

- *Normal lymph nodes*, usually with transverse diameter less than 8 mm, but may be enlarged, with diameter up to 12–13 mm and longitudinal axis up to 25 mm, with normal internal structure: hyperechoic sinus, thin hypoechoic cortex, few/absent vessels in the hilum, absent pericapsular and cortical Doppler signal, and scoring 1 or 2 Ueno.

- *Histiocytic necrotizing lymphadenitis/benign histiocytosis*, the most frequent lymphadenomegalies: the lymph nodes present central hypoechoic medullary (sinus), with preservation of a peripheral hyperechoic medullary rim, surrounded by the intense uniform hypoechoic cortical zone. Doppler is normal with few vessels in the hilum, without cortical new vasculature. Sonoelastography corresponds to scoring 2 or 3 Ueno. The benign lymph node histiocytosis is usually associated with plasma cell mastitis, chronic galactophoritis, or rheumatoid arthritis.
- *Chronic granulomatosis*, non-suppurative such as sarcoidosis: the unspecific aspect preserves the benign features of the enlarged lymph nodes, with usually poor or undetectable vasculature. In suppurative chronic lymphadenitis the diffuse borders and perinodal infiltration may mimic malignancy, especially because of the presence of caseum or calcifications that increase the strain ratio. Patient history may be useful in the differential diagnosis. A specific pathology is referred to as silicone-induced granulomatous adenitis.
- *Acute lymphadenitis*, which is less frequent, is characterized by thickening of the cortex, increasing of the vasculature with centrifugal orientation of the benign type, and scoring 1 or 2 Ueno. The clinical signs are useful and patients present with pain and swelling of the small parts in the axilla. There may be an allergic reaction, an unspecific upper limb bacterial infection, cellulitis, lymphadenitis in viral infections, or specific lymphadenitis such as Lyme disease after a tick bite. Cat scratch fever and brucellosis may cause acute axillary lymphadenitis.
- *Other axillary small parts infections*: acute hidrosadenitis and cellulitis.
- *Breast tissue*: hypertrophy of the axillary prolongation of the mammary gland or supernumerary mammary gland.
- *Other axillary benign tumors*: lipomas, cysts, fibroadenoma.

B. *Malignant Armpit Lumps*

The differential diagnosis of malignant-type axillary lymph nodes must include the following:

- *Other metastases*: primary malignancy in ipsilateral arm with the start point from skin tumors, such as malignant melanoma (usually intense hypoechoic with hypervasculature), epithelioma, adenocarcinomas, or sarcoma; or more frequently from metastasis of distant tumors from the head and neck (larynx, thyroid, pharynx, etc.); or, rarely, from the internal thoracic, abdominal, or pelvic organs or other lymph nodes metastases with unknown primary origin.
- *Systemic malignancies*: leukemia, lymphomas. Usually the lymph nodes are small, less 10 mm in the short axis, with hypoechoic aspect, without significant vasculature, and may present reduced elasticity with scoring 4 Ueno.
- *Primary malignant tumors* with armpit involvement: osteosarcoma especially in young, angio-pericitosarcomas, liposarcoma, rhabdomyosarcoma, etc.

Sonoelastography is easier to perform than a biopsy and is more specific than MRI findings of lymph nodes. Thus, lymph node biopsy would become unnecessary, and, in the future, sonoelastography and higher-resolution probes will increase the precision.

Internal mammary lymph node (IMLN) metastases are one of the two most important pathways of lymphatic dissemination in breast cancer. Metastases to the IMLN occur in up to 20 % of patients with clinically operable malignant breast tumors [67]. Although dissection of the axillary nodes is still a widely employed staging strategy for breast carcinoma, staging of disease by dissection of the internal mammary lymphatic chain is rarely performed. Real-time ultrasonography with a high-frequency linear-array transducer has been used to localize the internal mammary artery and veins and to demonstrate lymphadenopathy.

The examination is easily to perform because the internal mammary artery and its two satellite veins are located just laterally of the right and left sternal borders, behind the cartilaginous transonic ending ribs, and, together with the surrounding tissues, are completely visualized with the Doppler technique. The normal IMLNs are not distinct, but pathological lymph nodes appear as round or oval-shaped, well-delineated hypoechoic nodules, usually infracentimetric in size, with the vasculature more or less salient.

IMLNs suspected by ultrasonography can be proven by ultrasound-guided fine needle aspiration cytology (US-FNAC), which is considered to be useful because the evaluation of metastasis to IMLNs is required in TMN classification by the UICC (2002). US-FNAC could be performed comparatively safely and easily, with low-risk of complications of neither pneumothorax nor bleeding.

Only ultrasonography and MRI mammography are able to detect IMLN, which is another limitation of mammography. Whether occurring alone or combined with axillary metastases, IMLN metastases have a substantial negative effect on long-term survival and disease-free interval. According to TNM staging, ipsilateral IMLN metastases are considered as stage 3b, which is accepted as inoperable. The presence of IMLN involvement also affects the area that should be irradiated.

(Figs. 8.1, 8.2, 8.3, 8.4, 8.5, 8.6, 8.7, 8.8, 8.9, 8.10, 8.11, 8.12, 8.13, 8.14, 8.15, 8.16, 8.17, 8.18, 8.19, 8.20, 8.21, 8.22, 8.23, 8.24, 8.25, 8.26, 8.27, 8.28, 8.29, 8.30, 8.31, 8.32, 8.33, 8.34, 8.35, 8.36, 8.37, 8.38, 8.39, 8.40, 8.41, 8.42, 8.43, 8.44, 8.45, 8.46, 8.47, 8.48, 8.49, 8.50, 8.51, 8.52, 8.53, 8.54, 8.55, 8.56 and 8.57).

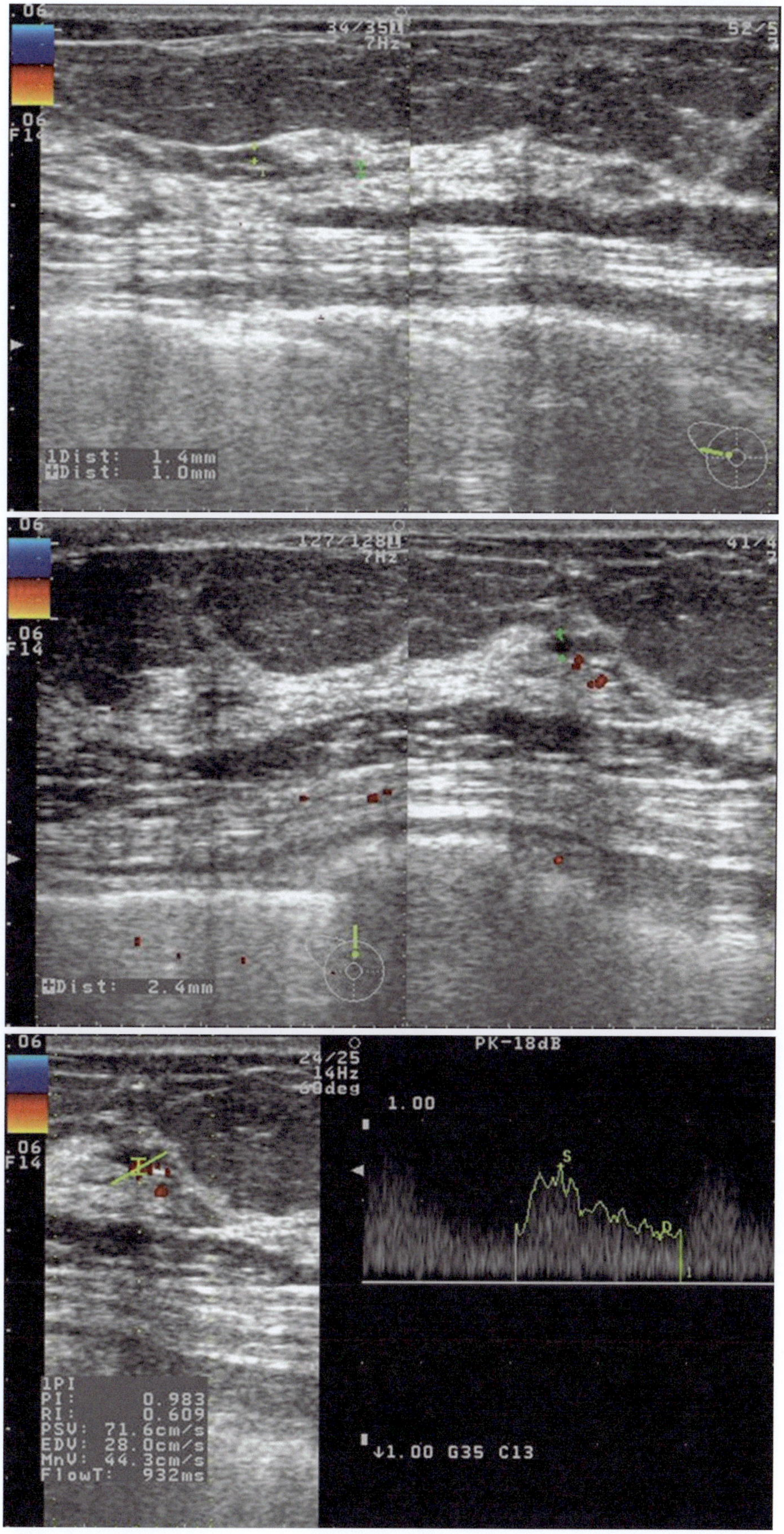

Fig. 8.1 Suspect lobular hyperplasia at R12:00 in a TDLU location in a dense breast of a 52–year-old patient whose mother had breast cancer. Doppler exam makes the differential diagnosis of these multiple lesions of focal ductal/lobular hyperplasia

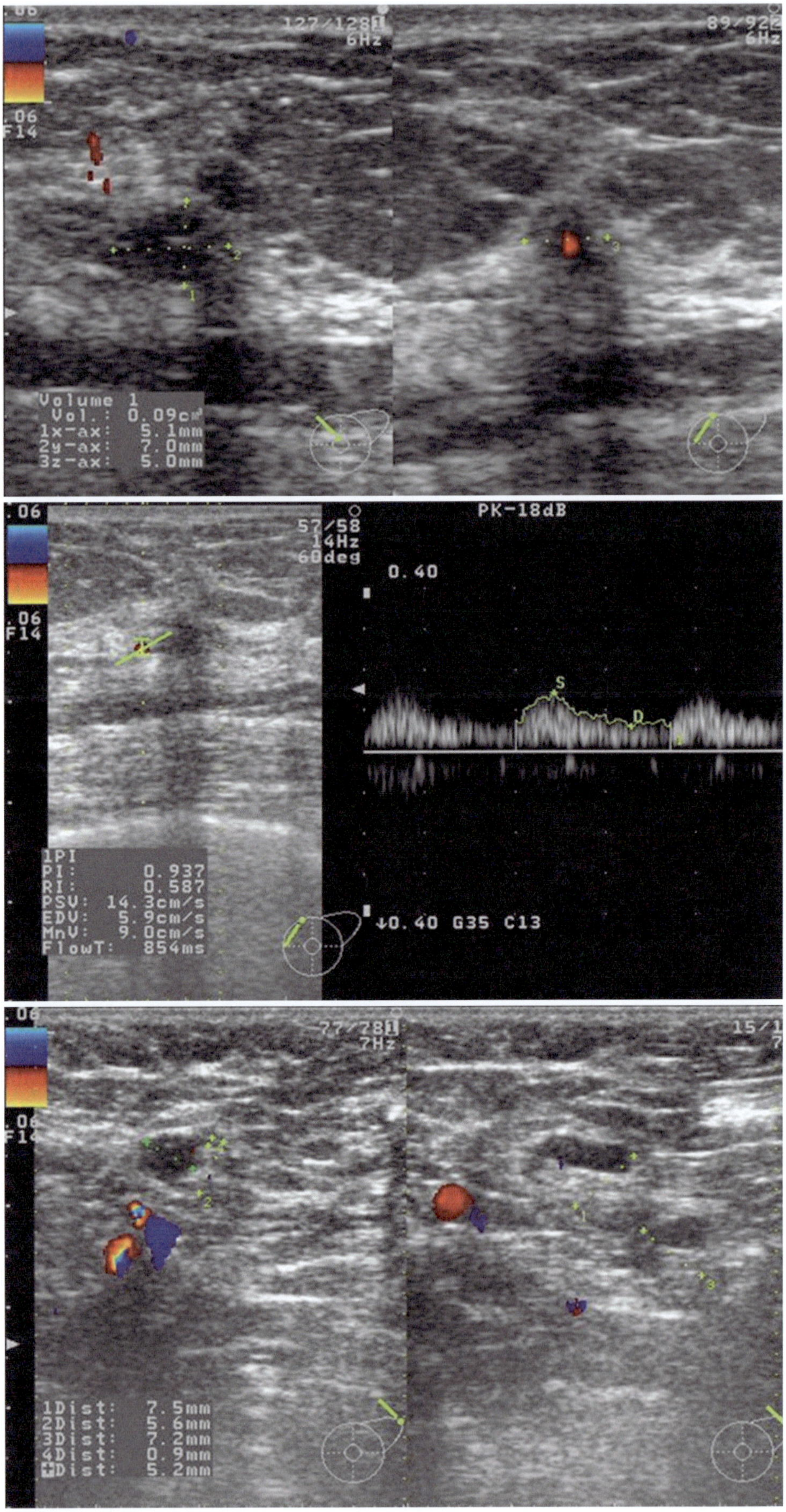

Fig. 8.2 Fifty-one-year-old patient who underwent ultrasound screening over 4 years for family history of breast cancer (mother). DE detected a 5/7 mm lesion in a TDLU localization, with irregular shape, heterogeneous hypoechoic structure, acoustic shadowing, and new vasculature in color and spectral Doppler. A few axillary lymph nodes presented focal cortical thickening, suggesting sentinel nodes. Ultrasound BI-RADS category 4C

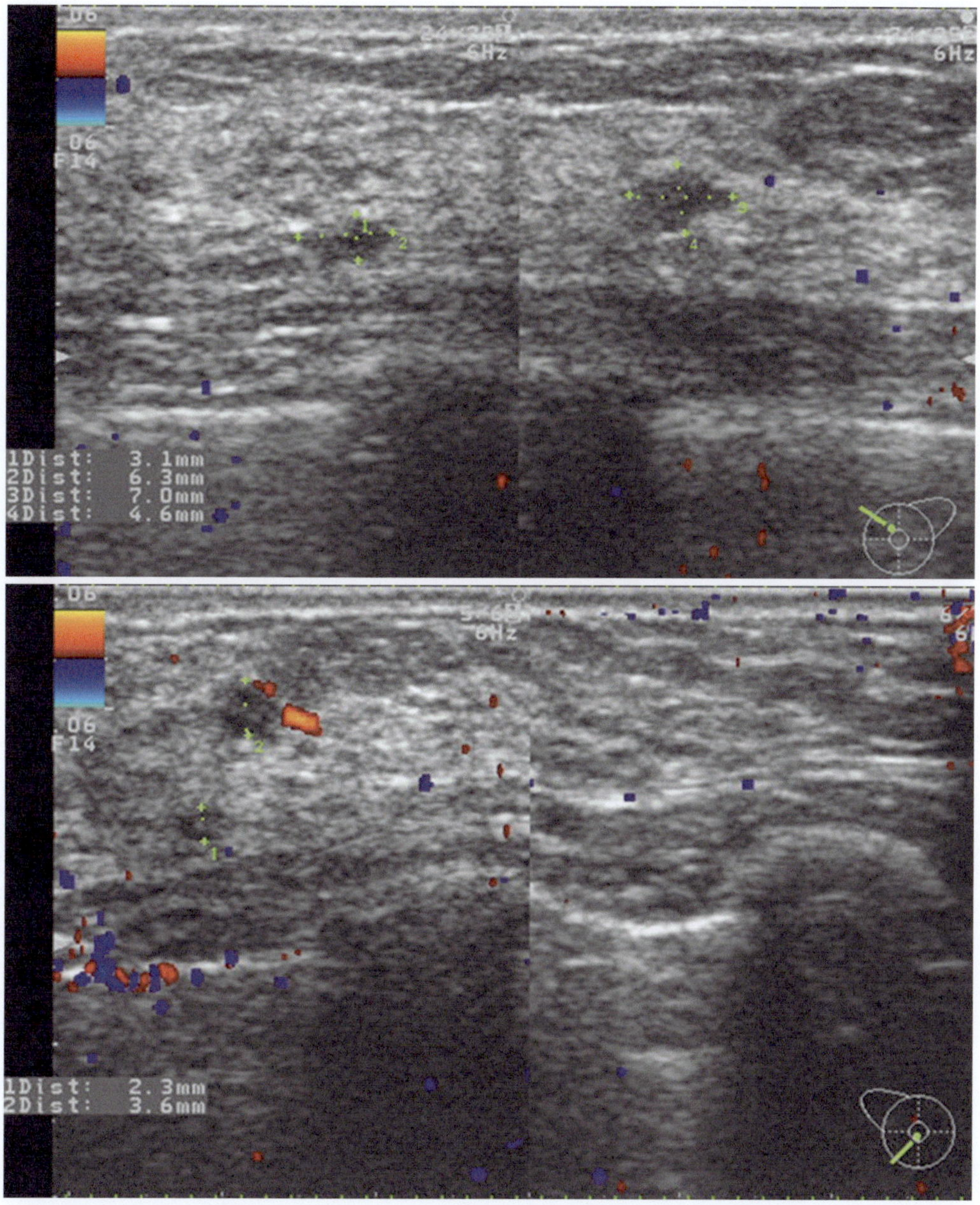

Fig. 8.3 Patient is 39 years old: Doppler DE presents at R7:00 a suspect micronodule less than 5 mm, with a double pole of new formation vasculature. It is similar in appearance, size, and aspect to L10:00 lobular hyperplasias but without salient vasculature. The suspect lesion was classified ultrasound BI-RADS category 4, and short-term follow-up was recommended. After 1 month the lesion doubled its diameter, increased its vasculature, and surgical biopsy confirmed DCIS

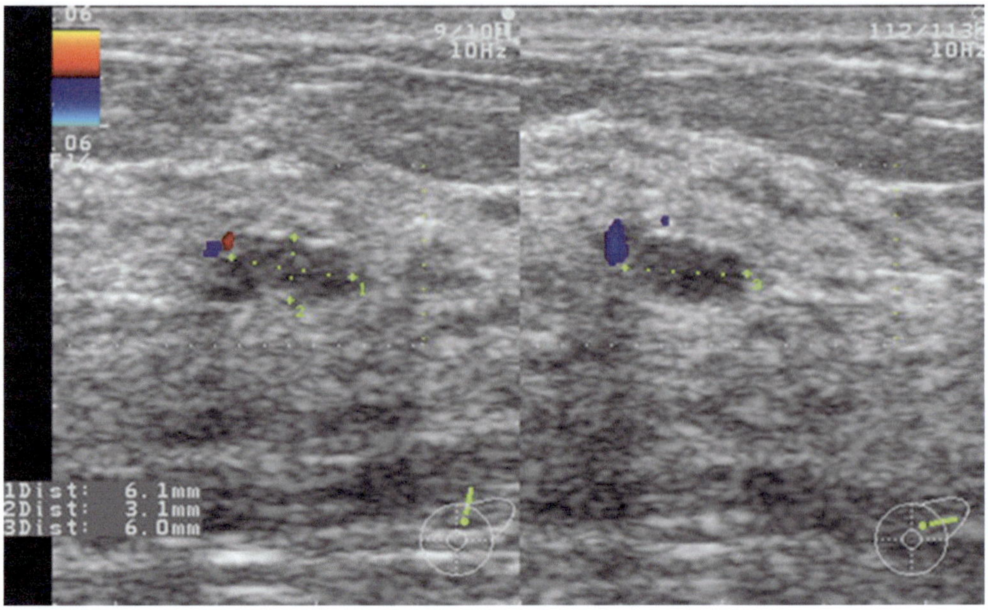

Fig. 8.4 Suspect infracentimetric lesion at Doppler DE: hypoechoic, with irregular shape and new formation vasculature. Radial and antiradial scans are used to demonstrate its ductal connection and to estimate its volume. U ltrasound BI-RADS category 4

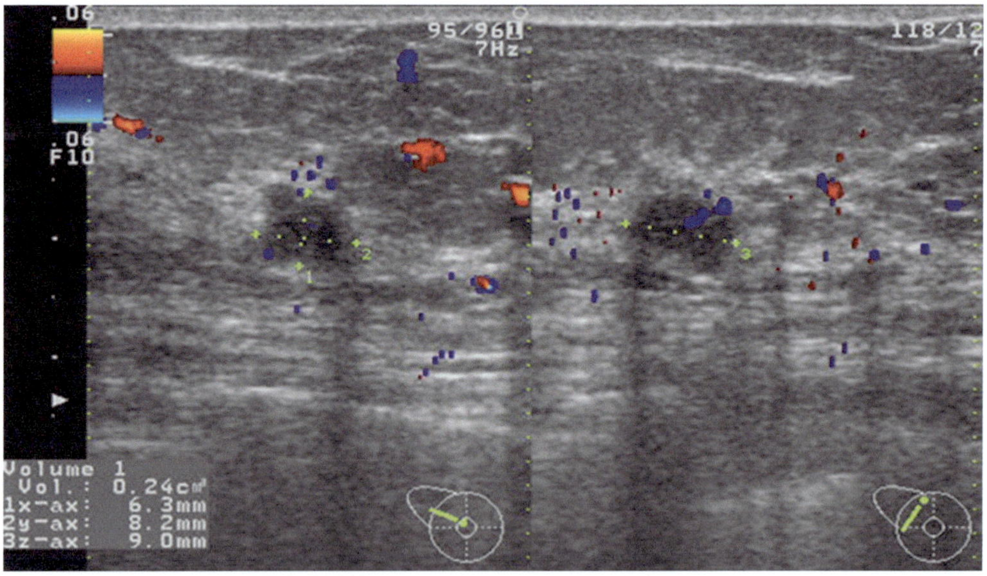

Fig. 8.5 Patient is 53 years old with a family history of breast disease (a sister died of breast cancer and her mother had breast dysplasia). DE detected an infracentimetric mass at R10:00 in a TDLU location, with polycyclic shape, hypoechoic texture, unequal lateral shadowing, and a centripetal vasculature. Adjacent small hypoechoic foci with shadowing suggest intraductal early spreading or multifocal malignancy. Without sonoelastography, the simple compression suggests a stiff lesion. The focal thickening of the cortical of an axillary lymph node is suggestive of a sentinel node. Based on the collateral history and the DE, the findings were assessed as ultrasound BI-RADS category 4. The pathological report presented lobular multiple micro-invasive carcinoma

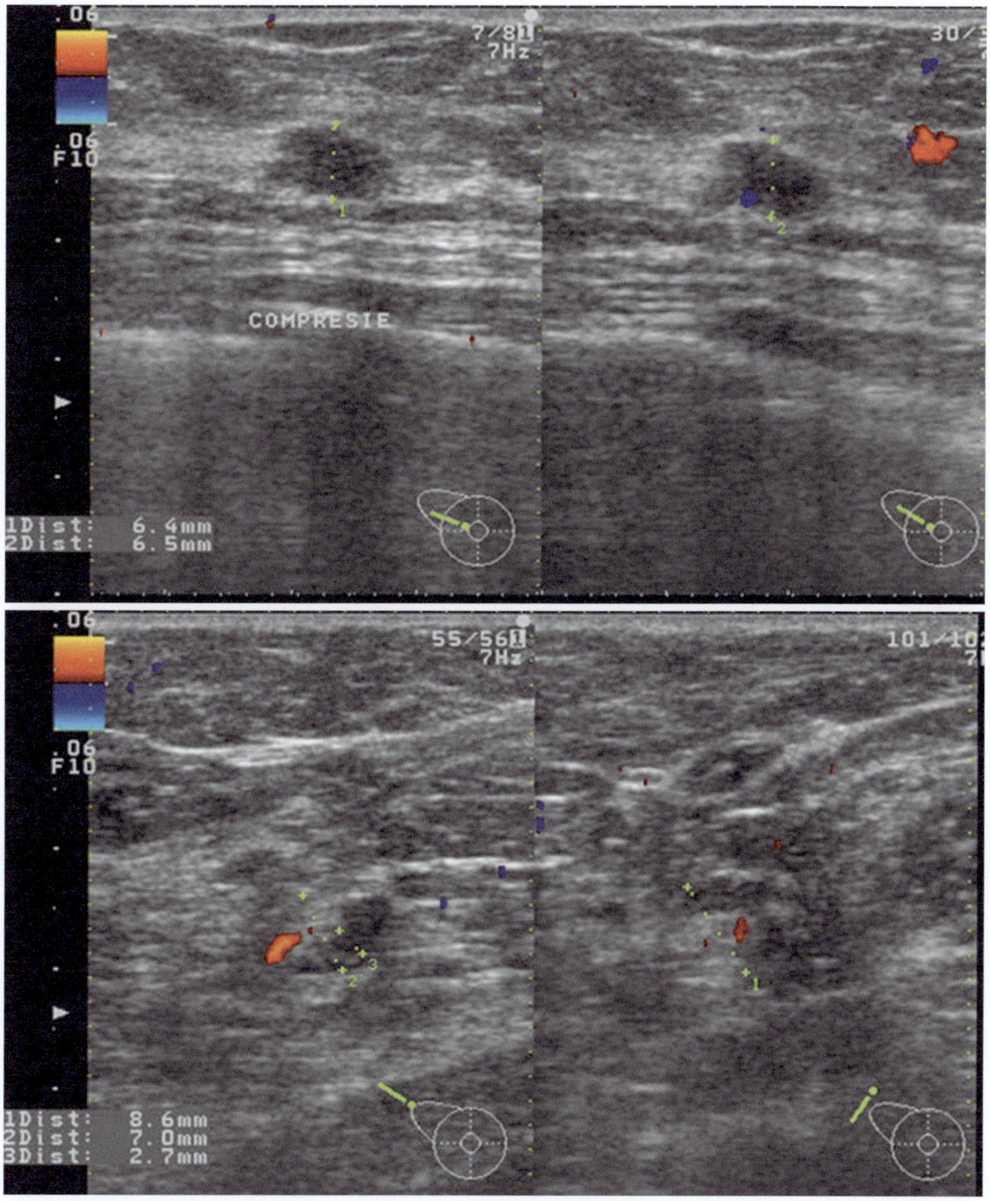

Fig. 8.5 (continued)

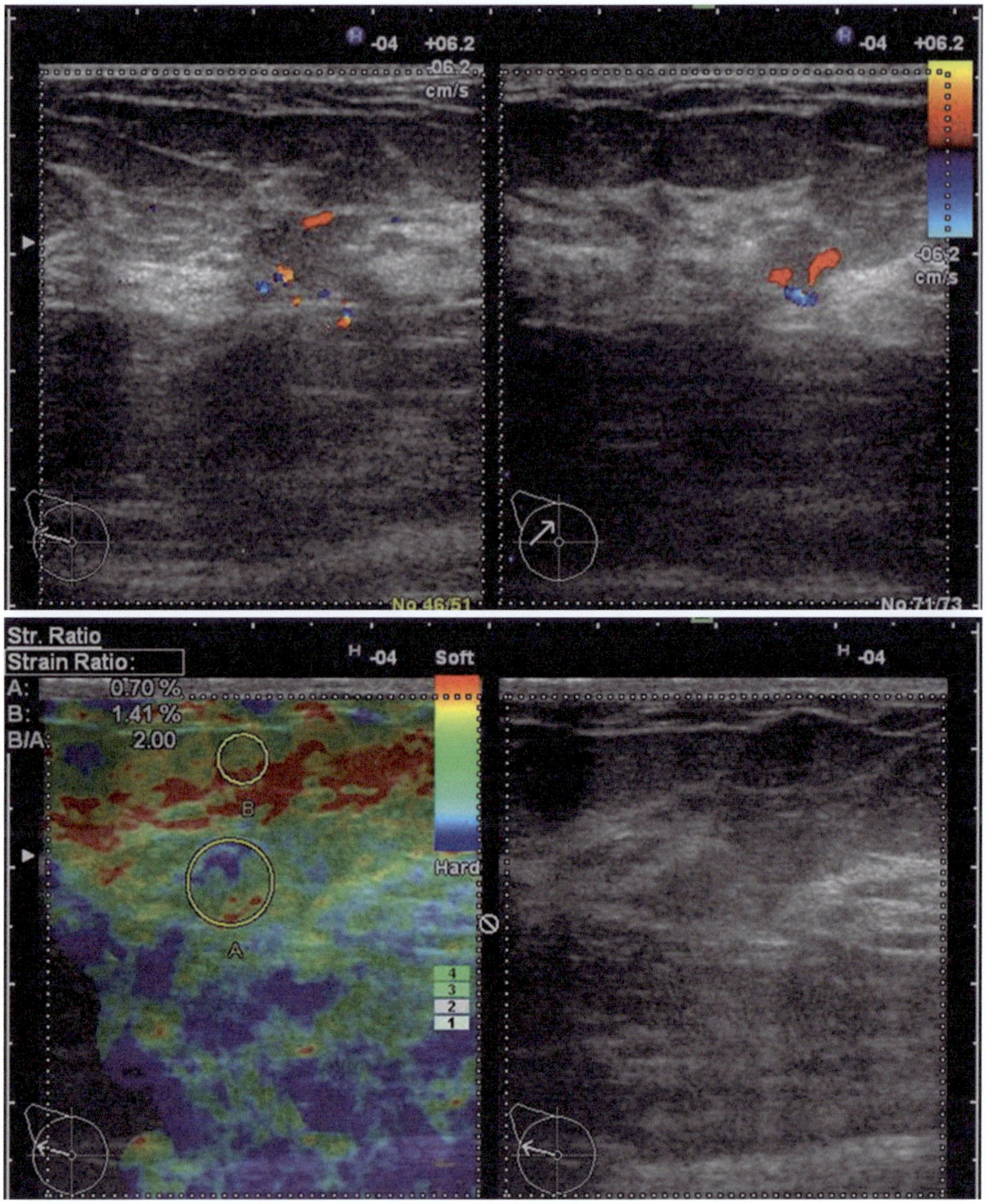

Fig. 8.6 Patient is 53 years old, with negative mammography 8 months earlier. A complementary FBU demanded for mastalgia demonstrated at R10:00 segmental ductal thickening without abnormal Doppler or sonoelastography. The same location developed in the interval an infracentimetric mass with isoechoic structure, no posterior effects, diffuse borders with irregular shape and thickened duct connections, and salient new formation vasculature but benign sonoelastography type BGR scoring. In this case, the sonoelastography is false negative, but the most important point is the local evolution and the verified new formation vasculature, which were concordant with an interval DCIS

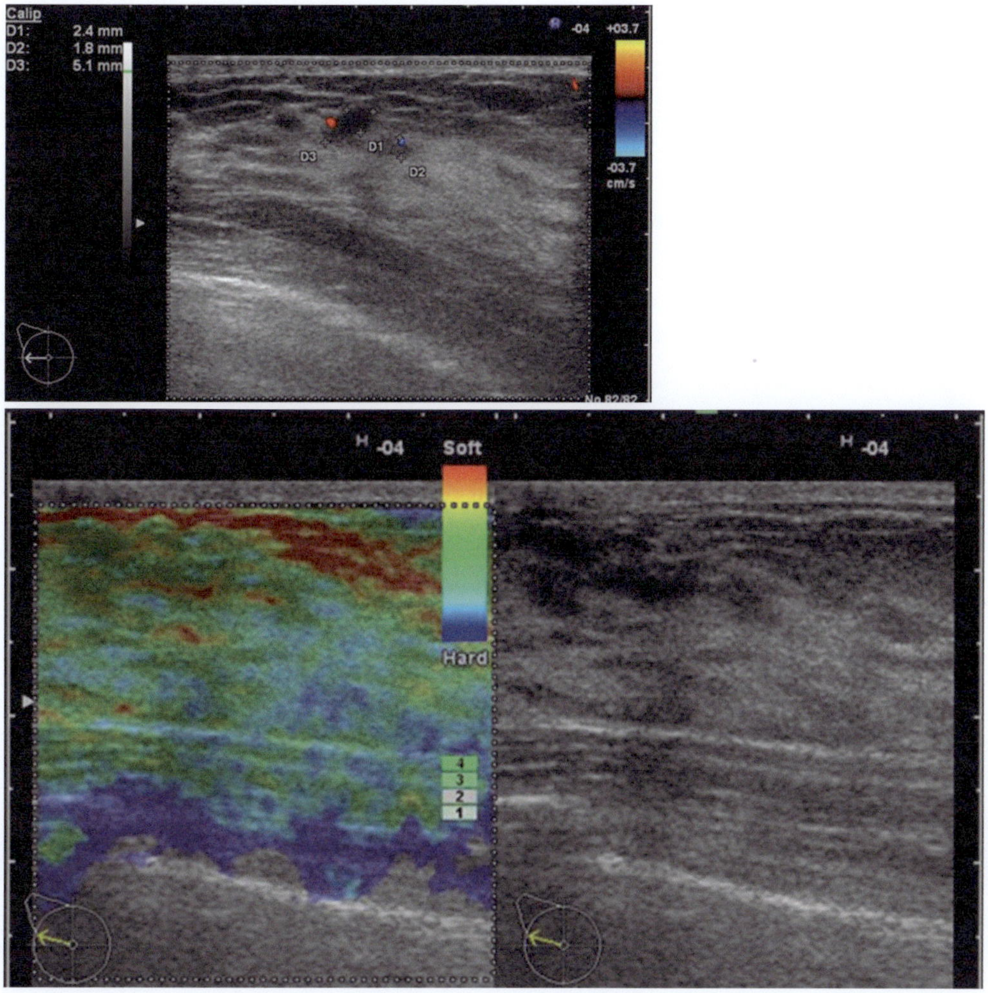

Fig. 8.7 The early stage of lobular carcinoma in FBU: multiple lobules enlarged up to 5 mm, with increased hypoechoic aspect and oblique orientation toward the ducts. The new formation of tiny vessels may be considered an alarm sign, but SE presents an initially benign score because of the small size of these lesions (false-negative sonoelastography)

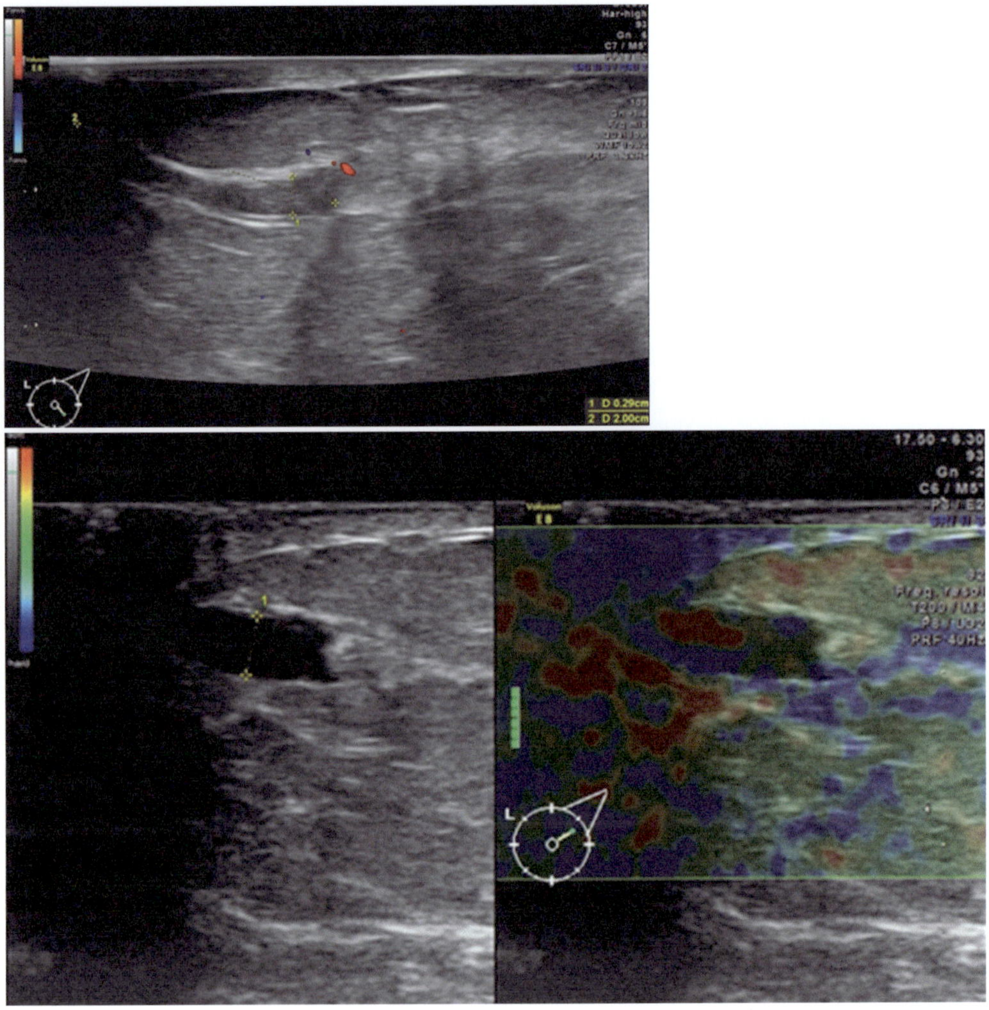

Fig. 8.8 Duct ectasia ended by an isoechoic intraductal mass, with nourishing vessel, suspect according to the small duct diameter and small mass, despite the benign SE. A short follow-up is recommended for the differential diagnosis of the ductal papilloma with a DCIS

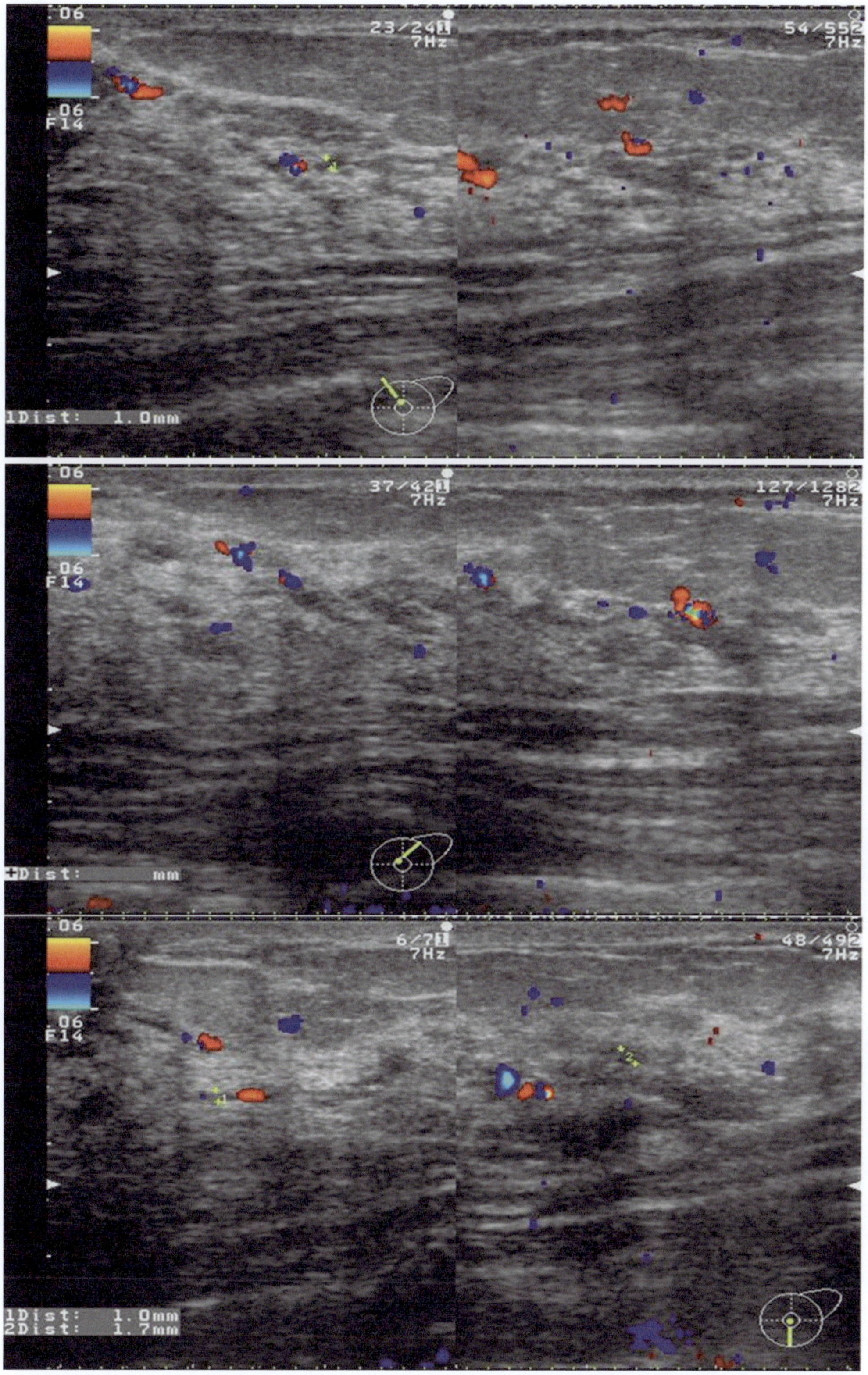

Fig. 8.9 Patient is 35 years old: the left breast stings and a lump is present on the upper-outer quadrant; mammogram is negative. The first important finding on Doppler DE is a gentle diffuse lobular hyperplasia with important periductal and perilobular hyper vasculature

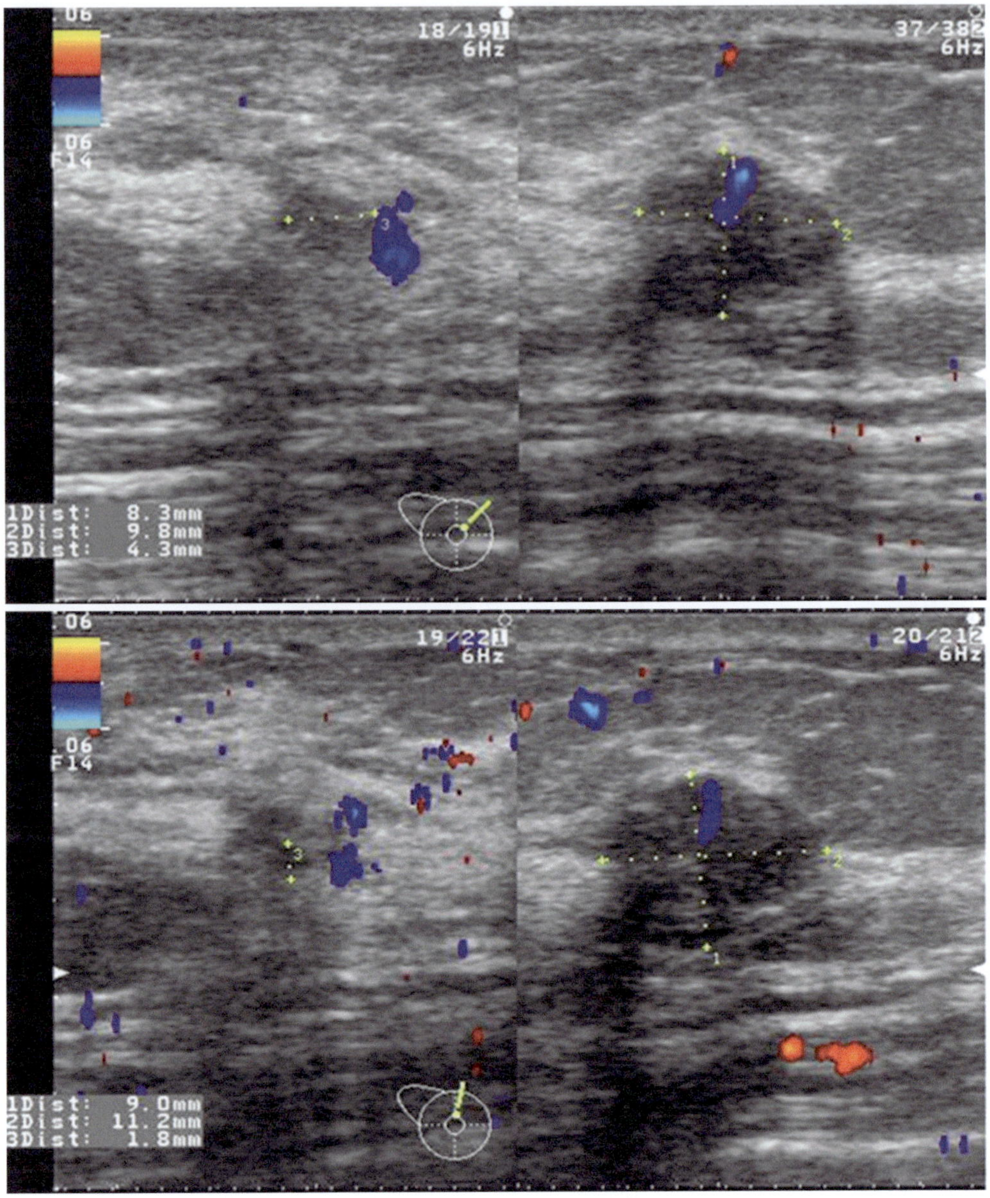

Fig. 8.10 Patient is 35 years old, same case as in Fig. 8.9: Doppler DE presents at R12:30-13:00 an impalpable 11 mm asymptomatic mass, polylobated, hypoechoic with posterior peripheral asymmetrical shadowing and centripetal plunging suspect vasculature. A second lesion, smaller and located centripetal to the nipple on the same radius, presenting similar characteristics including new vasculature, raises the suspicion of malignity. The qualitative color and power Doppler are more useful than the quantitative spectral Doppler because, in this case, with minimal stromal reaction the velocity indices are intermediate, as in the most benign masses (pulsatility index (PI) 0.927, resistive index (RI) 0.619). "Knobby carcinoma" type assessed as ultrasound BI-RADS category 5

Fig. 8.10 (continued)

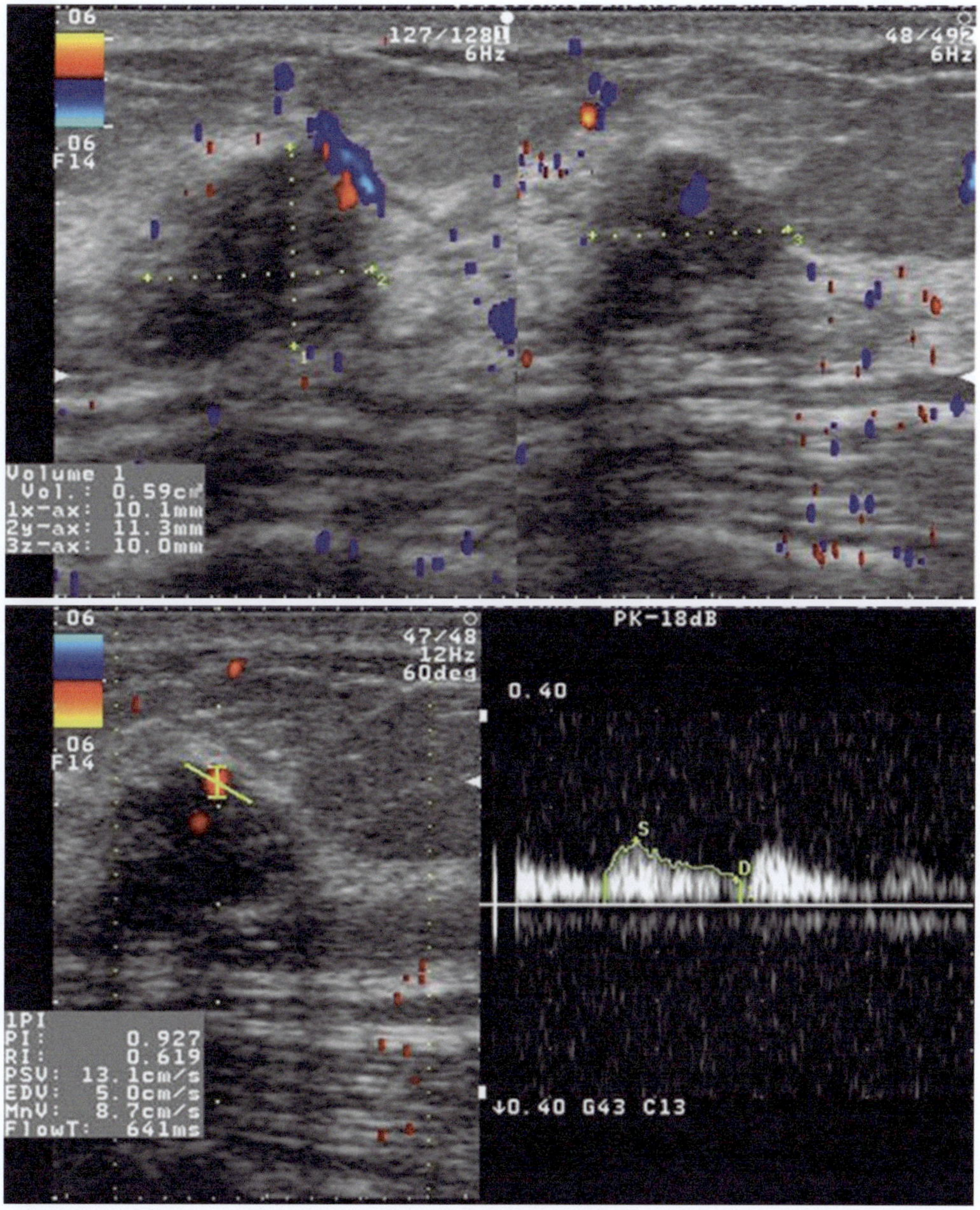

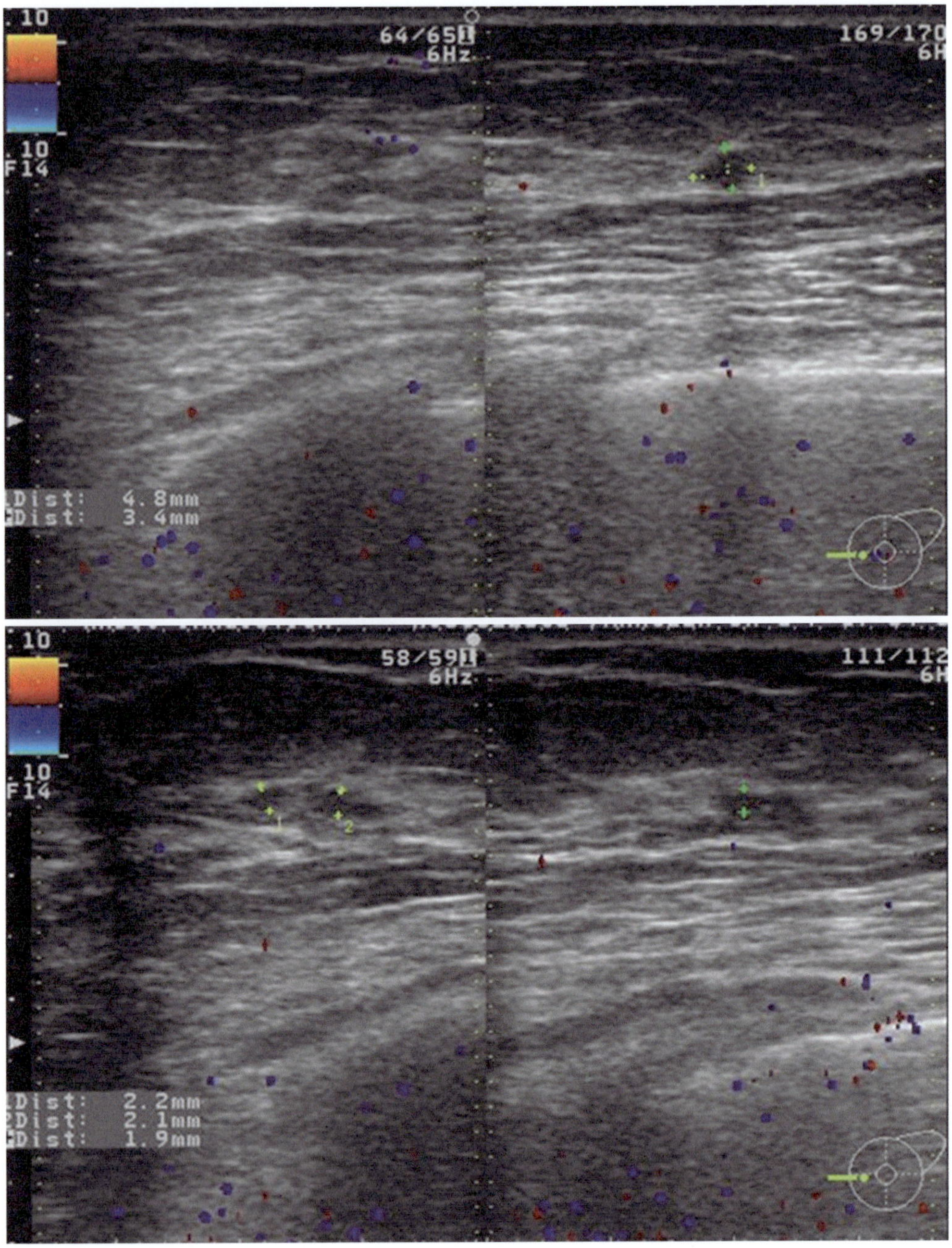

Fig. 8.11 A 67-year-old patient: predictable breast cancer or high-risk breast cancer may be assumed based on the dense breast in advanced menopause, with lobular hyperplasia as pseudo-nodules, some with acoustic shadowing, suggesting small sclerosing adenosis lesions. No abnormal vasculature maintains a benign characterization

Fig. 8.11 (continued)

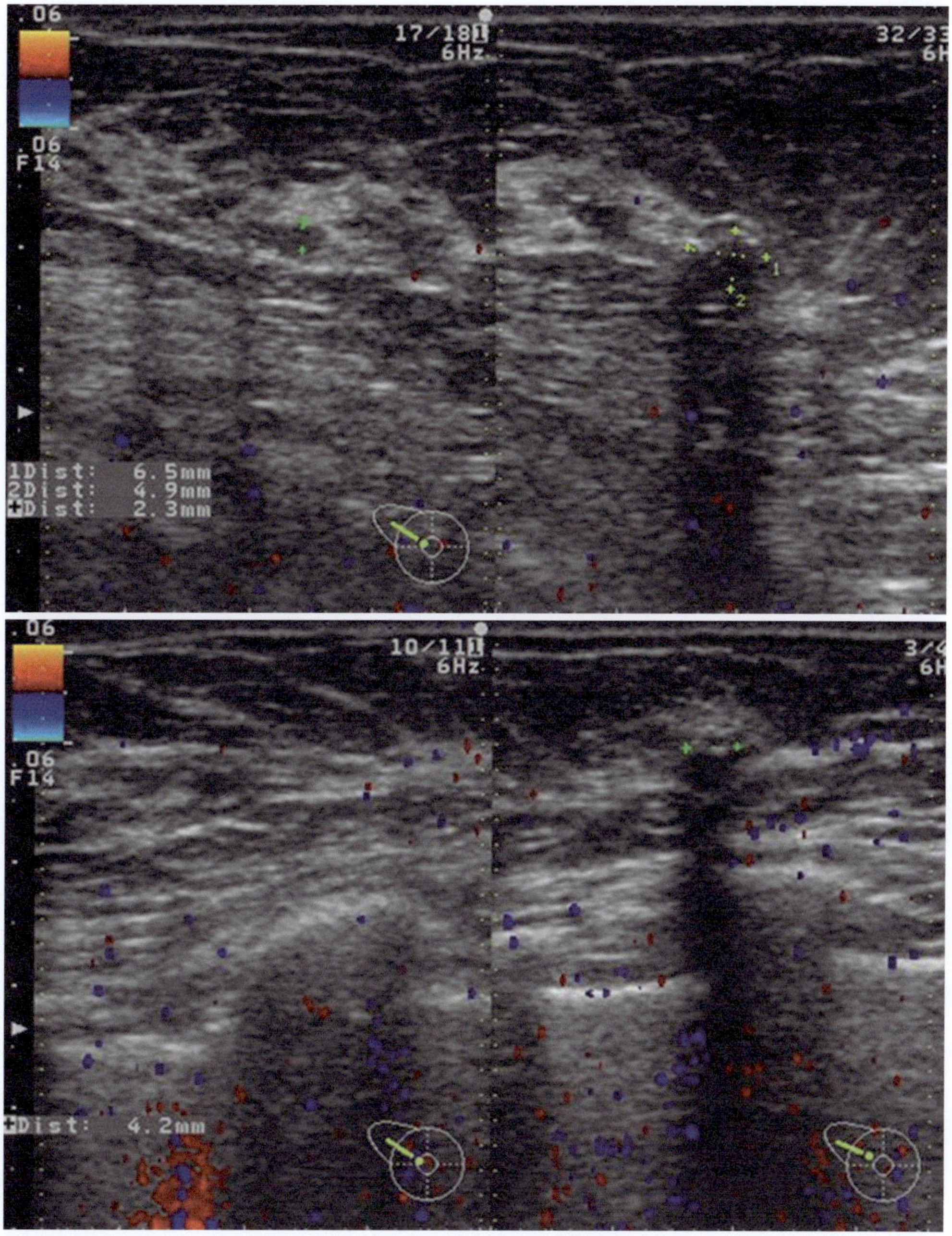

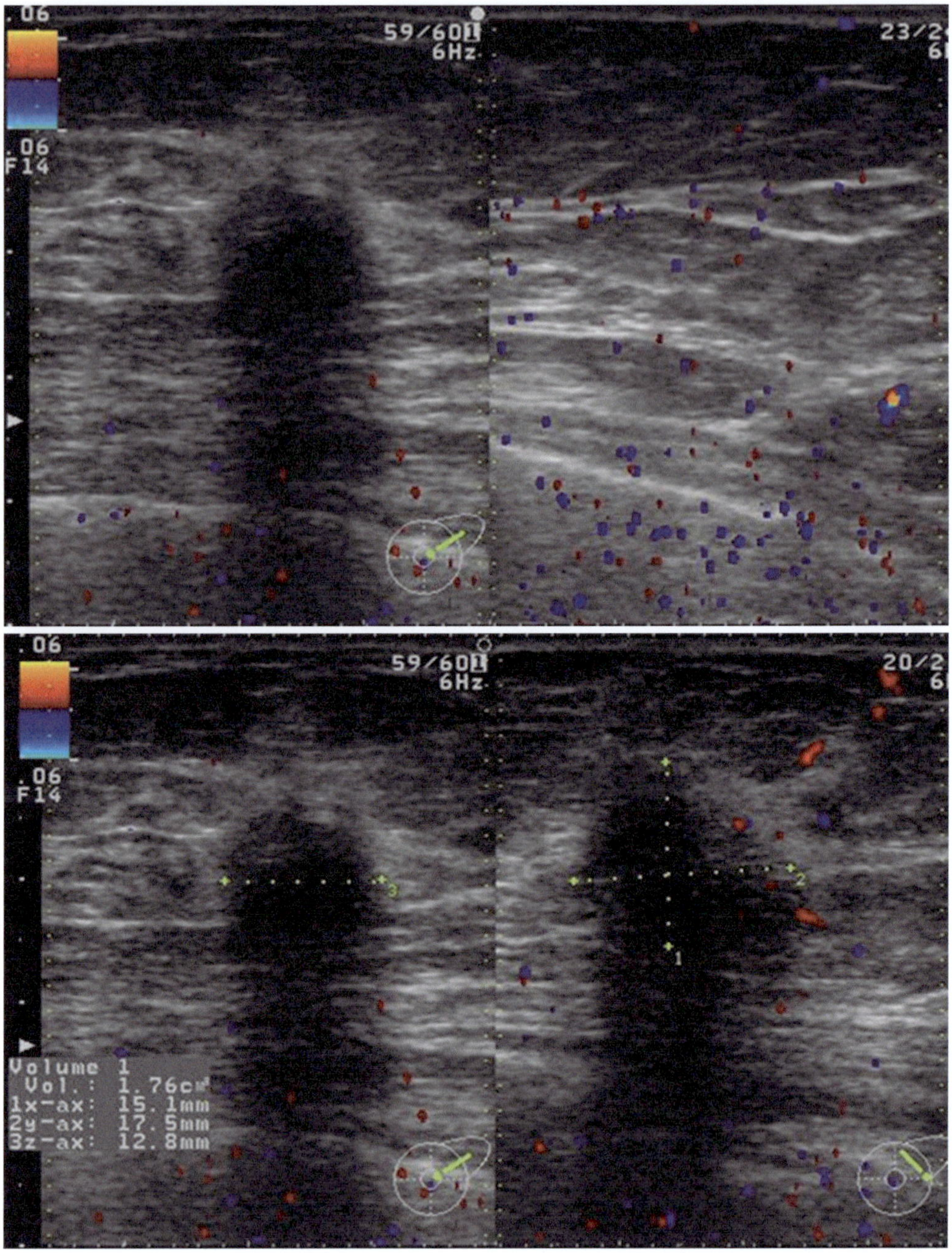

Fig. 8.12 The same patient as Fig. 8.11: L13:00 breast cancer less than 2 cm diameter with typical malignant descriptors after Stavros, acoustic shadowing and malignant-type new vasculature, with multipolar vessels having an incident plunging angle. "Stellate" carcinoma-type

Fig. 8.12 (continued)

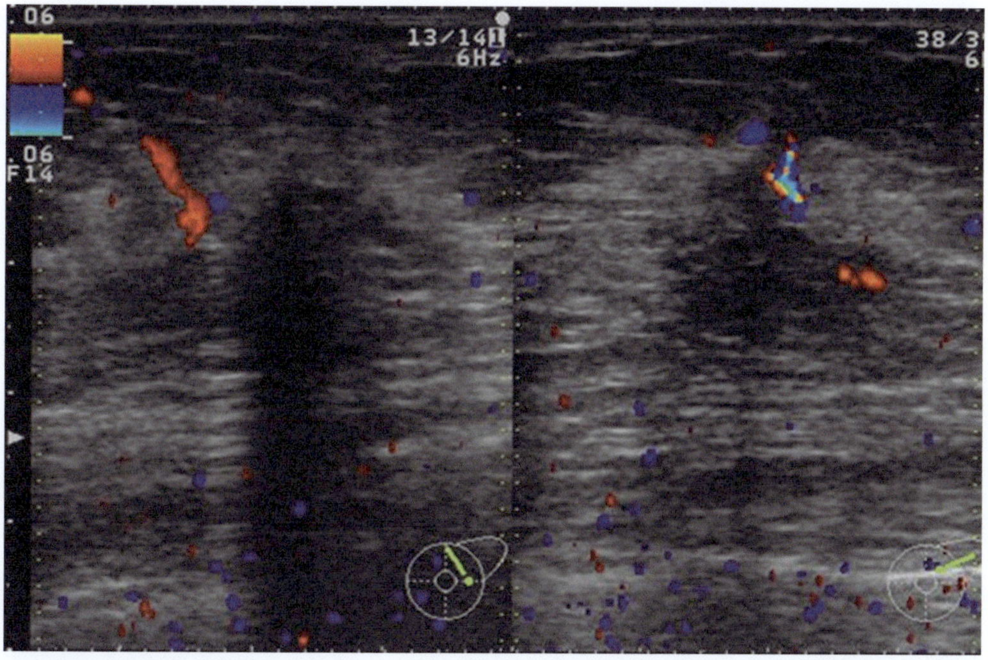

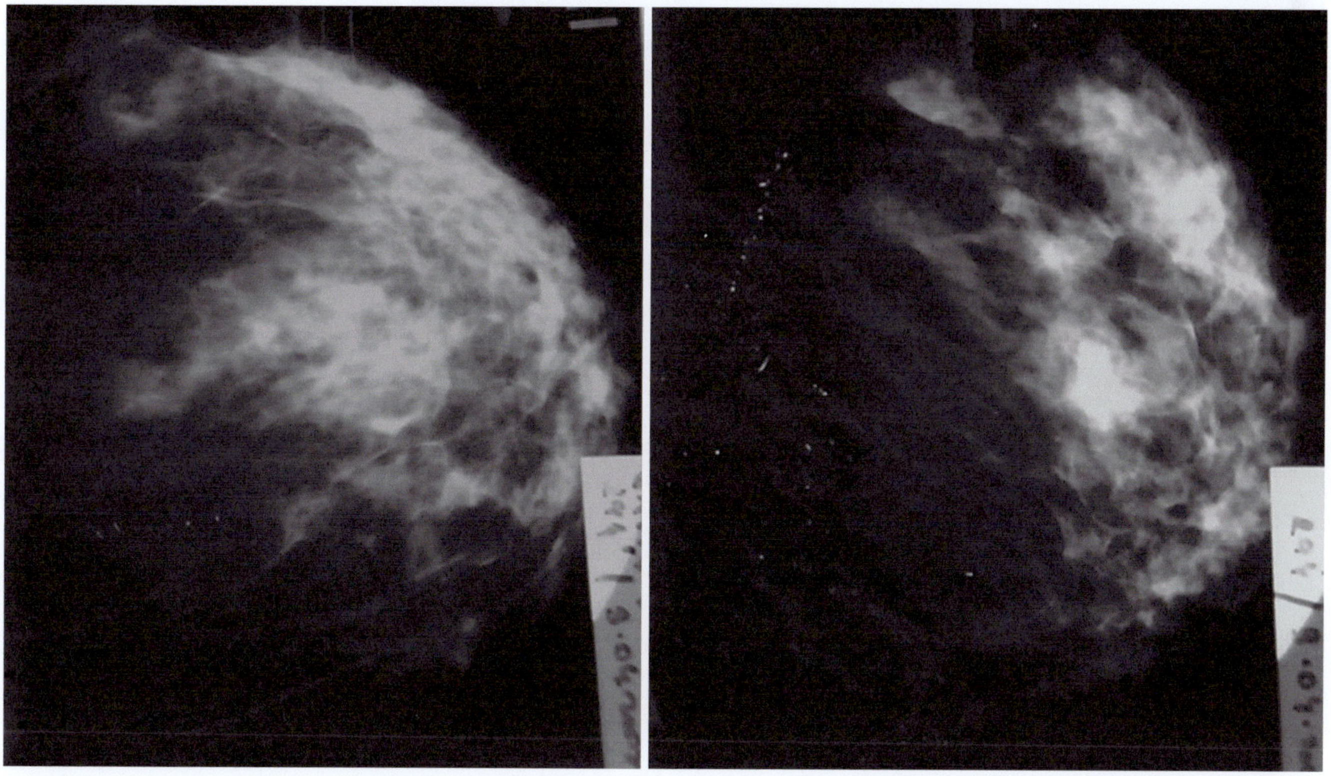

Fig. 8.13 Patient is 57 years old: follow-up mammograms 4 years (*upper*) and 5 years (*below*) after right breast cancer, treated with mastectomy, chemotherapy and radiotherapy. Large left dense breast post hormonal therapy for primary infertility, without significant changes on mammography, classified as BI-RADS category 2.3. We will not comment on the quality control of these films

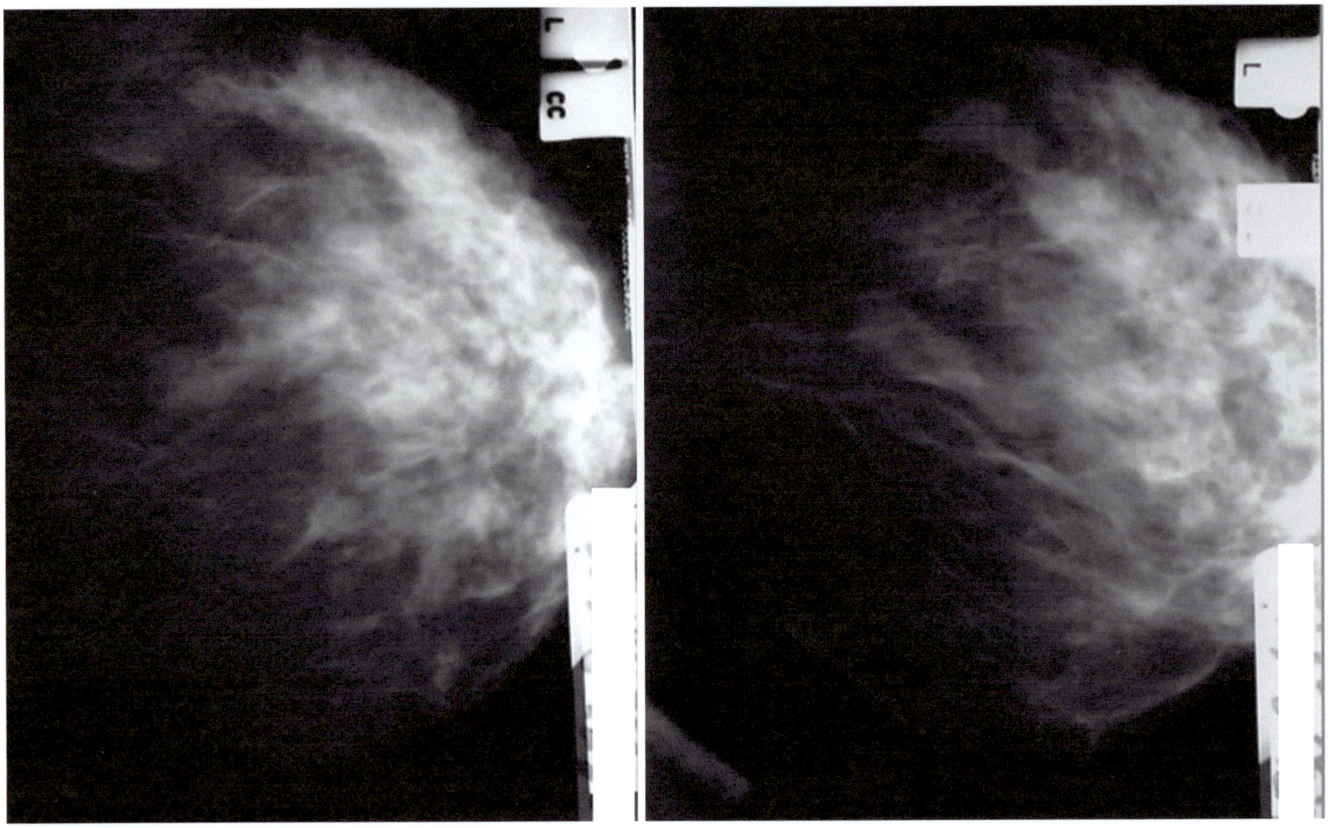

Fig. 8.13 (continued)

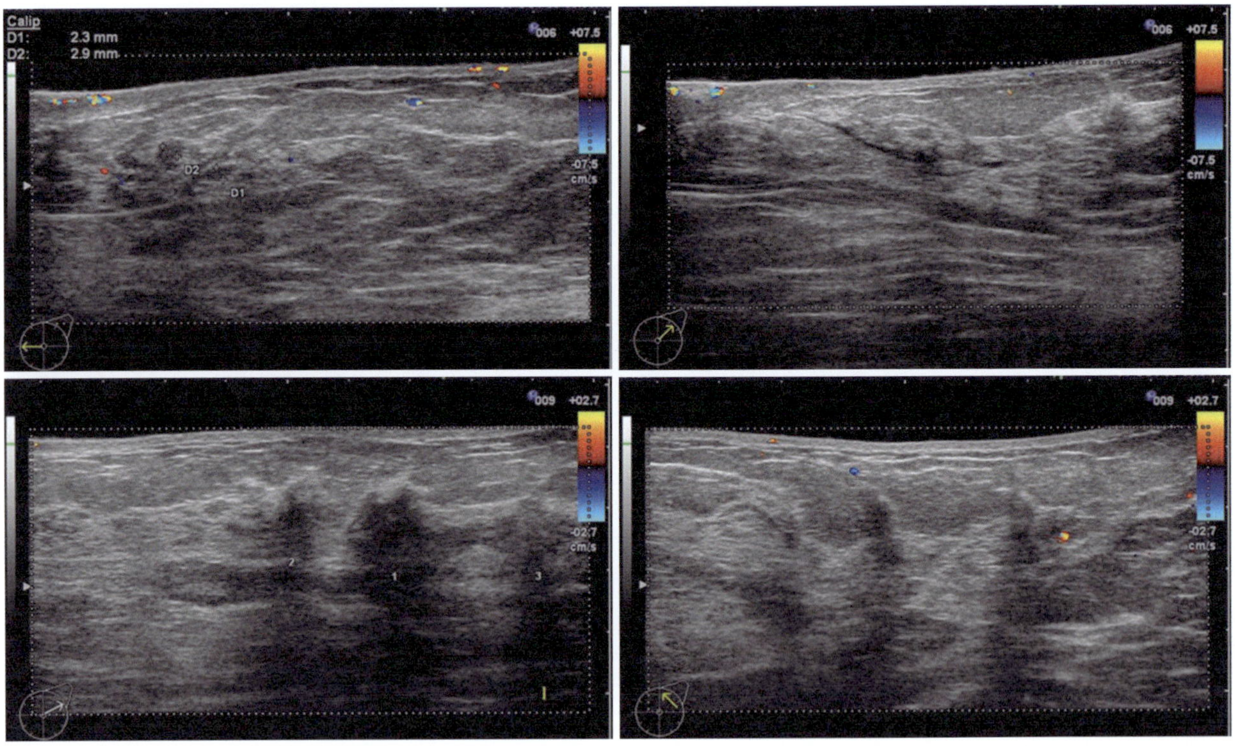

Fig. 8.14 Patient is 57 years old, same case as in Fig. 8.13: DE with long probe shows lobular hyperplasia and ductal ectasias, as remnant marks of the hormonal treatment of infertility. L1:00-2:00 multifocal cancers on radial and antiradial large scans, with malignant descriptors after Stavros (less salient vasculature with 7 MHz long probe, especially after chemotherapy)

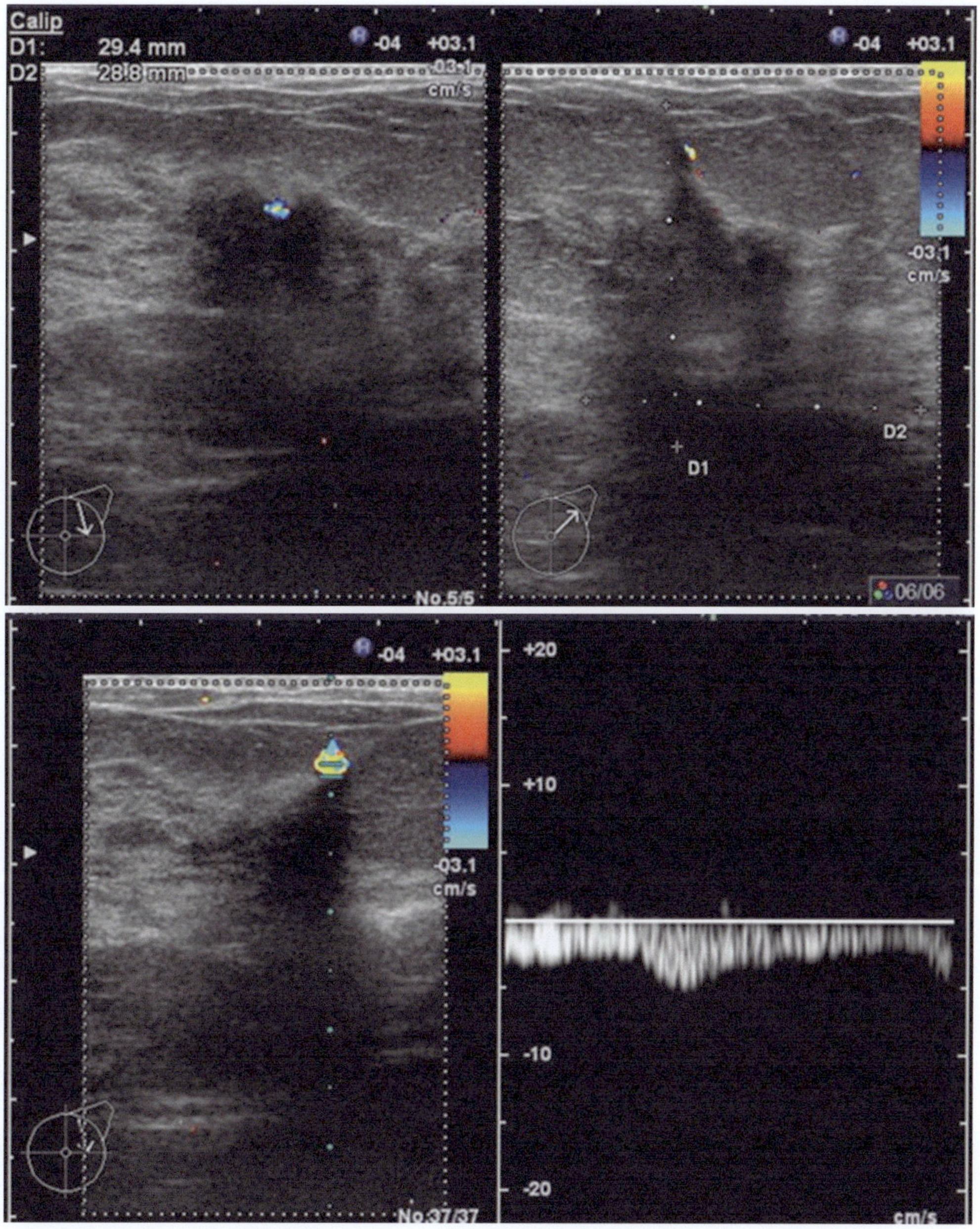

Fig. 8.15 Patient is 57 years old, same case as in Fig. 8.13: FBU demonstrates the spreading of the cancer by infiltration of the Cooper's ligament, with new vasculature on Doppler, and a desmoplastic reaction illustrated by a score 5 Ueno. The high stiffness is suggested by the black artifact and the huge FLR, over 108.00. "Stellate" cancer type

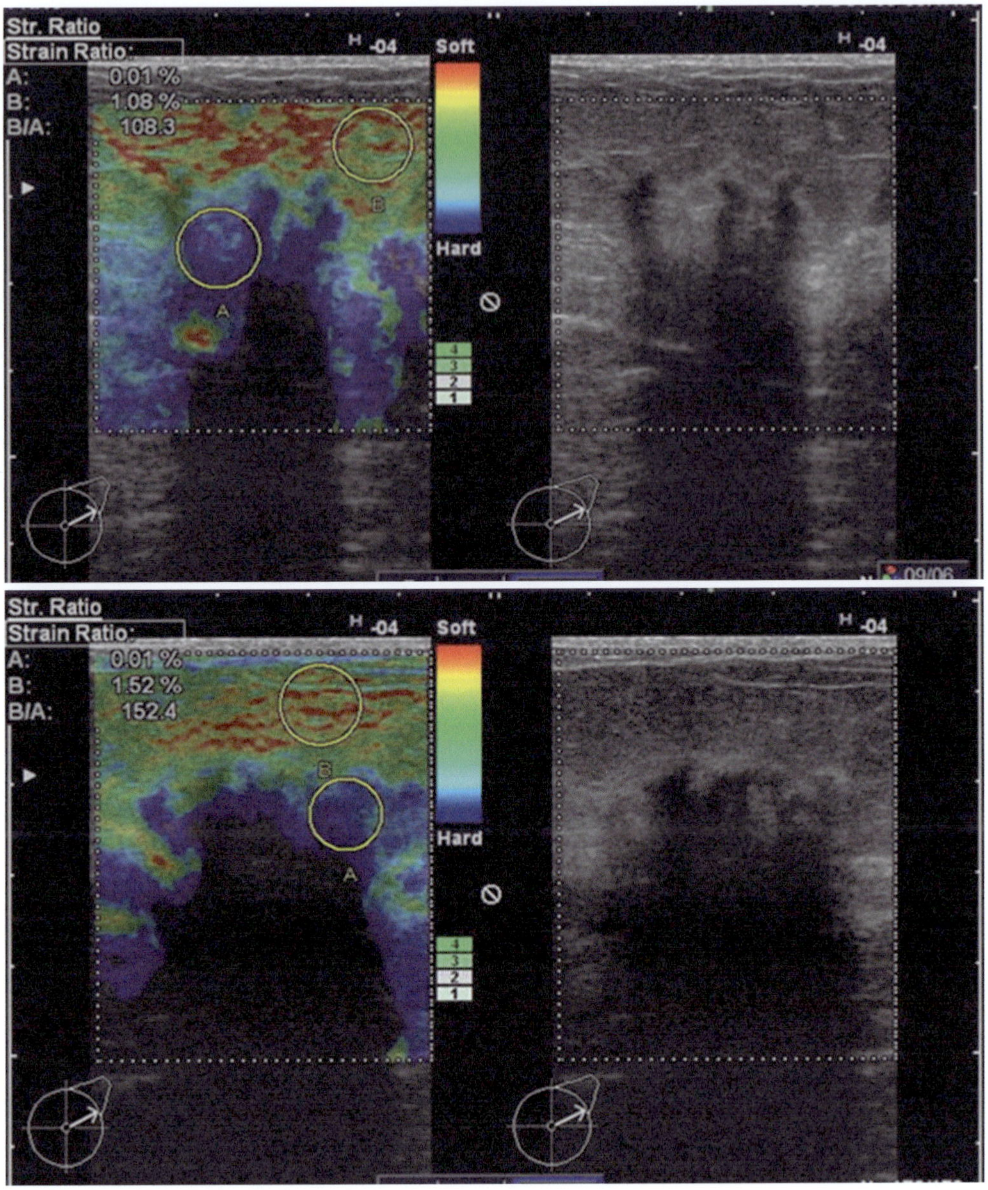

Fig. 8.15 (continued)

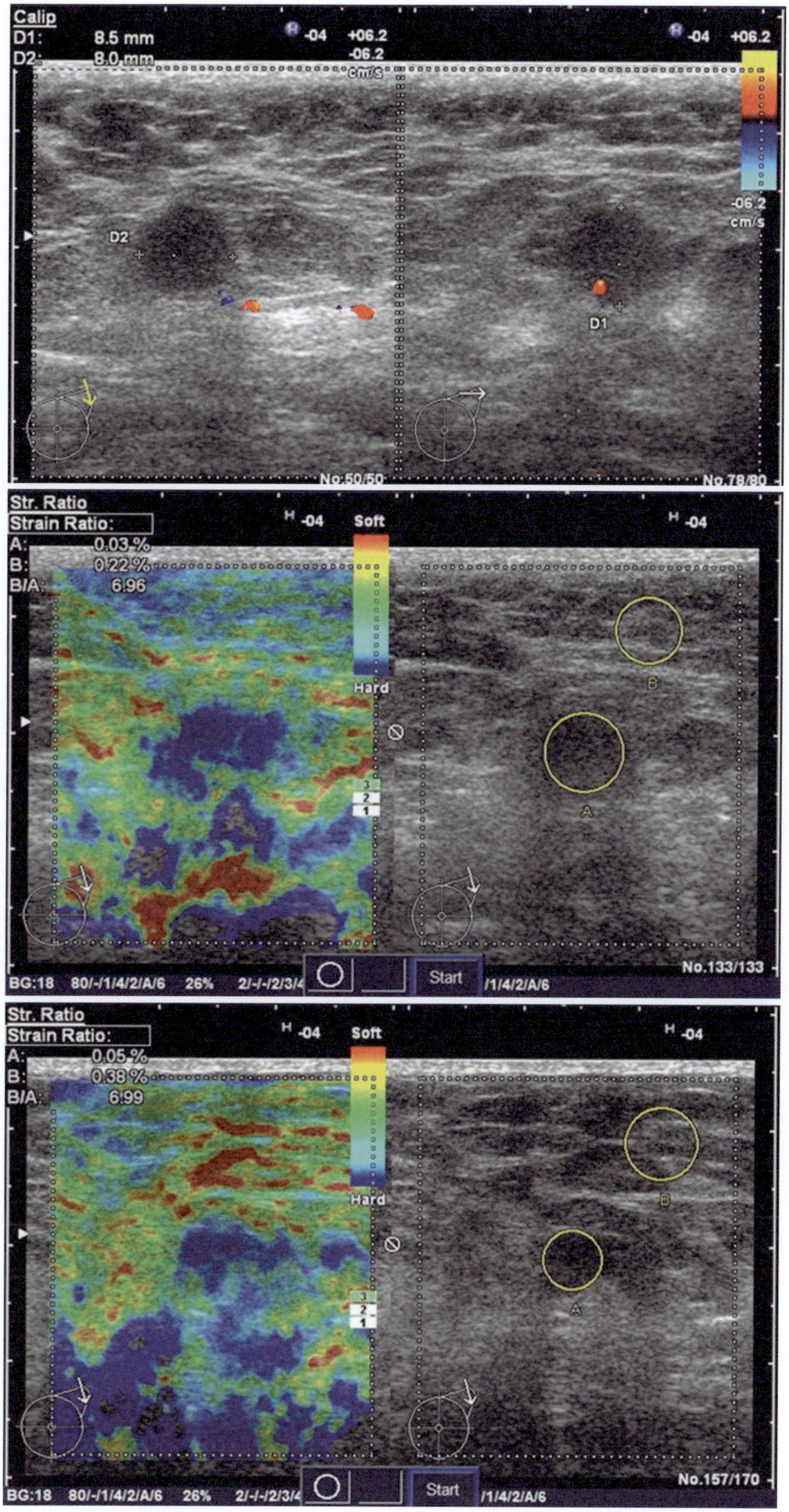

Fig. 8.16 Fifty-seven year, the same case: axillary lymphadenopathy, with hypoechoic cortical thickening, few vessels because of previous chemotherapy, but sonoelastography with a score 4 Ueno and FLR over 5.00 is high, suggestive of a sentinel node

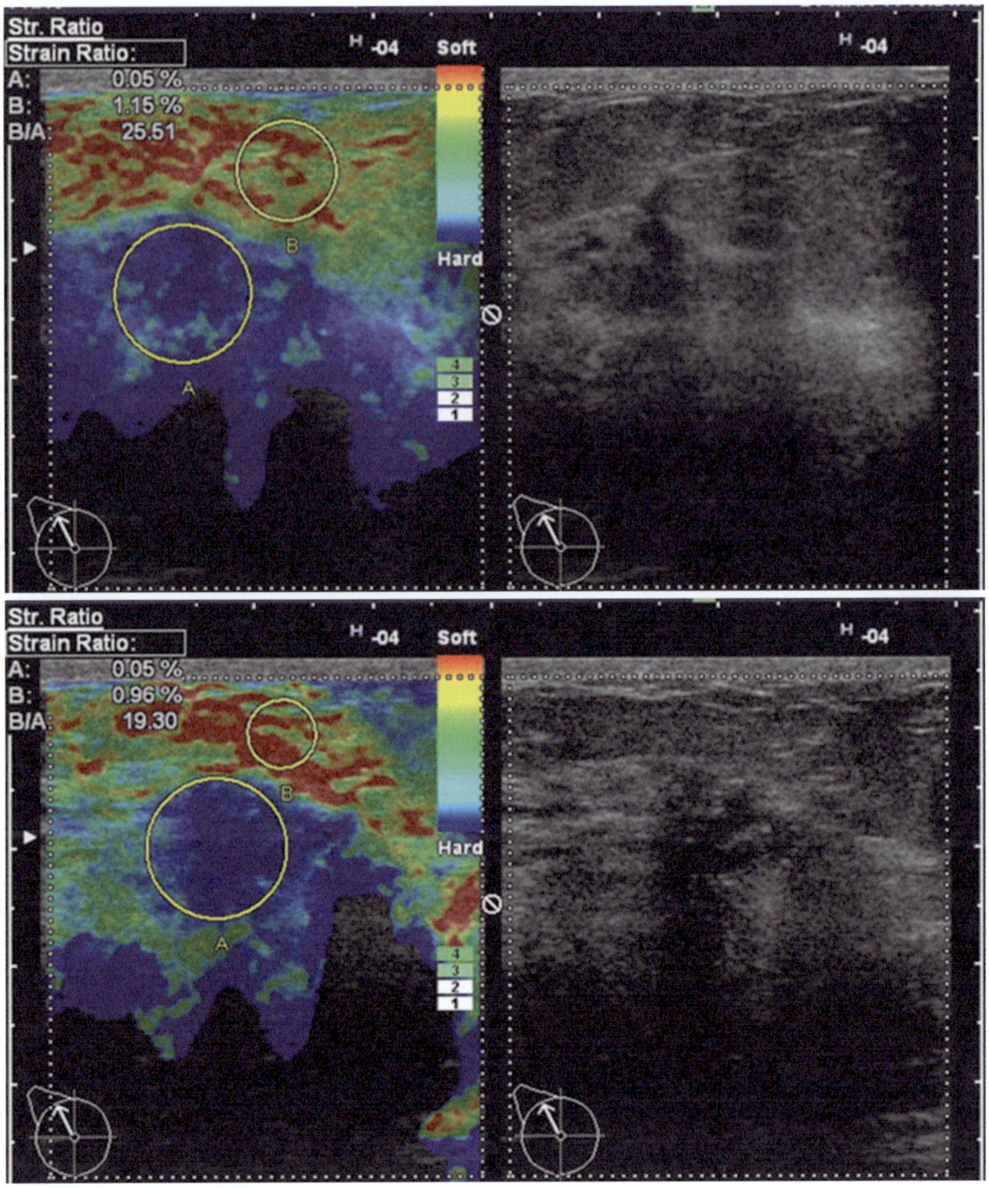

Fig. 8.17 Peripheral R: 11:00 "stellate" cancer, scored 5 Ueno, without axillary lymphadenopathy

Fig. 8.17 (continued)

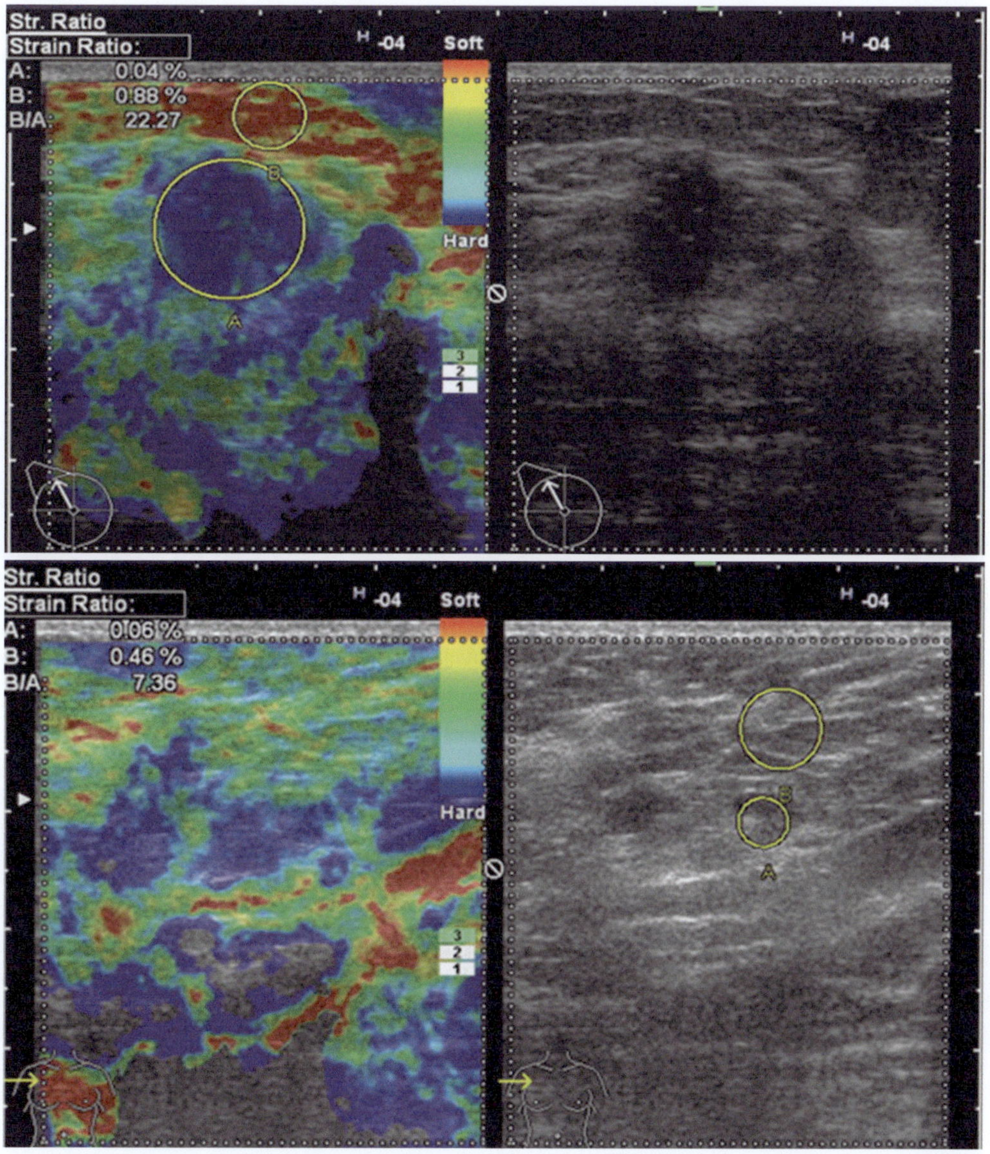

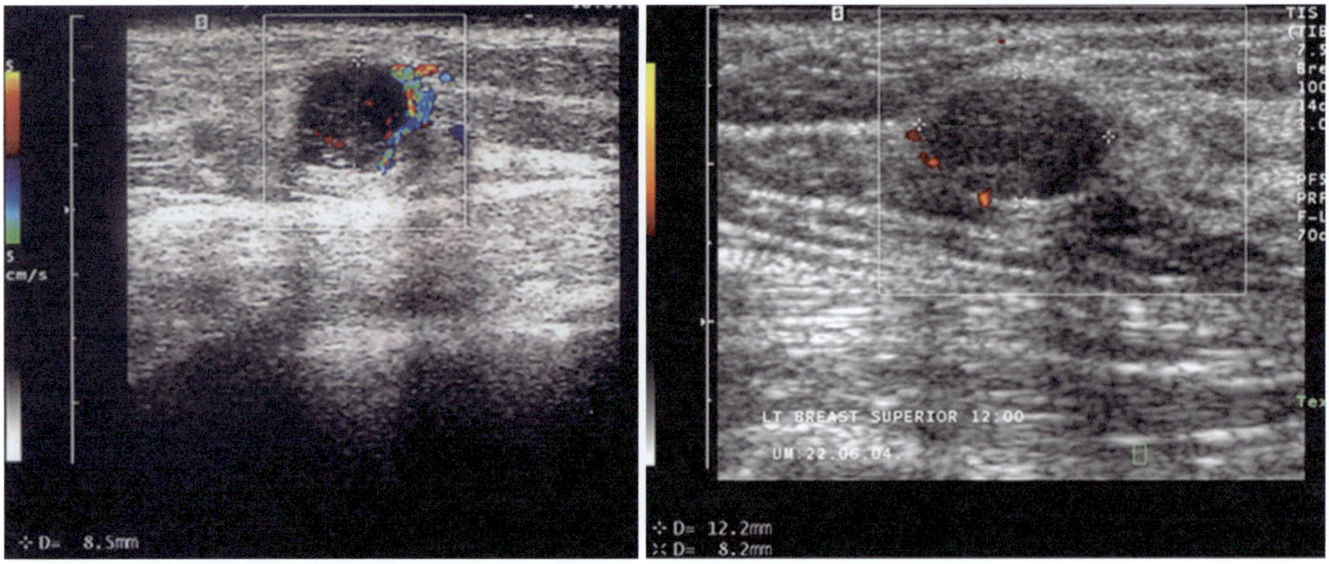

Fig. 8.18 Infracentimetric DCIS with pseudo-benign ultrasoundfeatures (*above*): posterior acoustic enhancement and marginal shadowing, similar to the fibroadenoma (*below*), but with peripheral and centripetal intense large new vasculature; otherwise, the malignant lesion is more hypoechoic. Both masses present adjacent hyperplasic lobule connected to the ductal tree

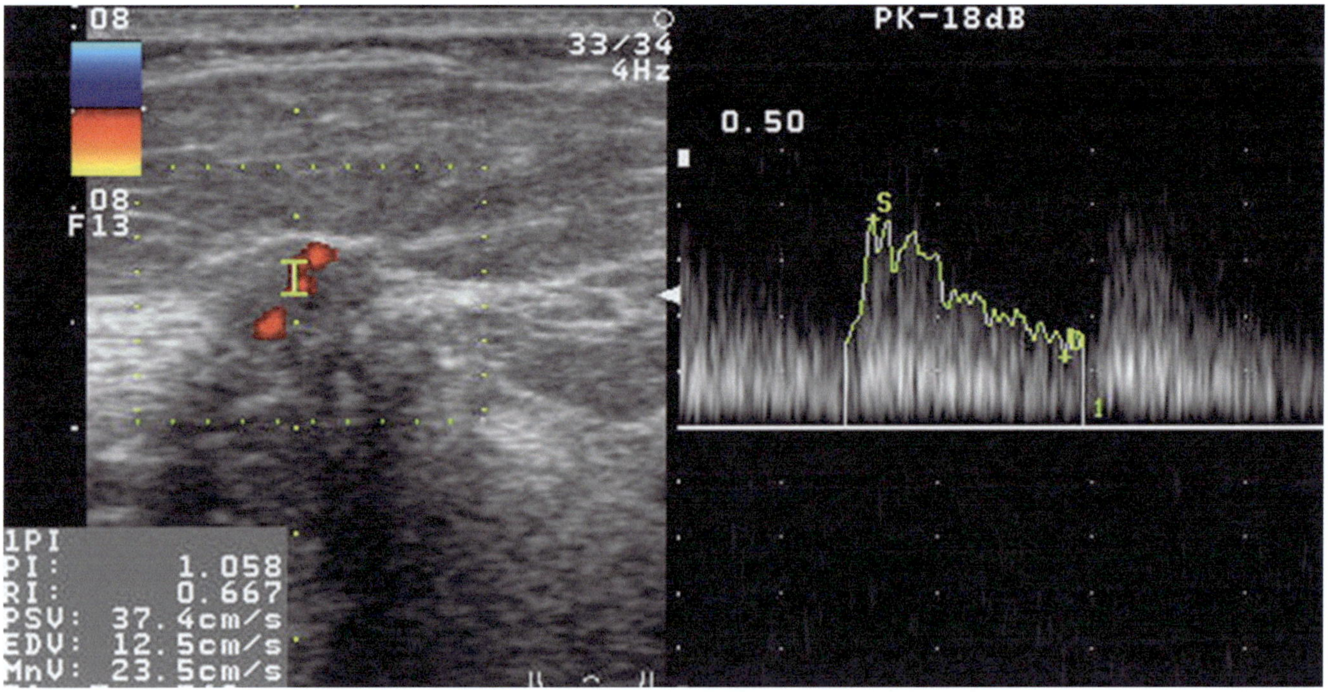

Fig. 8.19 Typical infracentimetric IDC, with ductal connection, spiculated irregular shape, acoustic shadowing, taller-than-wide, and with internal vasculature

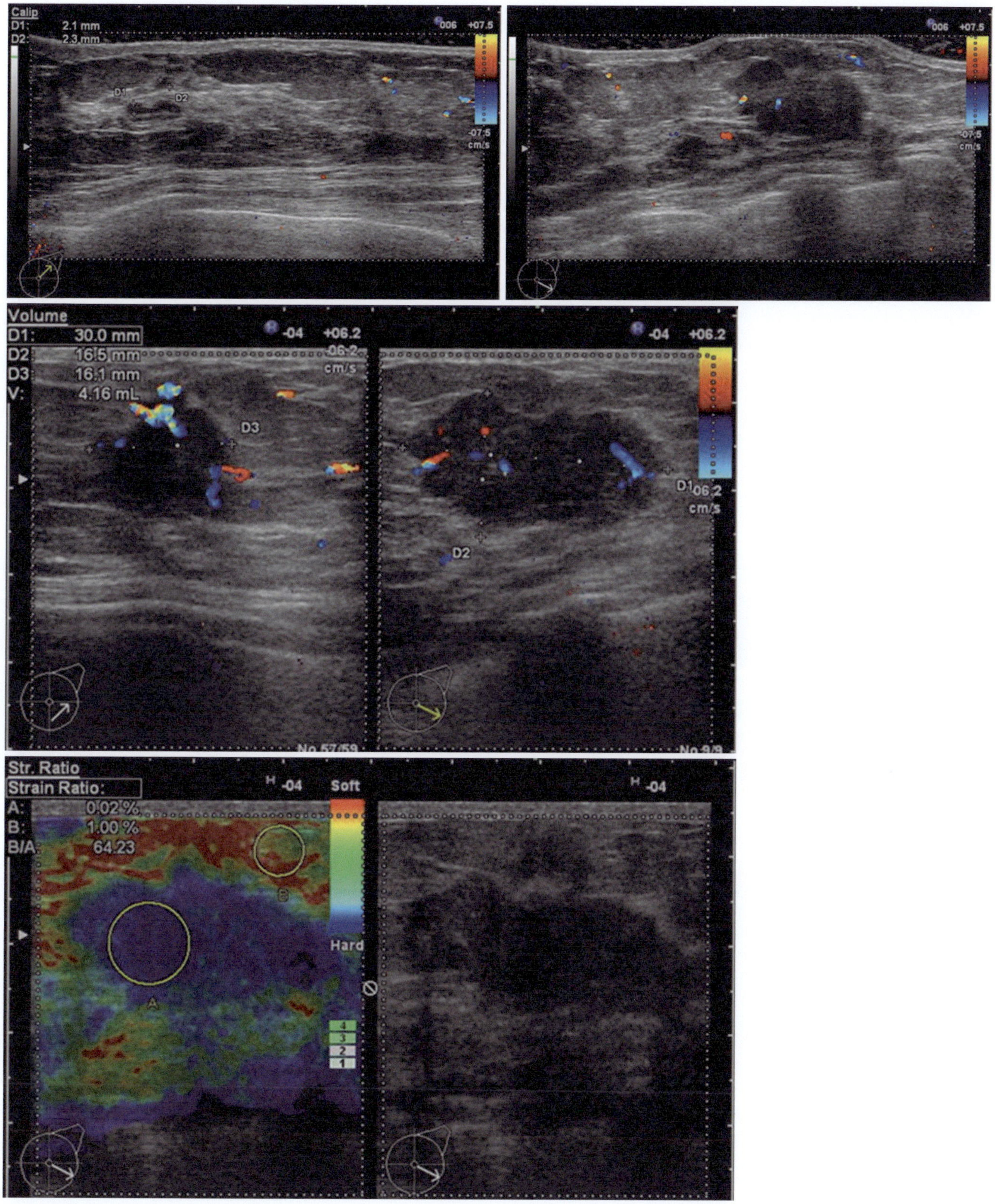

Fig. 8.20 Fourty-nine-year-old patient: presence of ductal-lobular hyperplasia with salient new vasculature is considered as a premalignant disease (upper), an "alarm sign" for possible associated malignancy, which must systematically be researched. At L:4:00 FBU illustrates a hypoechoic mass without significant acoustic shadowing, without hallo, the longer axis horizontal as in benign tumors. However, the irregular shape, with multilobulated contour, the Doppler malignant characters, and the sonoelastography scored 4 Ueno with high FLR are concordant with the presence of a medullary breast carcinoma, a rare tumor that demonstrates some pseudo-benign finding in classical ultrasound

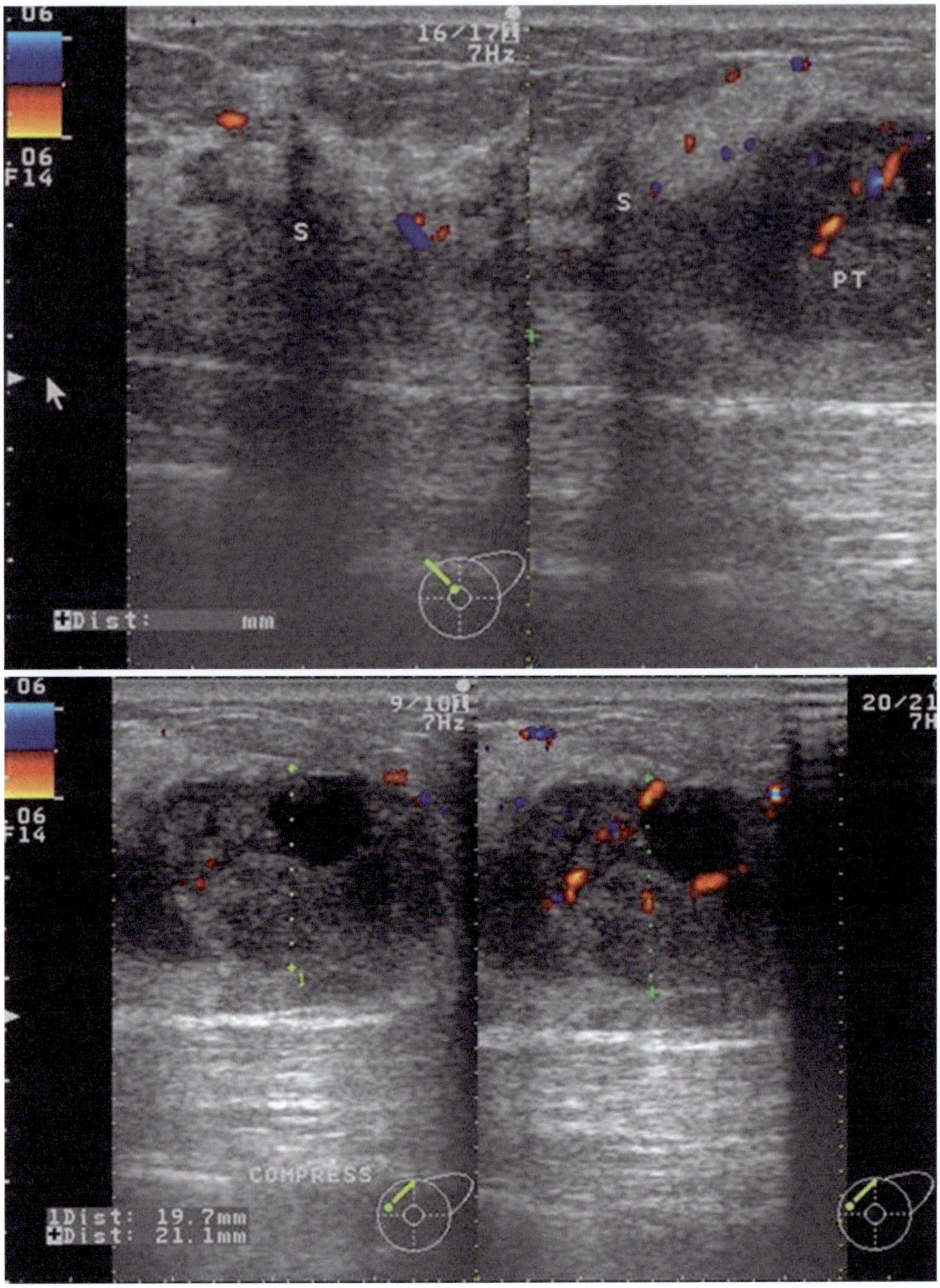

Fig. 8.21 Forty-year-old patient: palpable lump present for 2 years, enlarged in the last 3 months; Doppler DE visualizes the main pathological mass in the lobar periphery at L10:00, with pseudo-benign descriptors. and a cystic internal component, but with a few secondary centripetal lesions (s), and a new formation vasculature of malignant-type, originated from the internal mammary artery – multifocal cancer

Fig. 8.21 (continued)

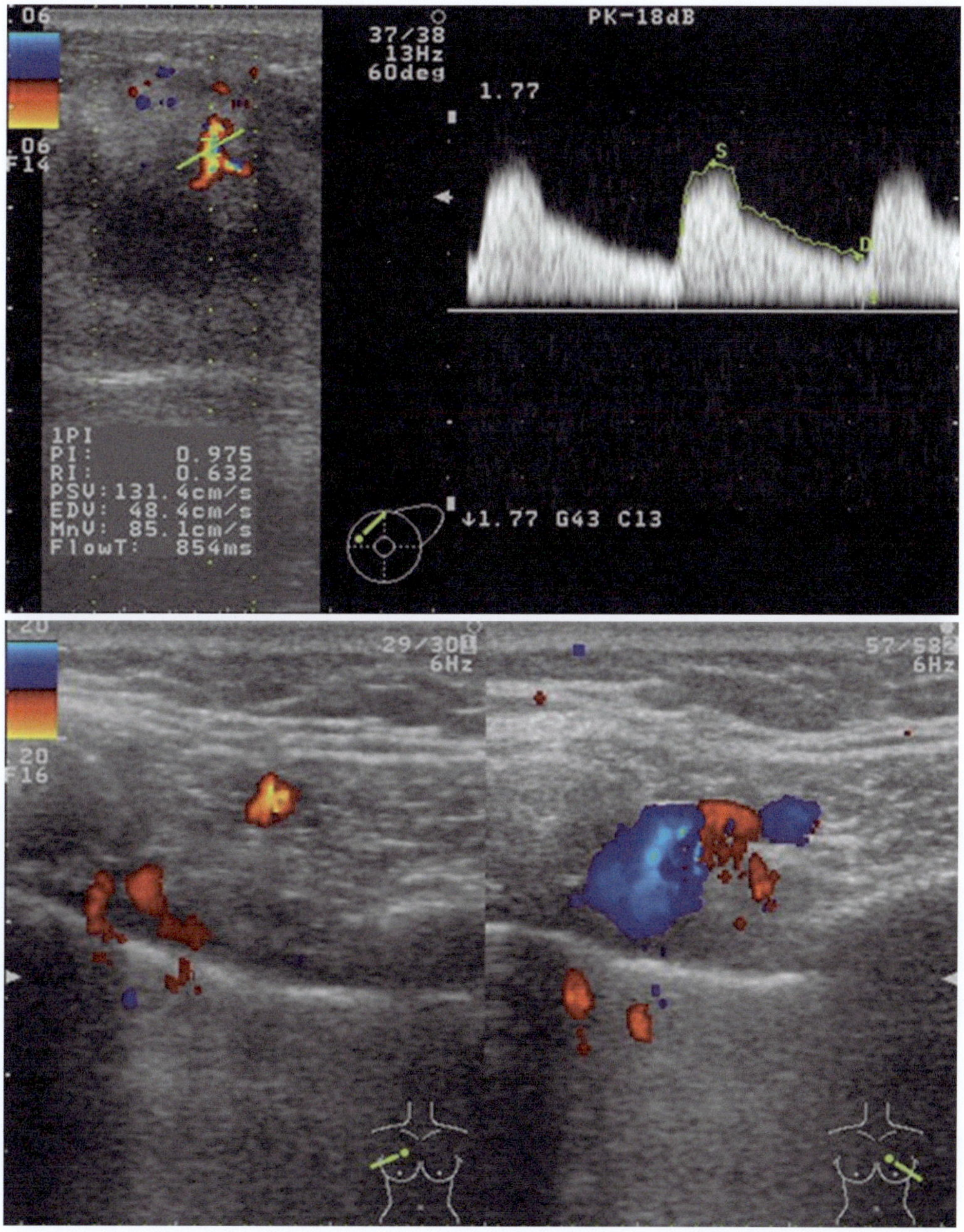

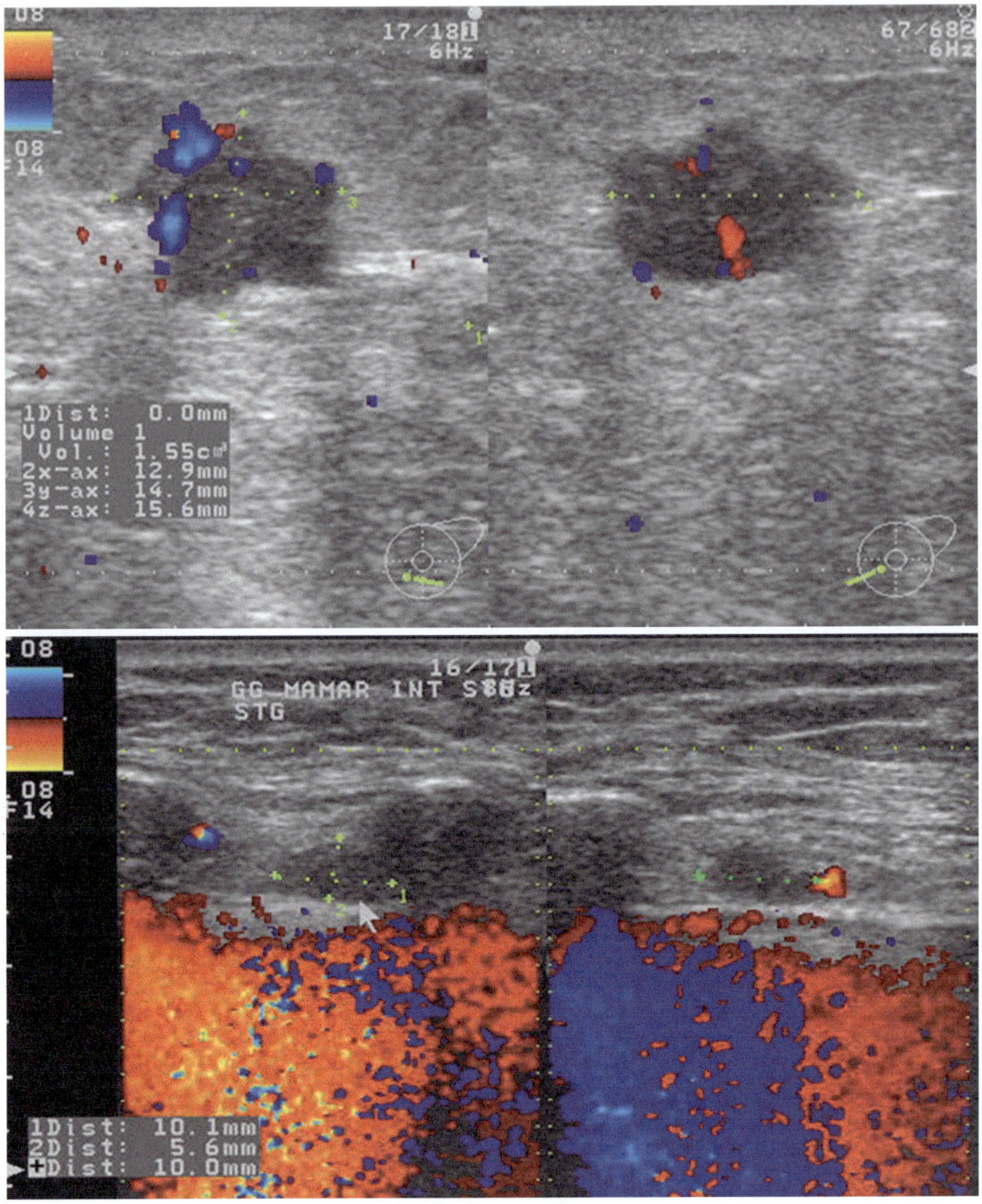

Fig. 8.22 Doppler DE: L8:30 "knobby" carcinoma less 2 cm in size, in a TDLU location, with angular malignant shape, hypoechoic but with posterior enhancement and marginal shadows (Kobayashi benign signs), and malignant new vasculature with incident plunging angle. The malignancy is confirmed by the pathological lymph nodes in the internal mammary chain (more frequent in inner quadrant cancers), and easy to explore by US [68], and axillary and subclavicular adenophaties (see Fig. 8.23). The absence of malignant shadowing and of the hallo is pathologically correlated with absence of any desmoplastic reaction, but the presence of multiple stations of adenophathies is suggestive of high-grade malignancy of this IDC

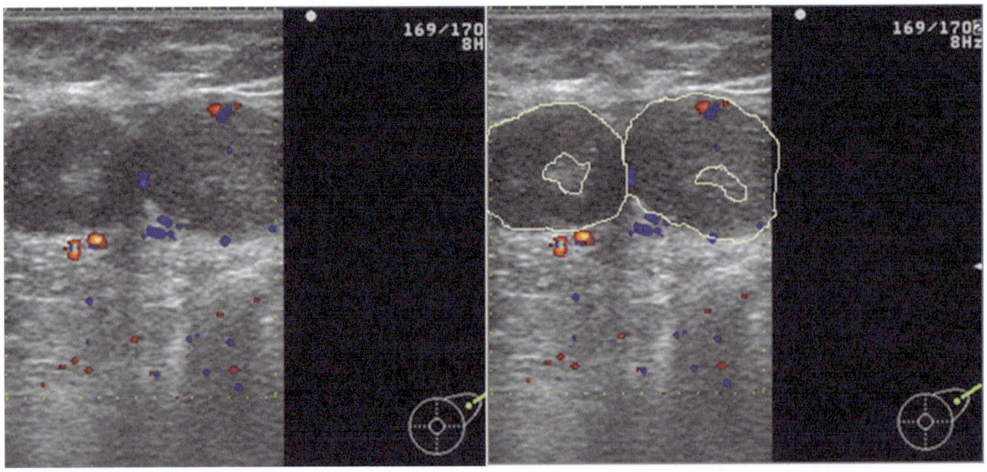

Fig. 8.23 The same case: A few axillary lymph nodes that are rounded-shaped and enlarged by increasing of the cortical hypoechoic thickness and with peripheral new vasculature are highly suggestive of lymph node metastasis

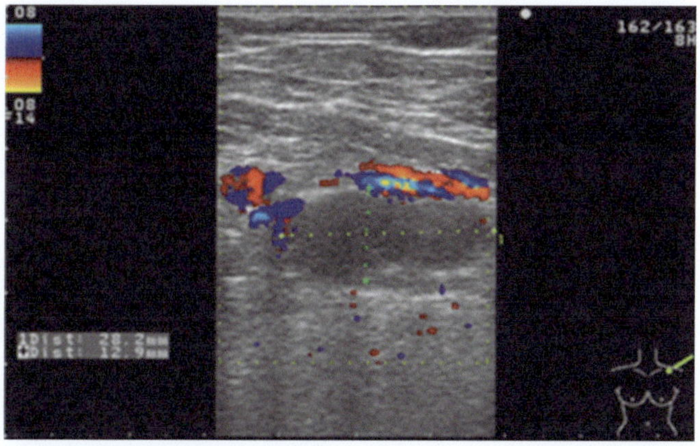

Fig. 8.24 The same case as in Figs. 8.22 and 8.23: supraclavicular lymph node with homogeneous hypoechoic internal texture and pericapsular vasculature. Differential diagnosis with other metastases or with leukemic lymphadenopathy is necessary when unknown breast cancer is present

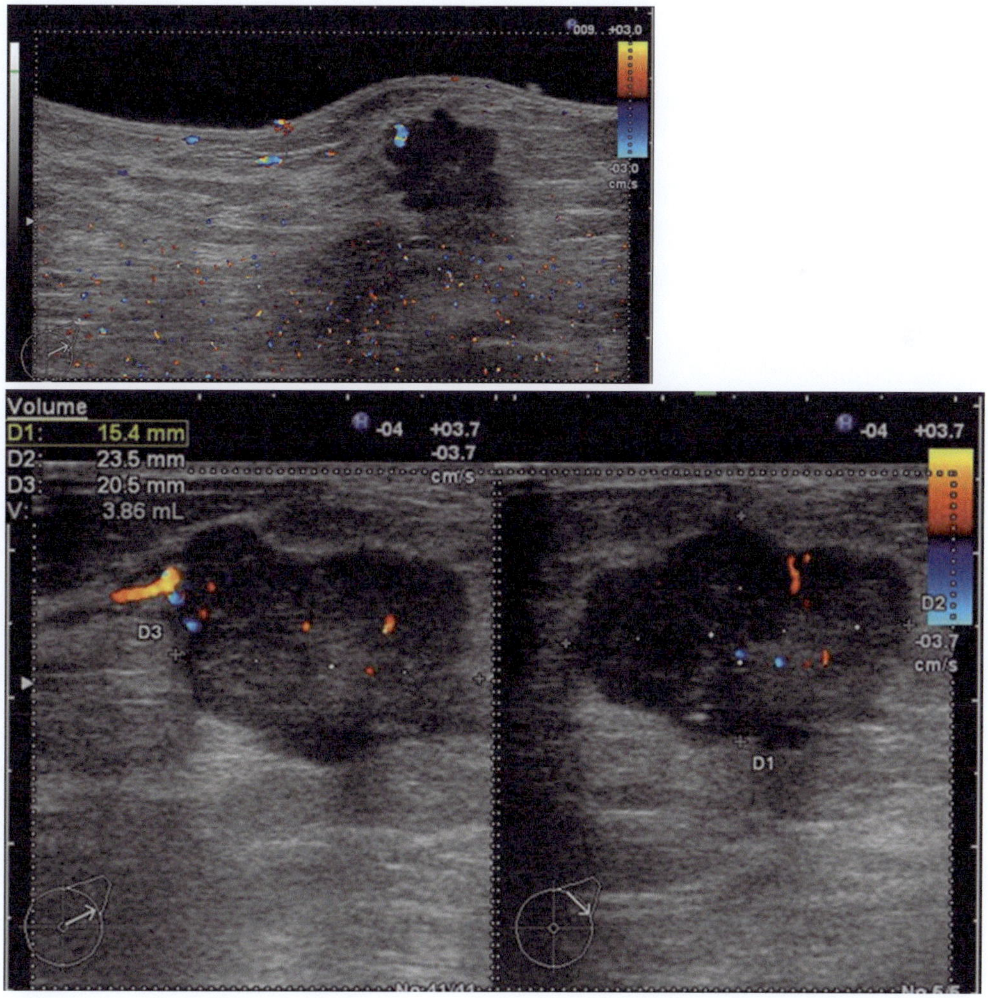

Fig. 8.25 L2:00 malignant mass with pseudo-benign features in 2D ultrasound in a 64-year-old patient, significant as it is a rare type of mucinous breast cancer. The benign findings, such as the largest diameter parallel with the skin and the posterior acoustic enhancement, are accompanied by the polycyclic shape, the incident angle of the plugging arteries, and the score 5 Ueno, all indicative of malignancy. Note the thickening of the emerging ducts with centripetal orientation and hypoechoic aspect, similar to the main tumor, indicative of intraductal spreading of the malignant cells. Sonoelastography and the salient vasculature confirm the associated ductal in situ malignancy, in concordance with the pathological report – “knobby” cancer

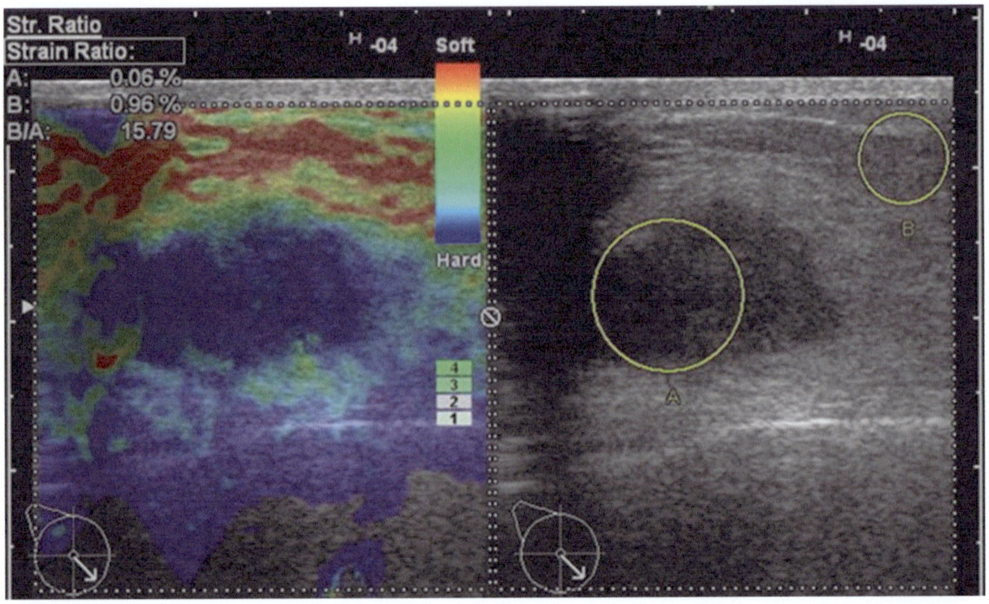

Fig. 8.25 (continued)

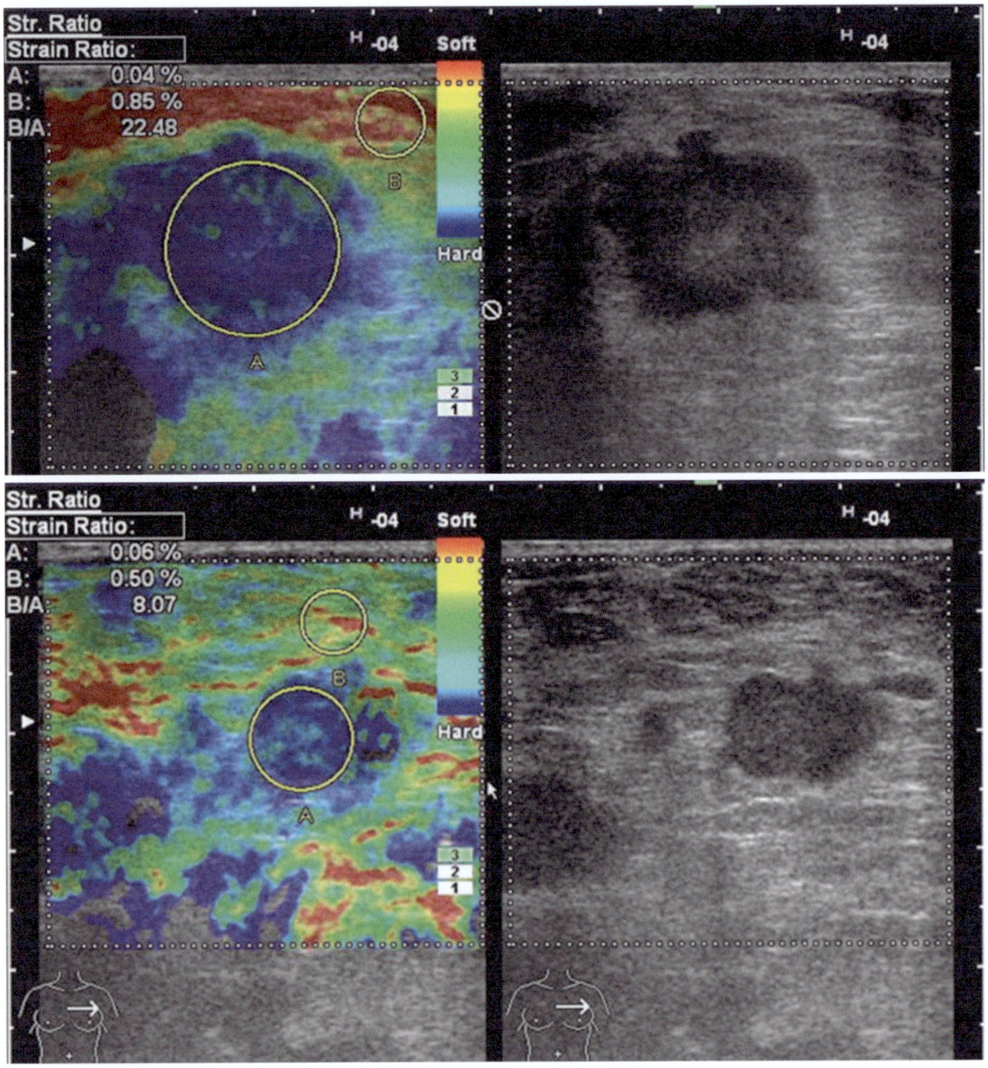

Fig. 8.26 The same case as in Fig. 8.25: note the similarity between the main tumor (*above*) and the multiple axillary lymph nodes metastases (below): polycyclic shape, posterior acoustic enhancement, score 4–5 Ueno with increased FLR

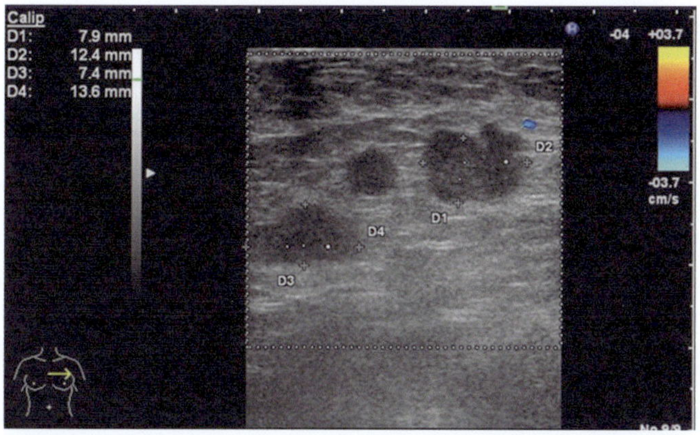

Fig. 8.26 (continued)

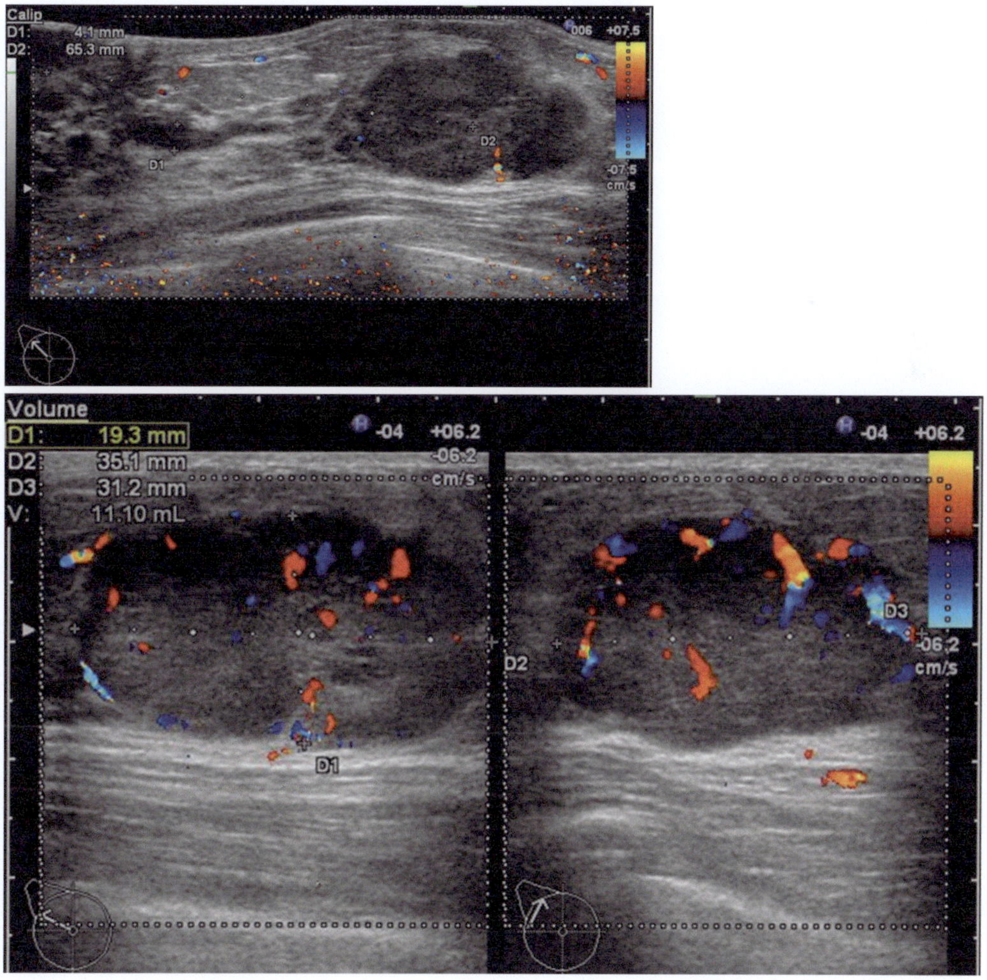

Fig. 8.27 Rare tumor in a 39-year-old patient with a pseudo-benign aspect after the classical criteria of Stavros. Doppler mapping is highly suggestive of malignancy, concordant with the score 4 Ueno and increased FLR over 10.00. The benign posterior features after Kobayashi show the aspect of a mucinous breast cancer

Fig. 8.27 (continued)

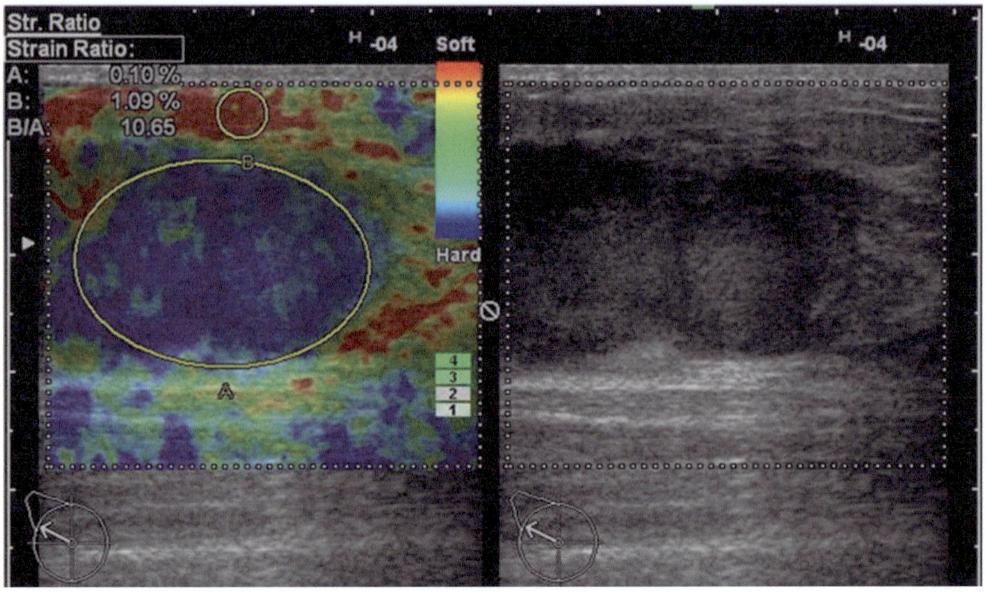

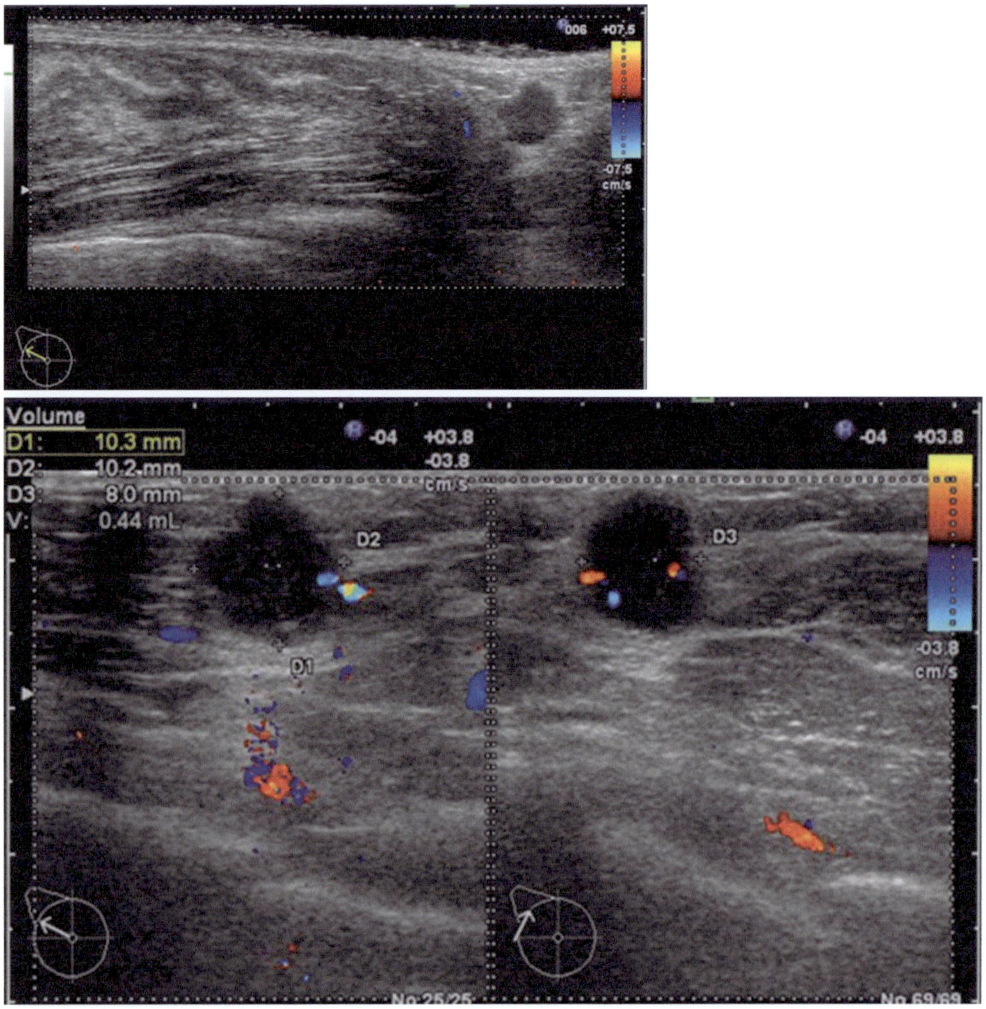

Fig. 8.28 Rare, small 10-mm tumor with both benign and malignant features in a 22-year-old woman. The score 4 Ueno is significant for rapid growth without desmoplastic reaction, concordant with an axillary sentinel node demonstrating thickened node cortex and with salient vasculature (bottom). The highly aggressive tumor is concordant with an undifferentiated cancer

Fig. 8.28 (continued)

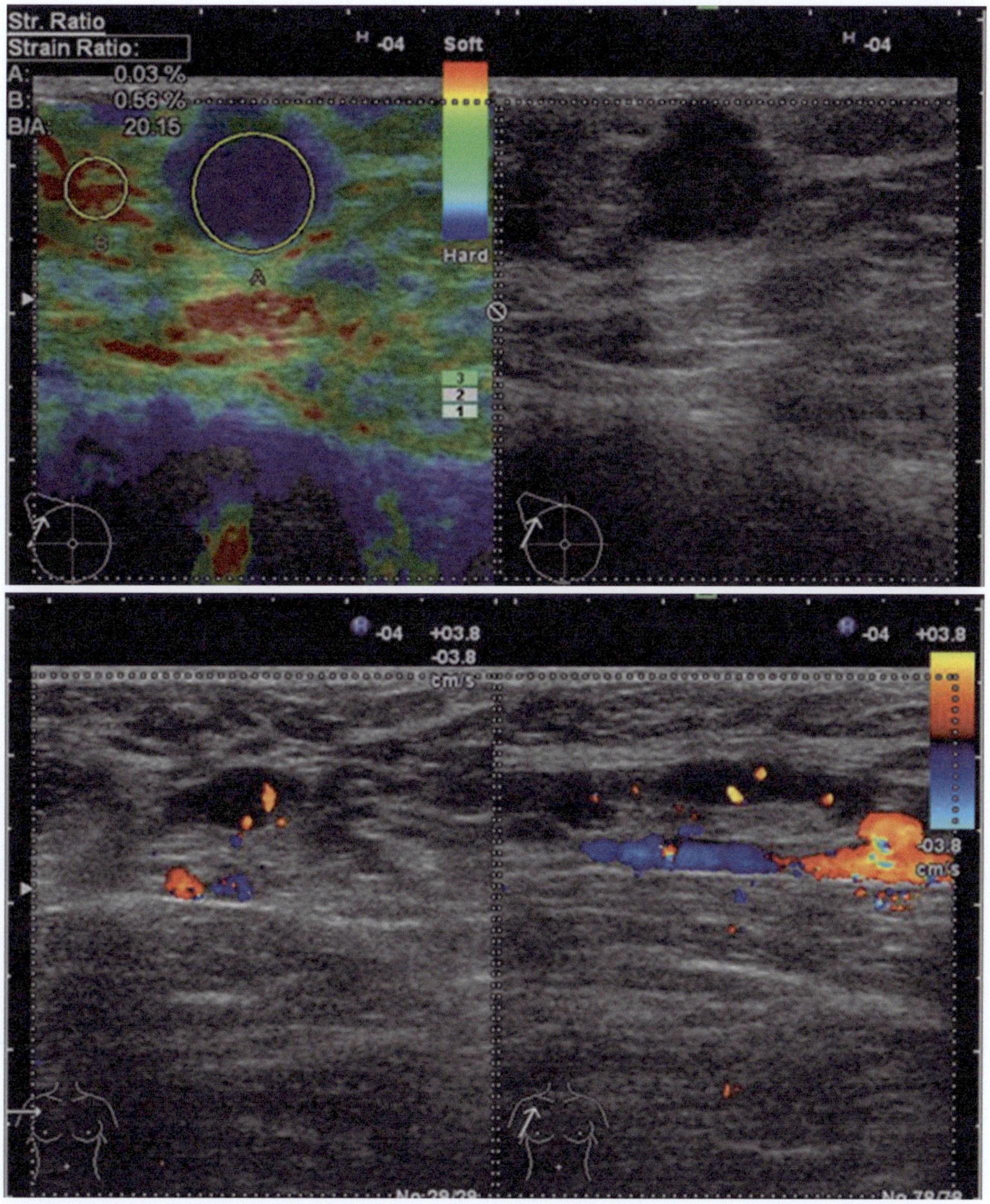

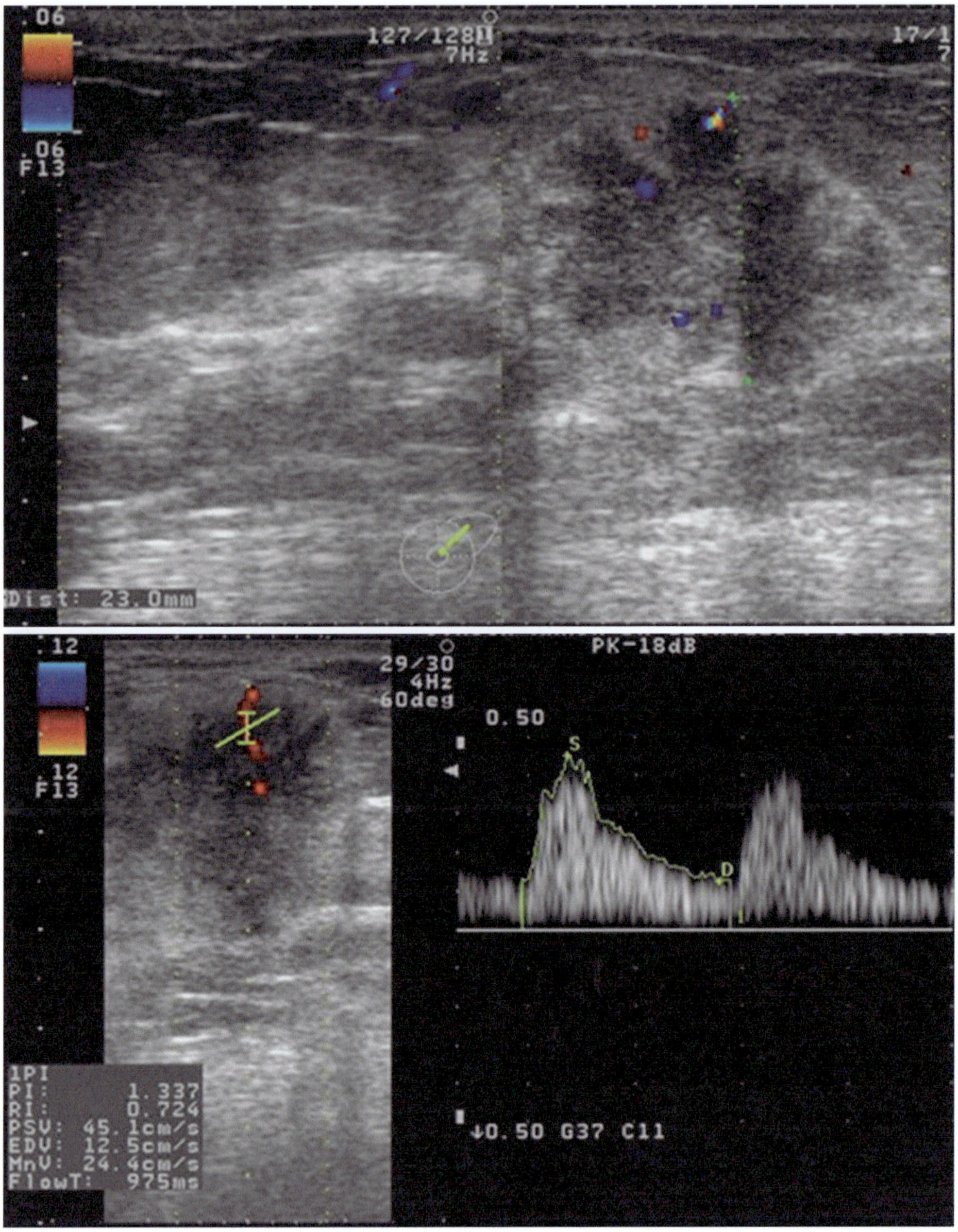

Fig. 8.29 Patient is 54 years old: 4D ultrasound acquisition of a "stellate" cancer with ductal extension. Note the illustration of the pathological architecture, despite the low resolution of the actual 4D transducersD dedicated improvements of the devices are mandatory

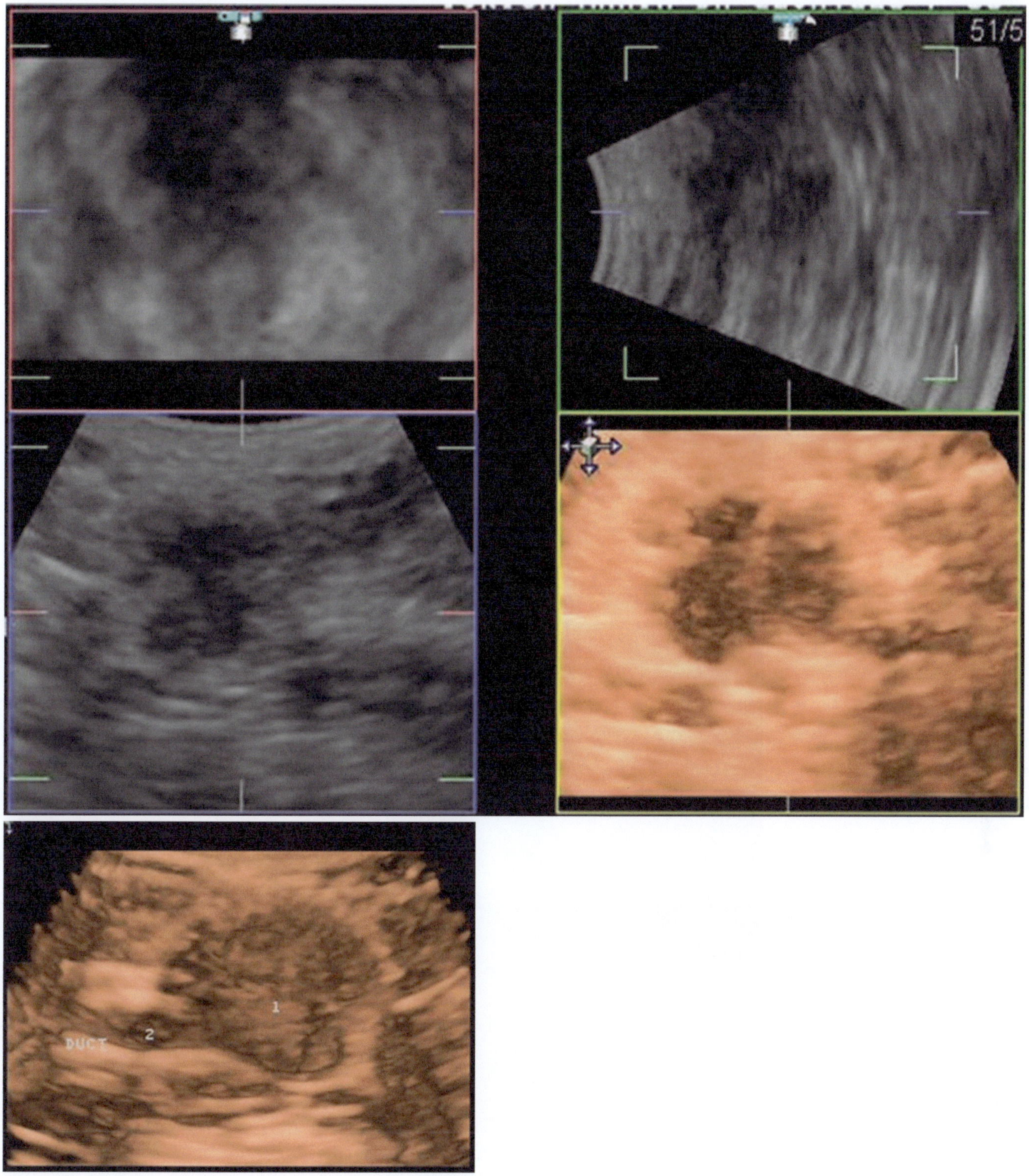

Fig. 8.29 (continued)

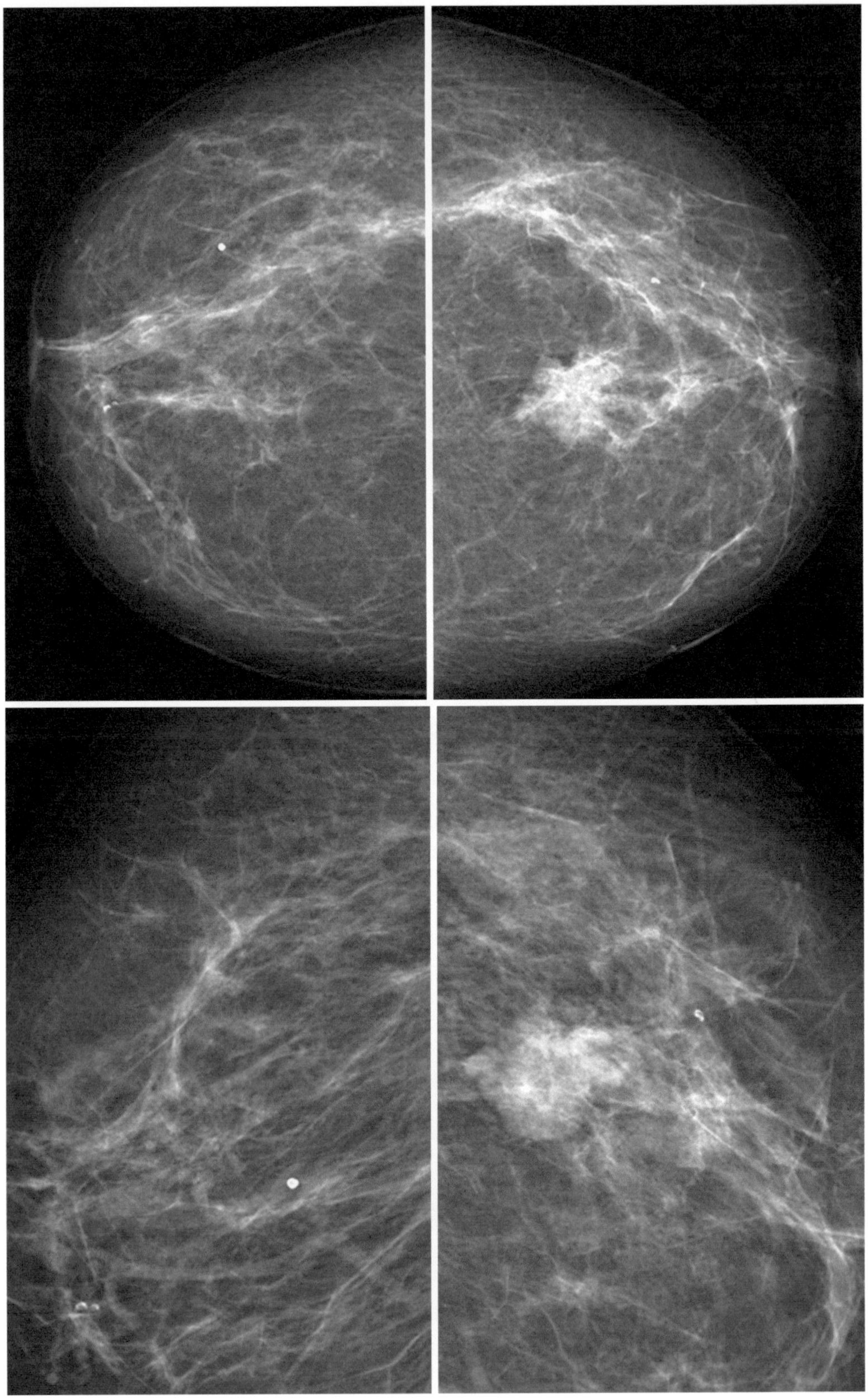

Fig. 8.30 "Stellate" cancer aspect on mammography. The digital mammography finally accepted after the improvement of the resolution cannot pass the limits of an analogue mammography, due to the radiological laws of absorption of the X-rays and the overlapping of the different tissues distributed in multiple layers of the whole breast. Thus, the gray-scale representation cannot distinguish the small associated lesions

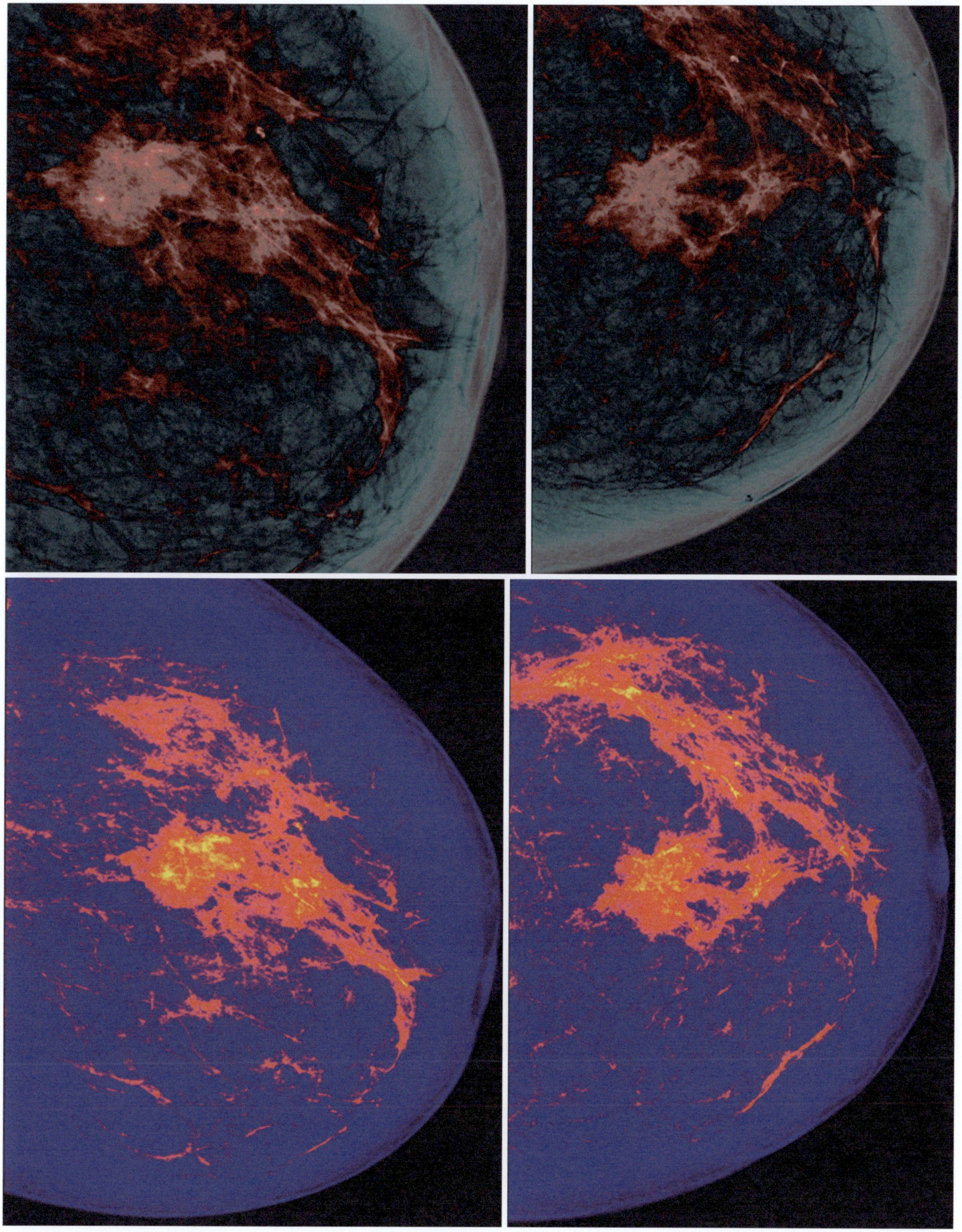

Fig. 8.31 The same case as in Fig. 8.30: by applying the Color Lookup technique, digital mammography allows better differentiation of the tissular densities, thus a multifocal breast cancer may be more easily suspected, changing the estimation of the extension of the malignancy and thus of the staging

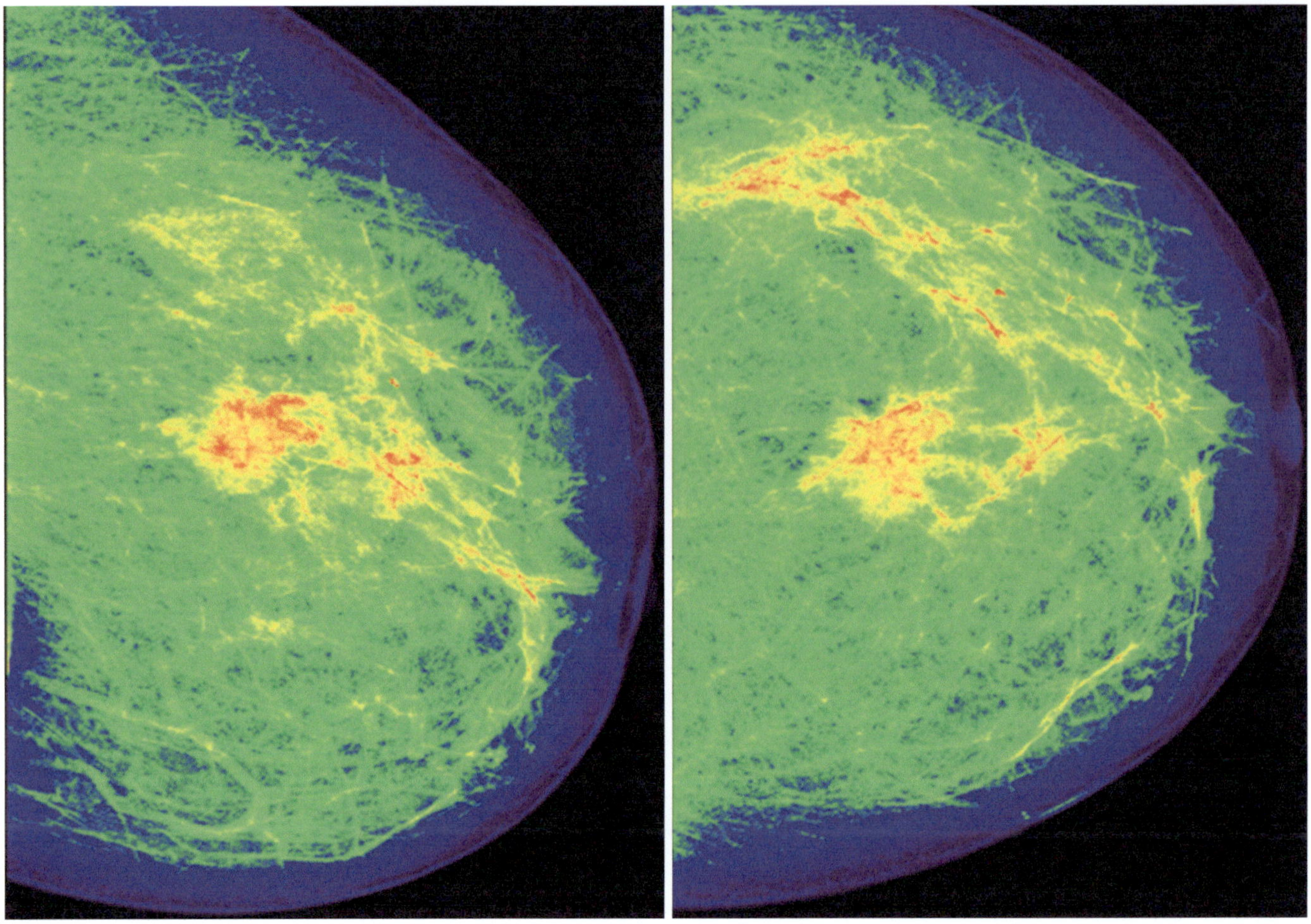

Fig. 8.32 The same case, different Color Lookup application, demonstrates the secondary centripetal lesion with increased density, and the upper-outer quadrant with increased diffuse glandular thickening, with radial orientation; however, the precise anatomy cannot be visualized, nor the precise location of the suspect masses. A more precise location, by eliminating the overlapping of the tissues, could be obtained by tomosynthesis, but the ductal branching anatomy remains unapparent and the differential diagnosis of multifocal from multicentric cancer is based on an arbitrary definition (different quadrants or more than 5 cm distance between the multicentric lesions)

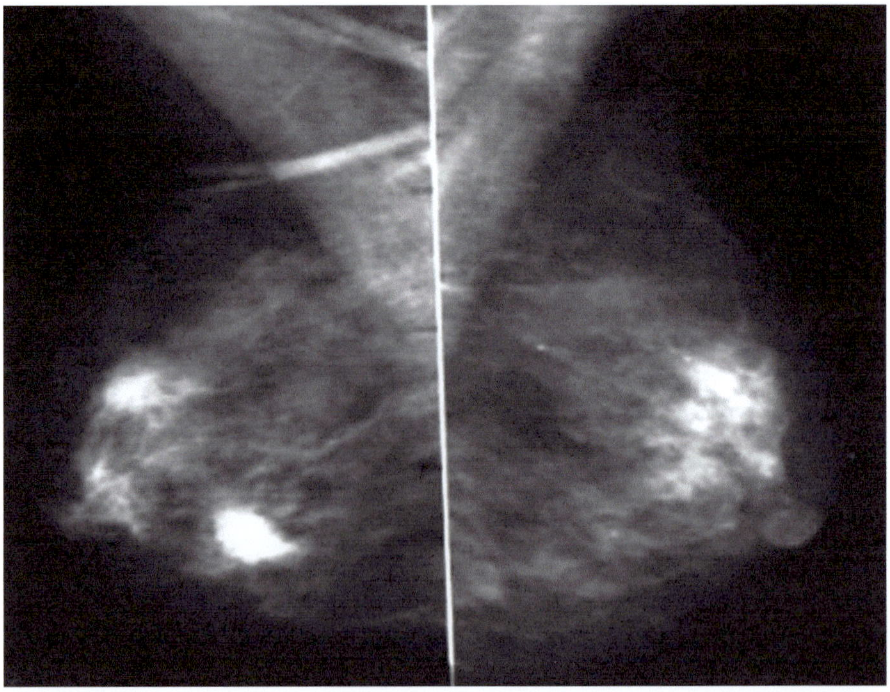

Fig. 8.33 Patient is 88 years old: mammography is first intention examination in the case of a patient with a sister with mucinous carcinoma confirmed 10 years earlier, illustrates in the MLO (mediolateral oblique view) incidence (CC (cranial caudal view) not shown): a mass with irregular borders but well delineated in the right lower (inner) quadrants, classified as BI-RADS category 4 and two spiculated masses in the right upper (outer) quadrants, classified as BI-RADS category 5

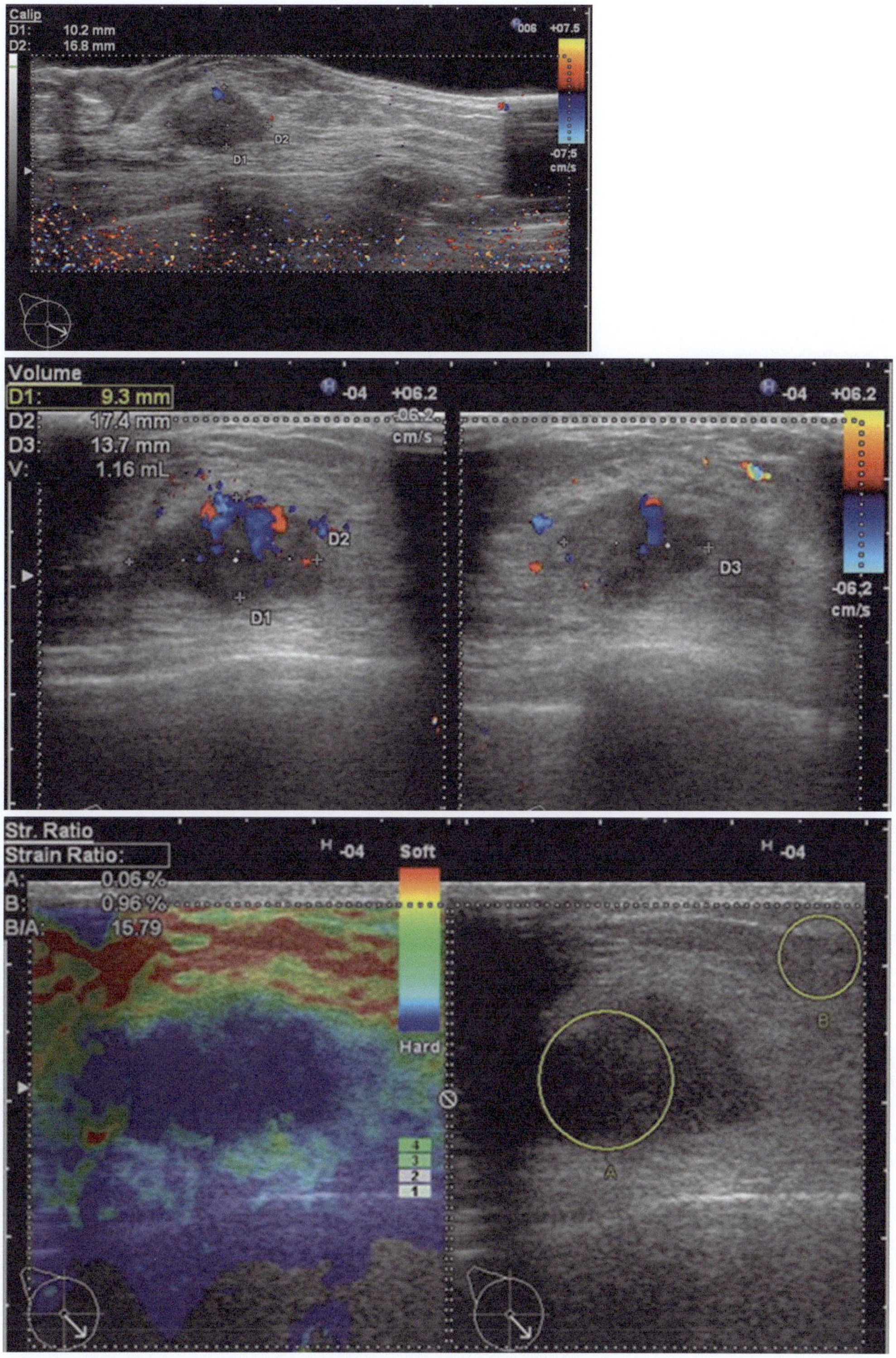

Fig. 8.34 Patient is 88 years old, same case as in Fig. 8.33: the lump in the lower-inner quadrant in FBU presents some benign 2D features (horizontal long axis, posterior acoustic enhancement) associated with malignant characters: hypoechoic, irregular borders, malignant vascular type, sonoelastogram of score 4 Ueno that suggests the absence of the stromal reaction and high FLR of 15.79, concordant with the pathological report of mucinous carcinoma. Ultrasound BI-RADS category 5

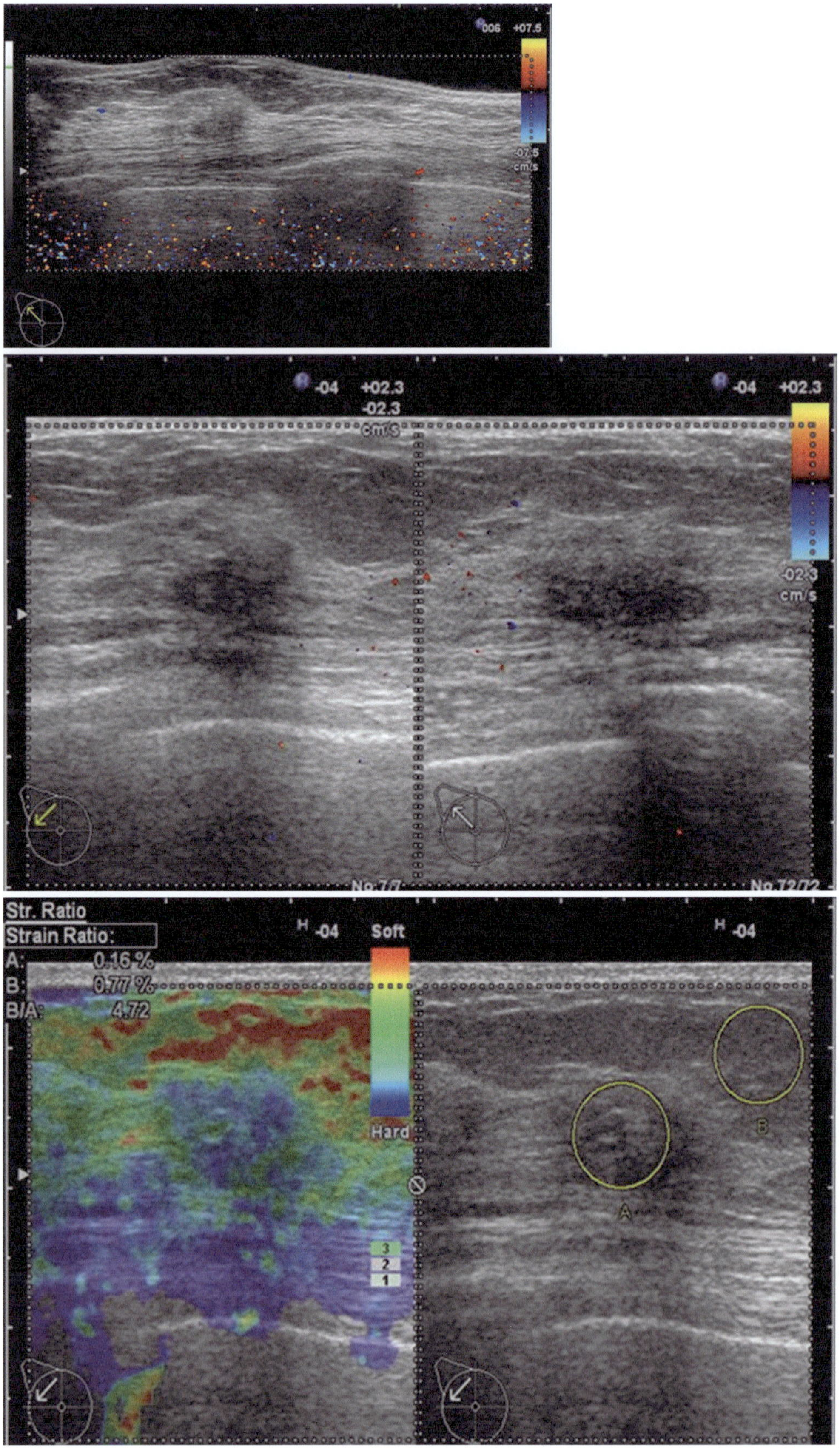

Fig. 8.35 Patient is 88 years old, same case as in Figs. 8.33 and 8.34: the upper-outer mammographic larger mass presented inhomogeneous ultrasound aspect, posterior acoustic shadowing, less vascular signal, and score 3 Ueno with borderline FLR of 4.72. The small mammographic spiculated mass with the same ultrasound features presented the score 2 Ueno with benign FLR of 1.76, despite the acoustic shadowing. These masses represented sclerosing adenosis

Fig. 8.35 (continued)

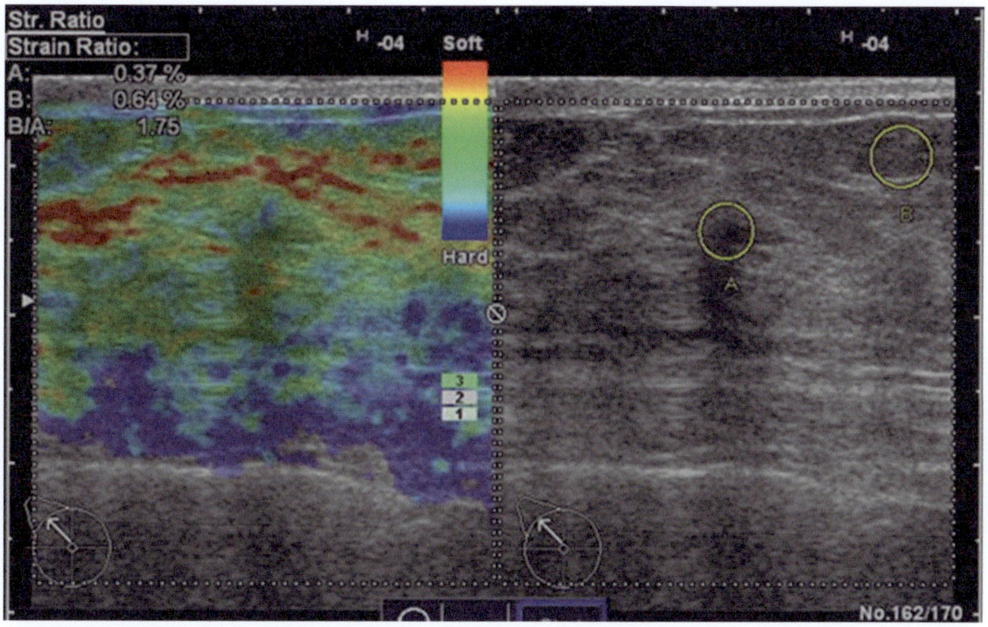

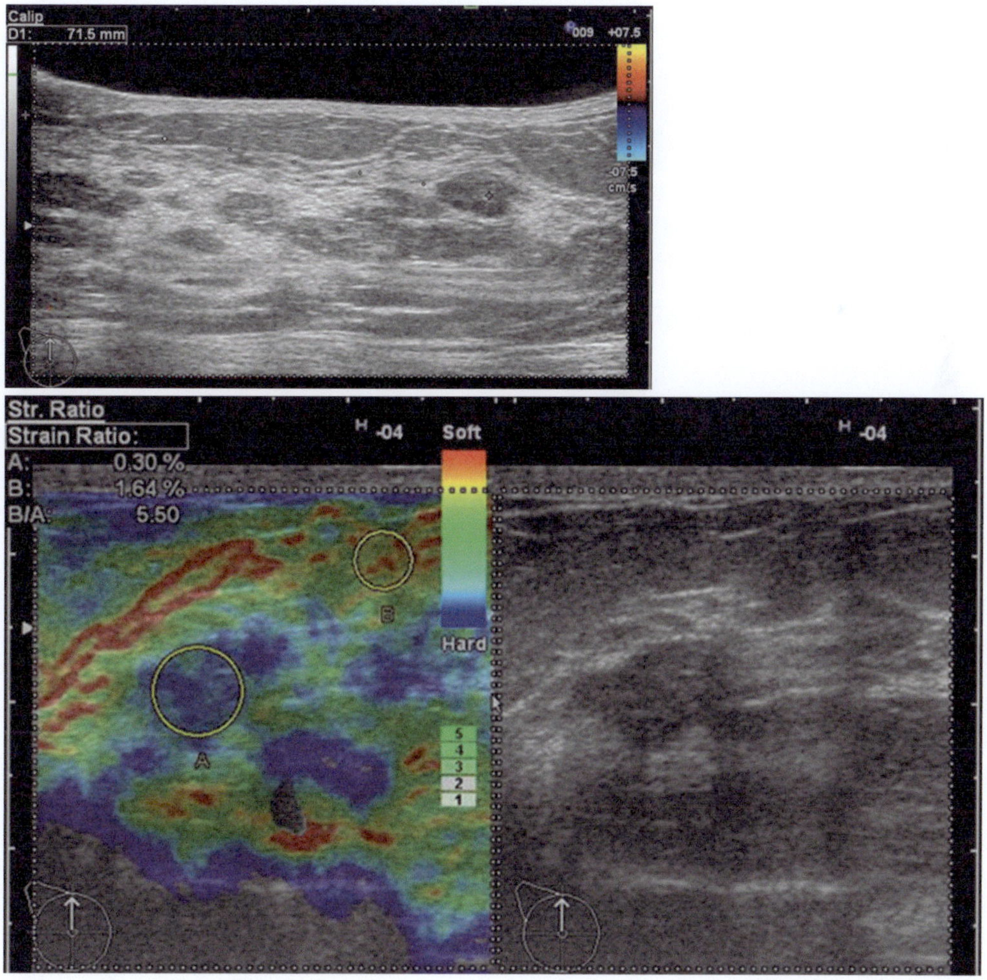

Fig. 8.36 A screening FBU was performed on a 43-year-old patient: bilateral nodular suspect lesions, with polycyclic shape, located in TDLU, with moderate new formation vasculature, scored 3 and 4 Ueno with FLR over 5.00. The connection with some thickened ducts is significant. In the right breast, the more important findings located at 12:00 and 2:30 radiuses are apparent as multicentric lesions

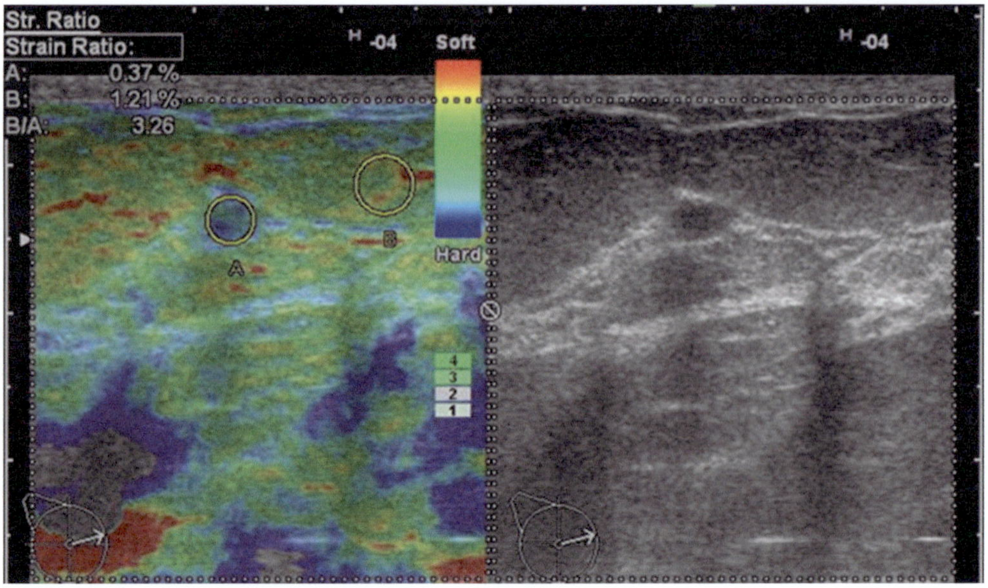

Fig. 8.36 (continued)

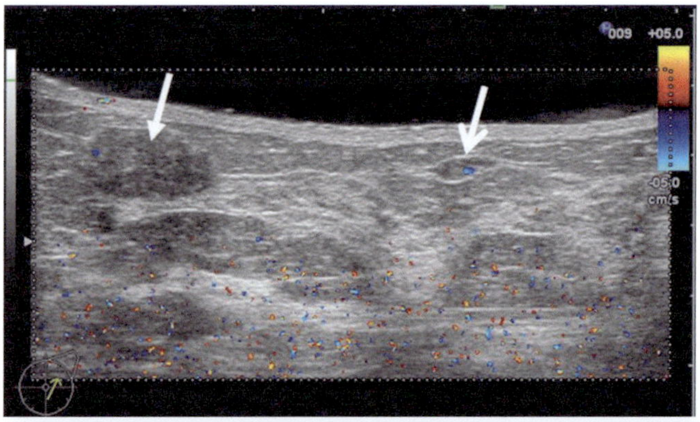

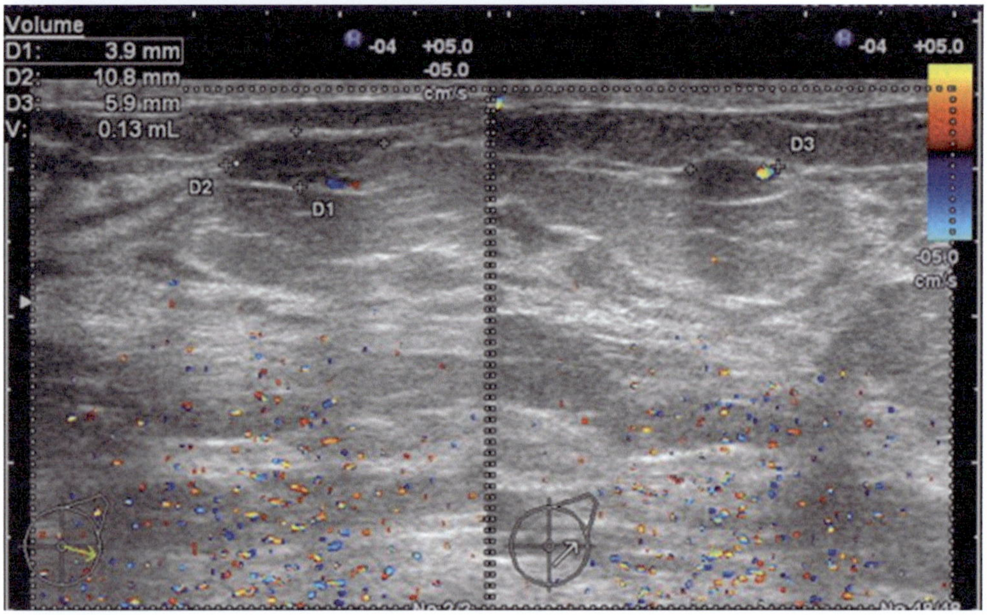

Fig. 8.37 Patient is 43 years old, the same case as in Fig. 8.36: the antiradial scan with the long probe illustrates a few lesions at L4:00 and L5:30 radius, with ductal evident interconnection, thus multifocal cancer (*white arrows*). Because of presence of other small, borderline lesions, a complementary breast MRI was recommended for the full cartography and therapeutical decision making (bilateral multicentric and multifocal cancer)

Fig. 8.37 (continued)

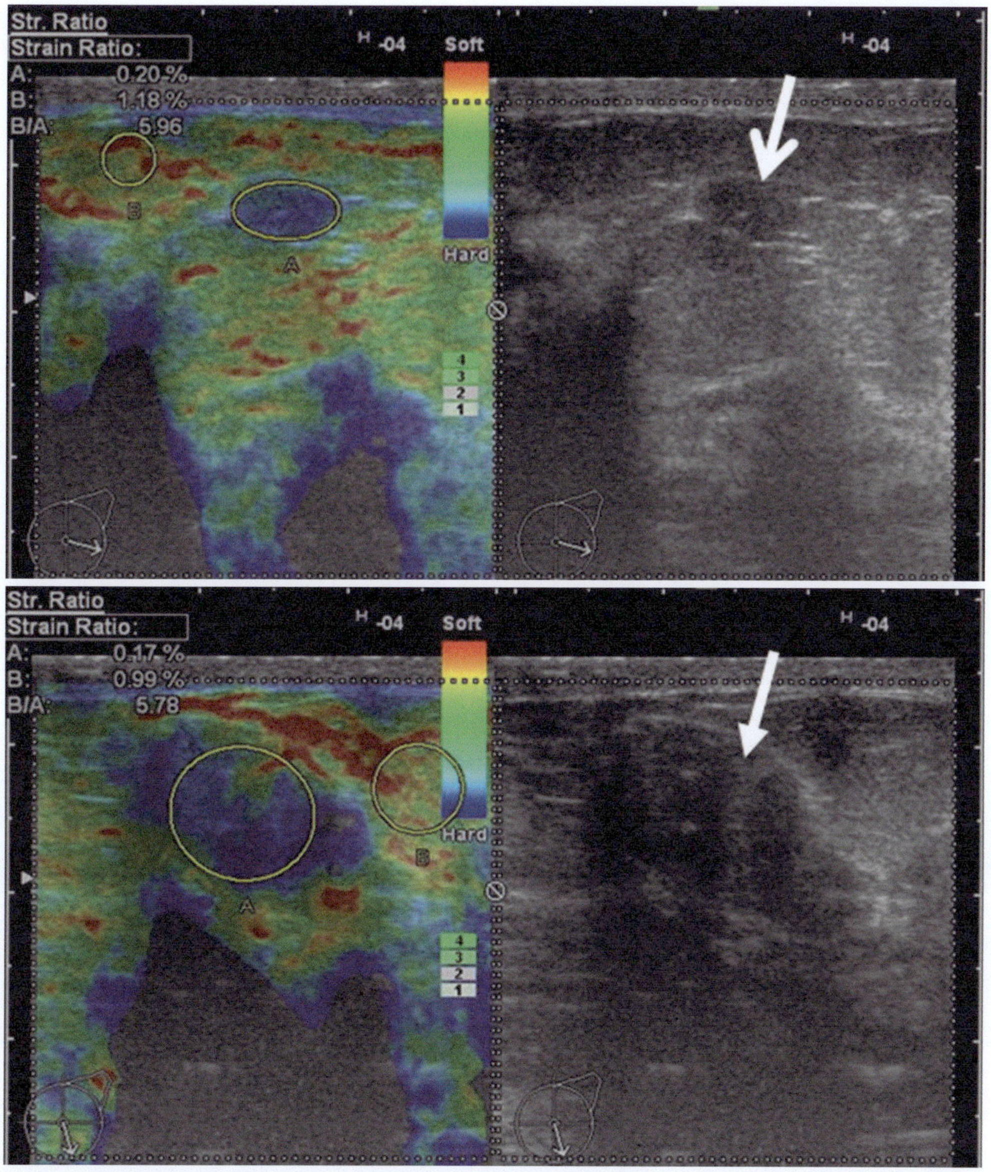

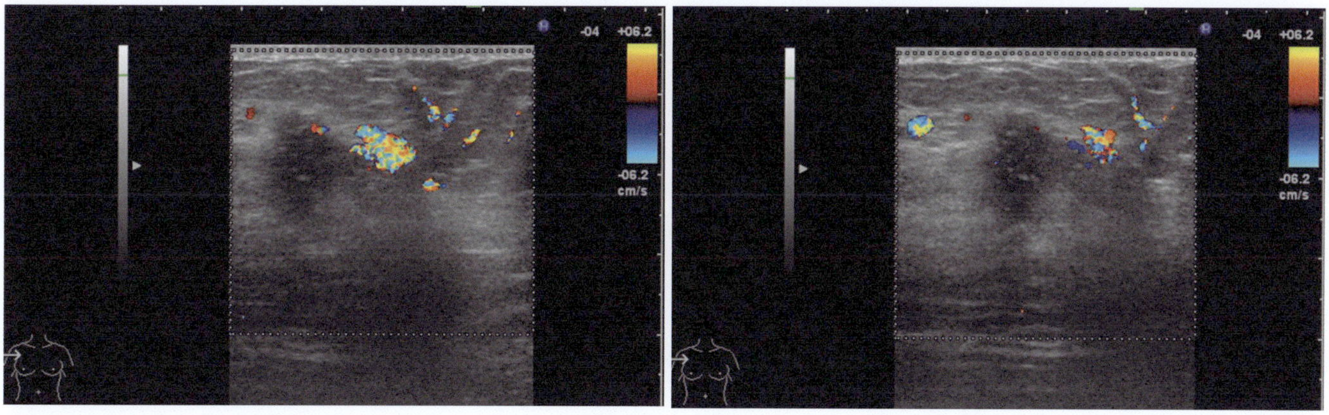

Fig. 8.38 Patient is 53 years old with breast cancer in the axillary prolongation of the R mammary gland (the Spence tail). The tumor architecture, type of vasculature, and extension along Cooper's ligaments differentiate this from the axillary lymphadenopathy

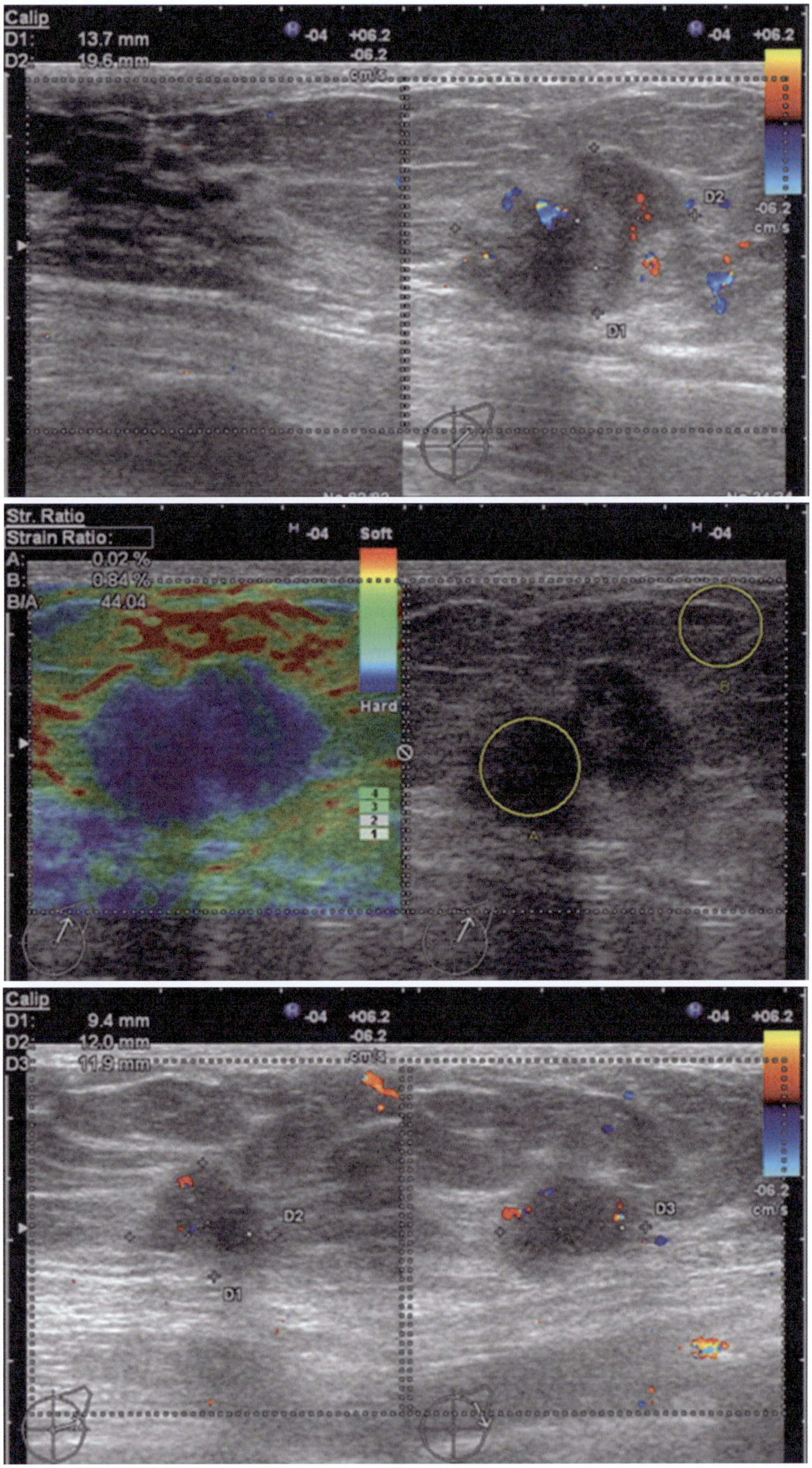

Fig. 8.39 Patient is 55 years old with L1:00 (double lesion) and L2:00 multifocal cancer, score 4 Ueno, ultrasound BI-RADS category 5

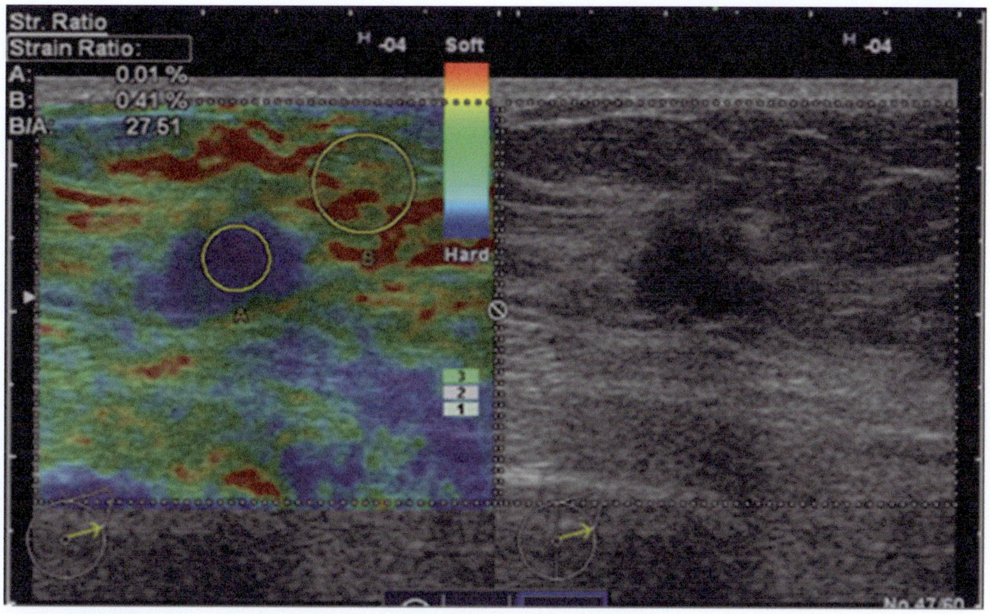

Fig. 8.39 (continued)

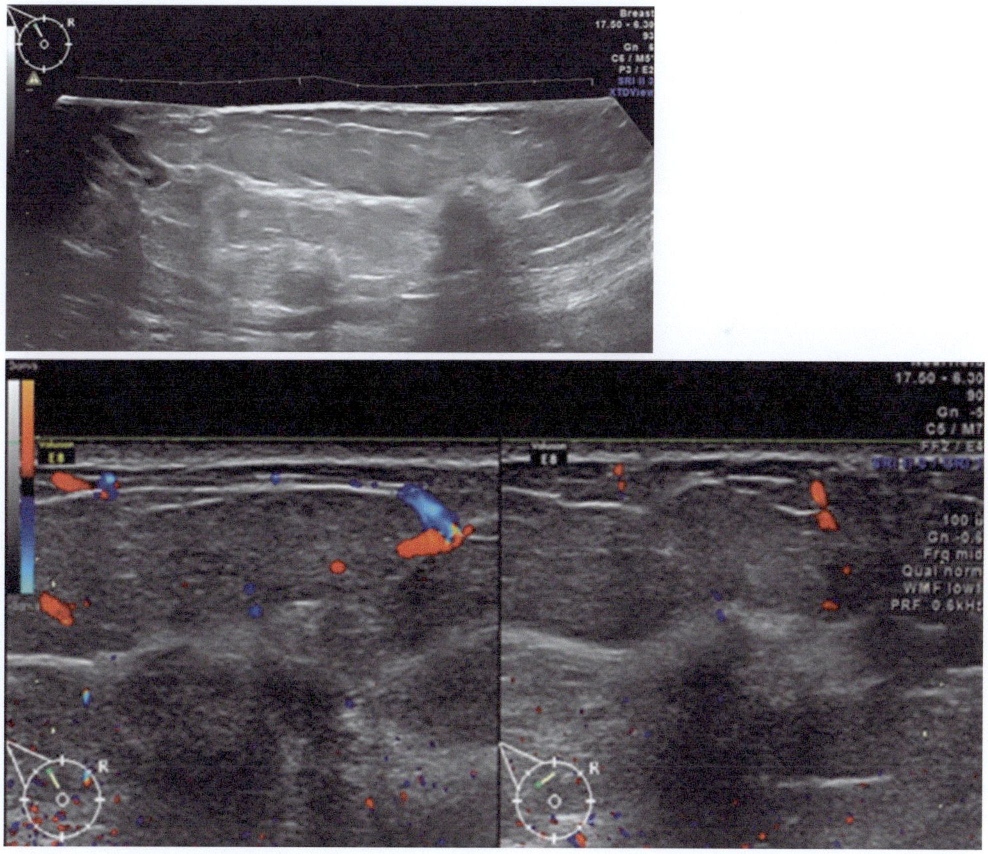

Fig. 8.40 Patient is 64 years old with fatty breasts and glandular atrophy, however, the lobar anatomy is recognizable. Multifocal breast cancer in R11:00 with new formation vasculature and score 5 Ueno. Note the central ductal-ampullary ectasia

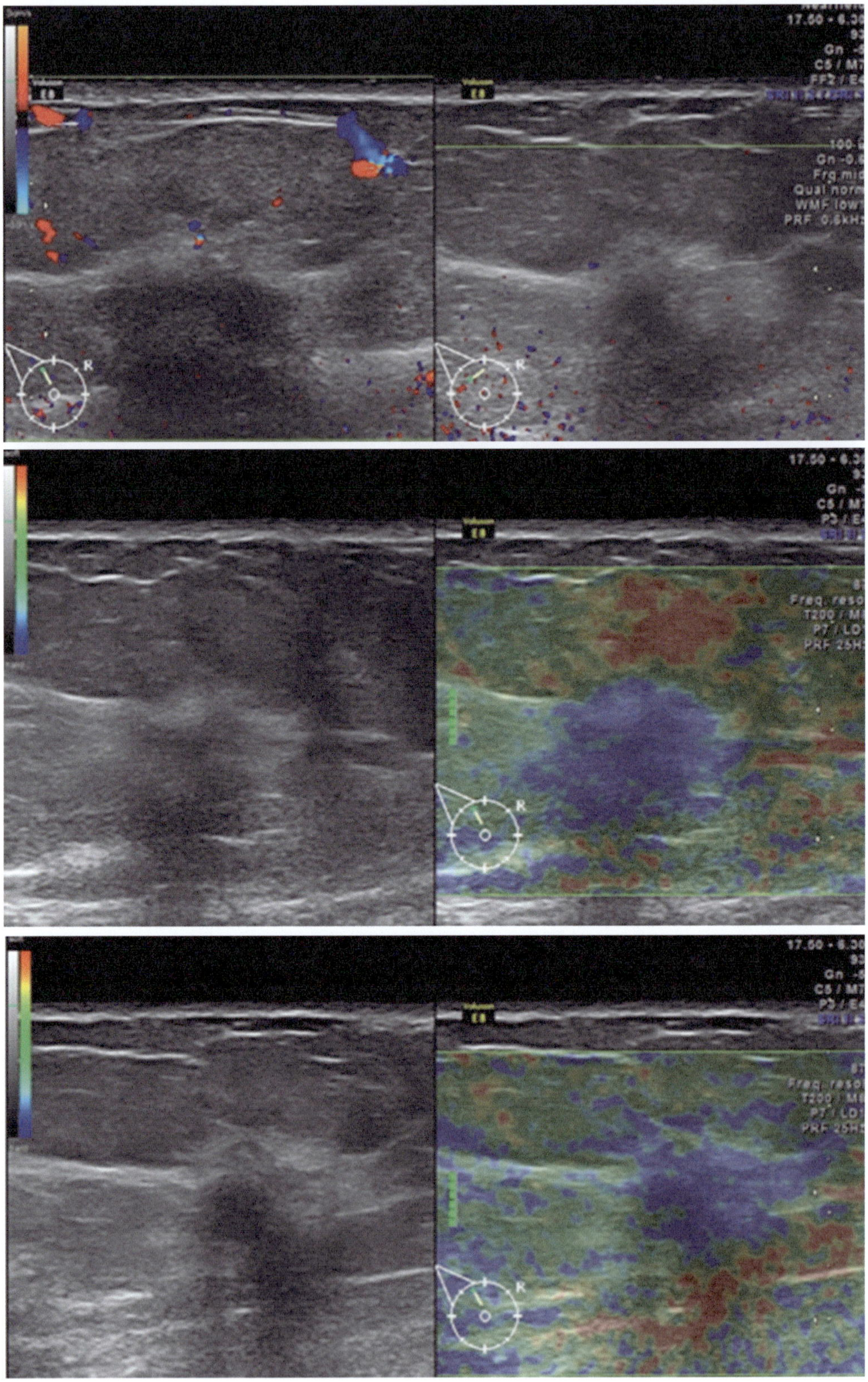

Fig. 8.40 (continued)

Fig. 8.40 (continued)

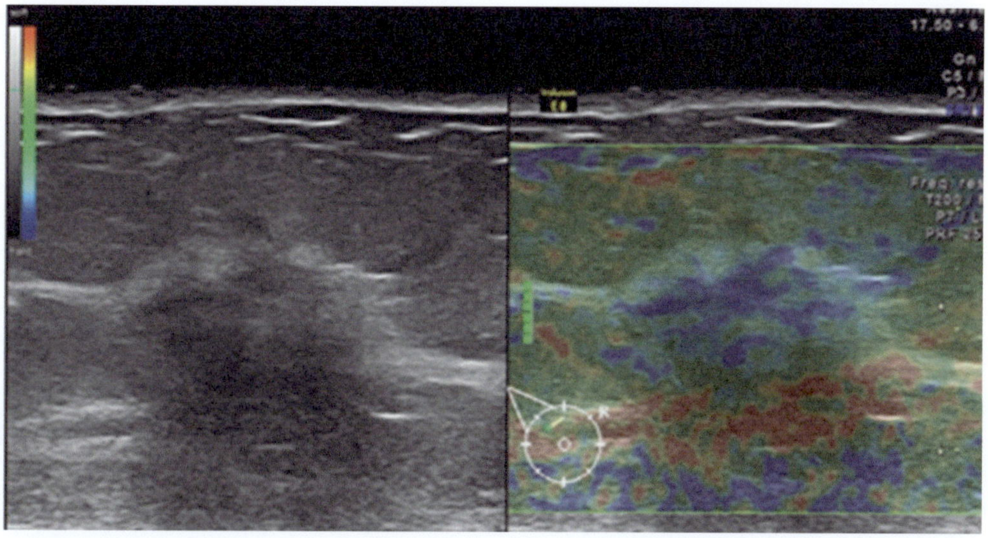

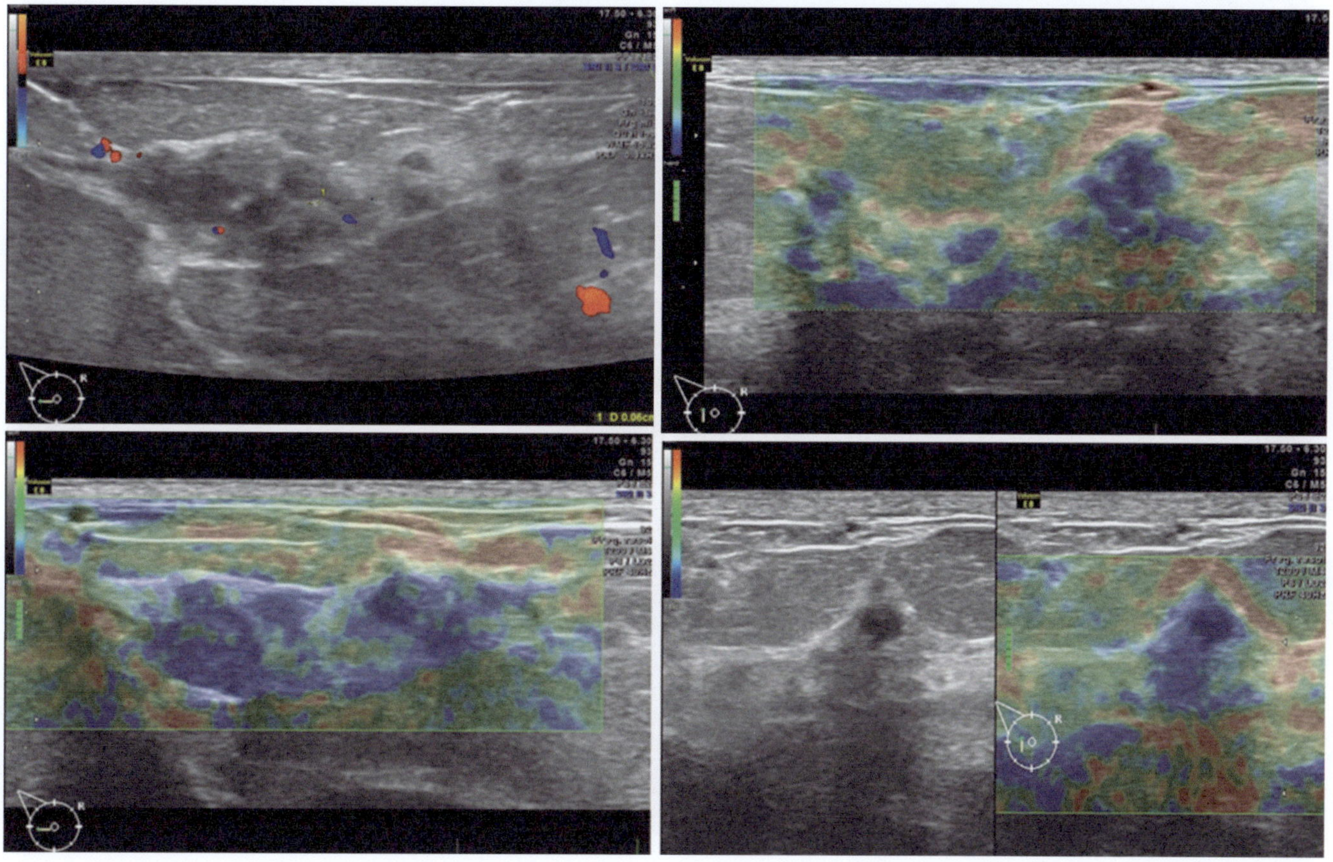

Fig. 8.41 FBU in a 42-year-old patient, after many miscarriages; lobar-type breast cancer, or diffuse, with typical shape of the lobe in the radial scan and with salient multifocal lesions in the anti-radial scans. Sonoelastography is mandatory, with scoring 4 and 5 Ueno, but the new vasculature just moderate. The axillary lymph nodes of benign-type, in the illustration with normal or hypoechoic hilum (*arrows*) and normal cortex, vasculature, and strain, are arguments for large, lobar extension of the malignancy but with reduced distant invasiveness

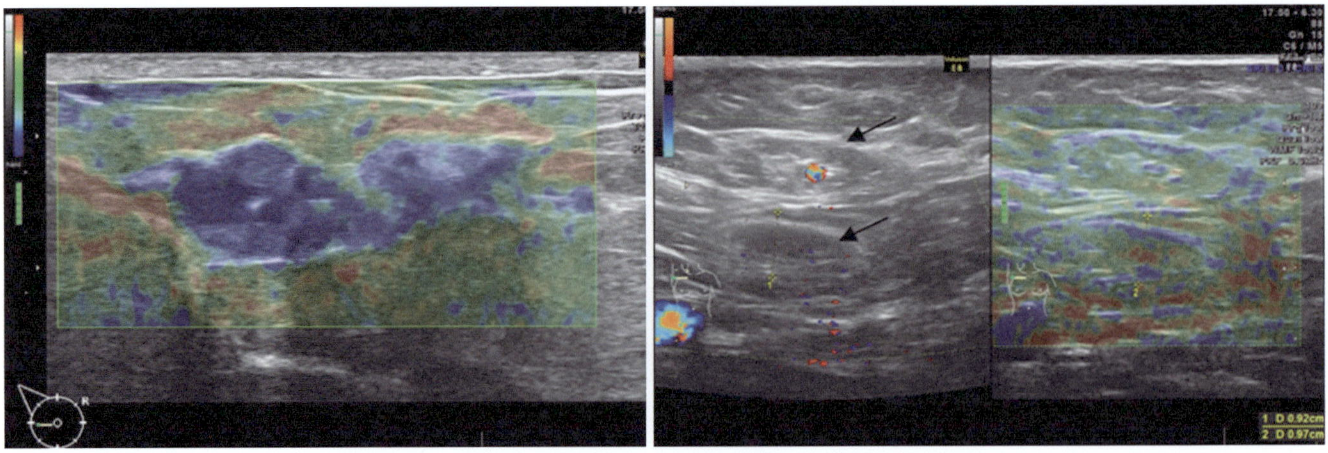

Fig. 8.41 (continued)

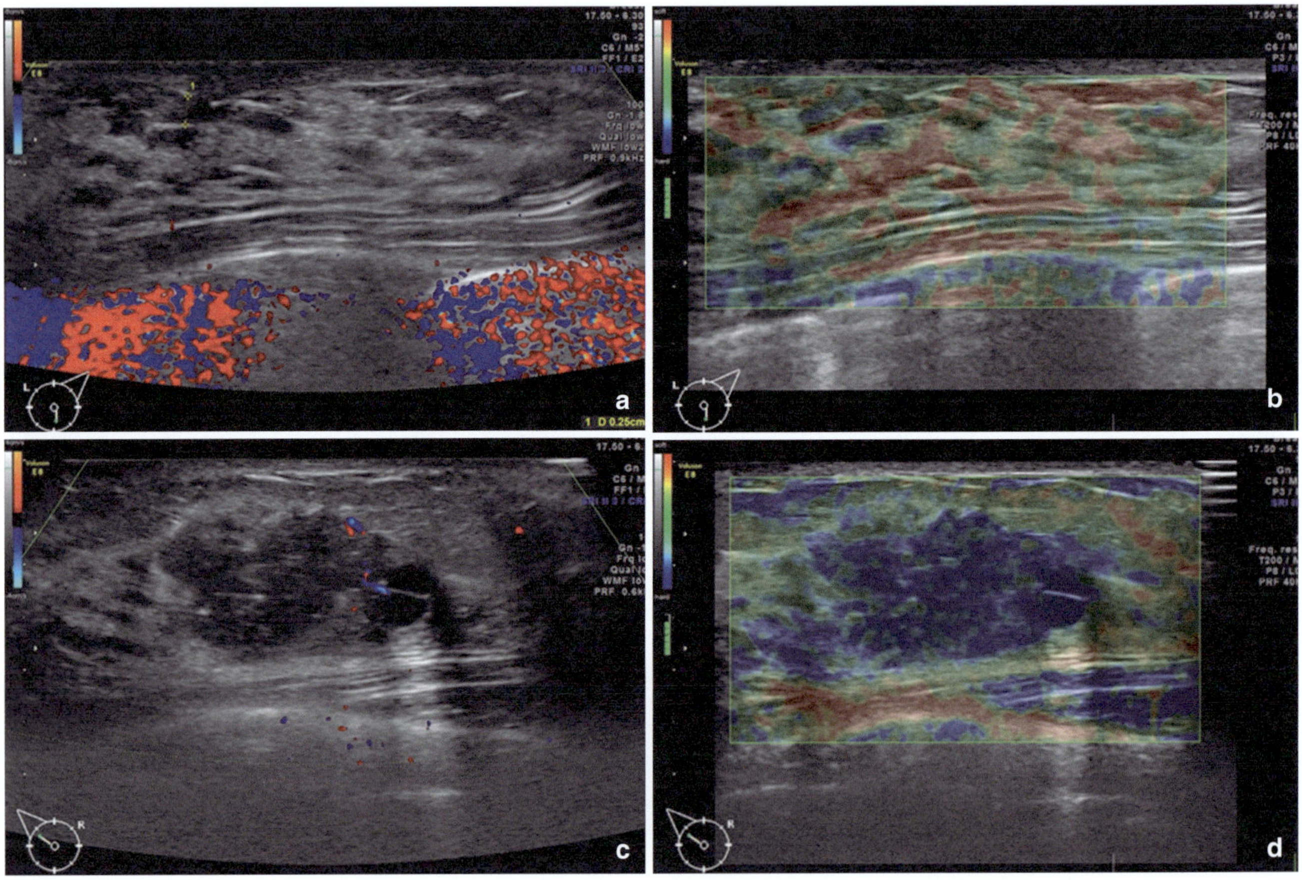

Fig. 8.42 FBU in a 31-year-old patient with dense breasts and "simple dysplasia" with focal ductal-lobular thickening, no abnormal vasculature, and benign-type sonoelastography illustrated at L6:00 (**a**, **b**). Diffuse malignancy with ill-defined palpable mass in the right upper-outer quadrant illustrates the breast parenchyma diffuse thickening with confluence in a mass strictly delimited by the Cooper's ligaments to the glandular volume, without extension to the fatty tissue. The pathological mass demonstrates salient new formation vasculature (**c**), increased stiffness with type 4 Ueno sonoelastogram both in the radial and antiradial scans (**d–f**). Note the abnormal score 4 Ueno of the cystic component (**d**), unusual in the nodular fibro-micro-cystic dysplasia. The malignancy is spreading ductally to the surrounding parenchyma, probably to the neighboring mammary lobes, such as demonstrated in the antiradial view (**f**)

Fig. 8.42 (continued)

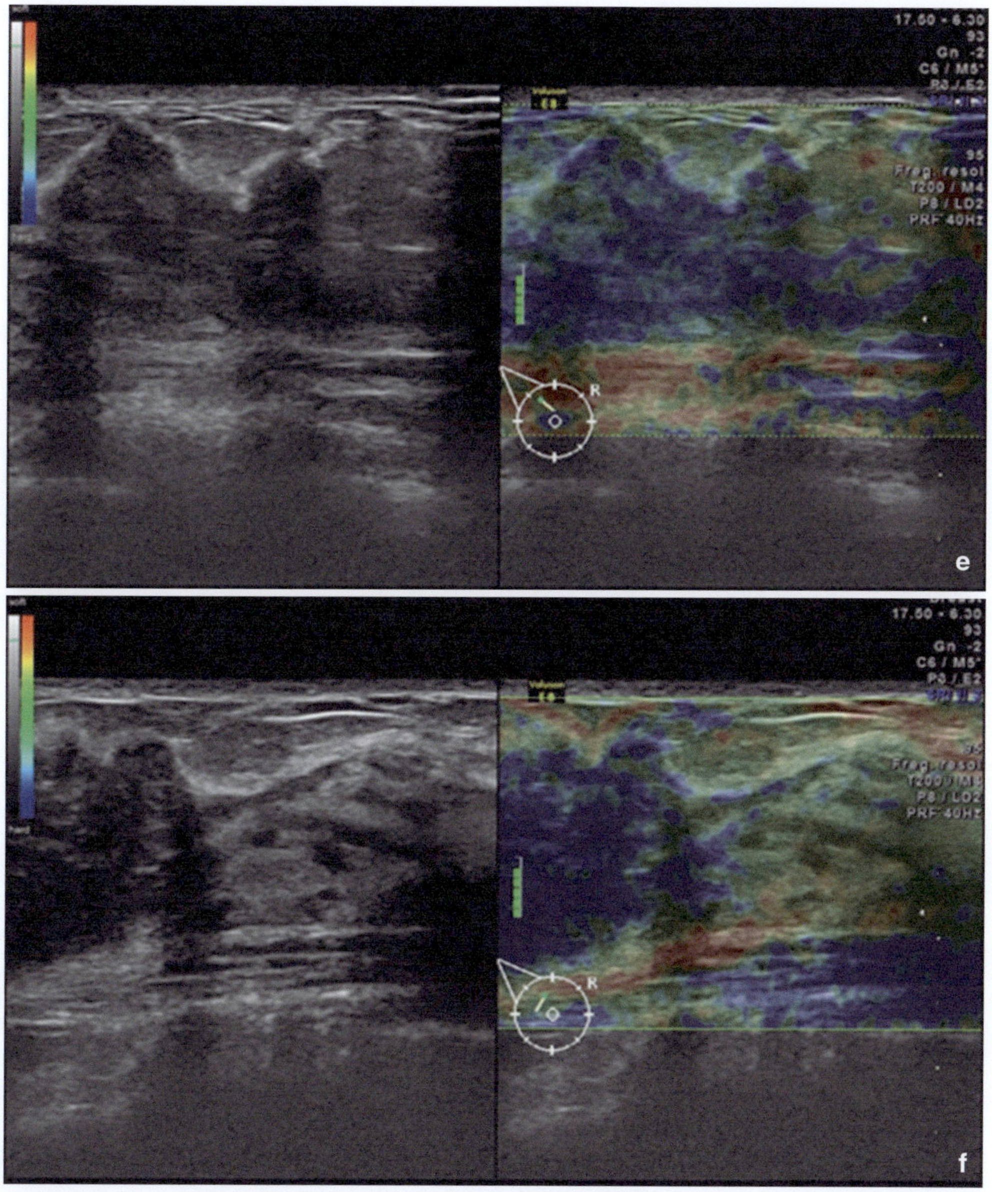

Fig. 8.43 Retroareolar malignancy; the mass has benign posterior effects after Kobayashi, but the new formation vasculature is significant; note the ductal-lobular segmental-associated hyperplasias

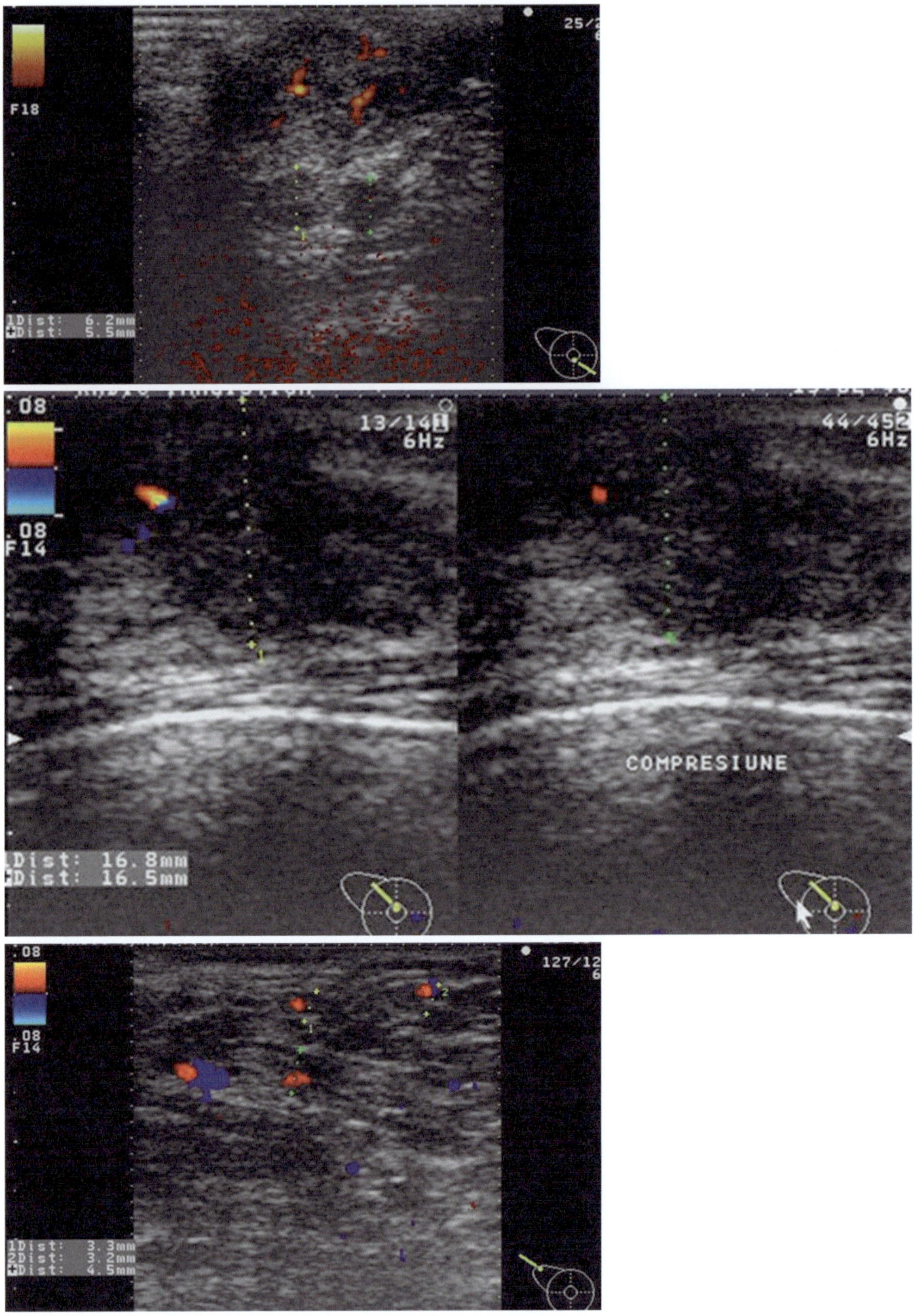

Fig. 8.43 (continued)

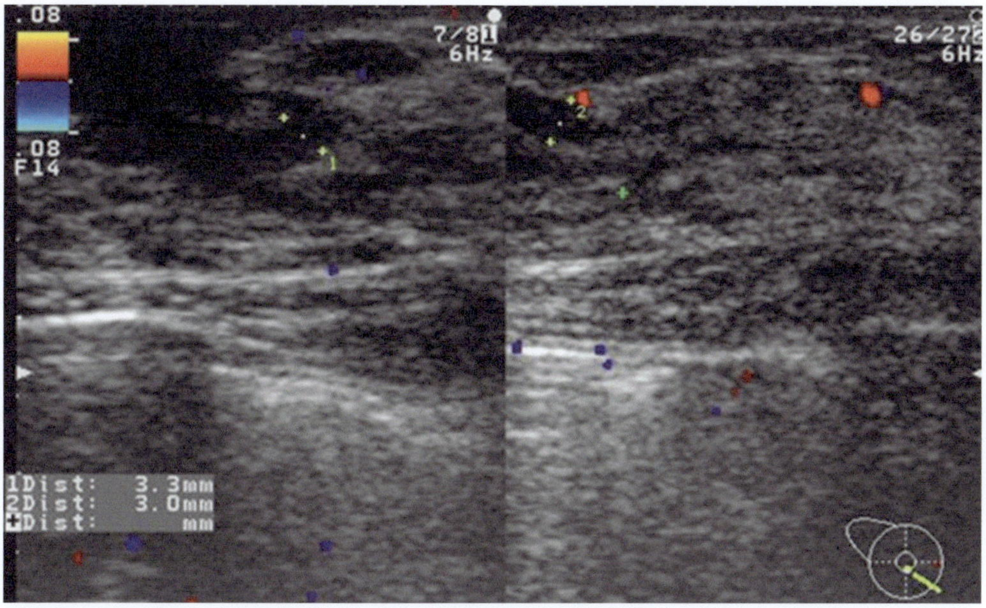

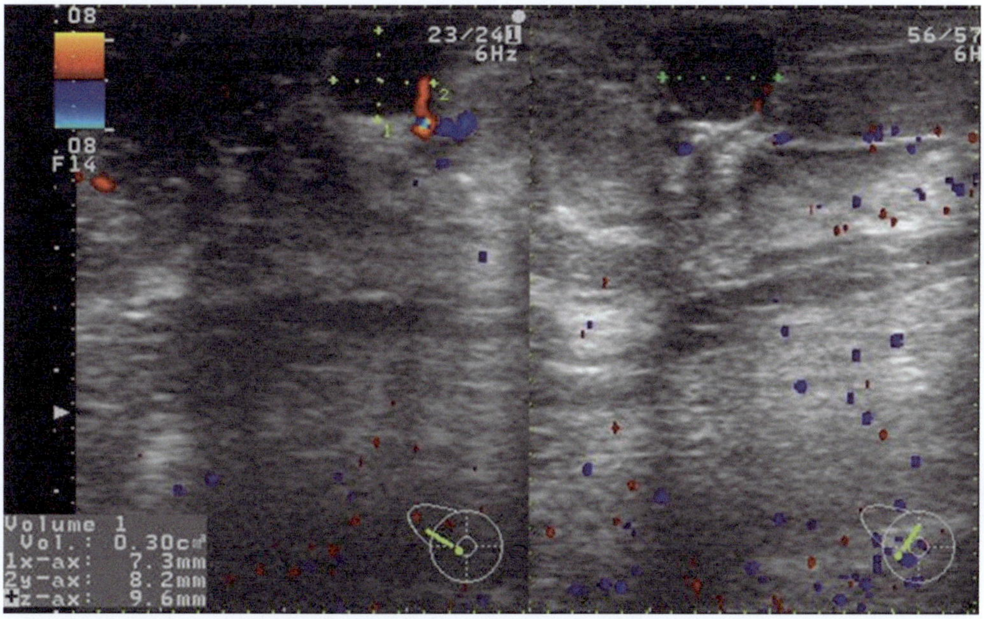

Fig. 8.44 Paget's disease with a retroareolar lesion less than 10 mm, suspect due its salient vasculature and its close relation with the nipple

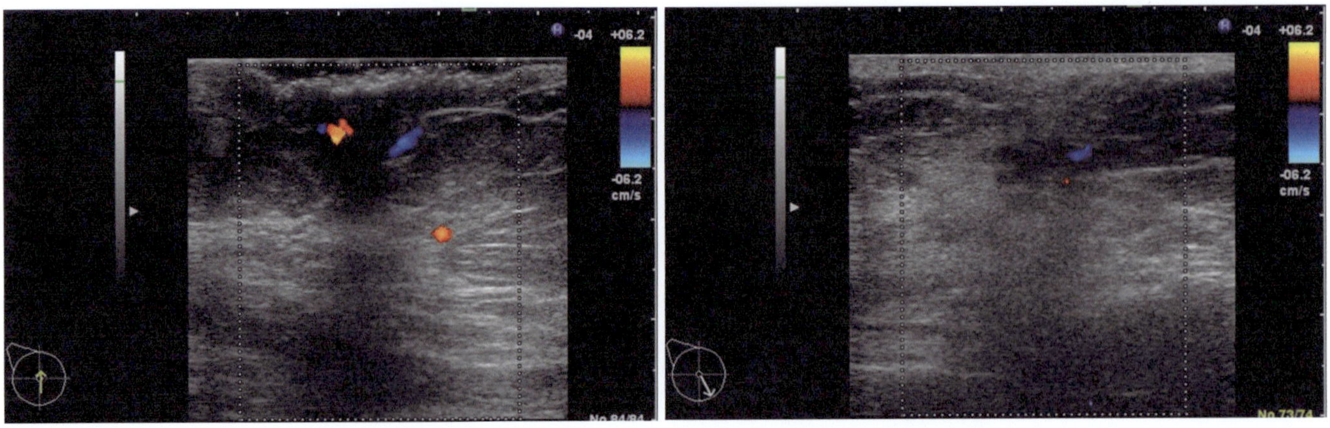

Fig. 8.45 Paget's disease with nipple and areola presenting a hypoechoic thickened aspect and salient vasculature (*upper image*); peripheral L5:00 infracentimetric mass with malignant descriptors: spiculated, with hallo, hypoechoic, acoustic shadowing, incident plunging artery (*below*)

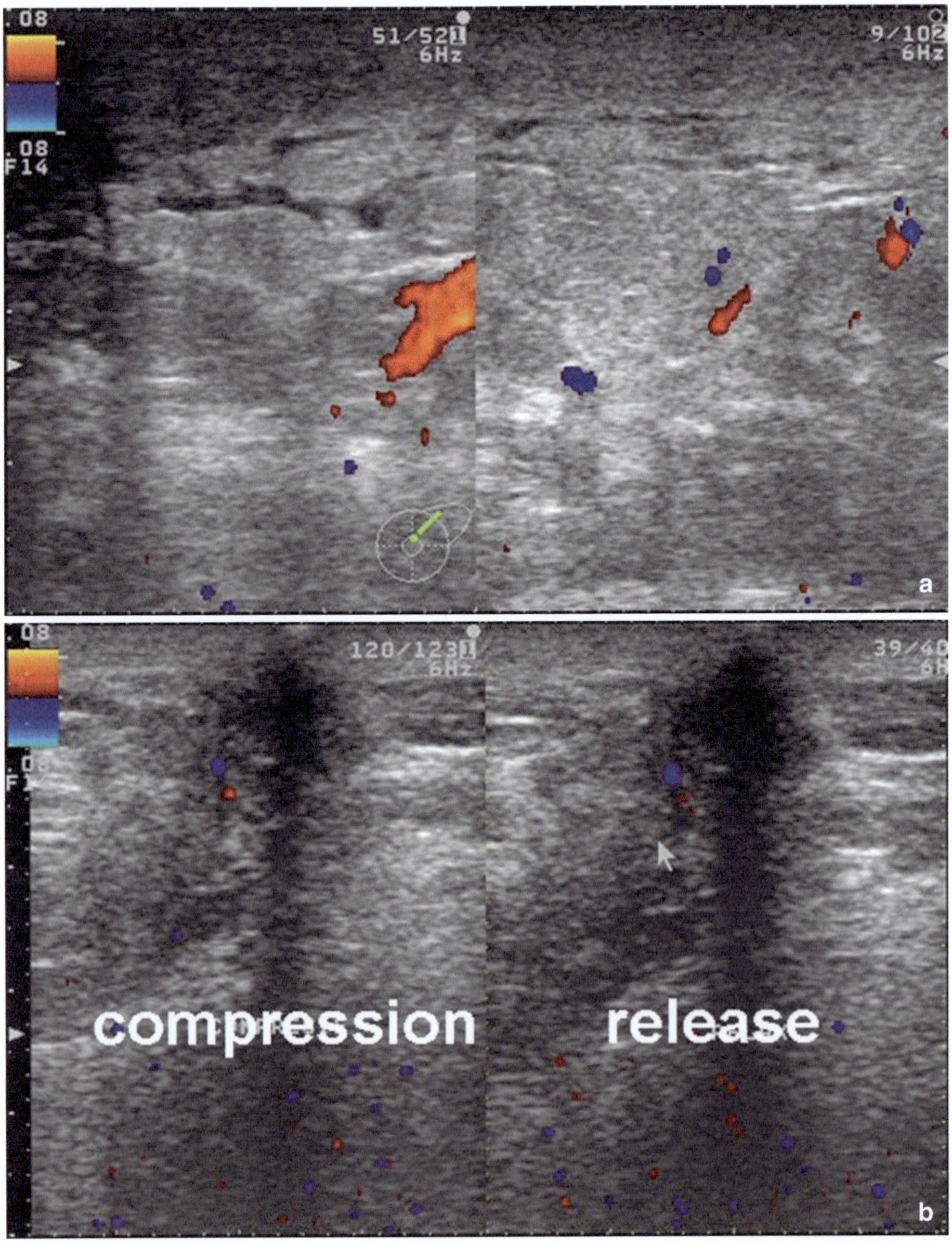

Fig. 8.46 Patient is 46 years old with left breast carcinomatous mastitis, dense breast in mammography without focal abnormality. Doppler DE illustrates lymphedema with superficial lymphatic spaces (**a**), increased vasculature in the glandular areas and a centimetric mass at L5:00, with malignant features after Stavros (**b**, **c**). In the absence of sonoelastography, a direct compression with the transducer may demonstrate low elasticity with persistent acoustic shadowing and no/small change in the vasculature. For ultrasound machines without a long linear probe, the double-screen option may help to realize a composed radial scan, suggestive of the anatomic relation between lesion and nipple (**c**)

Fig. 8.46 (continued)

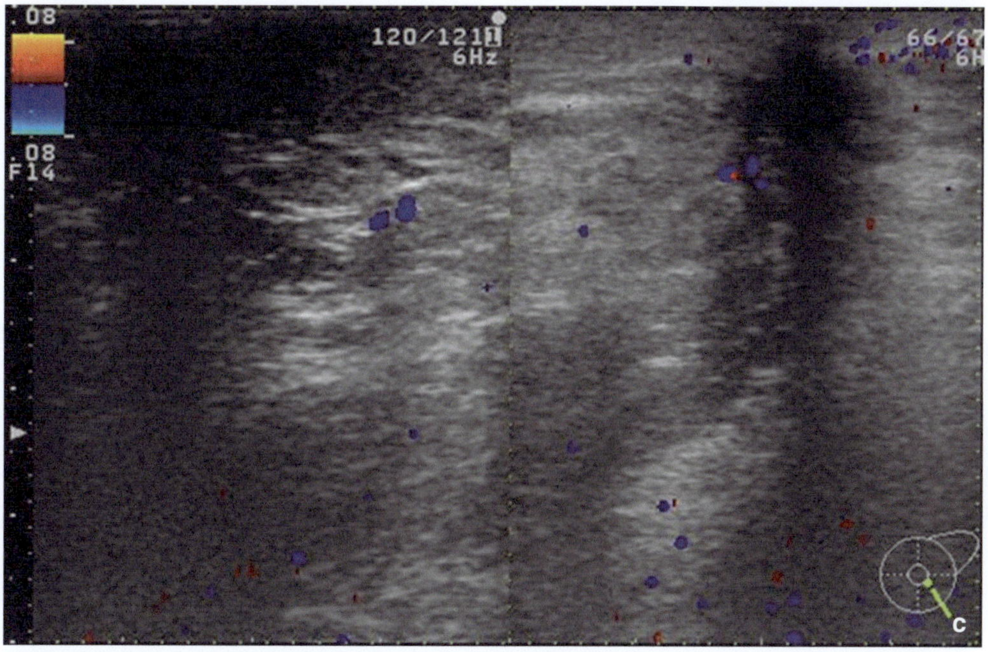

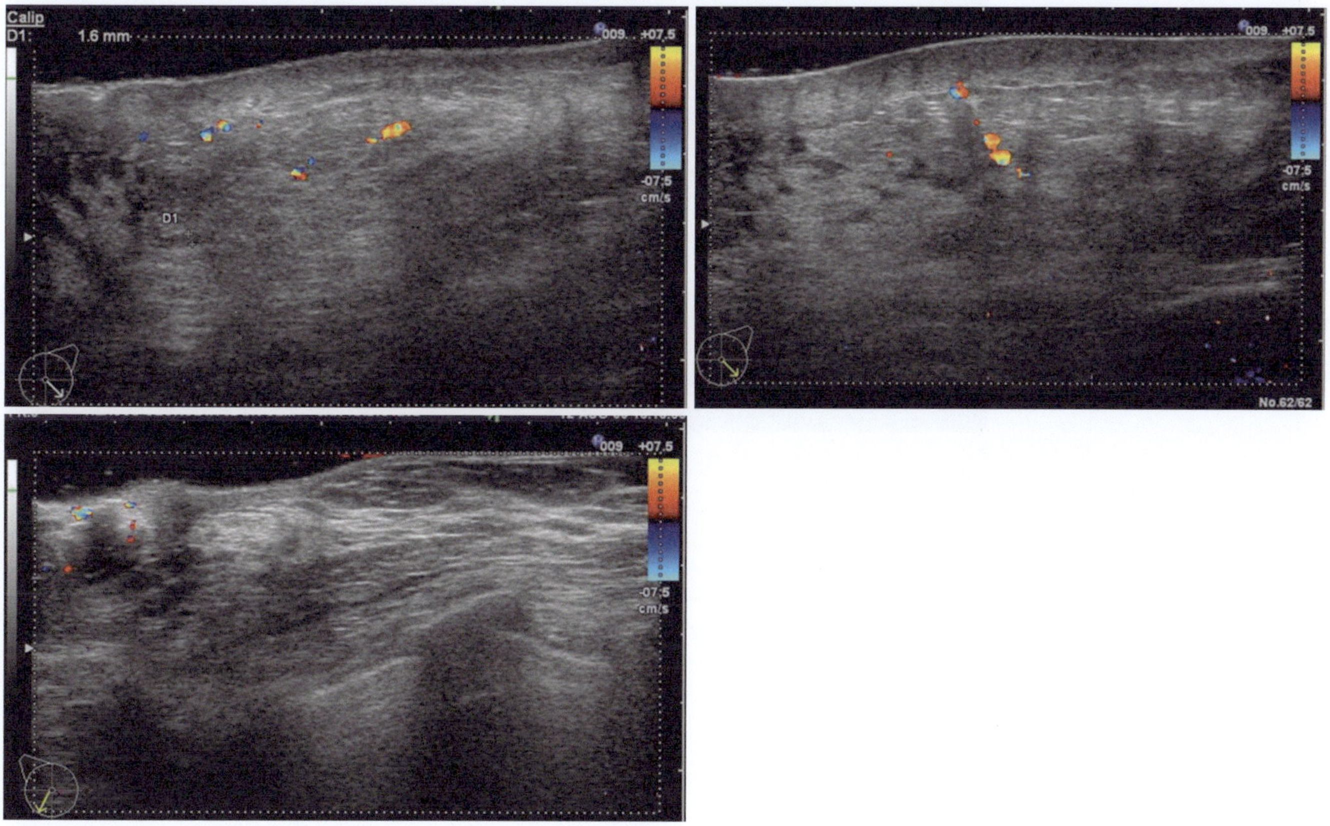

Fig. 8.47 Patient is 62 years old with left breast suspect carcinomatous mastitis, with skin thickening, loss of parenchymal differentiation, deep glandular hypoechogeneicity, and diffuse hyperemia. Comparative slices with the contralateral breast at the same radius scanning

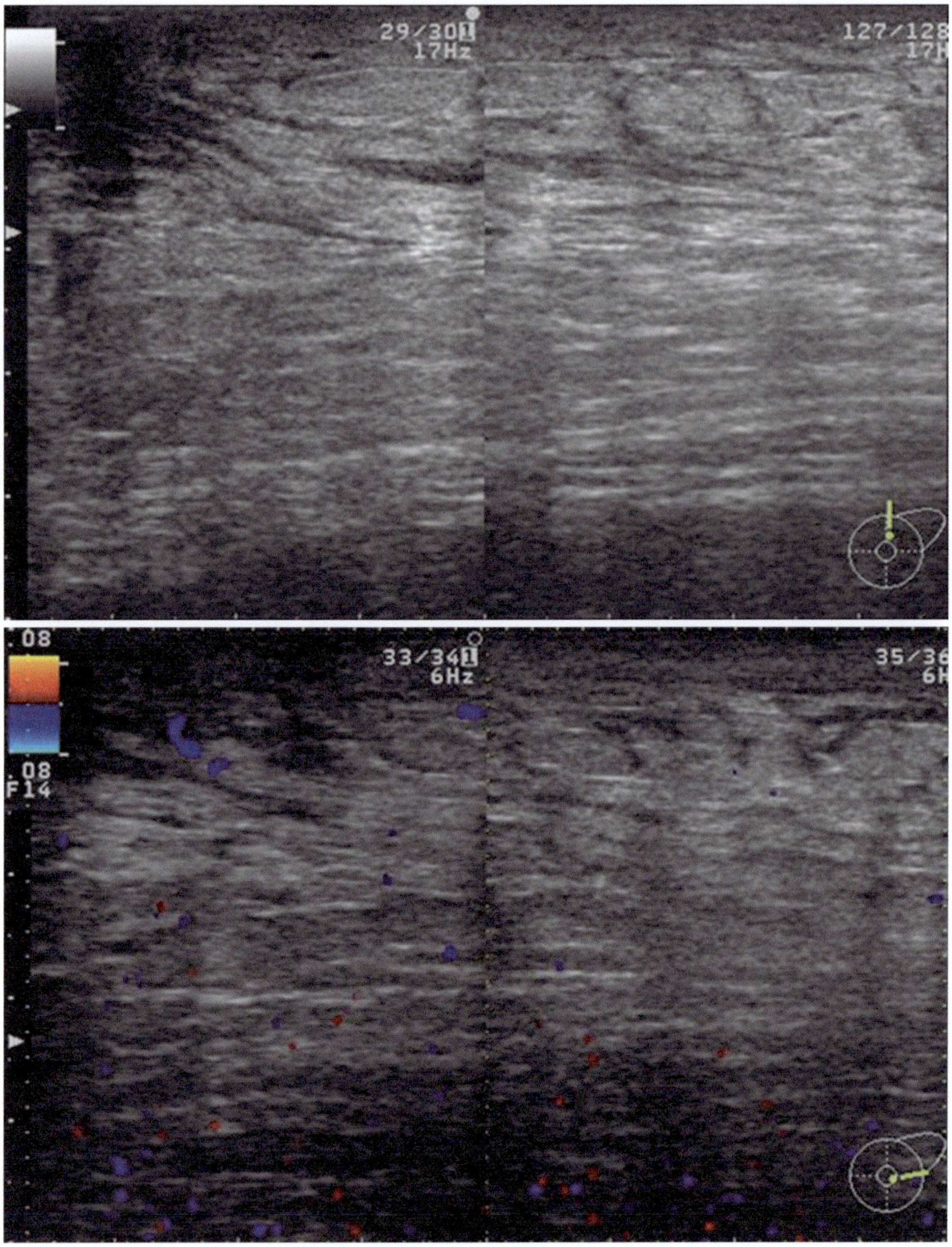

Fig. 8.48 Patient is 72 years old: left breast edema with normal vasculature of a patient with right shoulder fracture and cardiac insufficiency with bradycardia, arrhythmia, and pericardial effusion. No breast etiology was found for the breast edema, considered as secondary to the cardiac failure and the selective dorsal and left decubitus

Fig. 8.48 (continued)

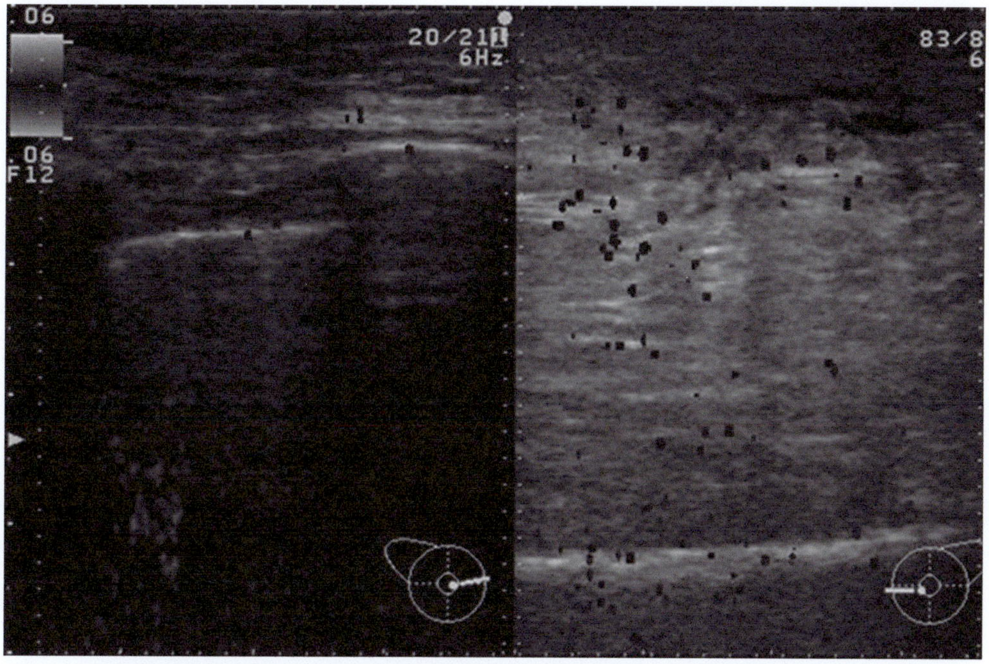

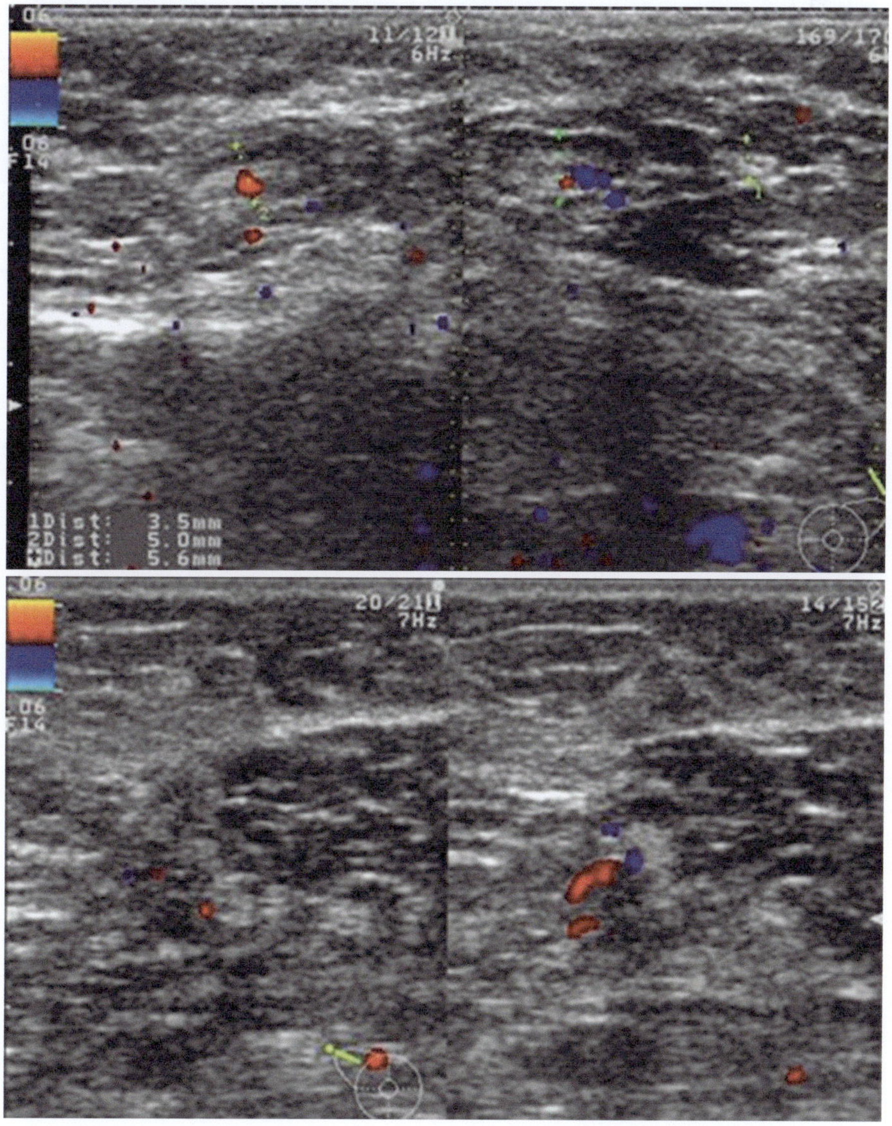

Fig. 8.49 Normal shapes of axillary lymph nodes. Their recognition is easier when using color Doppler acquisition, otherwise they are difficult to differentiate from the surrounding fatty tissue

Fig. 8.49 (continued)

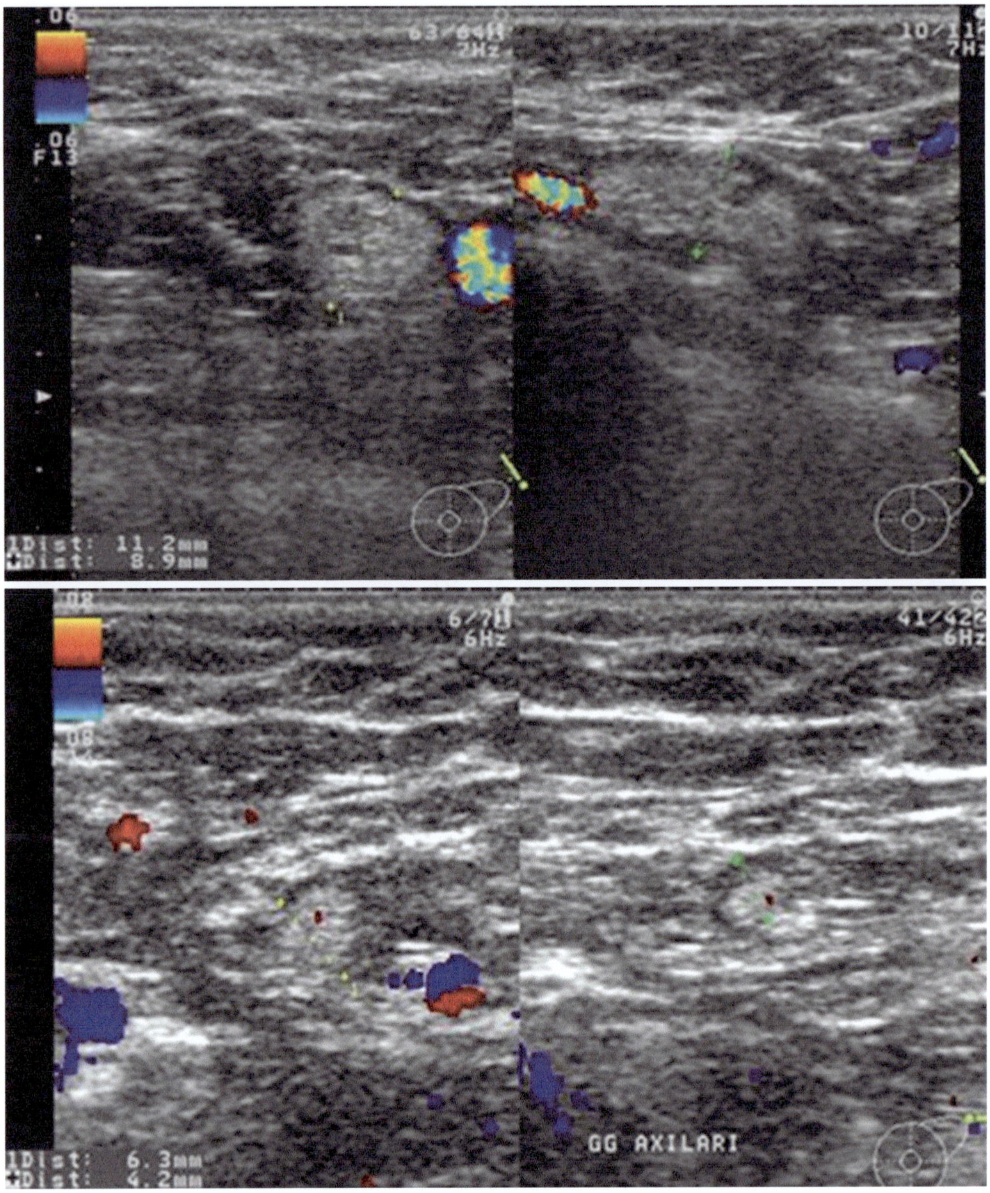

Fig. 8.50 Orthogonal slices of different axillary lymph nodes presenting ovoid shape, thin cortical zone, and peripheral hyperechoic medullary rim with central hypoechoic heterogeneous area. This aspect is suggestive of chronic inflammation and/or possible benign histiocytosis. The vascular aspect is of the benign type, with relative few and thin vessels arising from the hilum

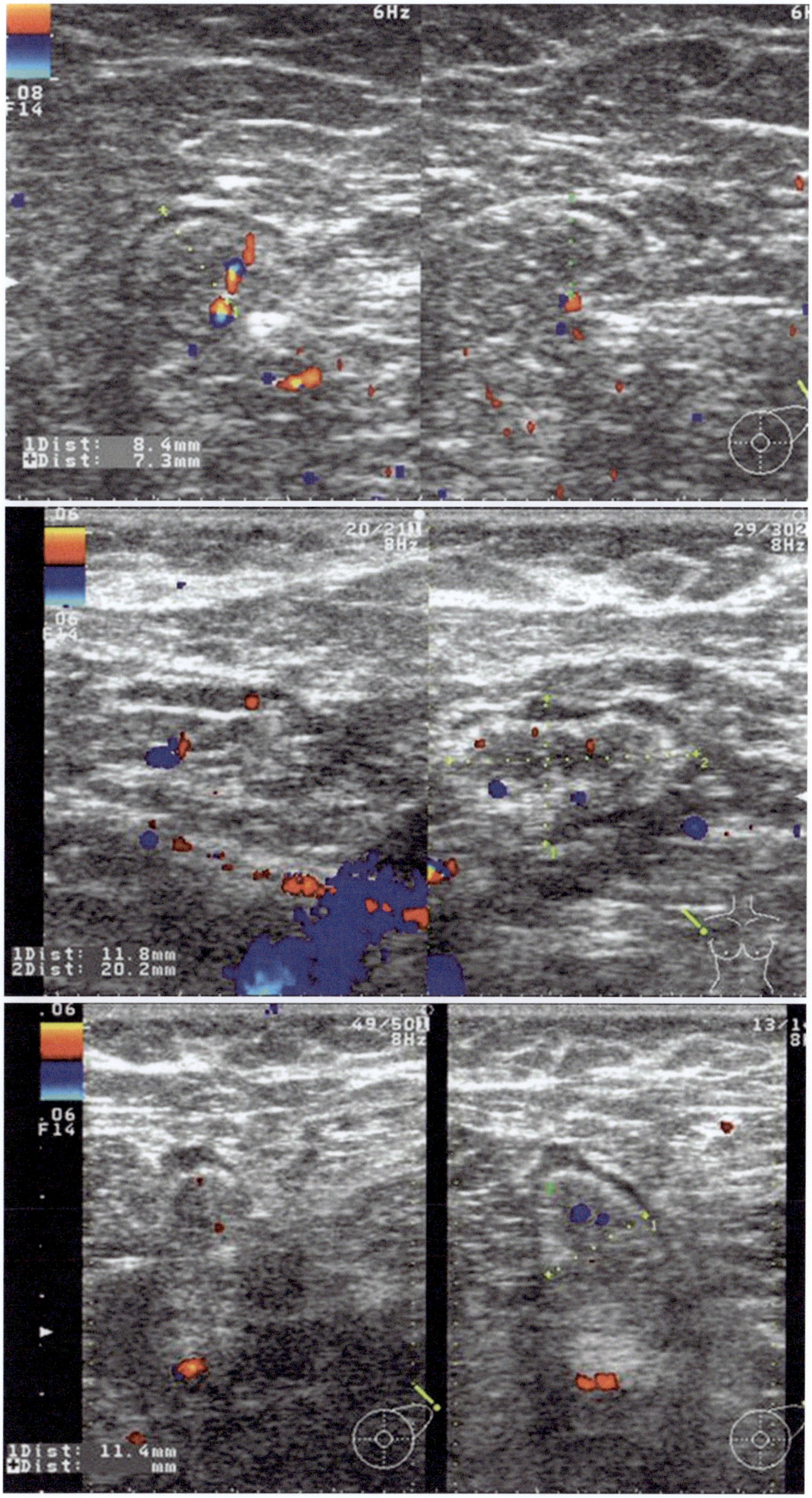

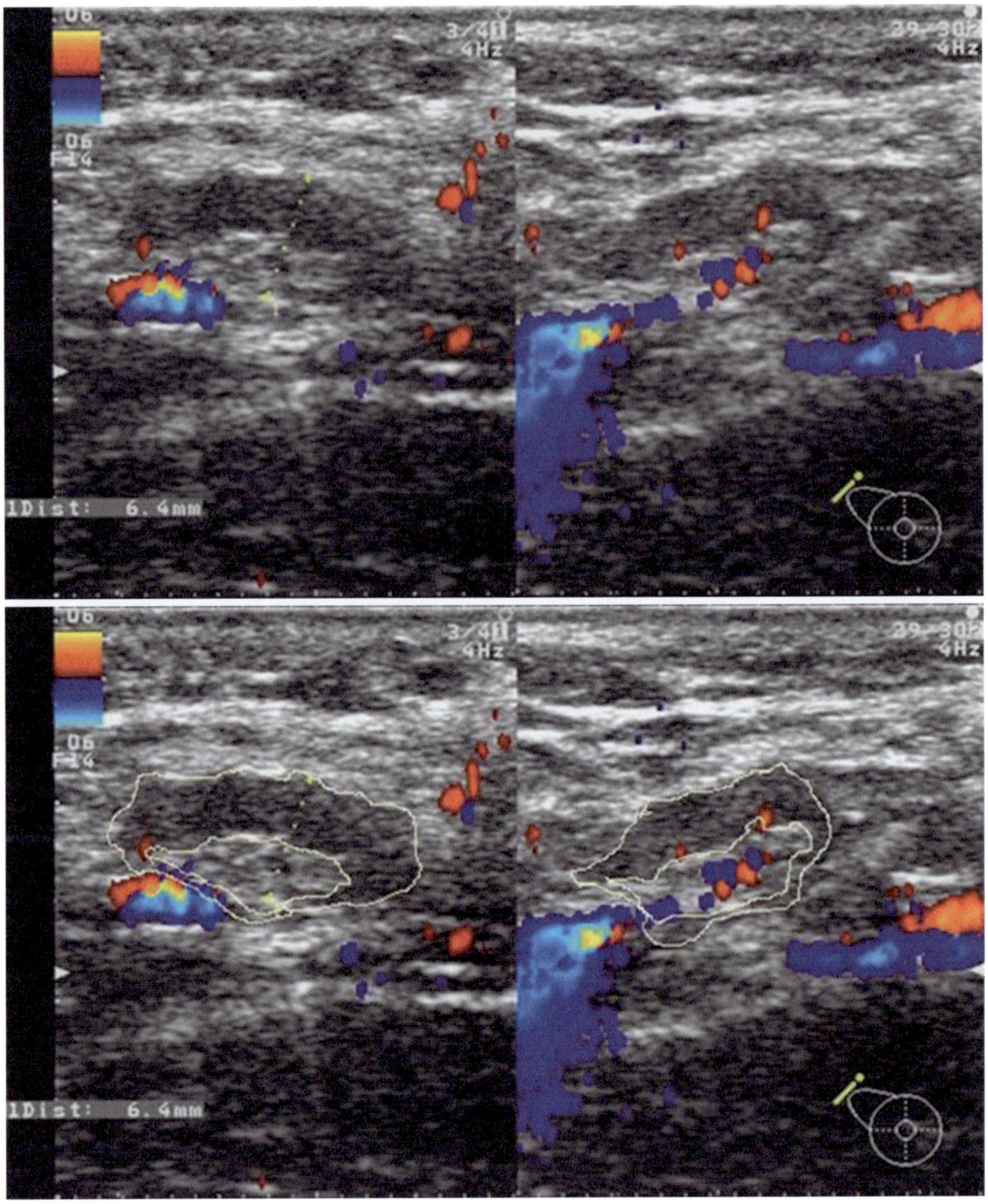

Fig. 8.51 Axillary enlarged lymph nodes with thickening of the cortex and moderate vasculature. This aspect is at least suspect and the biopsy is recommended

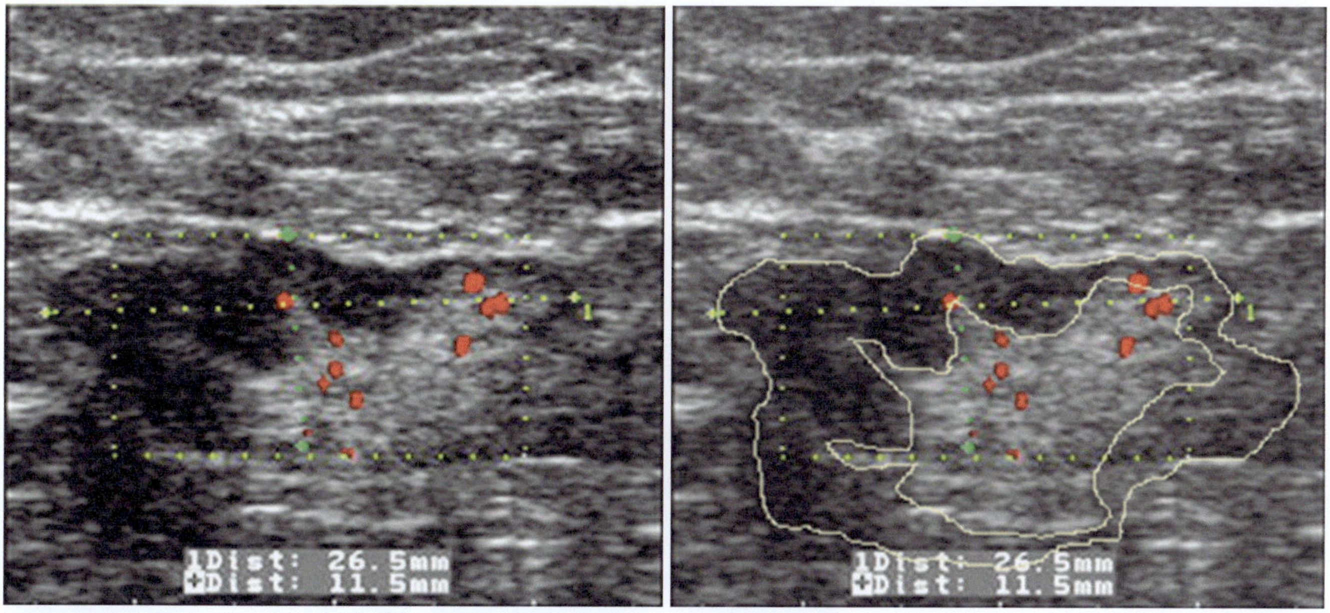

Fig. 8.52 Enlarged axillary lymph node with eccentrically thickened cortical region, more hypoechoic and moderately increased vasculature in power Doppler, in a patient with ultrasound BI-RADS category 4 breast lesion. This aspect, highly suspect for sentinel node, was confirmed by surgical biopsy

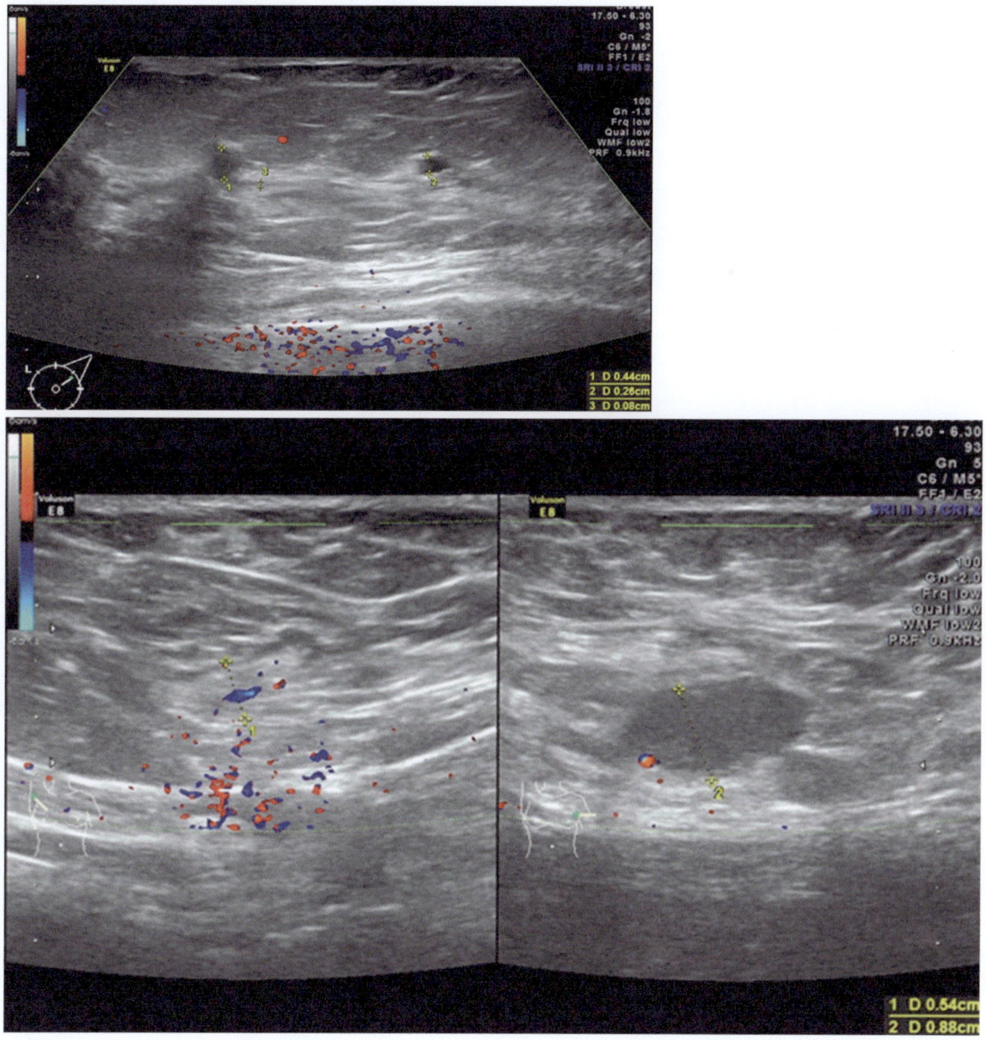

Fig. 8.53 Thirty-seven-year-old patient presents left enlargement of the axillary lymph nodes as compared with the opposite axilla, with cortical thickening and necrotic aspect with less vasculature in Doppler and BGR (Blue-Green-Red) score. The breast ultrasound detected only pseudonodular fibro-micro-cystic lesions in the upper-outer quadrant. Despite a possible etiology outside the breast area, the ultrasound BI-RADS assessment category 0 is mandatory

Fig. 8.53 (continued)

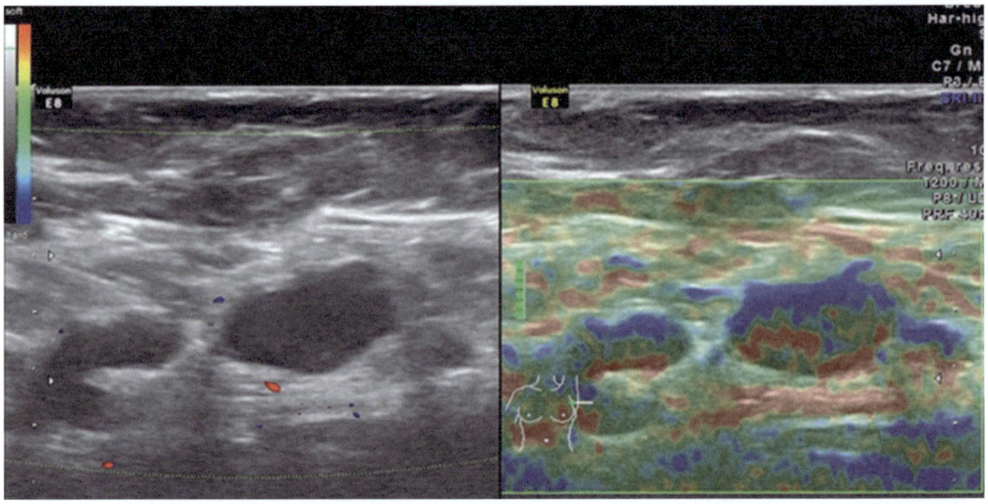

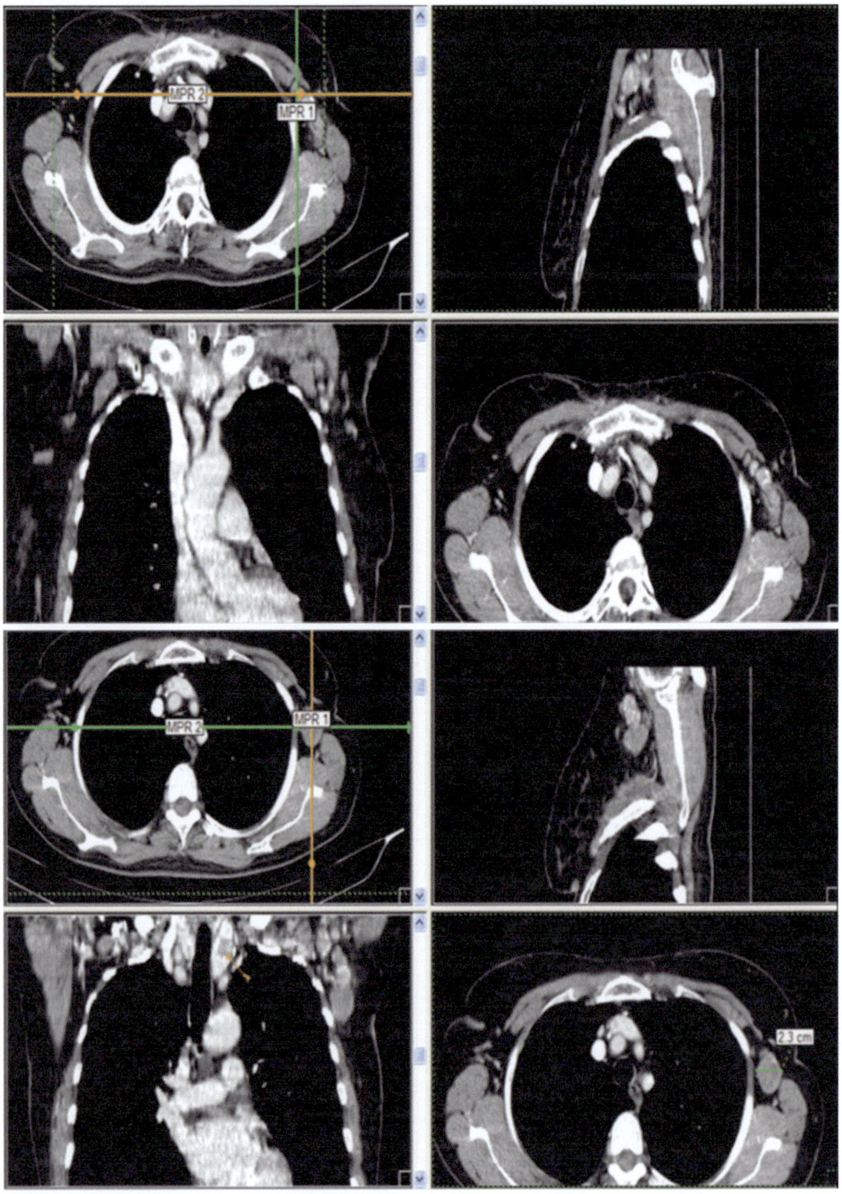

Fig. 8.54 The same case as in Figs. 8.4, 8.5, and 8.6 (Chap. 7): contrast multidetector CT illustrates left axillary adenopathy with and without calcifications in a patient with breast cancer. The MR (Multiplanar Reconstruction) illustrates the extent of the pathological lymph nodes under the lateral margin of the great pectoral muscle

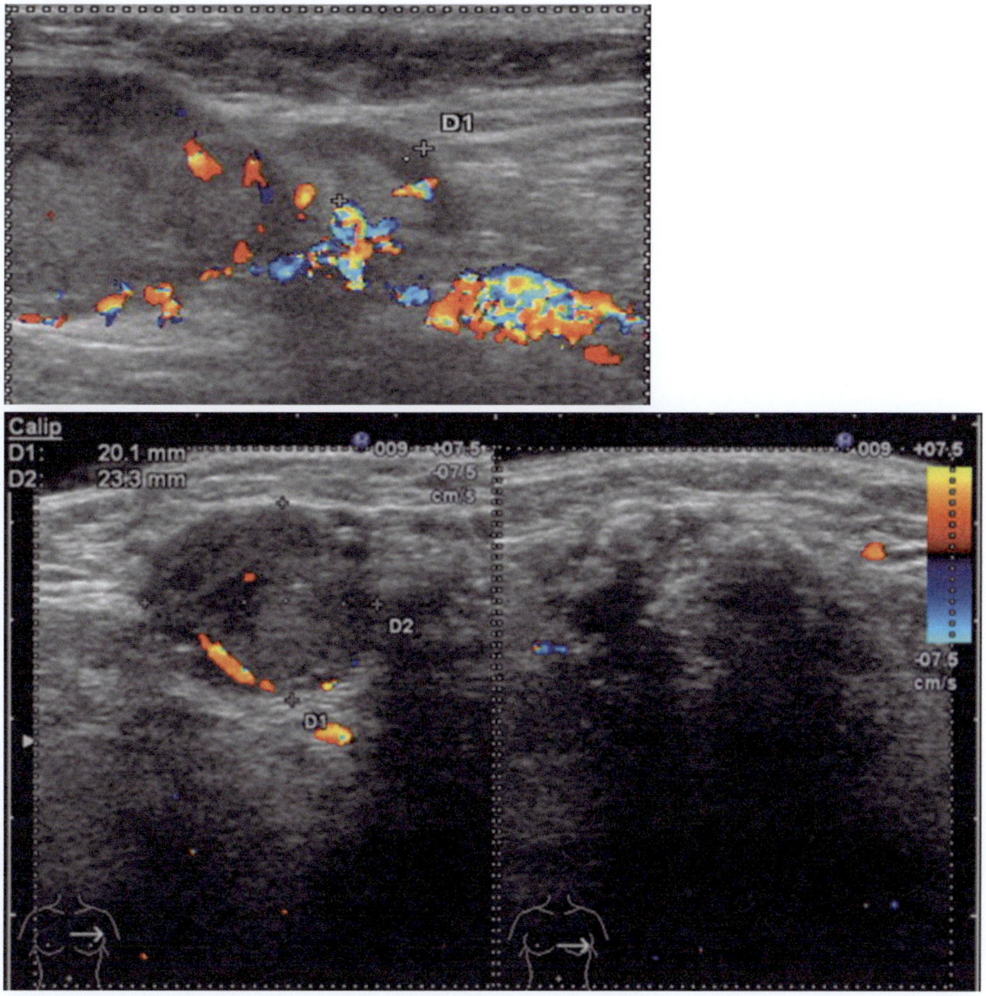

Fig. 8.55 The same case as in Fig. 8.54: Doppler ultrasound illustrates with better resolution and without contrast agent injection the left axillary adenopathy, with huge lymph node with structural changes and peripheral new formation vasculature near an almost normal node (*upper*); other pathological smaller nodes have various amount of microcalcifications (*below*)

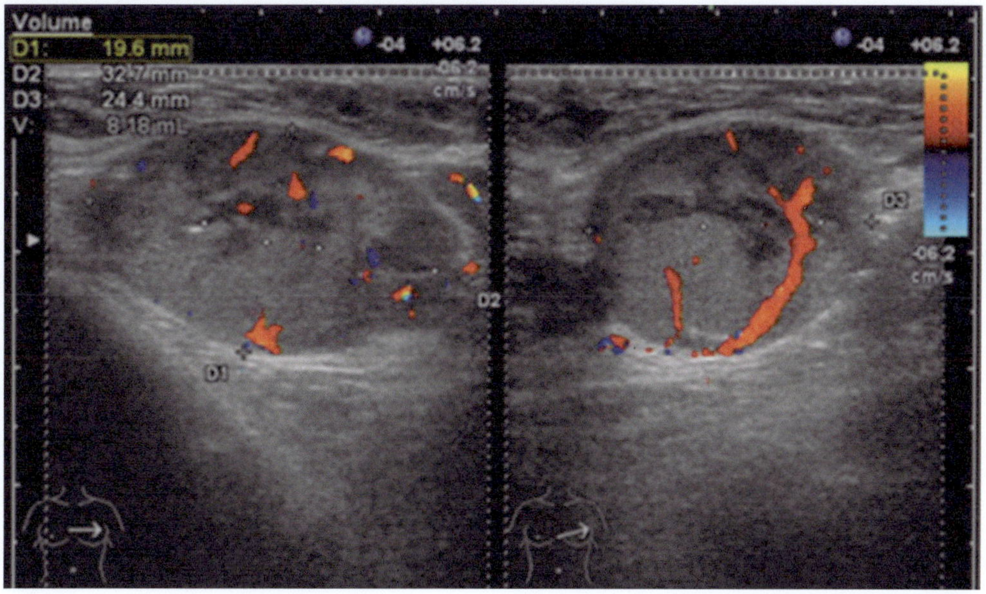

Fig. 8.56 The same case as in Figs. 8.54 and 8.55: FBU illustrates left axillary adenopathy, with and without calcifications. The main findings suggestive of malignancy are the new formation vasculature and increased strain. The sensibility and specificity are better than in classical ultrasound, but the limited field of view is inconvenient compared with computed tomography or MRI

Fig. 8.56 (continued)

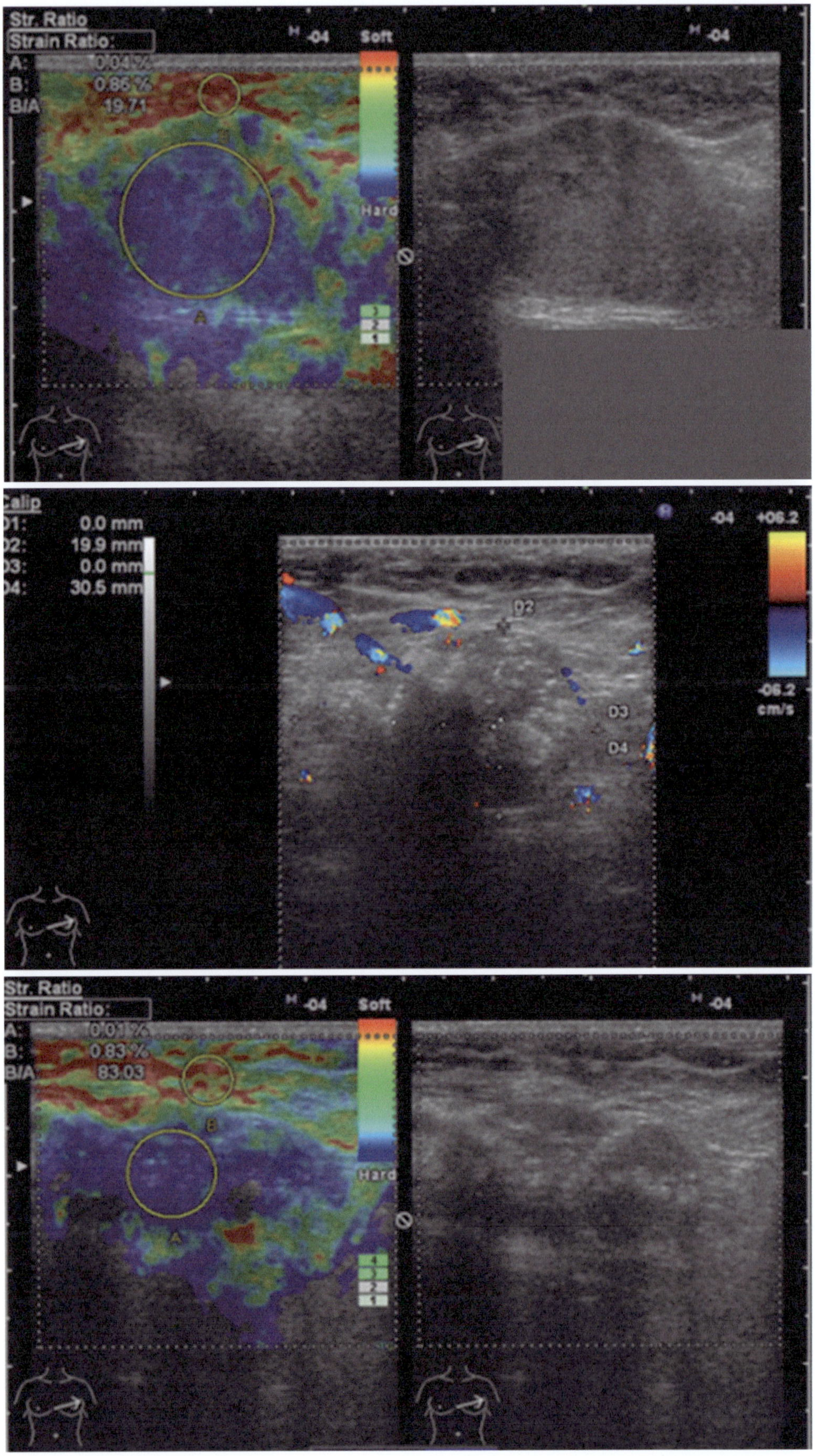

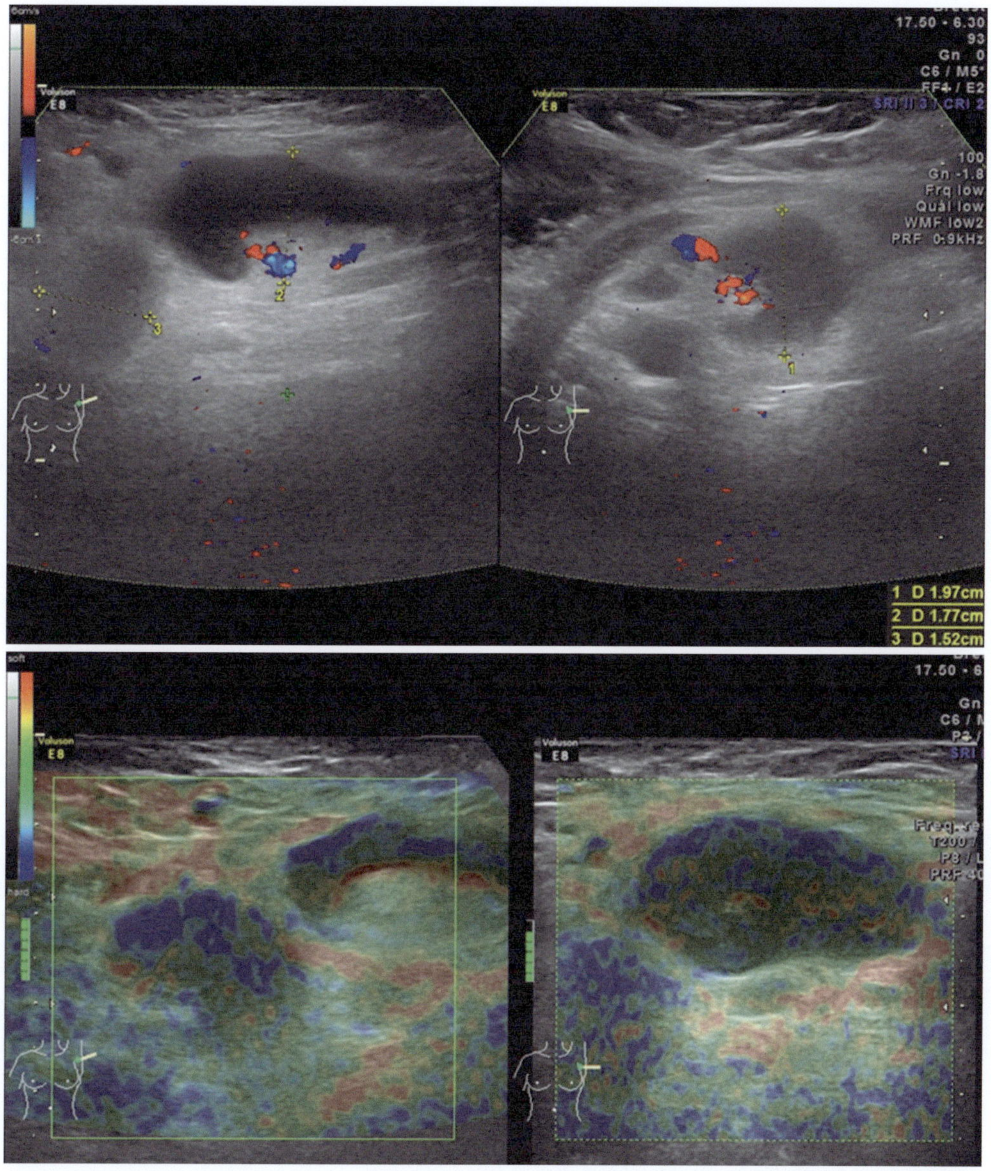

Fig. 8.57 Axillary adenopathy with increased transverse diameter and thickening of the cortical regions but normal vasculature in hilum. The BGR score, significant for either lymph nodes edema or necrosis, cannot eliminate the risk of malignancy, especially in qualitative SE. In this case, quantitative SE with FLR would be useful, but it is not yet implemented by all manufacturers

References

1. Tot T (2007) The theory of the sick breast lobe and the possible consequences. Int J Surg Pathol 1:68–71
2. Georgescu AC, Andrei EM, Enachescu V, Bondari S (2013) New horizons in breast Doppler ductal echography: the positive and differential diagnosis of ductal ectasia, with etiopathological correlations. ECR, Vienna, EPOS™. doi:10.1594/ecr2013/C-0667
3. Grio R, Cellura A, Germao R et al (1998) Clinical efficacy of tamoxifen in the treatment of premenstrual mastodynia. Minerva Ginecol 50(3):101–103
4. Fujimoto Y, Hatama M, Tezuka K, Otani H et al (2005) Ultrasonic screening of the thyroid in the patients with breast complaints. In: Research and development in breast ultrasound. Springer, Tokyo, pp 167–169
5. Fujimoto Y, Kato Y, Maekawa H et al (1988) Ultrasonic screening of thyroid in the patients with breast complaints. J Ultrasound Med 7:39–S283
6. Georgescu AC, Andrei ME, Manda A, Bondari S, Sendroiu I (2015) Contributions of imaging examinations in the diagnosis of the von Recklinghausen disease. ECR, Vienna, EPOS™. doi:10.1594/ecr2015/C-1014
7. Szymanowski K, Niepsuj-Biniaś J, Dera-Szymanowska A et al (2013) An influence of immunomodulation on Th1 and Th2 immune response in endometriosis in an animal model. Biomed Res Int 2013, Article ID 849492:7. doi:10.1155/2013/849492
8. Szymanowski K, Chmaj-Wierzchowska K, Yantczenko A et al (2009) Endometriosis prophylaxis and treatment with the newly developed xenogenic immunomodulator RESAN in an animal model. Eur J Obstet Gynecol Reprod Biol 142(2):145–148
9. Foschini MP, Baldovini C, Ishikawa Y, Eusebi V (2012) The value of large sections in surgical pathology. Int J Breast Cancer 2012, Article ID 785947:7. doi:10.1155/2012/785947
10. Cheatle GL (1906) Early recognition of cancer of the breast. Br Med J 1:1205–1210
11. Cheatle GL (1914) The relation between ducts and acini to cysts and cancer of the breast. J R Soc Med 7:241–244
12. Wellings SR, Jensen HM (1973) On the origin and progression of ductal carcinoma in the human breast. J Natl Cancer Inst 50(5):1111–1116
13. Foschini MP, Flamminio F, Miglio R et al (2007) The impact of large sections on the study of in situ and invasive duct carcinoma of the breast. Hum Pathol 38(12):1736–1743
14. Tot T (2010) Cost-benefit analysis of using large-format histology sections in routine diagnostic breast care. Breast 19(4):284–288
15. Tot T (2007) Clinical relevance of the distribution of the lesions in 500 consecutive breast cancer cases documented in large–format histologic sections. Cancer 110:2551–2560
16. Egan RL (1982) Multicentric breast carcinomas: clinical-radiographic-pathologic whole organ studies and 10-year survival. Cancer 49(6):1123–1130
17. Tot T, Gere M, Pekár G et al (2011) Breast cancer multifocality, disease extent, and survival. Hum Pathol 42(11):1761–1769
18. Martin JE (1988) Atlas of mammography. Histologic and mammographic correlations, 2nd edn. Williams & Wilkins, Baltimore, pp 69–268
19. Gallager HS, Martin JE (1969) The study of breast carcinoma by correlated mammography and subserial whole organ sectioning. Early observations. Cancer 23:855–873
20. Gallager HS, Martin JE (1969) Early phases in the development of breast cancer. Cancer 24:1170–1178
21. Teboul M (2010) Advantages of ductal echography (DE) over conventional breast investigation in the diagnosis of breast malignancies. Med Ultrason 12(1):32–42
22. Baldovini C, Foschini MP (2012) Multifocality of breast cancer. In: Proceedings of the 27th congress of the Adriatic Society of Pathology, June 2012
23. Cooper AP (1840) On the anatomy of the breast. London, Longman, Orme, Green, Brown, and Longmans. (special collections, Scott Memorial Library, Thomas Jefferson University, http://jdc.jefferson.edu/cooper/)
24. Sobin LH, Gospodarowicz MK, Wittekind C (eds) (2009) TNM classification of malignant tumors. 7th edn. Wiley Blackwell
25. Saslow D, Solomon D, Lawson H et al (2012) American Cancer Society, American Society for Colposcopy and Cervical Pathology, and American Society for Clinical Pathology screening guidelines for the prevention and early detection of cervical cancer. CA Cancer J Clin 62(30):147–172, Epub, Mar 14
26. American Cancer Society Guidelines for the Early Detection of Cancer (2014) www.cancer.org
27. Amy D (2010) Lobar Ultrasound of the Breast. In: Breast Cancer, 1.T. Tot (ed). © Springer-Verlag London Limited. doi:10.1007/978-1-84996-314-5_8
28. Amy D (2003) Sub-centimetric breast carcinoma. Echographic diagnosis. 13th International congress on the ultrasonic examination of the breast. International Breast Ultrasound School. The 10th meeting of Japan Association of Breast and Thyroid Sonology
29. Stavros AT, Rapp LC, Parker HS (2004) Breast ultrasound. Lippincott Williams & Wilkins, Philadelphia
30. Mendelson EB, Baum JK, Berg WA et al (2003) Breast imaging reporting and data system BI-RADS: ultrasound, 1st edn. American College of Radiology, Reston
31. JSUM guidelines for mass image-forming lesions (2005) In: Ueno E, Shiina M, Kuboto K (eds) Research and development in breast ultrasound. Springer, Tokyo. pp 78–84
32. Japan Society of Ultrasonics in Medicine and JABTS- (Draft) (2003) Diagnostic guideline for mass image forming lesions. 13th International congress on the ultrasonic examination of the breast. International Breast Ultrasound School. The 10th meeting of Japan Association of Breast and Thyroid Sonology
33. Chang R-F, Huang SF, Chen D-R, Moon WK (2003) Detection of spiculation in three-dimensional breast ultrasound. 13th International congress on the ultrasonic examination of the breast. International Breast Ultrasound School. The 10th meeting of Japan Association of Breast and Thyroid Sonology
34. Kujiraoka Y, Ueno E, Yohno E, Morishima I, Tsunoda-Shimizu H (2005) Incident angle of the plunging artery of breast tumors. In: Research and development in breast ultrasound. Springer, Tokyo, pp 72–75
35. LeCarpentier G (2008) 3D Doppler evaluation helps identify malignant breast lesions. Reuters Health. Radiology 249
36. Chou H-I (2003) Evaluation of periductal angiogenesis using contrast-enhanced ultrasound. 13th International congress on the ultrasonic examination of the breast. International Breast Ultrasound School. The 10th meeting of Japan Association of Breast and Thyroid Sonology
37. Ricci P, Cantisani V, Ballesio L et al (2007) Benign and malignant breast lesions: efficacy of real time contrast-enhanced ultrasound vs. magnetic resonance imaging. Ultraschall Med 28(1):57–62, PMID: 17304413 [PubMed – indexed for MEDLINE]
38. Drudi FM, Cantisani V, Gnecchi M (2012) Contrast-enhanced ultrasound examination of the breast: a literature review. Ultraschall Med 33(7):E1–E7. doi:10.1055/s-0031-1299408, Epub 2012 May
39. Watermann DO, Foldi M, Hanjalic-Beck A et al (2005) Three-dimensional ultrasound for the assessment of breast lesions. Ultrasound Obstet Gynecol 25:592–598
40. Vallone P, D'Angelo R, Filice S, Petrosino T, Rinaldo M, De Chiara A, Gallipoloi A (2005) Color-doppler using contrast medium in evaluating the response to neoadjuvant treatment in patients with locally advanced breast carcinoma. Anticancer Res 25:595–599, PubMed
41. Singh S, Pradhan S, Shukla RC, Ansari MA, Kumar A (2005) Color doppler ultrasound as an objective assessment tool for chemotherapeutic response in advanced breast cancer. Breast Cancer 12:45–51

42. Kumar A, Singh S, Pradhan S et al (2007) Doppler ultrasound scoring to predict chemotherapeutic response in advanced breast cancer. World J Surg Oncol 5:99. doi:10.1186/1477-7819-5-99
43. Chung SY, Yang I, Kim D, Shin SJ, Bae SH (2003) Characteristic US findings of inflammatory breast carcinoma: comparison with MR imaging. 13th International congress on the ultrasonic examination of the breast. International Breast Ultrasound School. The 10th meeting of Japan Association of Breast and Thyroid Sonology
44. Lee KW, Chung SY, Yang I, Kim HD et al (2005) Inflammatory breast cancer. Clin Imaging 29(1):22–25. doi:10.1016/j.clinimag.2004.03.006
45. Papotti M, Gugliotta P, Ghiringhello B, Busolati G (1984) Association of breast carcinoma and multiple intraductal papillomas: an histological and immunohistochemical investigation. Histopathology 8(6):963–975
46. Saad RS, Kanbour-Shakir A, Syed A, Kanbour A (2006) Sclerosing papillary lesion of the breast: a diagnosting pitfall for malignancy in fine needle aspiration biopsy. Diagn Cytopathol 34(2):114–118
47. Lefkowitz M, Lefkowitz W, Wargotz ES (1994) Intraductal (intracystic) papillary carcinoma of the breast and its variants: a clinicopathological study of 77 cases. Hum Pathol 25(8):802–809
48. Ueng S-H, Mezzetti T, Tavassoli AF (2009) Papillary neoplasms of the breast: a review. Arch Pathol Lab Med 133(6):893–907
49. Svane G (2005) Ductal Carcinoma in Situ (DCIS): incidence, prognosis, and diagnostic aspects on mammography, galactography, and needle biopsies. In: Research and development in breast ultrasound. Springer, Tokyo, pp 114–118
50. Takebe K, Izumori A (2005) The ultrasonographic diagnosis of nonpalpable DCIS without calcification on mammography and nipple discharge: advocacy of a new term, 3 non-DCIS. In: Research and development in breast ultrasound. Springer, Tokyo, pp 119–126
51. Tanaka K, Sakuma H, Sakamoto G et al (2005) Characteristic mammography and ultrasonography findings of ductal carcinoma in situ of the breast arising in sclerosing adenosis. In: Research and development in breast ultrasound. Springer, Tokyo, pp 135–140
52. Silverstein MJ, Recht A, Lagios M (eds) (2002) Ductal carcinoma in situ of the breast, 2nd edn. Silverstein/Lippincott Williams & Wilkins, Philadelphia
53. Kim EK, Oh KK, Shin HC (1996) Paget's disease of the breast: significance of mammographic findings. J Korean Radiol Soc 34(4):551–555
54. Choi SH, Chung SY, Lee KW et al (2001) Ultrasonography in Paget's disease of the breast: comparison with mammographic findings. J Korean Soc Med Ultrasound 20(20):137–142
55. Bacchetta J, Juillard L, Cochat P et al (2009) Paraneoplastic glomerular diseases and malignancies. Crit Rev Oncol Hematol 70:39–58
56. Kijima Y, Yoshinaka H, Owaki T et al (2004) Breast cancer with nephrotic syndrome: report of two cases. Surg Today 34(9):755–759
57. Valcamonico F, Ferrari V, Simoncini E et al (2004) Paraneoplastic nephrotic syndrome in advanced breast cancer patient. A case report. Tumori 90(1):154–156
58. Yoshizawa H, Akimoto T, Nishino K et al (2011) Nephrotic syndrome and renal failure in a patient with metastatic breast cancer. Clin Exp Nephrol 15(4):567–571. doi:10.007/s10157-011-0425-1, Epub 2011Mar 18
59. Oh KK (2003) The Paget's disease and pagetoid extension of the breast cancers: 3-D sonographic and pathologic correlation. 13th International congress on the ultrasonic examination of the breast. International Breast Ultrasound School. The 10th meeting of Japan Association of Breast and Thyroid Sonology
60. Sakita I, Yoshida T, Sohma I, Fukuchi N, Izawa H, Ebisui C, Hasuike Y, Ishizawa H, Kobayashi Y, Kotera I, Fujimoto T (2003) Determination of indication for sentinel lymph node biopsy using Doppler imaging. 13th International congress on the ultrasonic examination of the breast. International Breast Ultrasound School. The 10th meeting of Japan Association of Breast and Thyroid Sonology
61. Wisner ER, Ferrara KW, Short RE, Ottoboni TB, Gabe JD, Patel D (2003) Sentinel node detection using contrast-enhanced power doppler ultrasound lymphography. Invest Radiol 38(60):358–365
62. Britton PD, Goud A, Godward S, Barter S et al (2009) Use of ultrasound-guided axillary node core biopsy in staging of early breast cancer. Eur Radiol 19(3):561–569
63. Chung SY, Kim E-K, Oh KK (2003) Imaging findings of axillary abnormalities.13th International congress on the ultrasonic examination of the breast. International Breast Ultrasound School. The 10th meeting of Japan Association of Breast and Thyroid Sonology
64. Okamoto T, Horiuchi K, Kodama H et al (2005) Probability of axillary lymph node metastasis when sentinel lymph node biopsy is negative in women with clinically node negative breast cancer: a Bayesian approach. Breast Cancer 02/12(3):203–210. doi:10.2325/jbcs.12.203
65. Kusama M, Kawamoto A, Kaise H et al (2003) Ultrasound with tissue harmonic imaging in detection of axillary lymph node metastases in breast cancer patients. 13th International congress on the ultrasonic examination of the breast. International Breast Ultrasound School. The 10th meeting of Japan Association of Breast and Thyroid Sonology
66. Esen G, Gurses B, Ylmaz MH et al (2005) Gray scale and power doppler US in the preoperative evaluation of axillary metastases in breast cancer patients with no palpable lymph nodes. Eur Radiol 15(6):1215–1223
67. Rashmi S, Govardhan HB, Satyajt P et al (2014) Colour doppler – an evaluation tool for assessment of breast tumor size, axillary lymph node size and chemotherapeutic response. J Cancer Treat Res 2(2):9–15. doi:10.11648/j.jctr.20140202.11
68. Han SY, Kim HH (2003) Parasternal sonography of the internal mammary lymphatics in breast cancer. 13th International congress on the ultrasonic examination of the breast. International Breast Ultrasound School. The 10th meeting of Japan Association of Breast and Thyroid Sonology

9 Full Breast Ultrasonography as Follow-Up Examination After a Complex Treatment of Breast Cancer

9.1 Technique Particularities in Follow-Up Examinations by FBU*

The early diagnosis of a remnant or recidivated breast cancer is mandatory in long-term survival. The American Society of Clinical Oncology (ASCO) recommends only physical examination, breast self-examination, and posttreatment mammography, neglecting the remnant small parts after mammectomy/mastectomy and the remnant satellite lymph nodes. FBU has a great accuracy as a noninvasive follow-up examination of the whole region after complex treatment of breast cancer. This technique is safe, painless, and repeatable, with lower costs as compared with MRI, avoiding unnecessary biopsies and allowing early surgical reintervention.

FBU should be adapted in the follow-up examination of breast cancer, according to the type of the surgical treatment: conservative (quadrantectomy, lumpectomy) or curative (mammectomy, rarely mastectomy) with complete/incomplete axillary lymphadenectomy. By extension, any US could not be complete without Doppler characterization and (at least for the available applications) without sonoelastography, accomplishing the "full ultrasonography"; that results the US used for the breast evaluation will be generally named FBU, whatever type of breast surgery would be performed.

High-resolution linear transducers should be used for the anterior thoracic region including the axilla, supraclavicular fossa, and internal mammary artery, searching not only eventual tumor recidivate but also the surrounding small-part integrity, for the evaluation of the possibility of reparatory surgery. This analysis should be completed by Doppler and sonoelastography, avoiding unnecessary biopsies in suspect scars or local surgical complications: hematomas, seromas, suture granulomas, and remnant breast glandular tissue or remnant satellite lymph nodes with or without pathological changes.

Conservative surgery implies the examination of the remnant breast upon the DE technique, respecting the radial and antiradial scanning, with detailed explanations concerning the scars and the surrounding structures. In the last years, transducers were adapted with long scanning surfaces of 6–9 cm in lengths and/or water-bag devices, allowing the radial scans with better accuracy than the panoramic non-standardized view-type SieScape technique. Antiradial scans or even oblique scans along the scar axis may add useful information, as focused second step examinations after the radial comprehensive scanning, which is mandatory for avoiding "blind"/omitted regions of interest.

The DE technique is proving better sensibility than the classical US and a more objective reporting of the location of any abnormality benign or suspect over 0.4 mm upon the clockwise notation [2], which is already used by the clinicians and present in the pathological reports. When DE is completed by Doppler and SE upon the Ueno/Tsukuba scoring [3], whatever the ultrasonographic machine provider, then the FBU is achieved and the specificity of the diagnosis is increased up to 95–99 % [4, 5]. If available, strain ratio calculated as FLR can be assessed to be of malignant type if measuring over 4.70 (5.00) [6].

In cases with previous mastectomy/mammectomy, FBU should be applied to the *whole anterior thoracic region*, represented by:

- *The homolateral area* from the supraclavicular fossa to the submammary line and from the axilla and external thoracic artery to the presternal small parts and internal mammary artery, with systematic research of the scars and surrounding small parts, using axial, sagittal, and oblique scans, panoramic views, and high-resolution high-frequency transducers, according to the specific findings.
- *The contralateral breast* is examined upon the DE of Teboul accomplished as FBU, including the satellite lymph node stations, because of the risk of developing contralateral metachronous malignancy; moreover, the contralateral breast may provide information about the structural type of breast, with the dense breast being more susceptible to develop a malignant lesion. Any benign pathology should be mentioned in the remnant breast.

*(Chapter based on the author's presentation in collaboration with ME Andrei, at EPOSTM Vienna 2015, DOI:10.1594/ecr2015/C-0266 [1]).

A. Colan-Georges, *Atlas of Full Breast Ultrasonography*, DOI 10.1007/978-3-319-31418-1_9

In conclusion, in the follow-up of breast cancer, we should apply FBU to the whole anterior thoracic area, from the supraclavicular lymph nodes to the submammary sulcus and from the external thoracic artery and lymph nodes to the internal mammary arteries and node chain. For any adenopathy found in a lymph node station, the research area must be extended, for instant the presence of any suspect lymph node in the supraclavicular fossa push the limits to the deep lateral cervical nodes, up to the suboccipital spinal nodes, which are be found in advanced stages.

9.2 Findings in the FBU Follow-Up Examinations of Breast Cancer

The utility of the follow-up examination in breast cancer treatment is multiple, and full US could be the best noninvasive technique, with the following aims:

1. *To determine the remnant breast cancer, in the conservative therapy or radical mastectomy.* Indeed, there were reported at least 13.5 % positive margins at initial resection [7]; moreover, in a similar rate of positive margin, the local recurrence reported was very important, of 35.62 % cases, located in the intact breast, on the chest wall, in the axilla, in the supraclavicular fossa, and rarely in the internal mammary chain [8]. The authors did not mention the methods of diagnosis, but all these locations are available for FBU. There seemed to be no significant increased risk of second malignancies in patients undergoing conservative treatment (lumpectomy and radiation therapy) versus mastectomy without radiation [9, 10]; Obedian et al. [11] found in both cases 10 % rate of risk of second breast cancer at a 15-year survey. We think an earliest detection of the remnant cancer in the breast, the chest wall, or the satellite lymph nodes is possible after 3 weeks from the surgical treatment, and this is essential before completing the oncological protocol; any incomplete follow-up diagnosis will increase the risk of tumor recidivate. A six-month-interval follow-up FBU may be useful in the screening of breast cancer after complete or during the complex treatment, at least up to 5 years of survey; the malignancies detected may have different etiologies, according to the time from the first cancer: "forgotten" (missed tumors, either the main tumor if small in dense breast or associated lesions in multifocal cancers), "recidivate" (incomplete resection, usually malignant scar or developing adenopathies), and new malignancy (metachronous, multicentric, others).
2. *To differentiate a benign keloid from a malignant scar:* 2D US and SE may be similar in both scar types, but Doppler signal was increased in recidivate to the surgical positive margin; the initial negative margin on frozen examination may turn in positive margin with intraductal carcinoma on the permanent pathology, while the frozen positive margin at initial resection may be significantly associated with lobular histology [7]; in our experience, the initial lobular cancer was frequently multifocal, so the risk of remnant malignant foci from the same mammary lobe is increased in incomplete lobar resection, as was assumed by "the theory of the sick lobe" of Tot [12].
3. *To estimate the risk of metachronous breast cancer in the same or in the contralateral breast:* in FBU, it is possible to examine any abnormality of the ducts and lobules in the dense breast, to discriminate the ductal and lobular hyperplasia with premalignant increased risk, especially in postmenopausal patients, from duct ectasia or nodular fibro-micro-cystic dysplasia, with low potential for developing breast cancer.
4. *To illustrate the benign associated lesions*, usually neglected in patients with breast cancer, but with significant impact on the quality of life and sometimes on the treatment protocols; the chronic overinfected galactophoritis and the fibrocystic dysplasia were the most frequent associated lesions. Another usual "complications" reported in breast surgery are local infections, lymphedema, and suture granuloma; the rates of infections in breast and axillary incisions are reported between 1 and 20 % [13]; therefore, we think that the presence of the pathogen Staphylococci is wrongly attributed to the contamination from the skin during surgical or postoperative maneuvers, but we found it in the preoperative nipple surge. Other pseudomalignant findings may be chronic seroma/hematoma, inspissated cysts, benign tumor especially with periareolary location (papilloma, fibroadenoma), and nodular fibro-micro-cystic dysplasia.
5. *To precise the imaging distinction of the multifocal from the multicentric breast cancer* [14]: that is better illustrated by FBU, because the multifocal cancer is connected to the same lobar branching duct, it is decreasing in size with the distance from the main tumor, with salient abnormal Doppler signal present in the first 3–4 mm of any malignant lesion, while the strain ratio is according to the size and the malignancy, too; otherwise, multicentric cancers are located in different mammary lobes, without ductal interconnection as demonstrated by Cooper since 1840 [15], without correlation in size, and with possible differences in their malignant characters.

In a retrospective analysis of 142 (11.07 %) examinations in 87 patients after surgical radical or conservative therapy and partial/complete oncological treatments (chemotherapy, hormonal therapy, radiotherapy) of breast cancer, which were included in total 1283 random FBU (Jan. 2009–Feb. 2014), we found [1]:

- *17/142 cases of remnant/recidivate cancers*, most of them in the first year of follow-up, usually in the same breast after conservative/radical breast cancer surgery, in satellite "forgotten" lymph nodes, or in the contralateral breast and axilla; the high rate of the remnant/recidivate breast cancer of 11.97 % is similar to the values found in literature, and most patients studied after surgery were previously investigated using the worldwide accepted diagnostic tools: mammography, complementary classical US or FBU, biopsy, and rarely breast MRI. Except for FBU and MRI, other methods are considered not accurate in multifocal or multicentric breast cancer [14]; DE was useful in detecting small multiple malignant lesions because it is an anatomical imaging technique and almost all malignancies are related to the ductal tree. The advantage of the FBU was the early detection in the first year of almost all remnant/recidivate cancers, with the risk being less than 5 % after 2 years.

- *Up to two synchronous and up to four metachronous breast cancers in the same/contralateral breast* were found after an initial breast cancer with conservative/radical surgery, usually with different cellularities (multiclonal), proving multicentric cancer. From 3 cases, with initial ductal carcinoma in situ, one patient with conservative surgery followed by radiotherapy developed invasive ductal carcinoma in the same breast in the next 14 months.
- *Edema: Benign lymphedema* had less vascular pattern on Doppler, and the strain of the glandular structures was reduced as compared with the thickening skin and the premammary fatty tissue, while *carcinomatous mastitis* presented more salient vasculature and a reduced elasticity of the glandular part. In some cases, upper limb edema was proved to be undetermined by the axillary lymph node excision, but secondary to the axillary vein thrombosis, with increased incidence after intravenous chemotherapy; venous Doppler examination proved the venous valve with echogenic content and the laminar or absent blood velocity of the central lumen.
- *Biopsied tumors:* Malignant tumors could be too large at the first presentation and the surgical treatment was delayed; follow-up examination was demanded after biopsy and preoperative chemotherapy, and the imaging sonographic diagnosis proved essential complementary information related to the size, vascularity, and surrounding tissue alterations; as a positive response, the size diminished, the vascular pattern was according to the size, the acoustic shadowing if present diminished, and a better delineation with the pectoral fascia could be demonstrated.
- *In 4 cases, we found remnant cancers* missed by the initial diagnosis by mammography and classical US and omitted by the surgical treatment because of the *peripheral location* of the tumors, such as the submammary sulcus (2p), parasternal area (1p), and the outer breast border on middle axillary line (1p). These locations had the greatest risk to be omitted by screening mammography and US, and breast MRI was not recommended as routine examination. Moreover, after mammectomy, preferred for a radical surgery, we frequently have found mammary remnants of the peripheral glandular tissues without pathological changes or with benign aspects such as fibrocystic dysplasia;
- The most *"forgotten" axillary lymph nodes* were benign, with normal architecture or inflammatory changes, some of them presenting further malignant evolution at the follow-up FBU. In most cases, malignant remnant lymph nodes were found in the homolateral axilla, especially in the retropectoral and apical group; in the contralateral axilla, metastatic lymph nodes were rarely found especially after initial massive invasion of the homolateral axillary lymph nodes.
- *Other lymph node stations*: The internal supraclavicular lymph nodes and the deep lateral cervical and spinal chain involvement were exceptionally found. The internal mammary lymph node chain was detected by Doppler US in only one patient from 87 cases, with primary breast cancer located in an upper-inner quadrant; the integrity of this chain in the rest of cases was verified by the Multidetector Computed Tomography performed as routine follow-up examination at 6 months interval during the oncologic treatment; the accuracy of the Doppler US for the internal mammary lymph nodes was proved in the literature [8], but the incidence of their involvement was not so important as it was expected.
- The most difficult diagnosis in FBU was the assessment of the remnant enlarged *lymph nodes presenting necrosis* with a BGR scoring upon Ueno; the strain ratio or FLR may be reduced under 4.00 as in benign cases, the vasculature may be increased pericapsular specific for malignancy or appears normal, while MRI diagnosis is confusing, too; FNAB may be unuseful because of the necrosis. In our experience, the oncologists preferred to recommend a supplementary radiotherapy instead of repeated surgery, with good results.
- *The differential diagnosis* of a remnant/ recidivate breast cancer from other malignancy with the same location was possible by FBU in skin tumors (epithelioma, malignant melanoma), lymphoma, and sarcomas.
- *Early postsurgical complications:* In the first 6 months of follow-up, we found 51 (35.91 %) postsurgical "benign" abnormalities (seroma, hematoma, suture granuloma, lymphedema).
- 74 (52.11 %) cases presented *additional primary benign breast pathology*: ductal-lobular hyperplasias, ductal ectasias, papillomas, fibrocystic dysplasia, etc.
- Benign scars had sometimes pseudomalignant aspects in classical US or SE alone, but FBU made the differential diagnosis. FBU offered a good management of benign associated abnormalities, useful for the differential diagnosis and treatment, thus resulting in an improvement of the quality of life.

Most cases presented various association of findings, benign, postsurgical, and eventually malignant, determining a complex evaluation and a personalized treatment. Nodular fibro-micro-cystic dysplasia was the best mimicker of malignancy on mammography and 2D US, but the absence of new vasculature and the summation-BGR score in SE allowed positive diagnosis.

In conclusion, screening FBU at the mastectomy site proved useful, safe, painless, and cheaper than any other techniques. US is also recommended for the diagnostic of surgical involvements or for radiotherapy side effects, as well as for the control of the remaining breast structures after lumpectomy or partial breast excision or after aspiration biopsy or cryoablation. Radiotherapy may be harmful, and US offers the best imaging evaluation because of the highest resolution and of the possibility to estimate the vitality based on the vasculature presence. Breast reconstruction (implants, slipped muscular-cutaneous flaps) after mammectomy can be accurately examined by FBU (Figs. 9.1, 9.2, 9.3, 9.4, 9.5, 9.6, 9.7, 9.8, 9.9, 9.10, 9.11, 9.12, 9.13, 9.14, 9.15, 9.16, 9.17, 9.18, 9.19, 9.20, 9.21, 9.22, 9.23, 9.24, 9.25, 9.26, 9.27, 9.28, 9.29, 9.30, 9.31, 9.32, 9.33, 9.34, 9.35, 9.36, 9.37, 9.38, 9.39, 9.40, 9.41, 9.42, 9.43, 9.44, and 9.45).

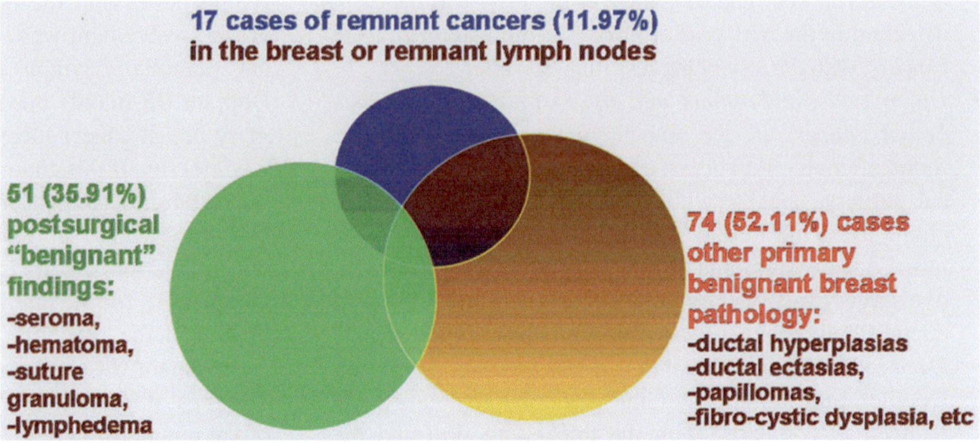

Fig. 9.1 Possible associations of the pathological findings found in breast cancer follow-up using FBU (upon [1])

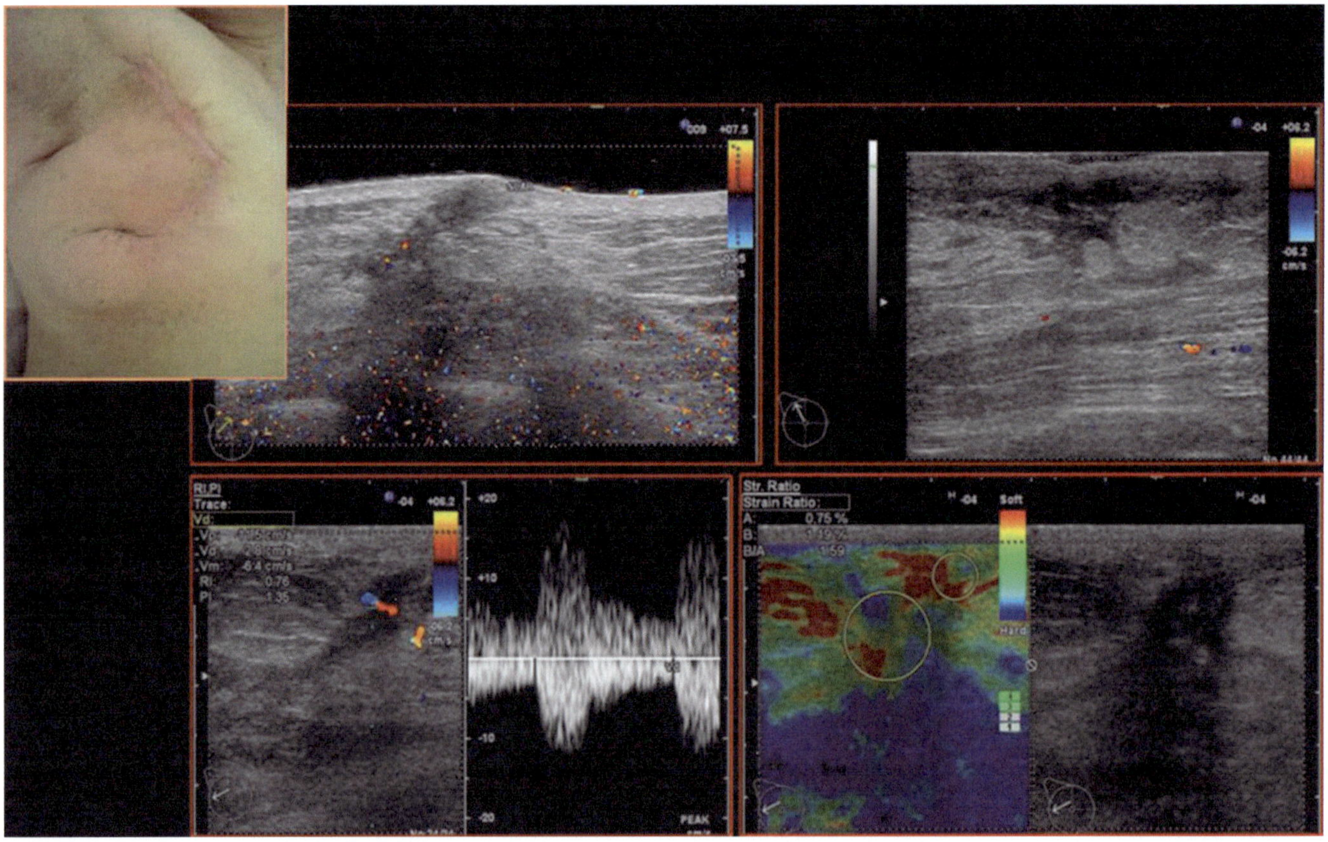

Fig. 9.2 FBU in a 45-year-old patient: benign scar with deep pseudomalignant keloid (upon [1])

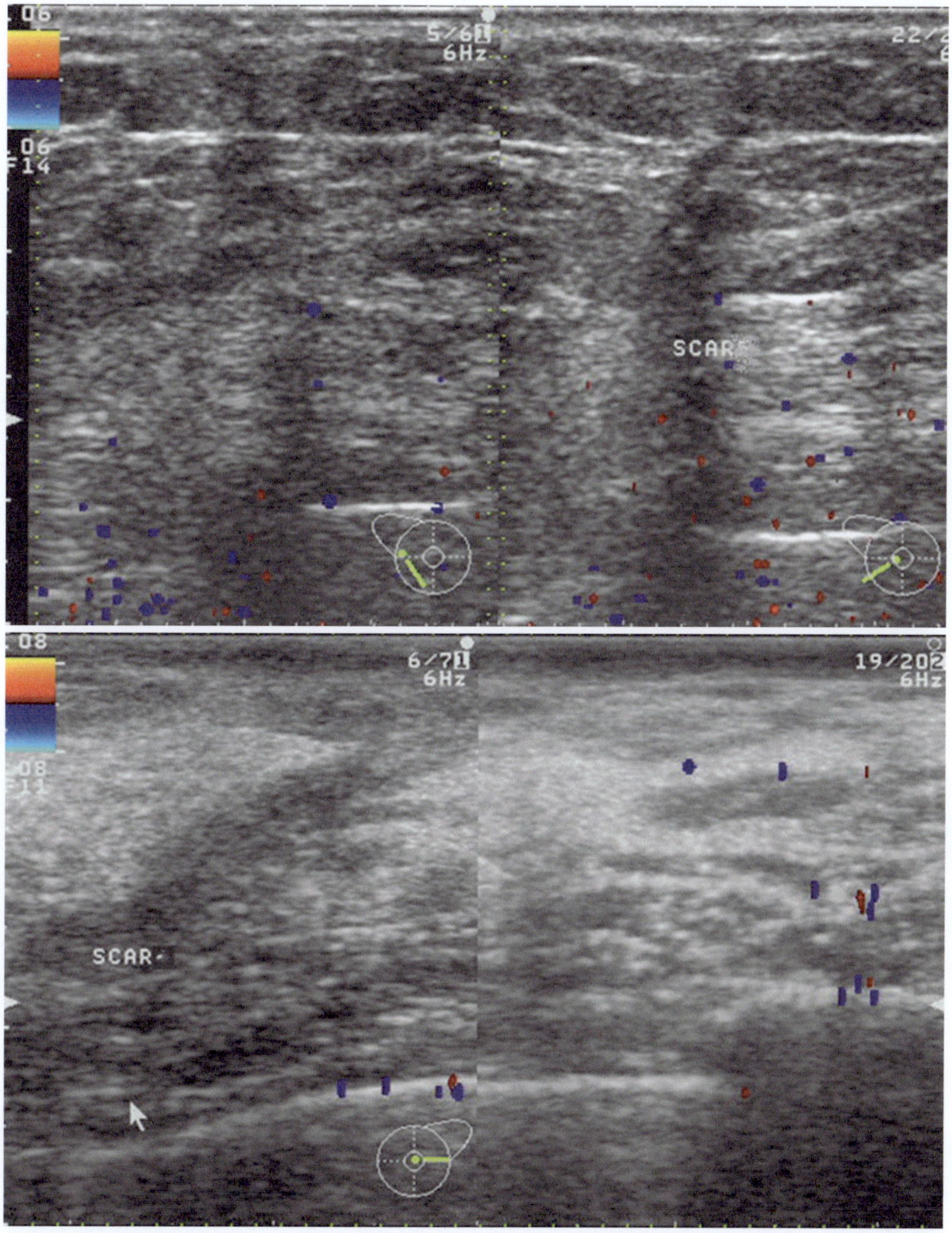

Fig. 9.3 Different shapes of scars, mimicking malignant lesions: history, real-time multiplanar scans, and absence of Doppler signal are usually sufficient argues for the diagnosis; sonoelastography could be used as a complementary tool

Fig. 9.3 (continued)

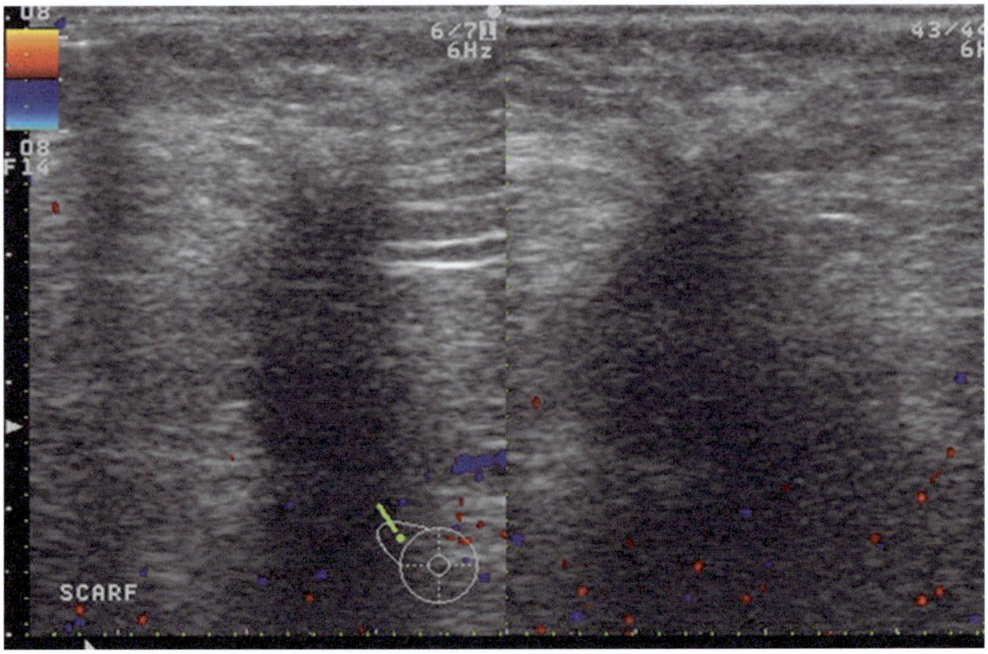

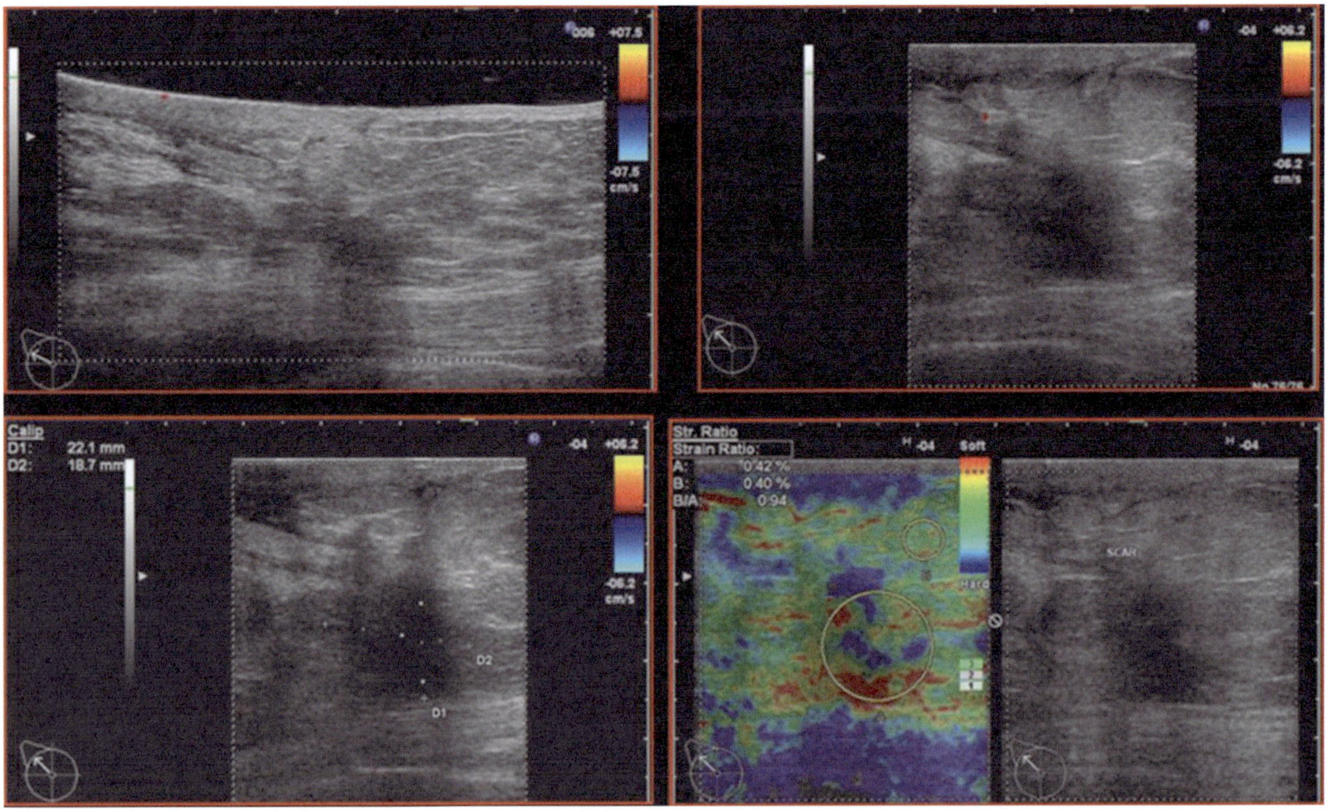

Fig. 9.4 A 48-year-old patient with R 10:30 pseudotumor on mammography and 2D US after conservative breast cancer surgery. FBU demonstrates benign scar without salient vasculature and with a complex BGR score in a chronic seroma (upon [1])

Fig. 9.5 A 60-year-old patient with left mammectomy: R 9:00 pseudomalignancy located in a TDLU, with angular margins, salient peripheral vasculature, irregular acoustic shadowing, and BGR score at sonoelastography, suggesting nodular fibro-microcystic dysplasia (upon [1]). A short-time FBU follow-up is recommended

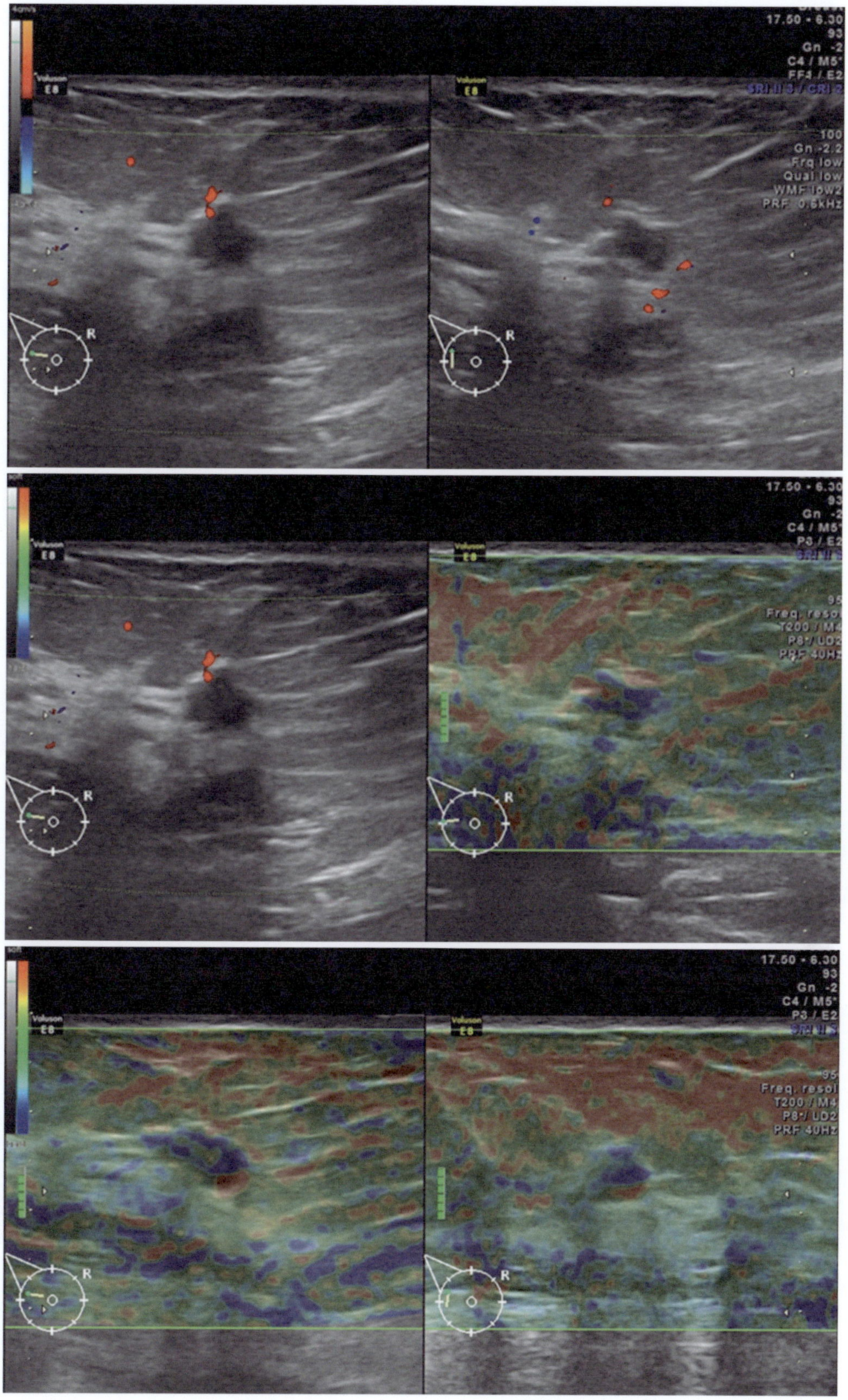

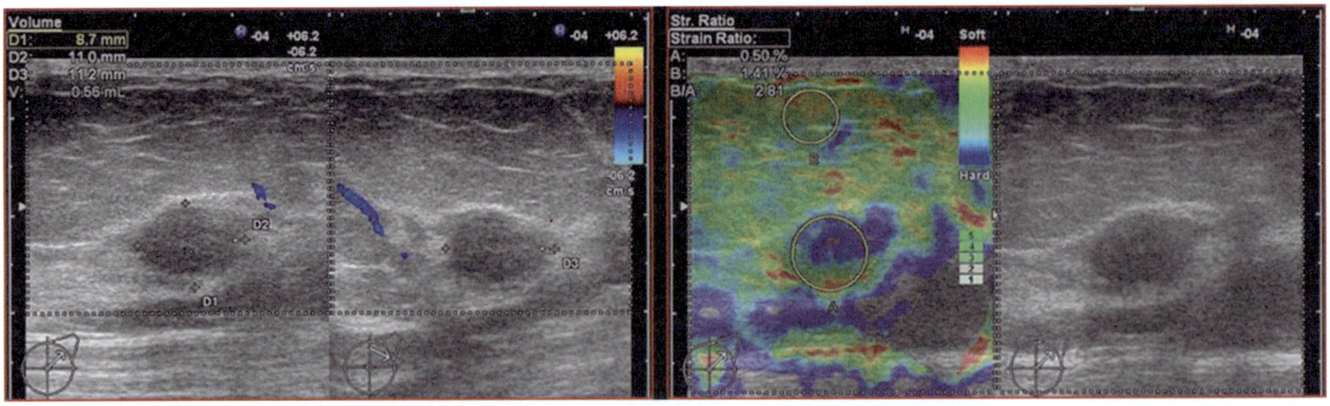

Fig. 9.6 FBU in a 51-year-old patient: remnant pseudotumor—inspissated cyst in the vicinity of the scar, with BGR scoring (upon [1])

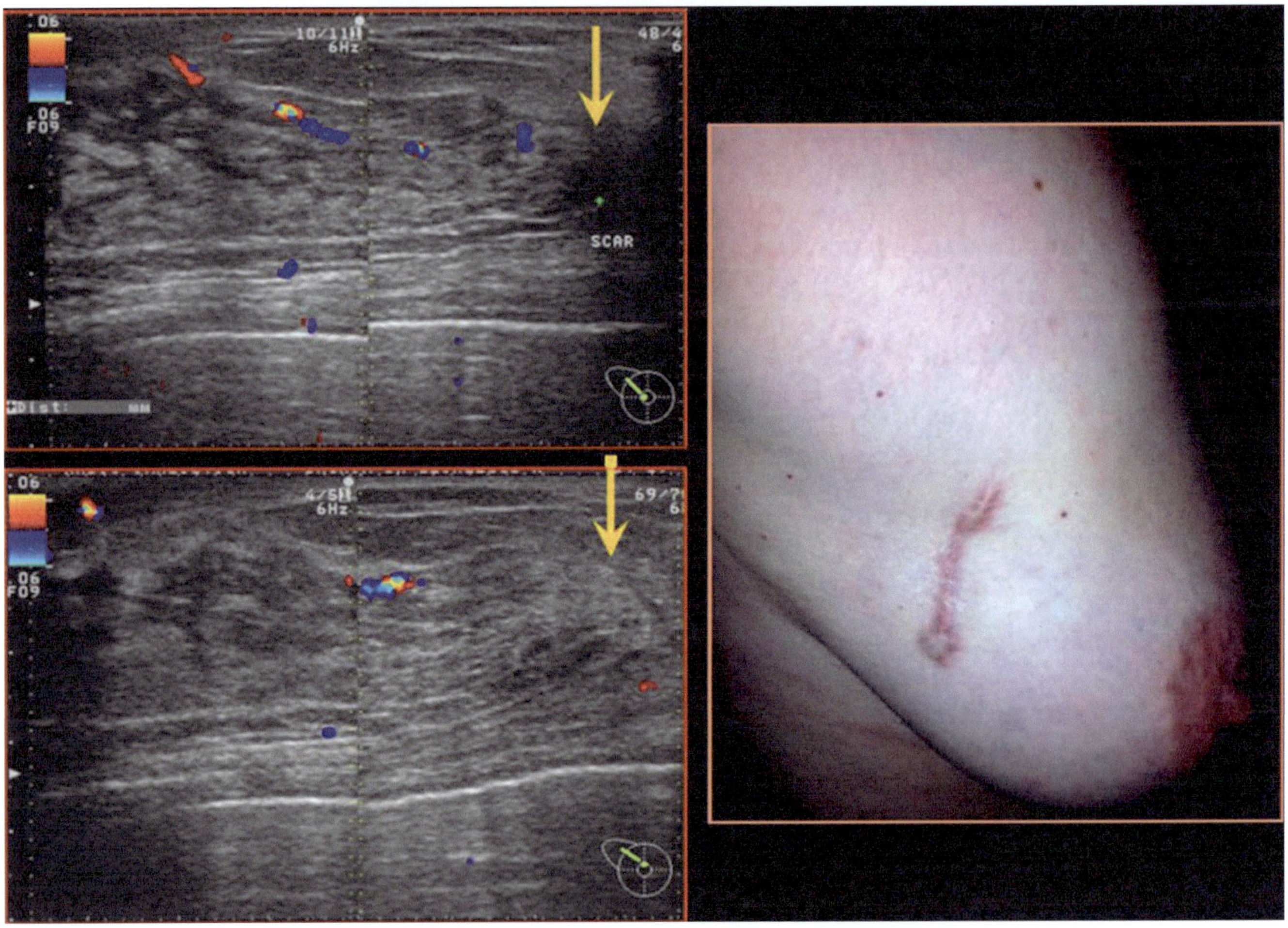

Fig. 9.7 DE in a 34-year-old patient with breast cancer in dense breast with benign scar (*arrow*): illogical lumpectomy instead of lobectomy, with increased risk of intraductal spreading; salient centripetal vasculature recommends a short-time follow-up (upon [1])

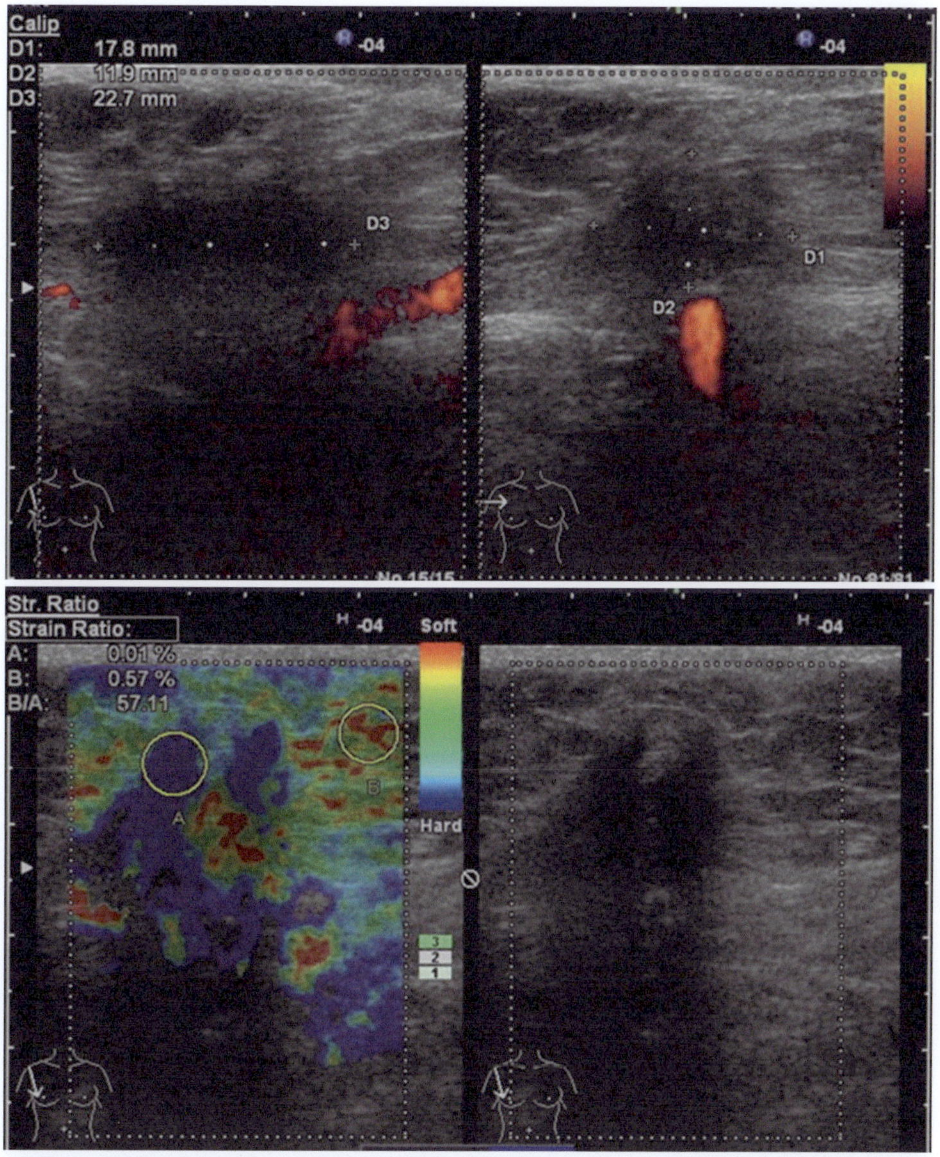

Fig. 9.8 A 43-year-old patient with benign axillary scar presenting a spiculated shape on CT and 2D US, but a complex score type 3 Ueno combined with BGR; the absence of any new formation vasculature inside the lesion reinforces the differential diagnosis with a malignant scar

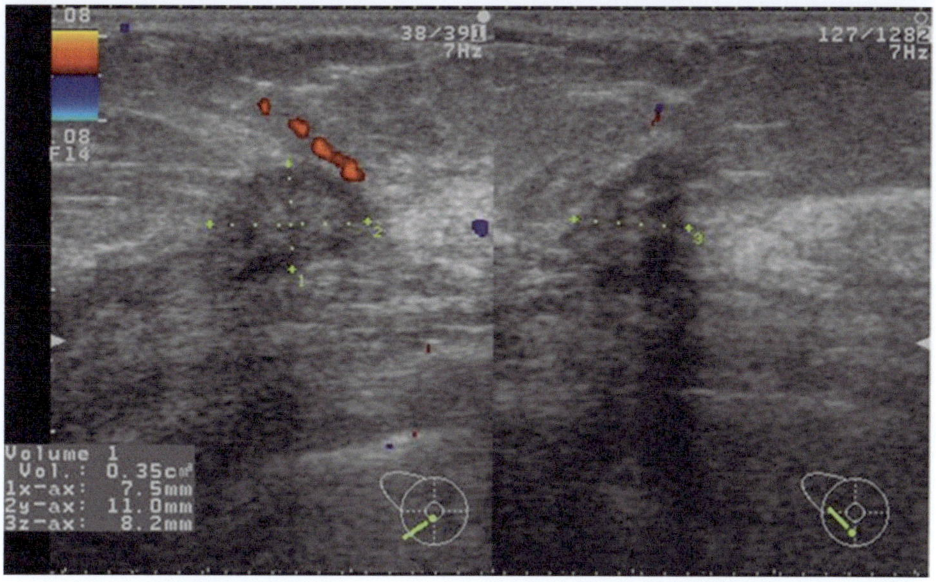

Fig. 9.9 Pathological scar: nodular inhomogeneous lesion, irregularly shaped, with posterior asymmetrical shadowing, may represent a suture granuloma; because of the peripheral new vasculature, a sonoelastography and short-time US follow-up are recommended instead of biopsy

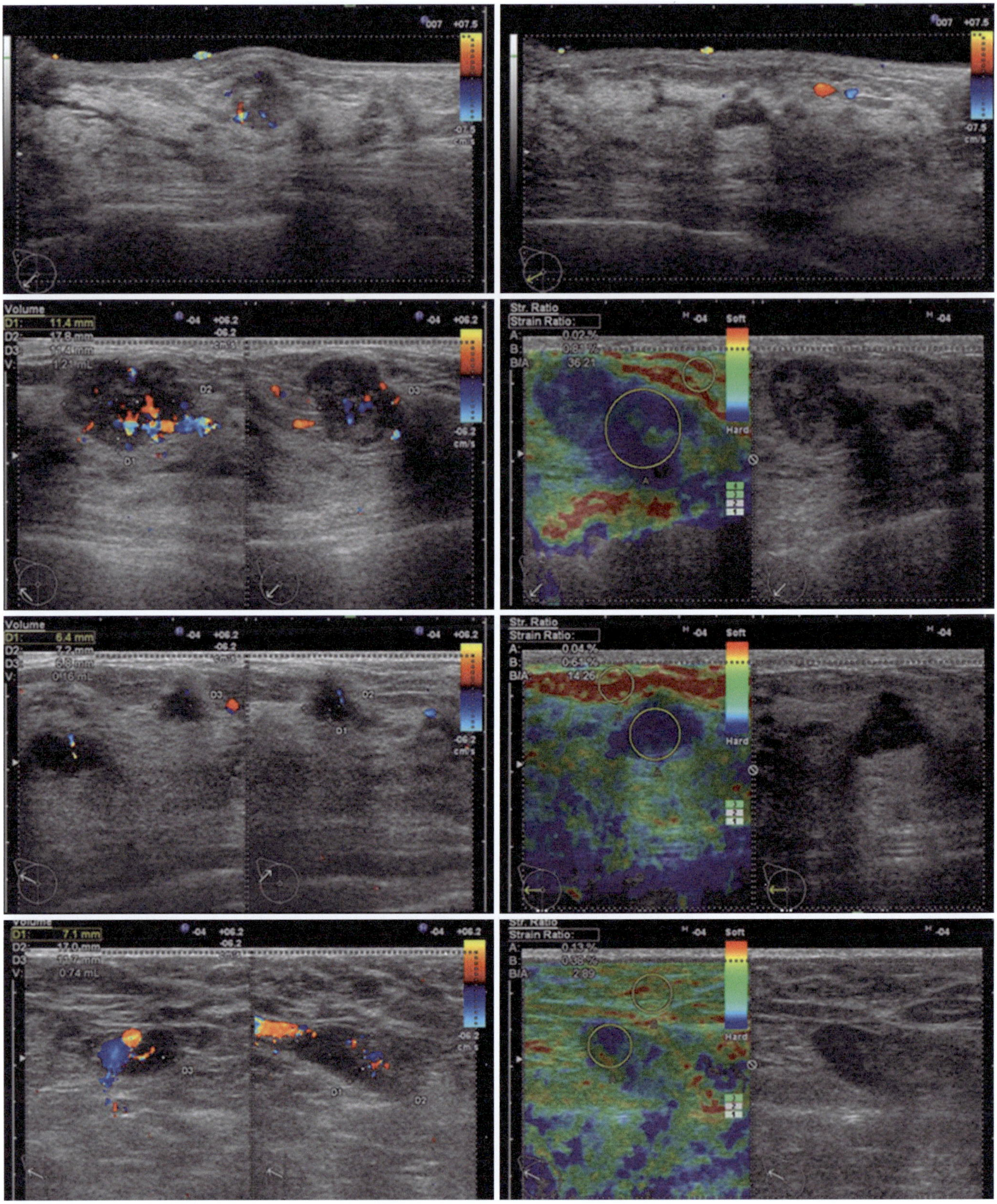

Fig. 9.10 "Multicentric" cancer in the R breast outer (different) quadrants, upon the arbitrary definition; "multifocal" cancer from the R 8:00 to R10:00 radius, according to the morphological characters, ductal connection and decreasing size from the lower tumor to the upper one, the nearest to the axilla, in the spreading way of the malignancy. The risk of "forgotten" tumor is increased if the real extension of the disease is misdiagnosed, in this large mammary lobe partially extended in 2 different quadrants (EPOS™ Vienna 2015, doi: 10.1594/ecr2015/C-0266 [1])

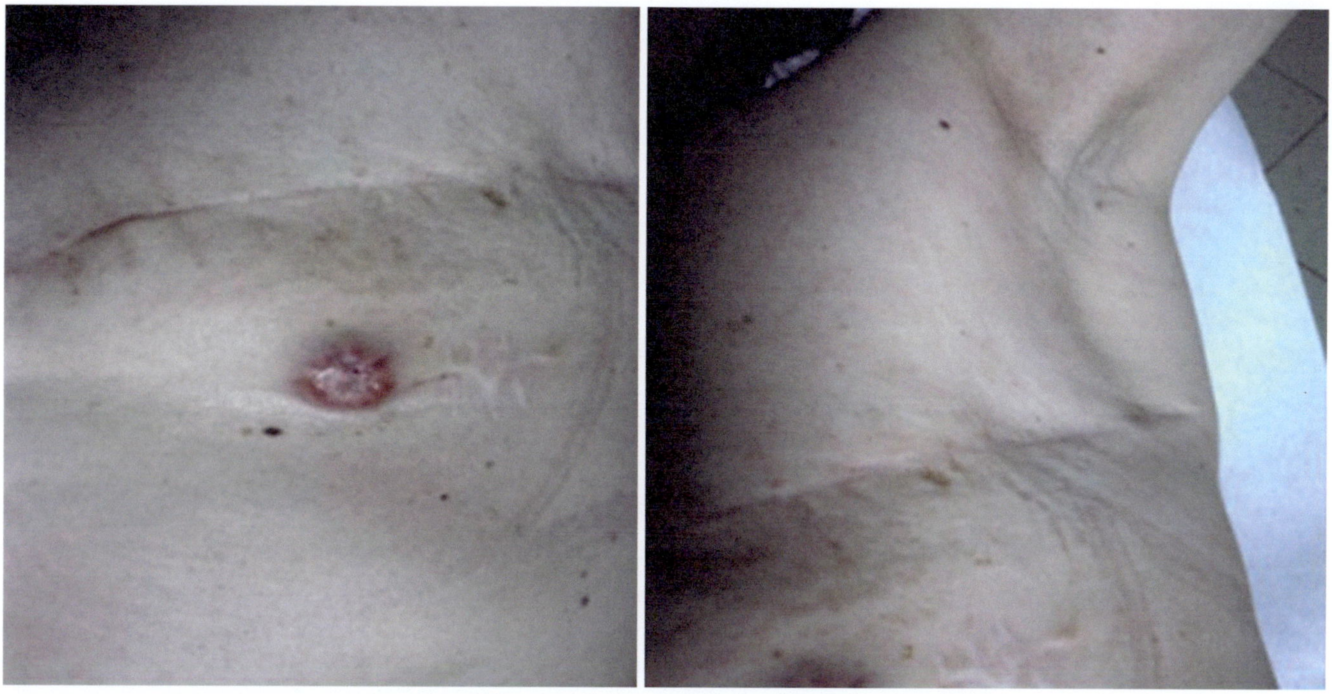

Fig. 9.11 A 64-year-old patient: mammectomy without any breast cancer findings on the specimen, but 7/15 left axillary lymph nodes were found with metastases from breast carcinoma. Aspect after 10 months, following chemotherapy, without radiotherapy (EPOS™ Vienna 2015, doi: 10.1594/ecr2015/C-0266 [1])

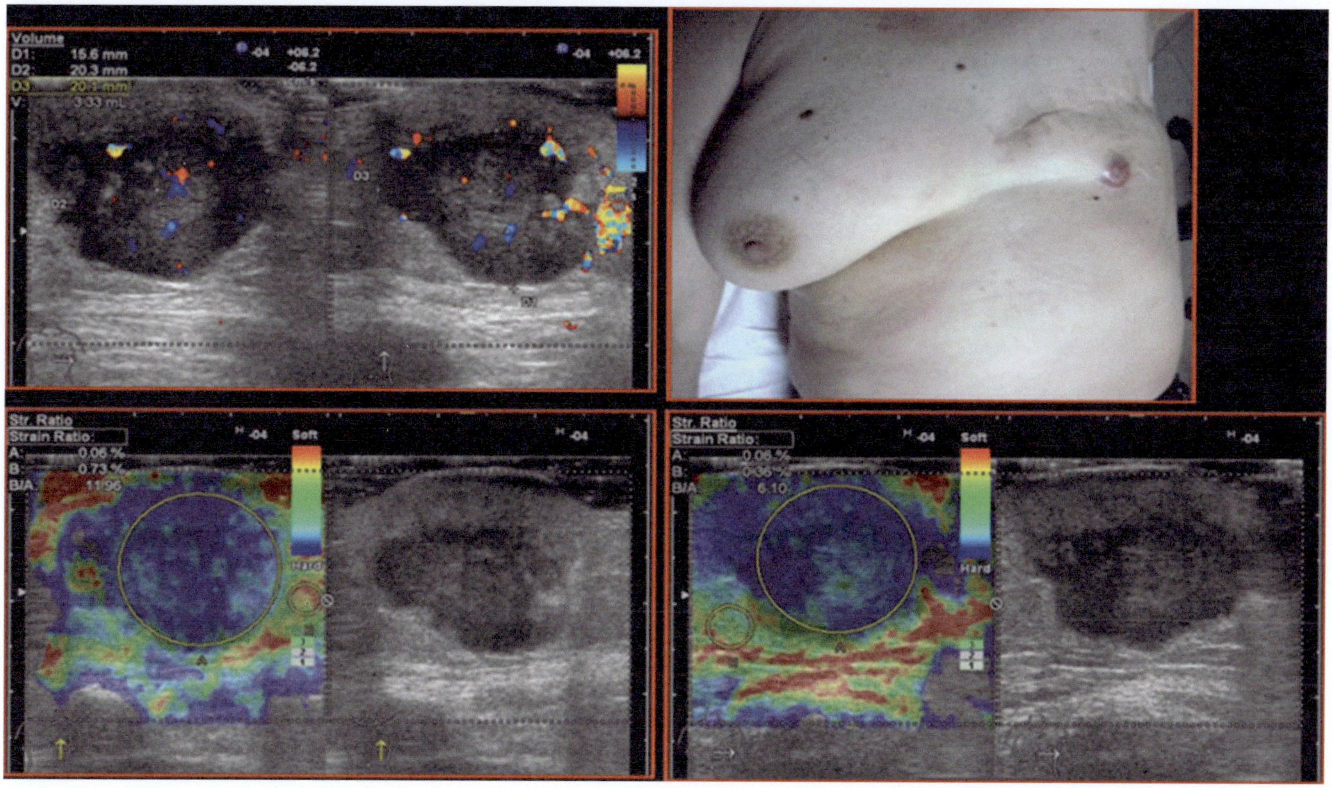

Fig. 9.12 The same case: remnant primary malignancy or recidivate? The tumor location corresponds to the submammary sulcus. Remember no cancer was found in the specimen of mammectomy (EPOS™ Vienna 2015, doi: 10.1594/ecr2015/C-0266 [1])

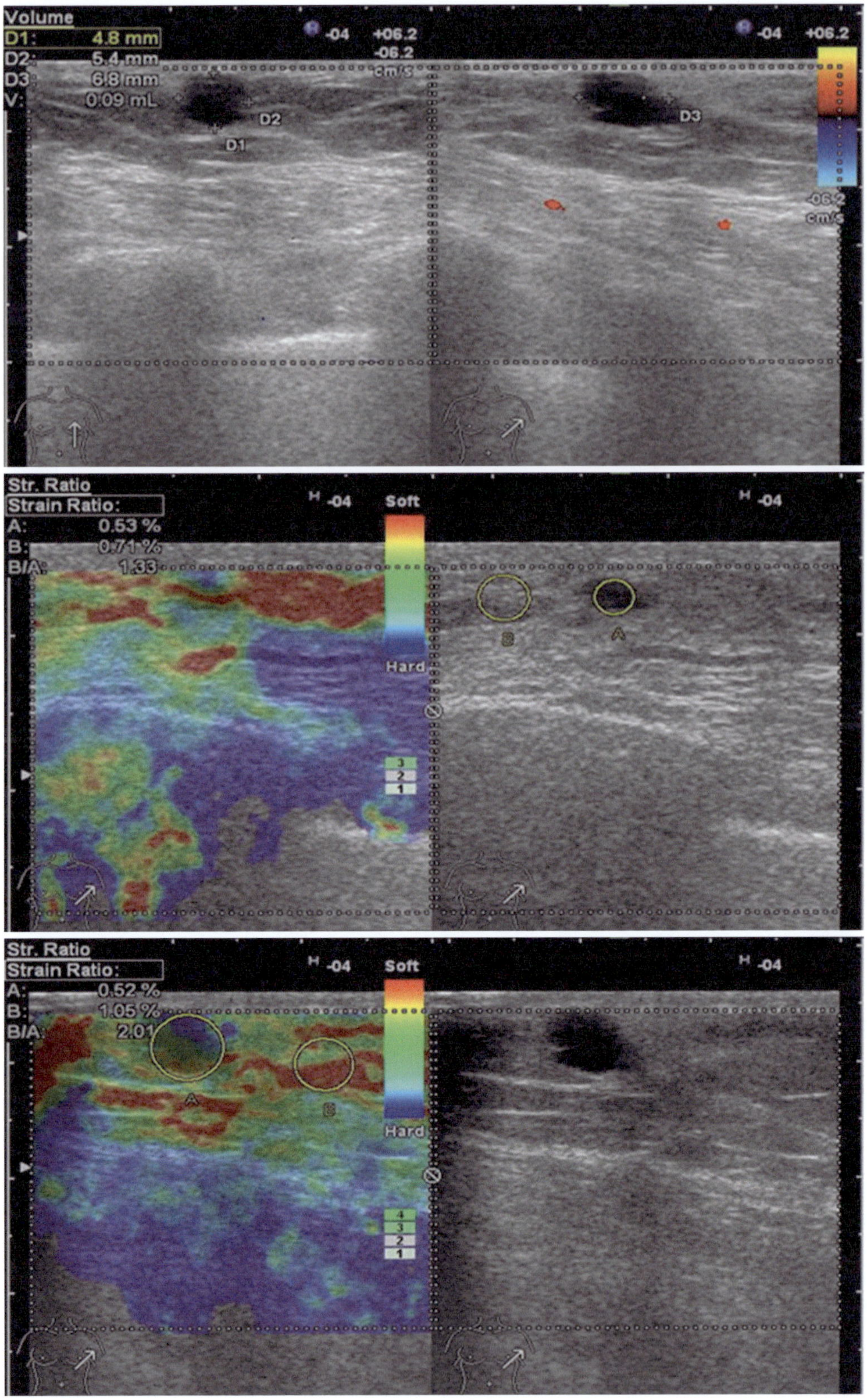

Fig. 9.13 The same case: FBU illustrates suture granulomas with cystic appearances—transonic with irregular borders, without vasculature, and with BGR score of low FLR (EPOS™ Vienna 2015, doi: 10.1594/ecr2015/C-0266 [1])

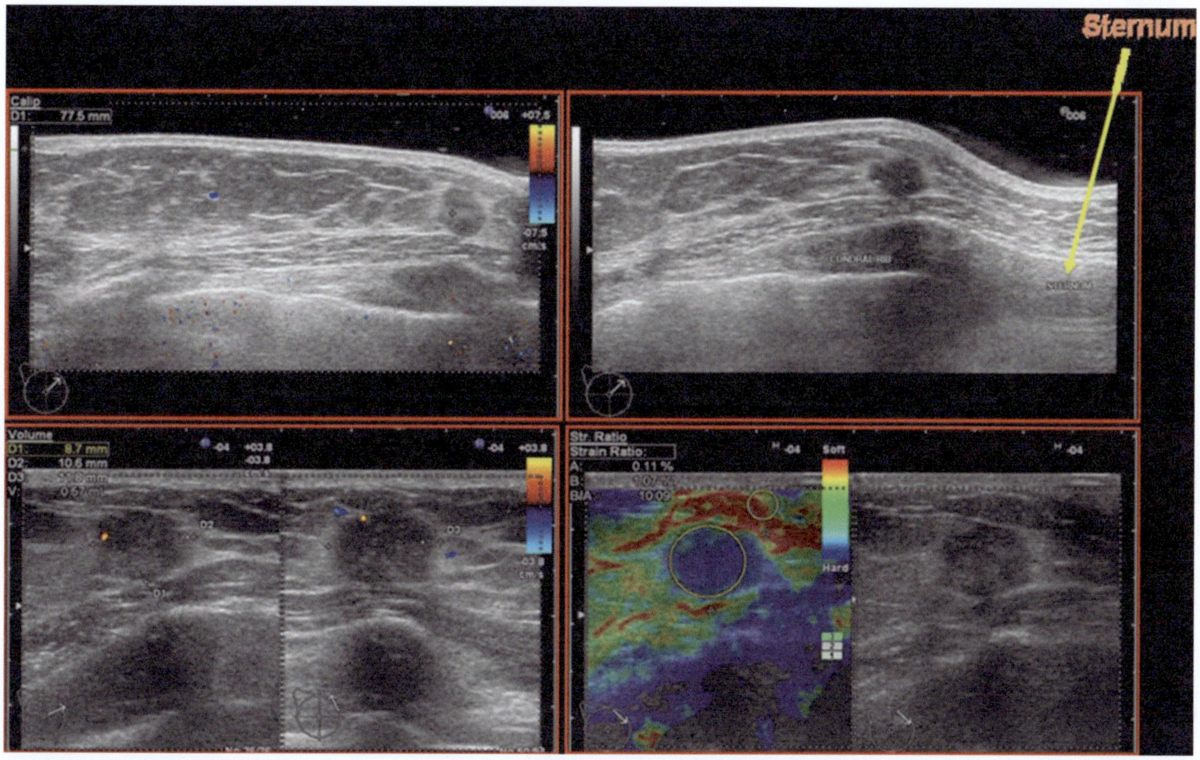

Fig. 9.14 A 64-year-old patient: recent lumpectomy in the right UIQ for palpable lesion, mammographically visible. FBU illustrates remnant parasternal IDC: "recidivate" or missing cancer? (EPOS™ Vienna 2015, doi: 10.1594/ecr2015/C-0266 [1])

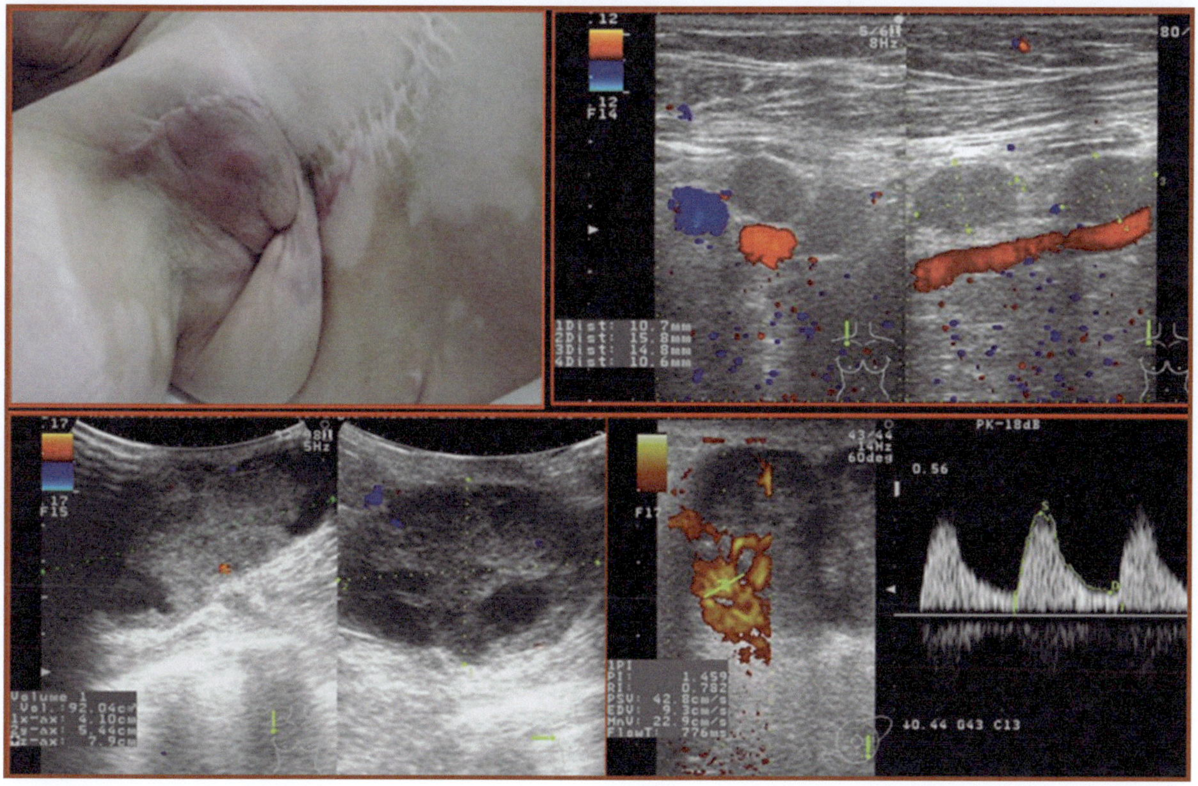

Fig. 9.15 Huge breast tumor in a 56-year-old female treated in other service by tumorectomy without lymphadenectomy; with pathological reports proving malignancy, it was followed by mammectomy with axillary lymphadenectomy and chemotherapy. Actual presentation has secondary axillary recidivism and supraclavicular adenopathy. We have to answer many questions: Why tumorectomy? What was the initial diagnosis? Why incomplete lymphadenectomy and secondary adenopathy? The Doppler US aspect is similar to the findings in malignant cystosarcoma phyllodes that may explain the evolution (EPOSTM Vienna 2015, doi: 10.1594/ecr2015/C-0266 [1])

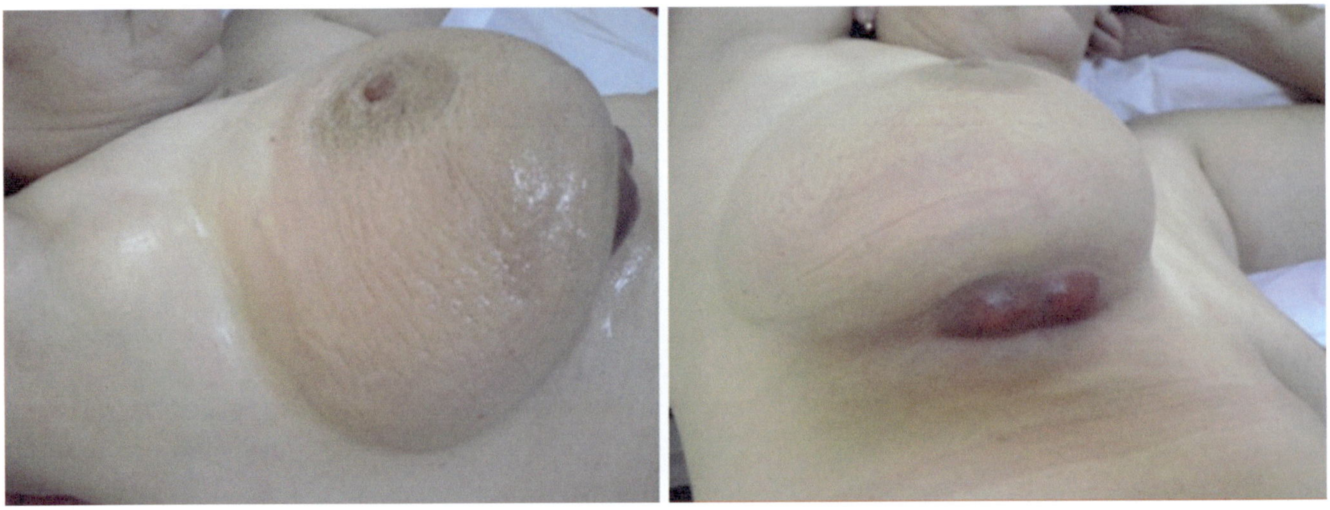

Fig. 9.16 A 58-year-old patient: huge breast malignant tumor with malignant cytology both in mammary and axillary lymph node aspirates; follow-up after preoperative chemotherapy (EPOSTM Vienna 2015, doi: 10.1594/ecr2015/C-0266 [1])

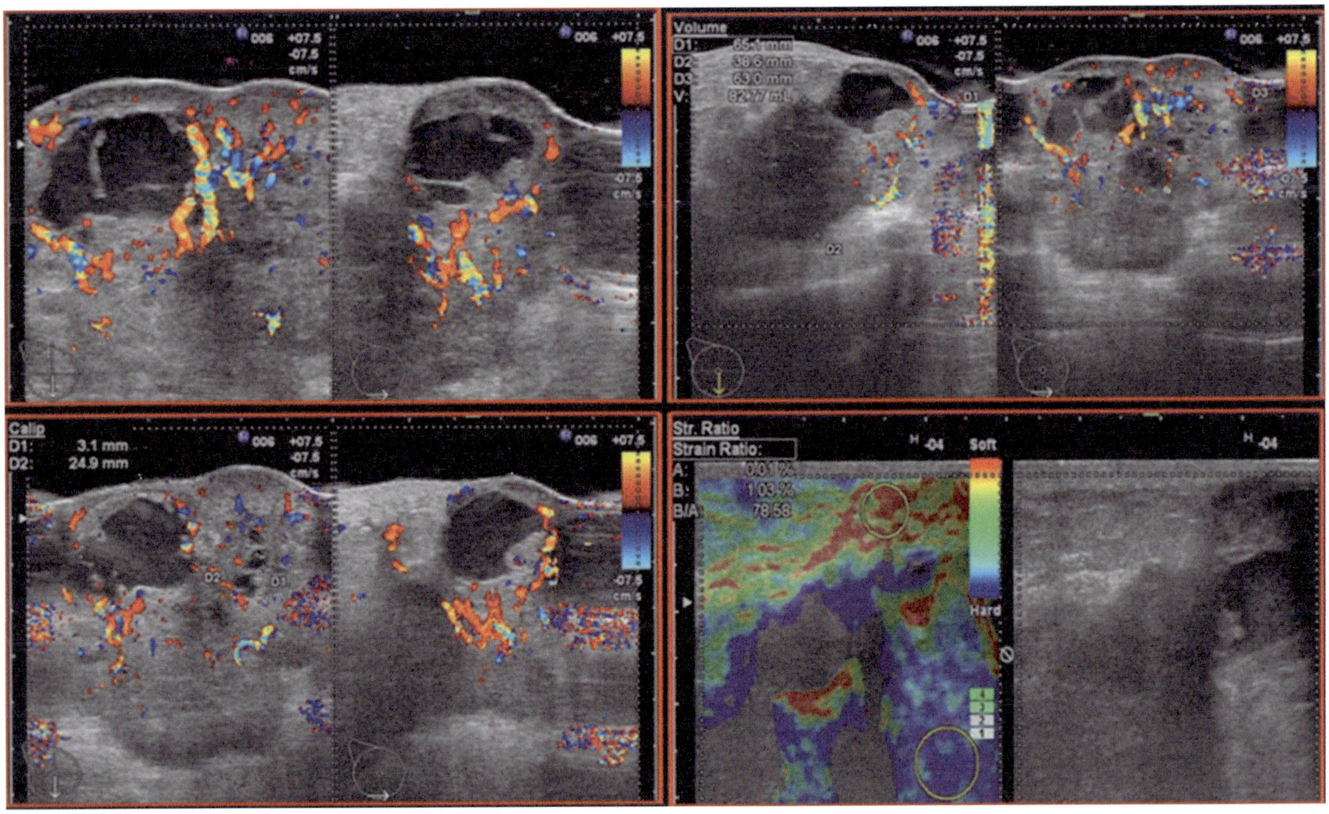

Fig. 9.17 The same case, FBU aspect: huge breast tumor with solid and cystic areas, malignant-type vasculature, and high FLR. Malignant cystosarcoma phyllodes was suspected (EPOSTM Vienna 2015, doi: 10.1594/ecr2015/C-0266 [1])

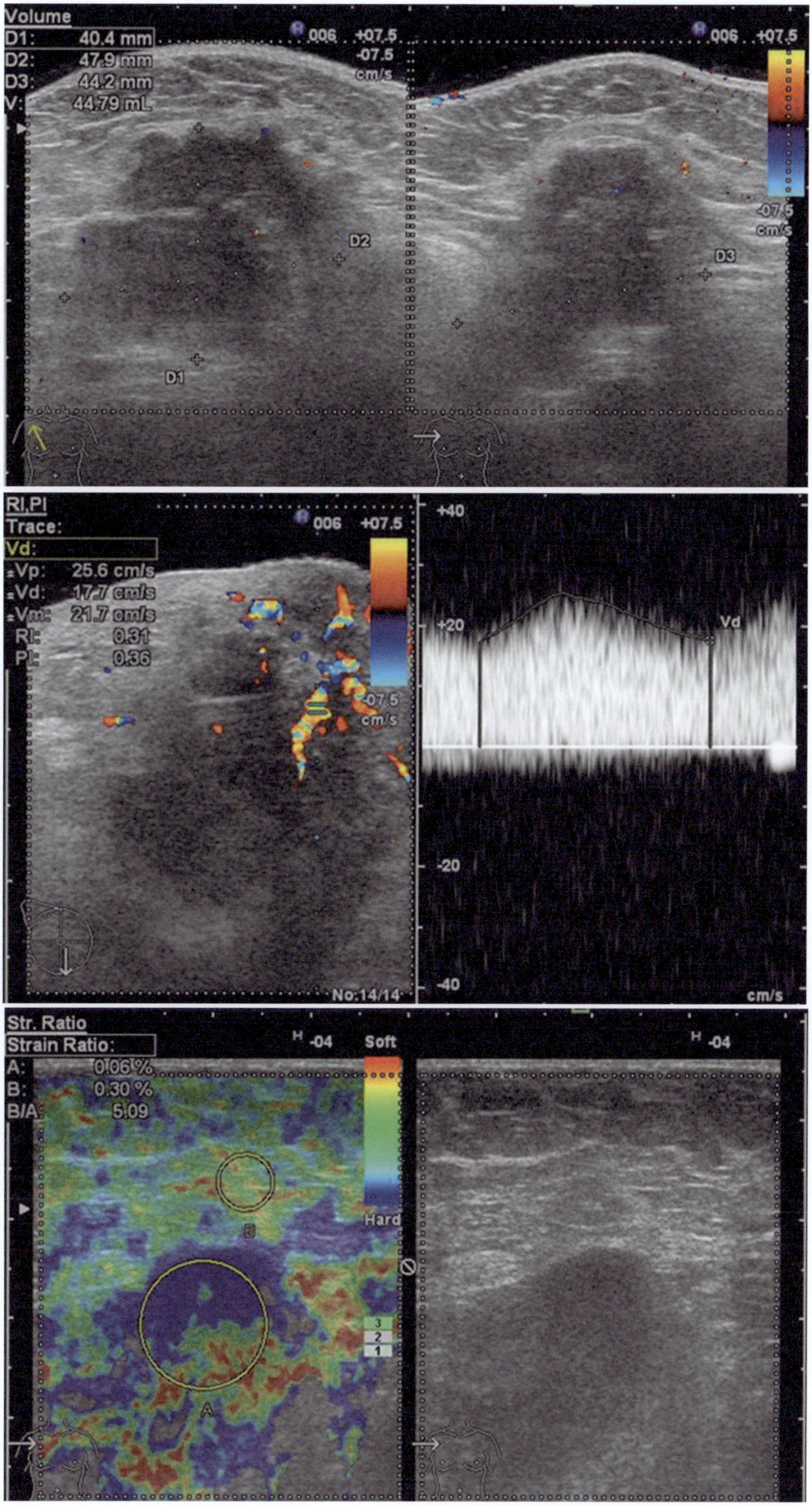

Fig. 9.18 The same case: axillary metastatic lymph nodes with similar internal structure, low-resistance blood flow indices, and BGR score of moderate increased FLR up to 5.09 ("true benign" BGR is usually less than 2.50). Malignant cystosarcoma phyllodes was confirmed (EPOS™ Vienna 2015, doi: 10.1594/ecr2015/C-0266 [1])

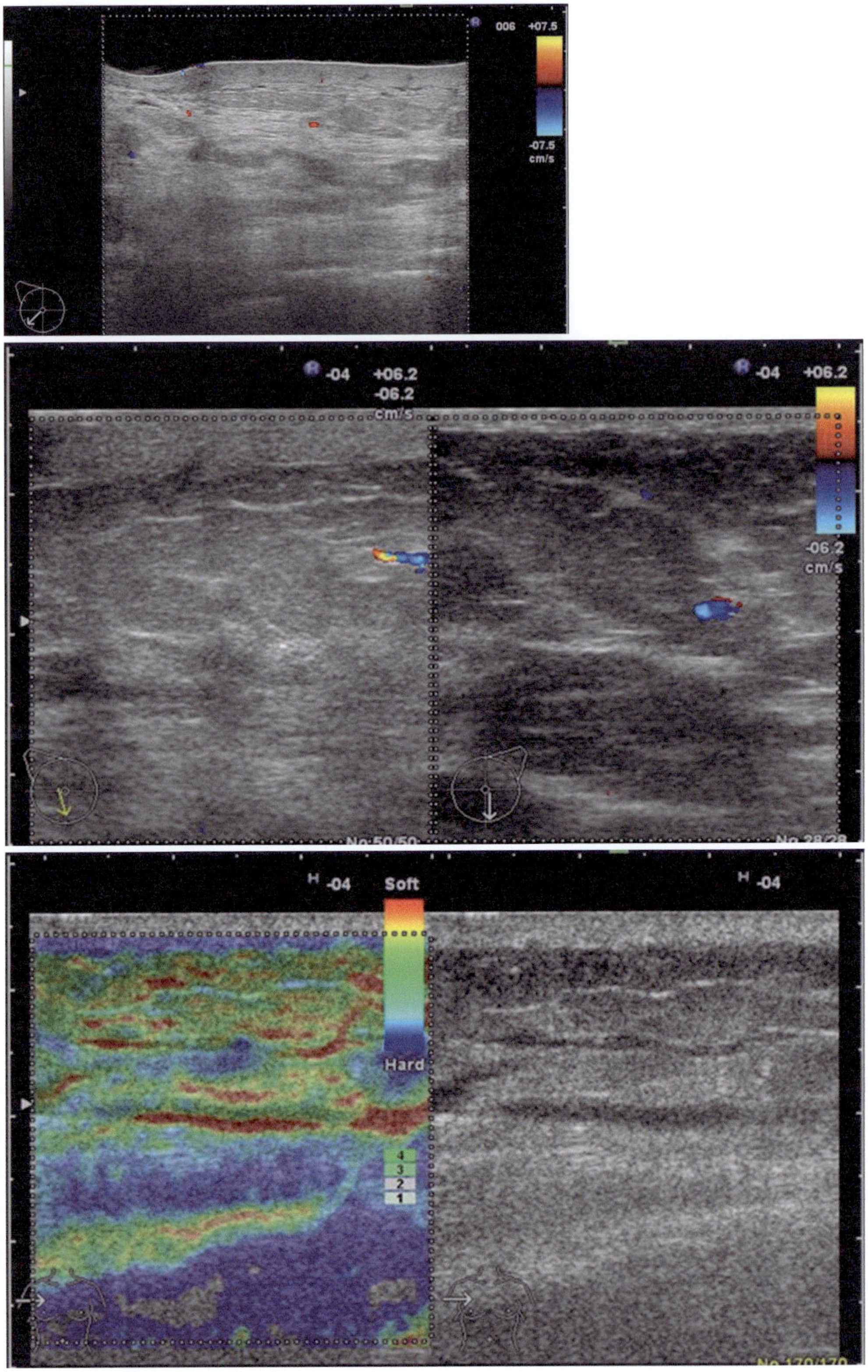

Fig. 9.19 The same case: malignant-type lymphedema in the breast outside the tumor, due to the axillary lymph node involvement; note the salient diffuse vasculature and the relative increased hardness at sonoelastography of the glandular layers as compared with the premammary fatty tissue (EPOS™ Vienna 2015, doi: 10.1594/ecr2015/C-0266 [1])

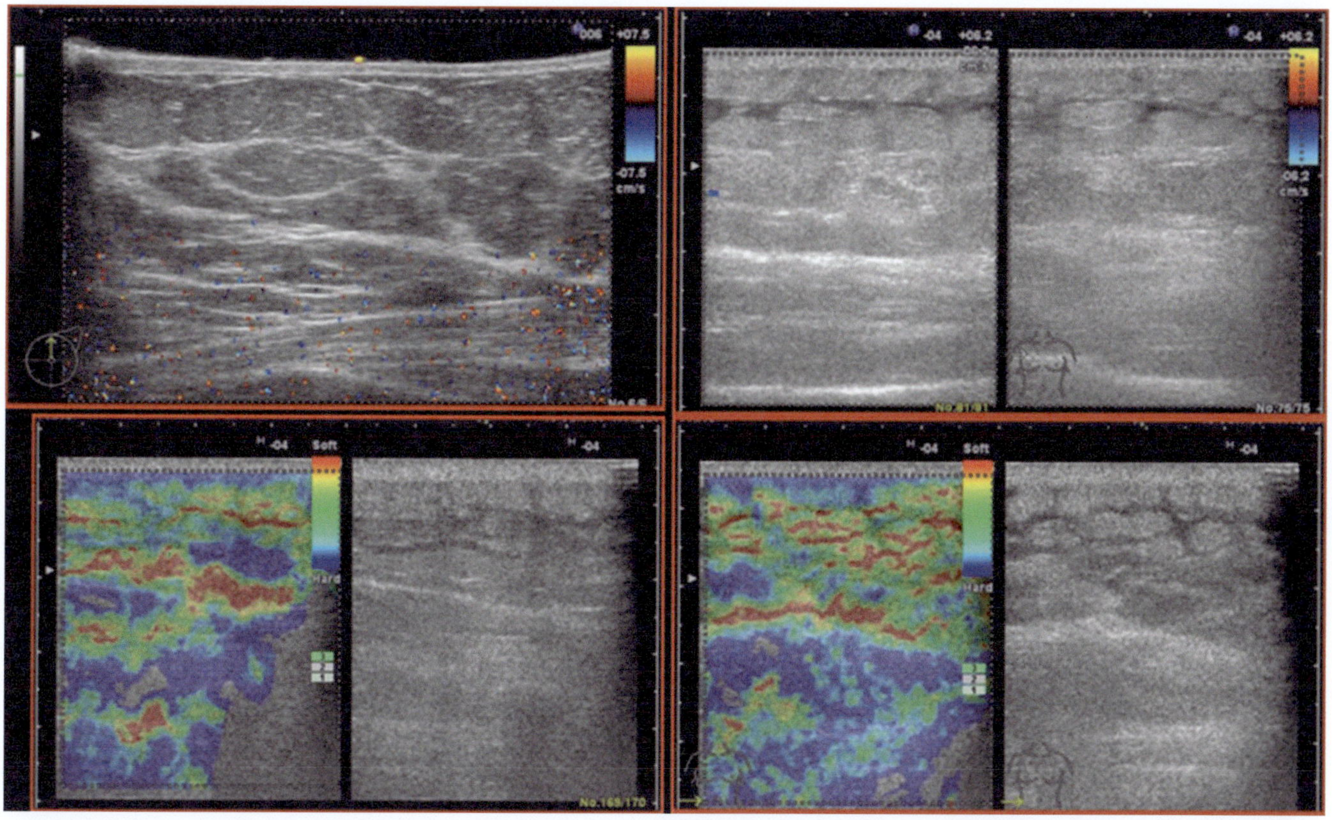

Fig. 9.20 A 58-year-old patient: fatty breast on the left side and benign lymphedema of the right breast postsurgical treatment and radiotherapy (EPOSTM Vienna 2015, doi: 10.1594/ecr2015/C-0266 [1])

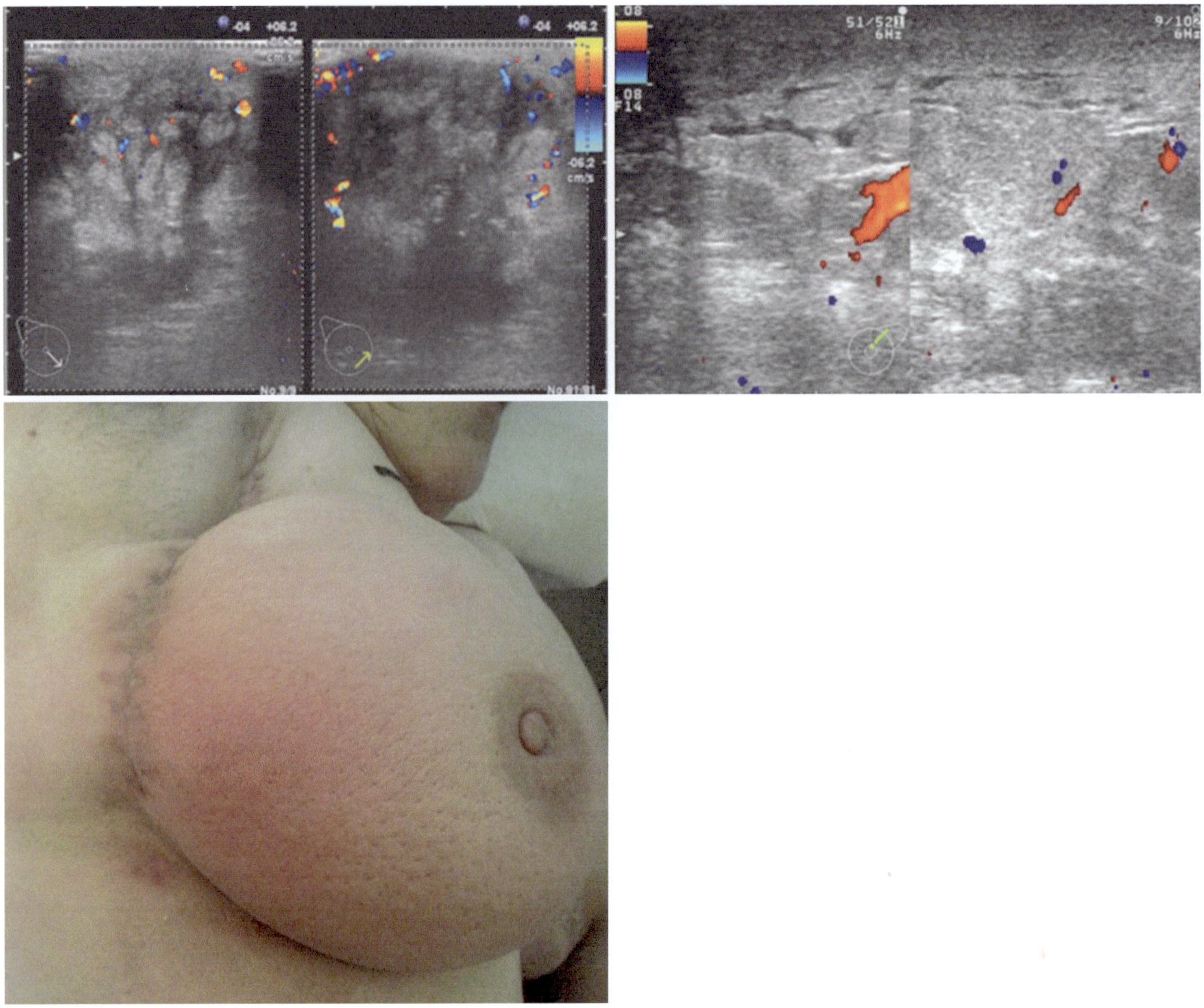

Fig. 9.21 Carcinomatous mastitis: large, irregular lymphatic spaces with significant new vasculature and acoustic shadowing (*left*) as compared with benign lymphedema, parallel to the skin lymphatics, with diffuse hyperechogenicity, and with moderate Doppler signal (*right*) (EPOSTM Vienna 2015, doi: 10.1594/ecr2015/C-0266 [1])

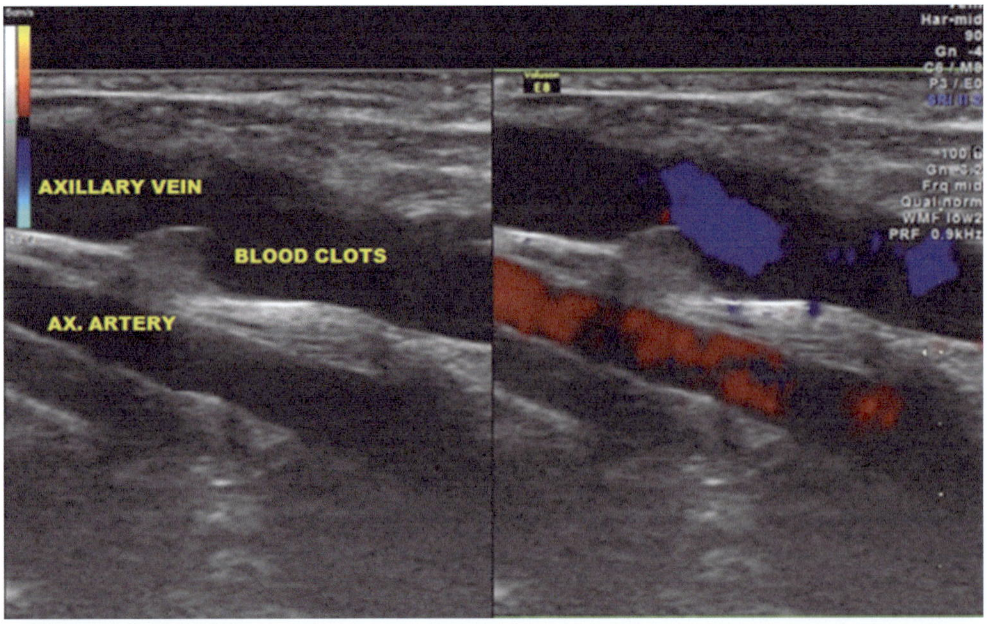

Fig. 9.22 Postsurgical upper limb edema and partial thrombosis of the axillary vein: the initial/starting location near the venous valves (EPOSTM Vienna 2015, doi: 10.1594/ecr2015/C-0266 [1])

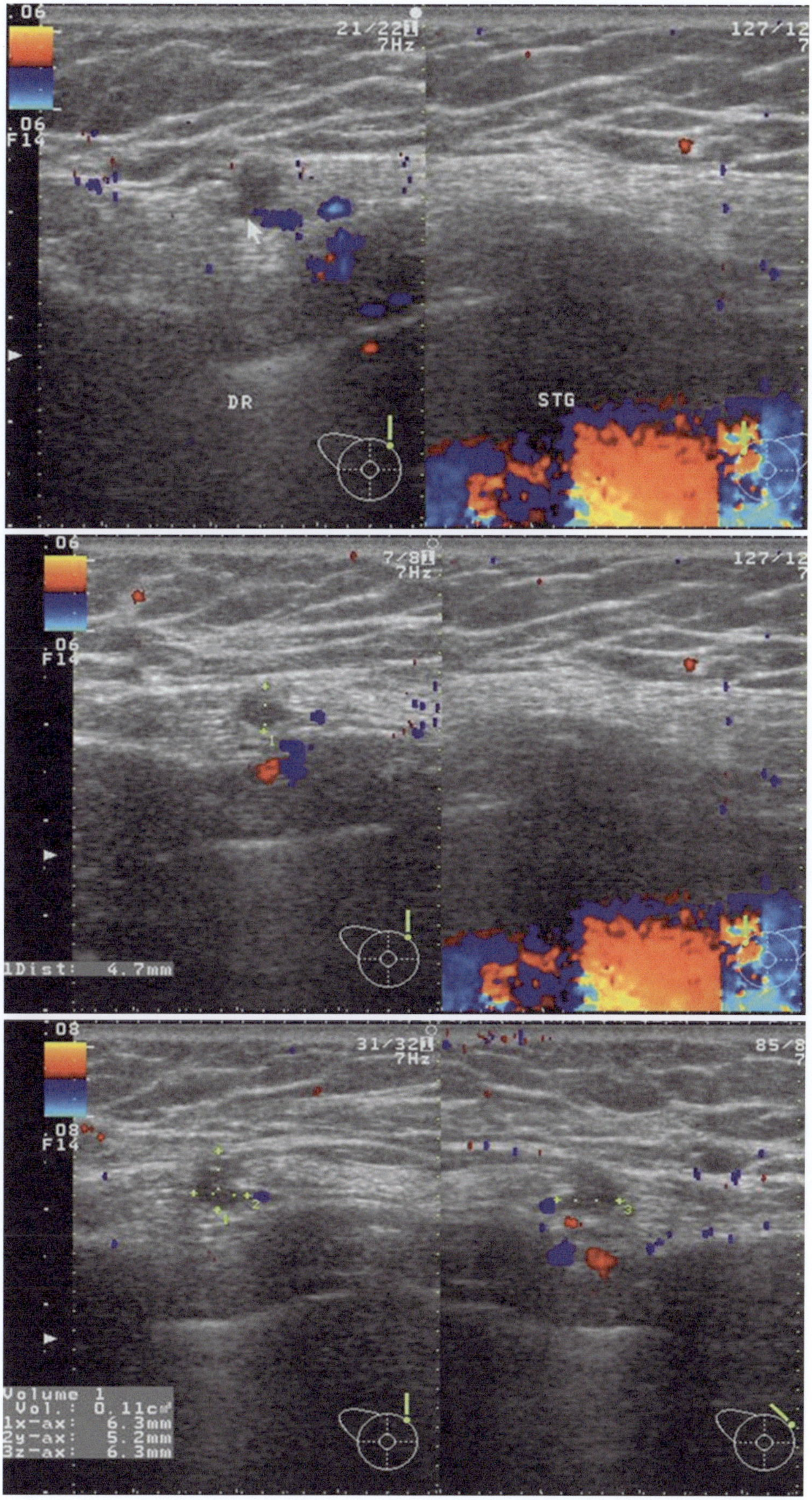

Fig. 9.23 Local recurrent carcinoma in the upper-inner quadrant, located in the parasternal pectoral muscle; the aspect is easy to confirm when compared with the contralateral region, and the malignancy is better characterized by the new vasculature with deep connections

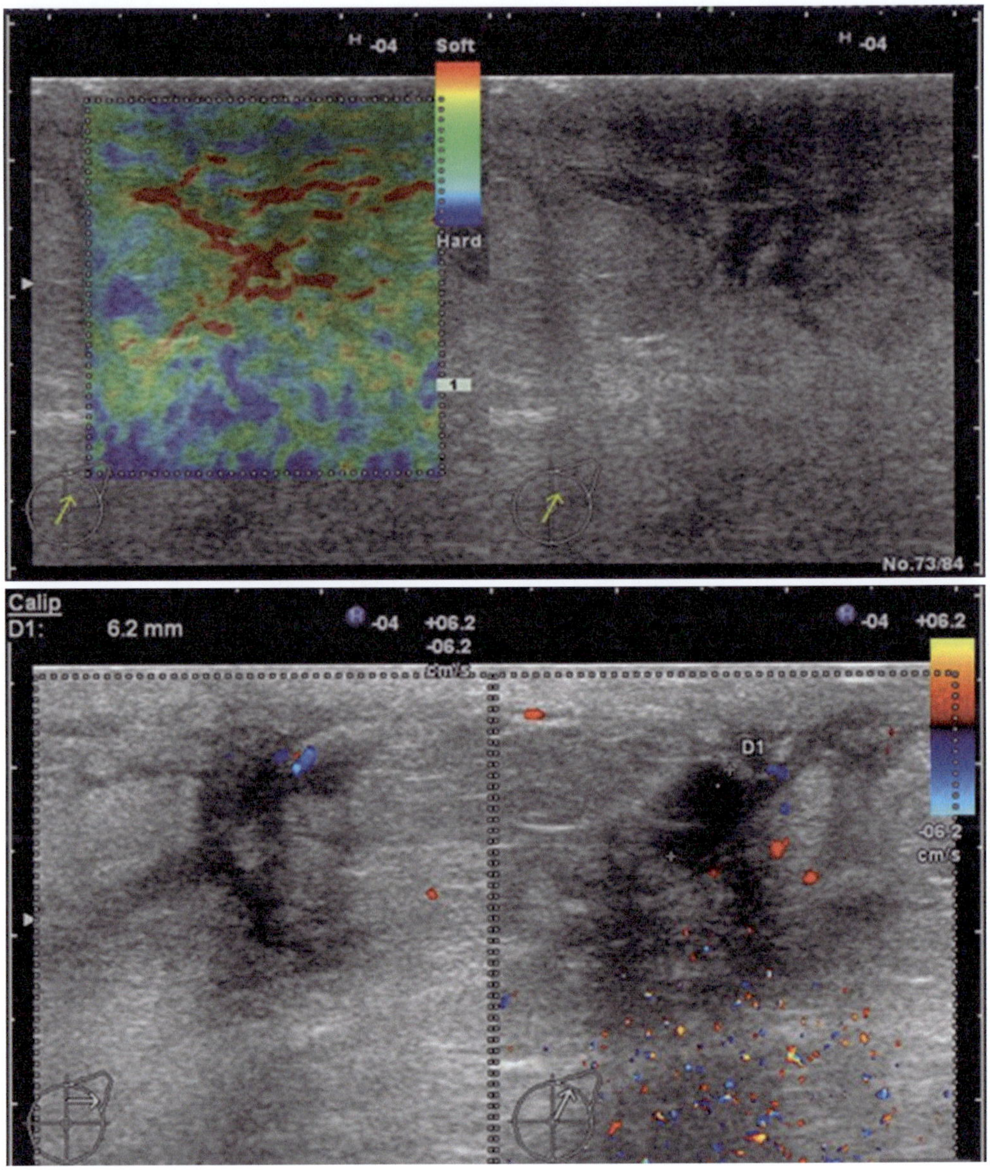

Fig. 9.24 A 62-year-old patient: retroareolar lymphedema (upper), benign scar, and granuloma, better differentiated from malignancy with FBU, despite the equivoque aspect in 2D US. A short-term follow-up is recommended

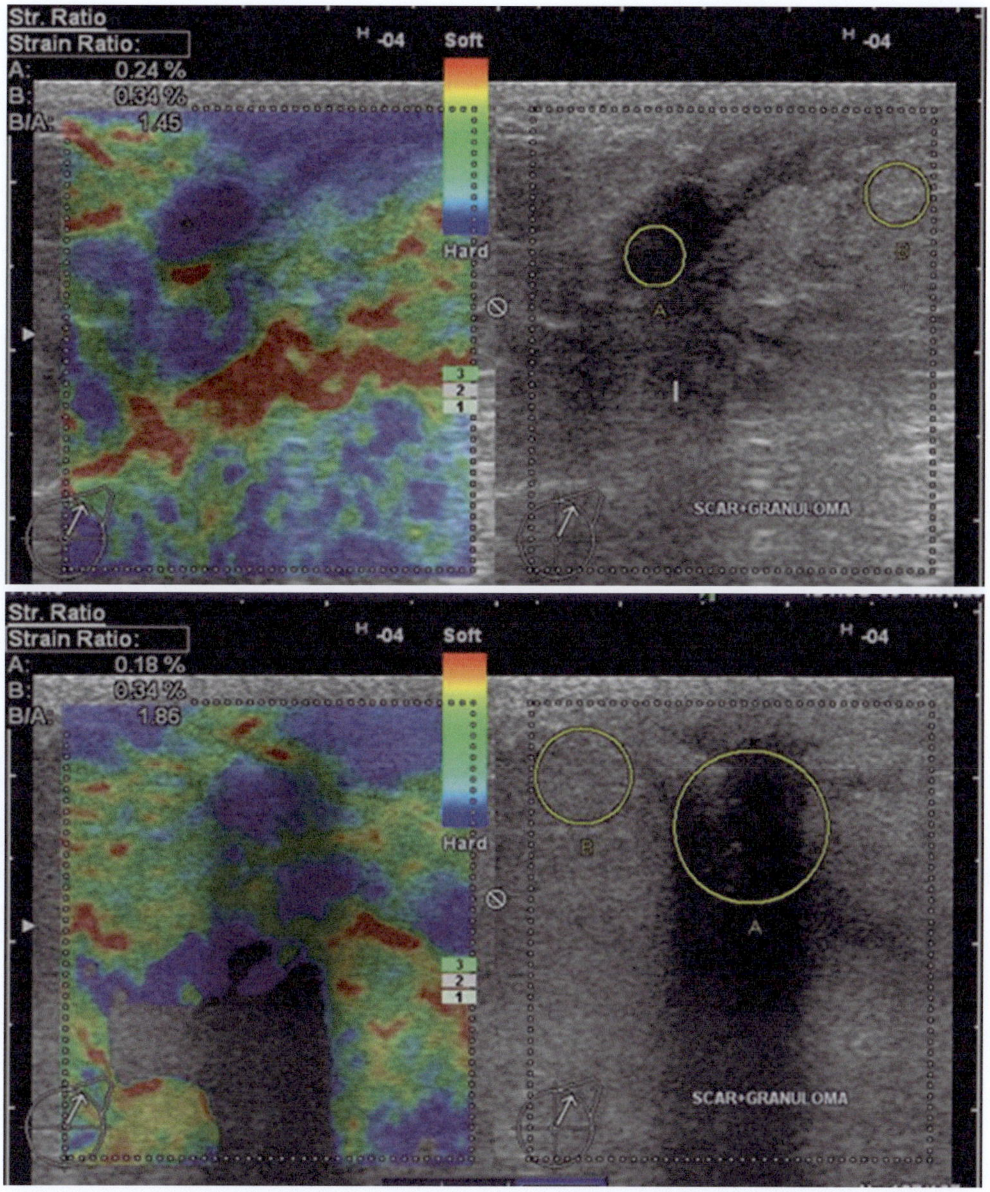

Fig. 9.24 (continued)

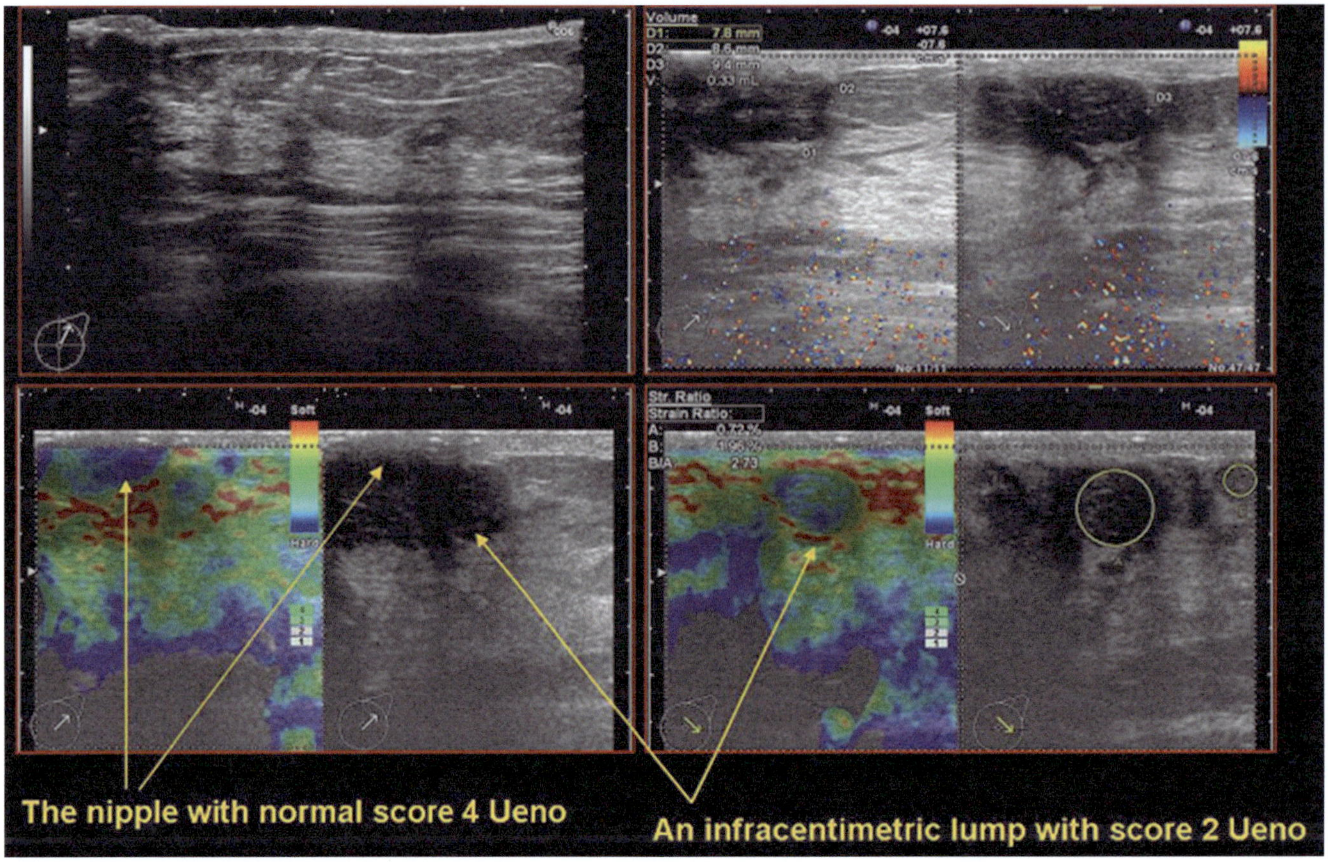

Fig. 9.25 A 44-year-old patient with remnant periareolary tumor: FBU illustrates a "solid", benign-type tumor (EPOSTM Vienna 2015, doi: 10.1594/ecr2015/C-0266 [1])

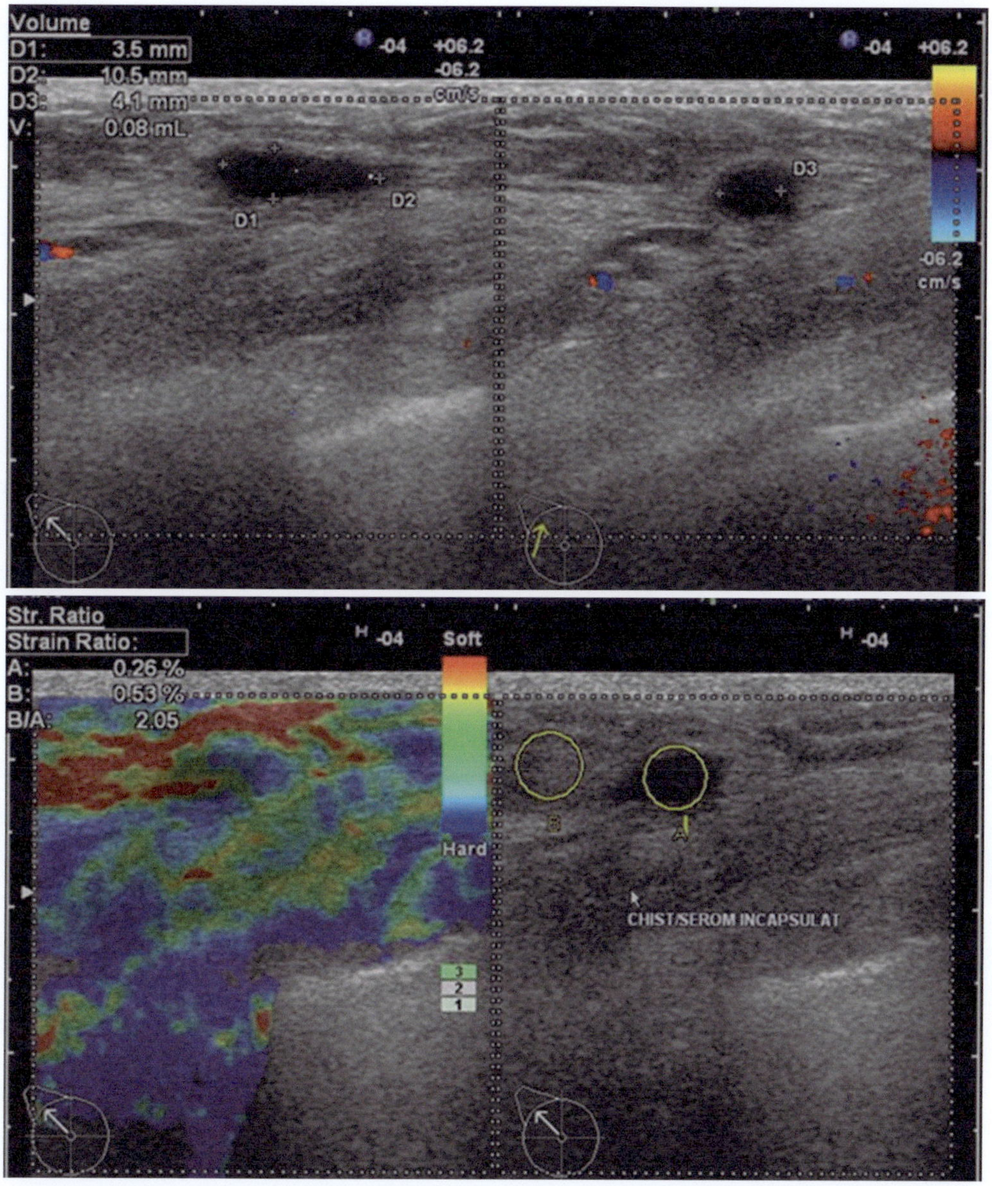

Fig. 9.26 A 35-year-old patient: residual seroma 14 months postmammectomy, with BGR score in sonoelastography; the thickened wall is secondary to the radiotherapy and long-term evolution

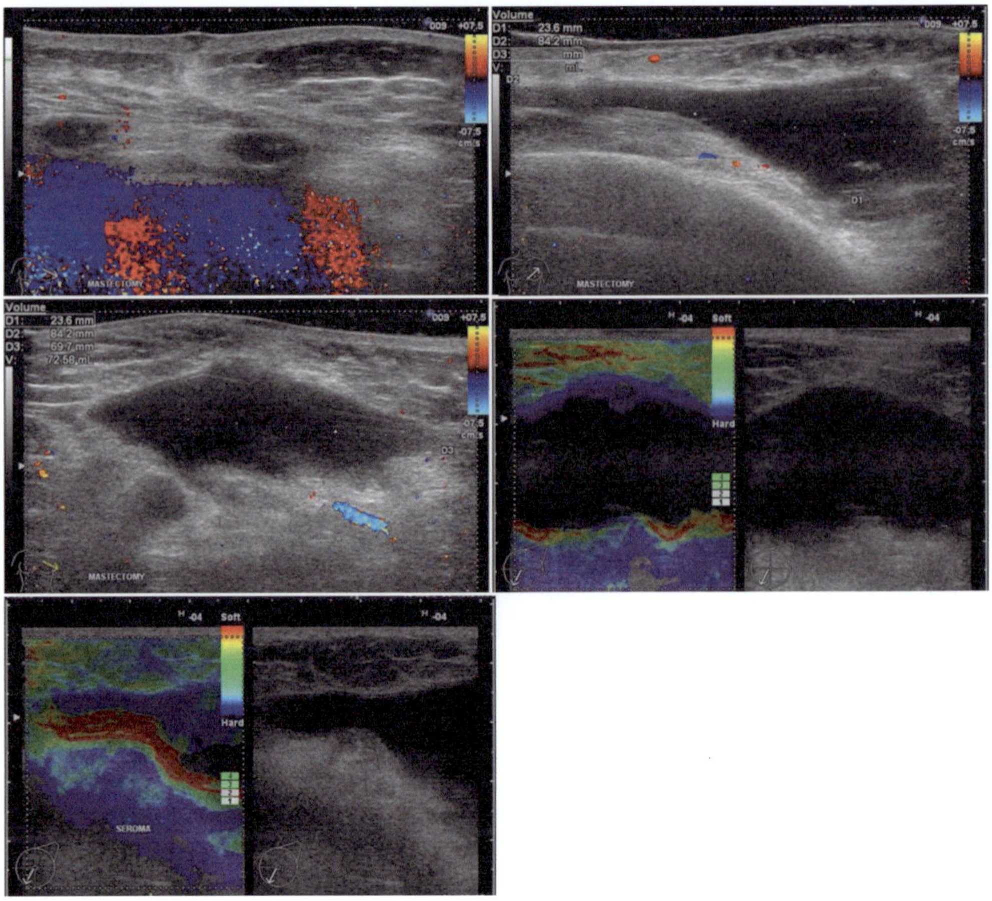

Fig. 9.27 A 48-year-old patient: large seroma post left breast conservative surgery, on radial and antiradial scans with a water-bag 9 cm length transducer; RTSE with short high-frequency transducer on the central region presents artifact because of the great diameters, but at the periphery demonstrates the typical BGR score for fluids

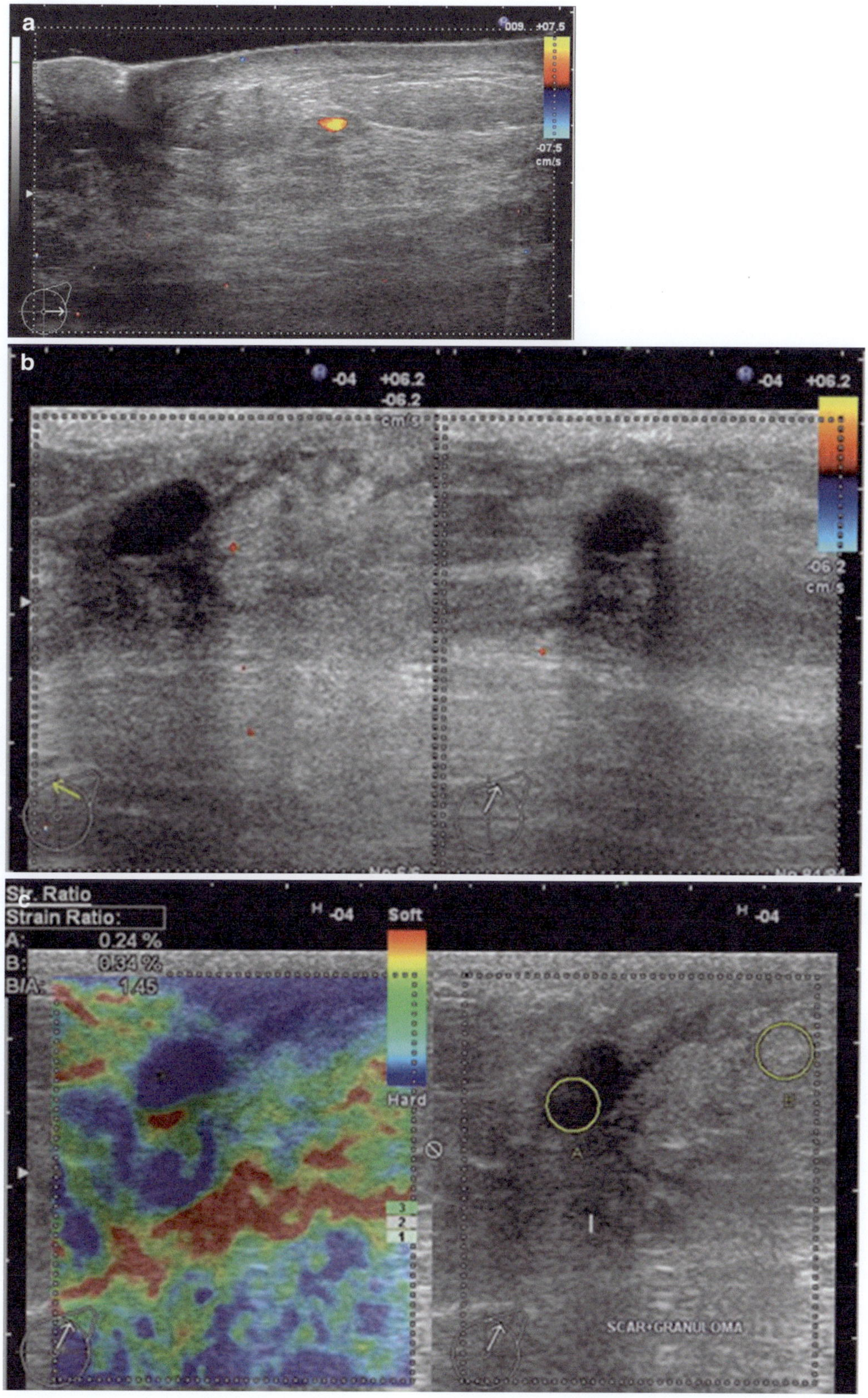

Fig. 9.28 A 62-year-old patient with a scar post conservative surgical treatment of breast cancer in the upper-outer left quadrant, followed by radiotherapy, associated with complex changes: follow-up FBUS illustrates breast edema with skin thickening and hyperechoic premammary fatty tissue (**a**), a cystic lesion in the scar area with BGR score (**b**, **c**), a suspect segment of the scar with classical US features of malignant type (**d**) but presenting a score 3 Ueno with low FLR (1.86) and retroareolar edema (**e**)

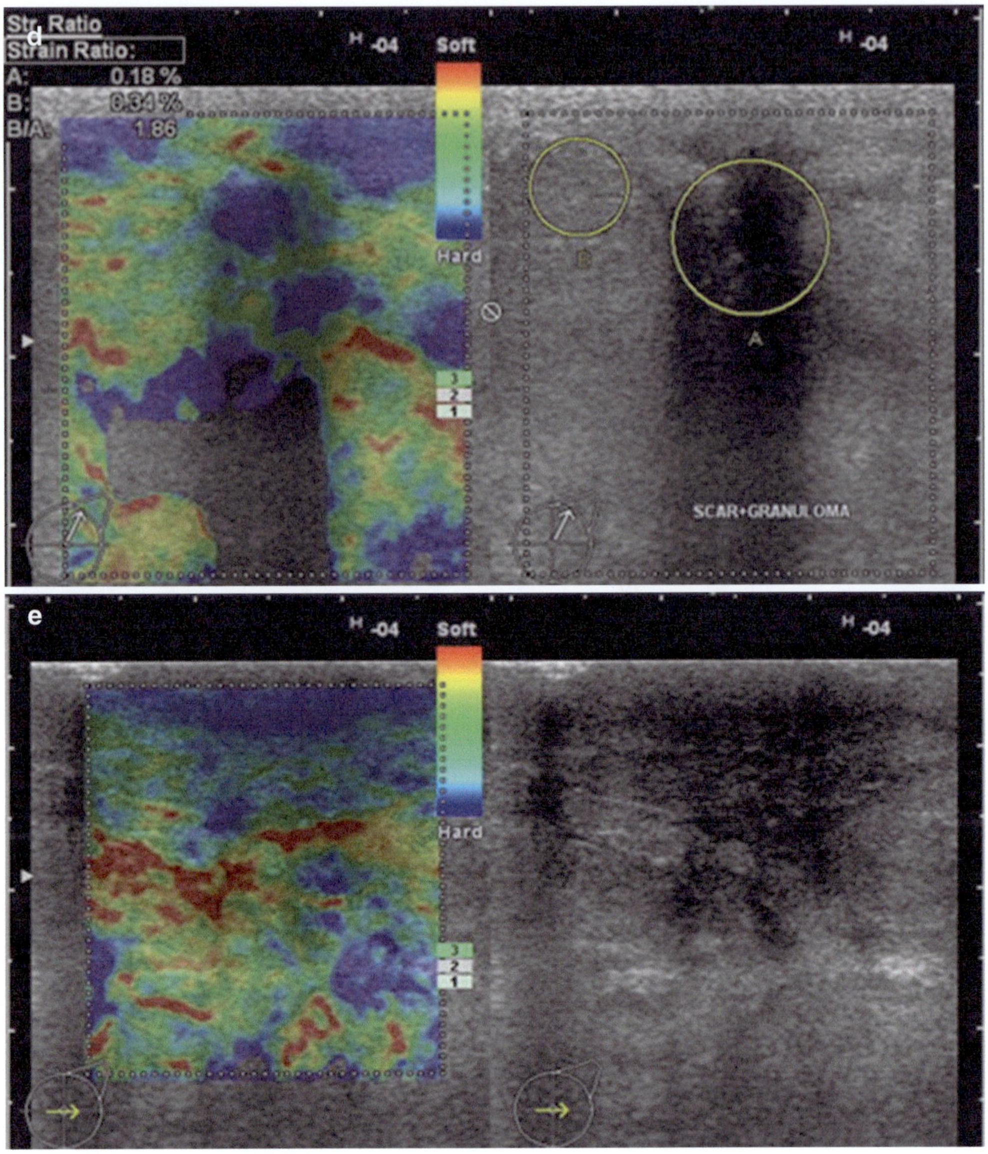

Fig. 9.28 (continued)

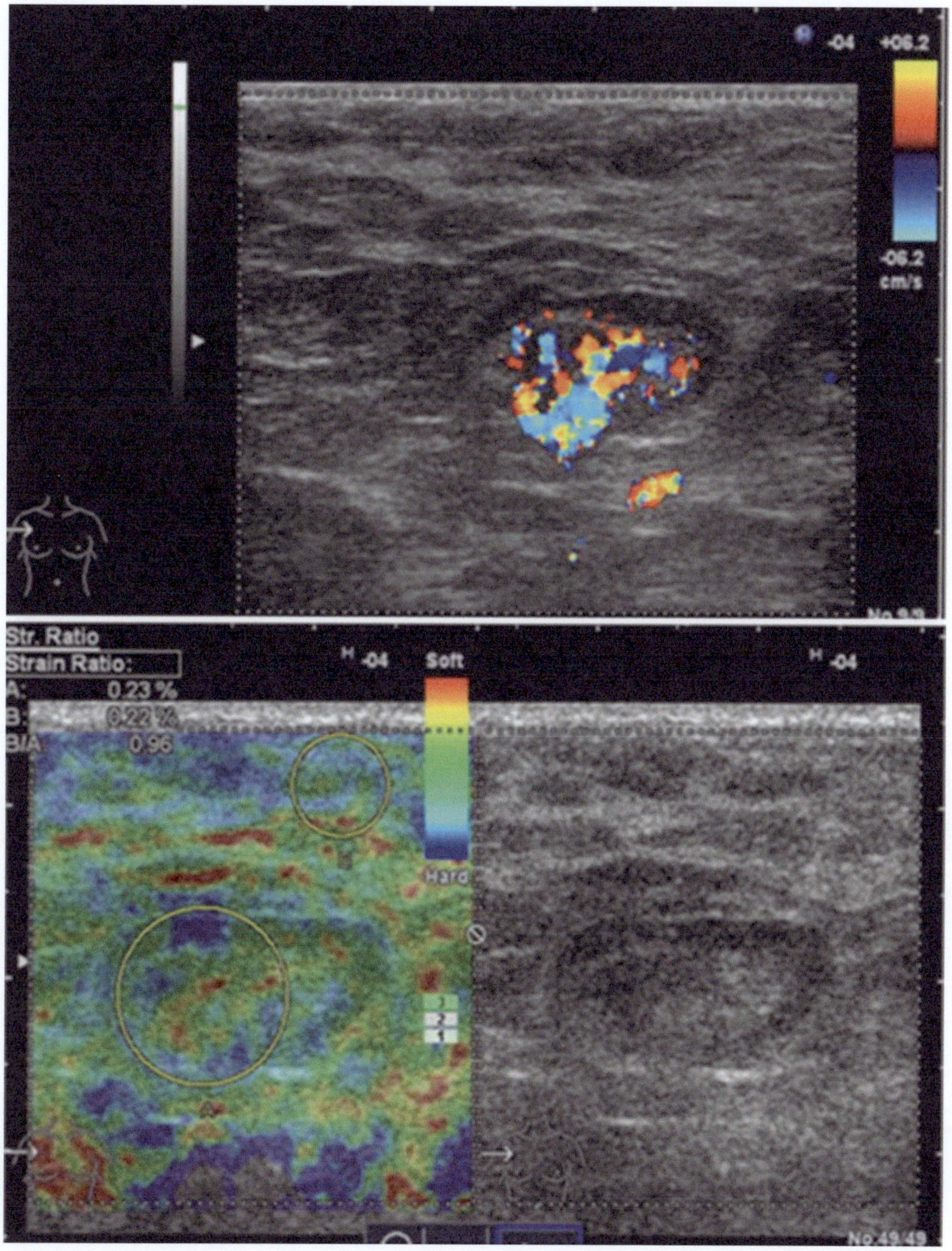

Fig. 9.29 FBU in benign-type remnant lymph nodes: when the vasculature is increased in the sinus, without cortical changes, an acute inflammation is present, while a hypoechoic aspect of the central part of the sinus is correlated with benign histiocytosis in chronic lymphadenitis (EPOSTM Vienna 2015, doi: 10.1594/ecr2015/C-0266 [1])

Fig. 9.29 (continued)

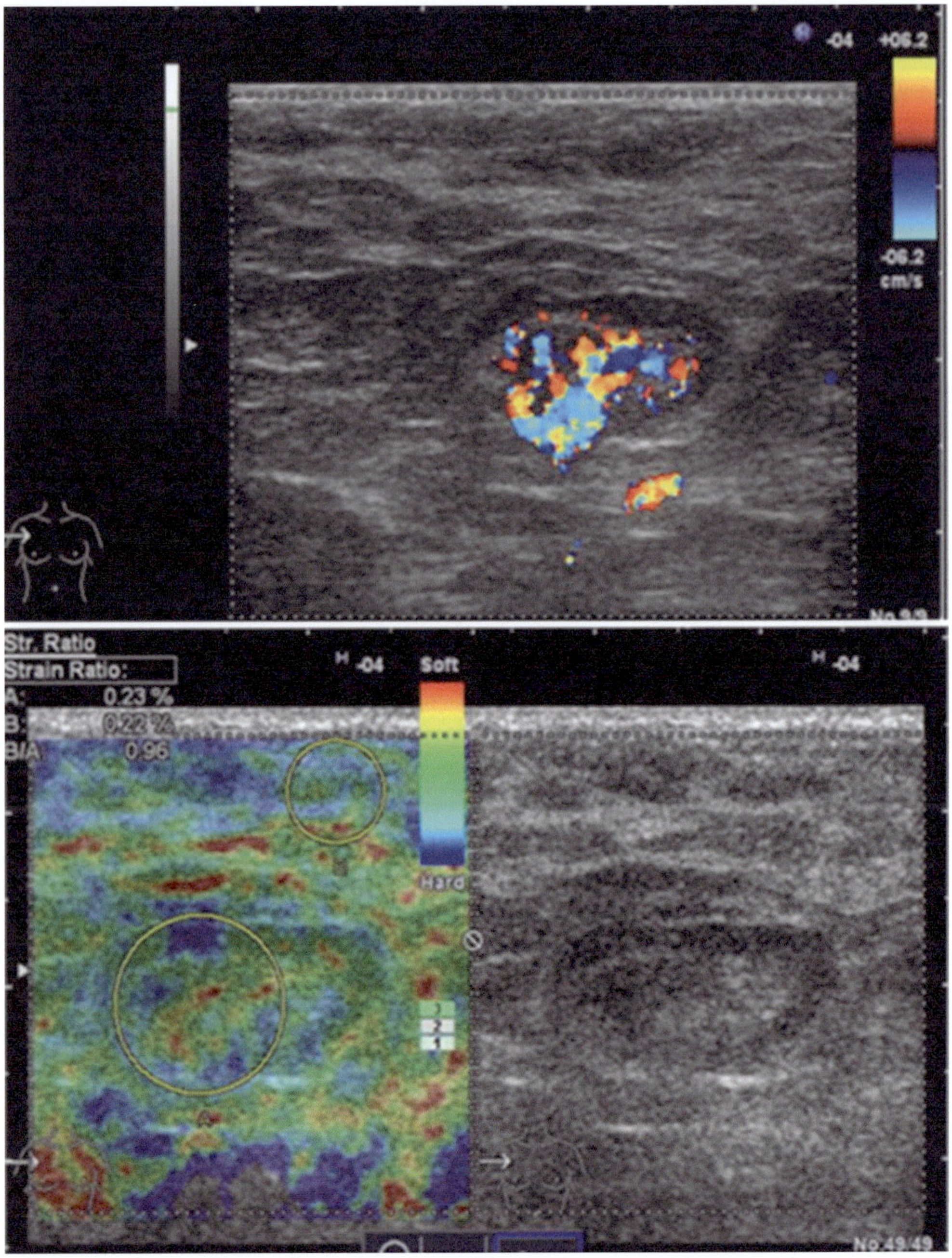

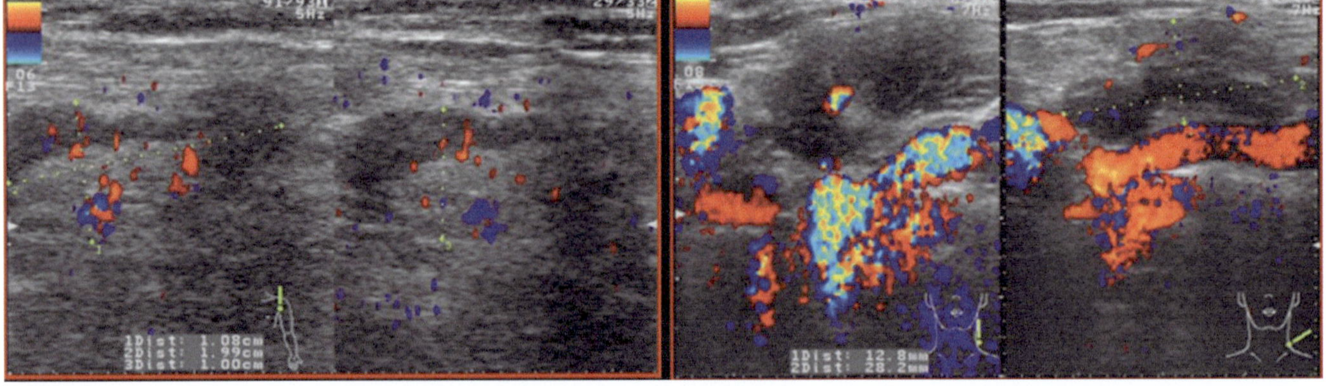

Fig. 9.30 A 38-year-old patient: remnant axillary borderline lymph nodes with increased cortical thickness and focal cortical new vasculature; more salient changes in the supraclavicular nodes (EPOSTM Vienna 2015, doi: 10.1594/ecr2015/C-0266 [1])

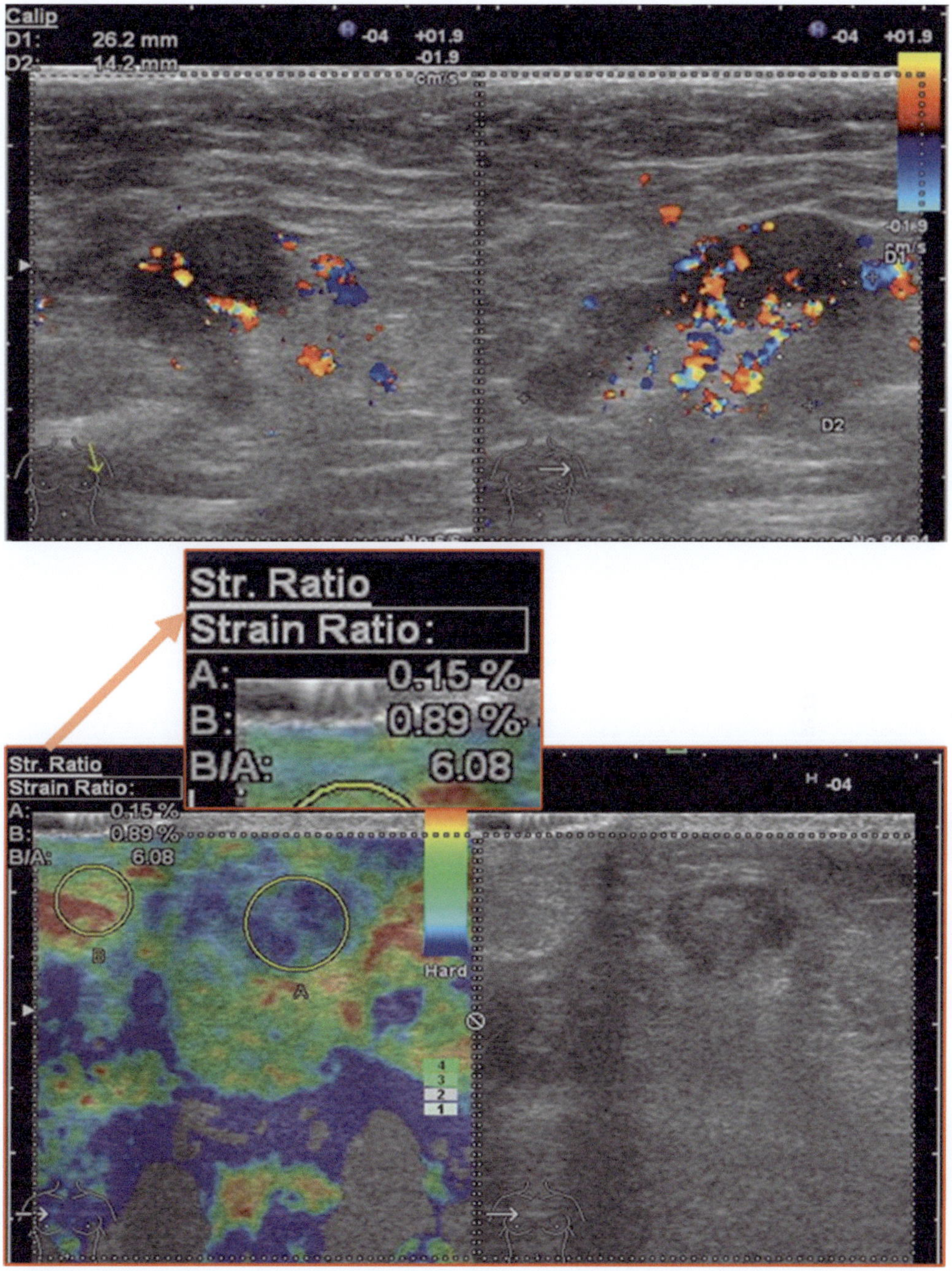

Fig. 9.31 A 65-year-old patient: remnant malignant lymph node after 6 months (radical mammectomy followed by chemotherapy); the excised nodes were normal. The late salient node metastasis had full resolution after supplementary radiotherapy (EPOSTM Vienna 2015, doi: 10.1594/ecr2015/C-0266 [1])

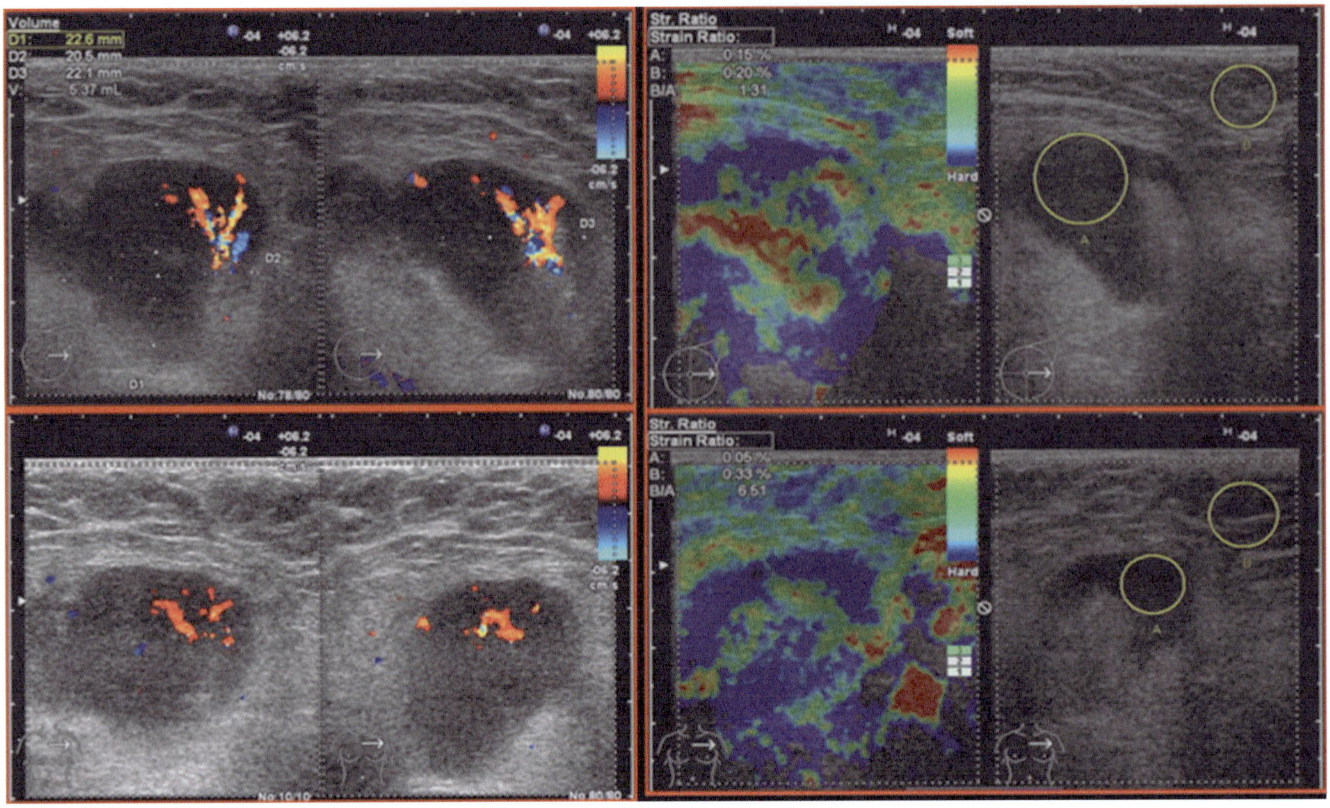

Fig. 9.32 A 64-year-old patient: remnant malignant lymph node with necrosis, complex BGR score, but high FLR; lymph nodes necrosis may be frequently present after chemotherapy or after previous biopsy (EPOSTM Vienna 2015, doi: 10.1594/ecr2015/C-0266 [1])

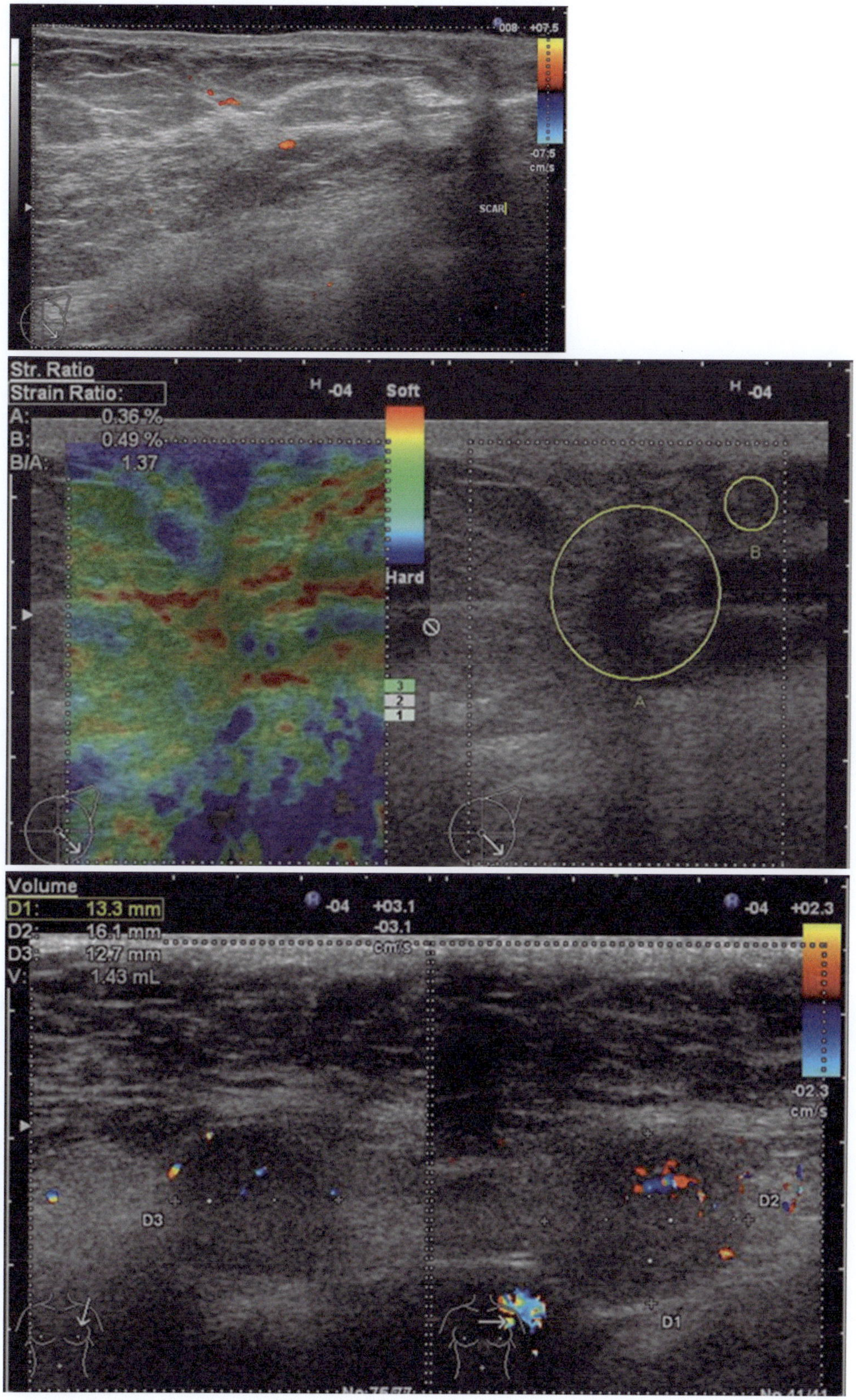

Fig. 9.33 A 66-year-old patient with bilateral medullary breast carcinoma; conservative surgical treatment in the left breast 2 years ago, with follow-up FBU that illustrates benign breast scar, but with a remnant axillary lymph node, with loss of architecture, new vasculature, and score 4 Ueno with high FLR of 126.6, concordant with the contrast CT findings (EPOSTM Vienna 2015, doi: 10.1594/ecr2015/C-0266 [1])

Fig. 9.33 (continued)

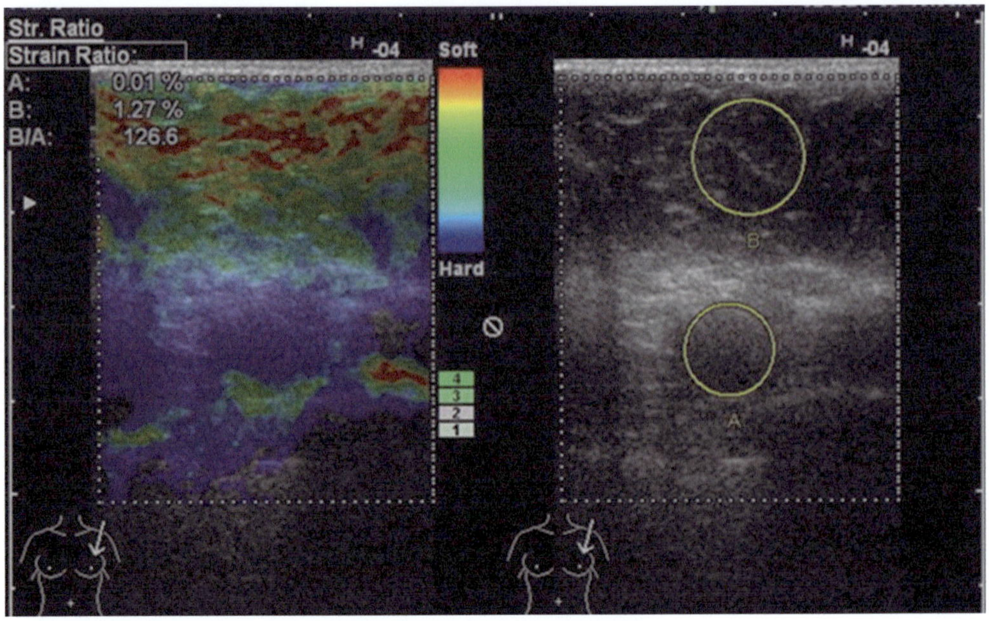

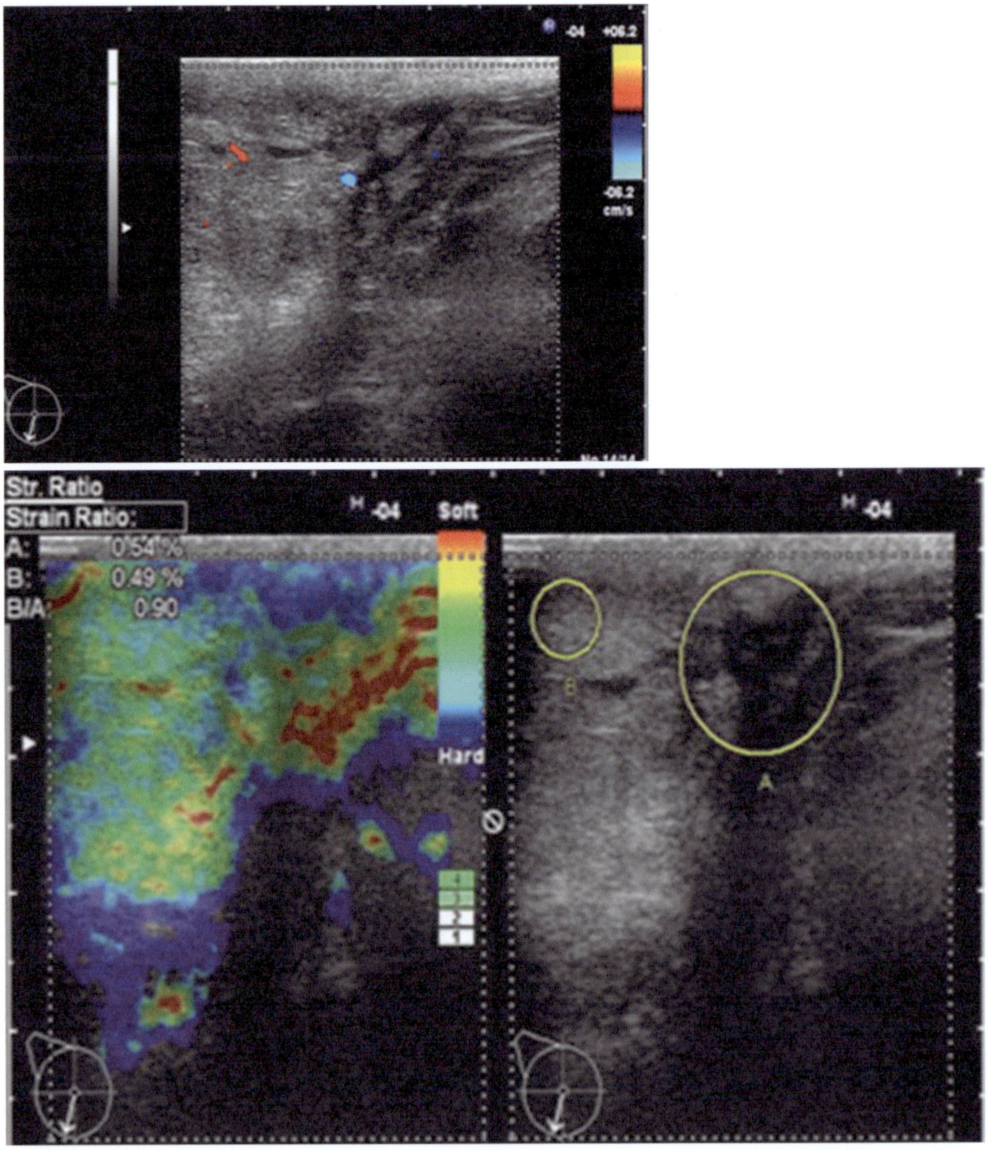

Fig. 9.34 A 66-year-old patient, the same case: conservative surgical treatment 10 months ago in the right breast; FBU presents benign aspect both of the breast scar (*upper* scans) and of the hypertrophic axillary scar (*bottom*)

Fig. 9.34 (continued)

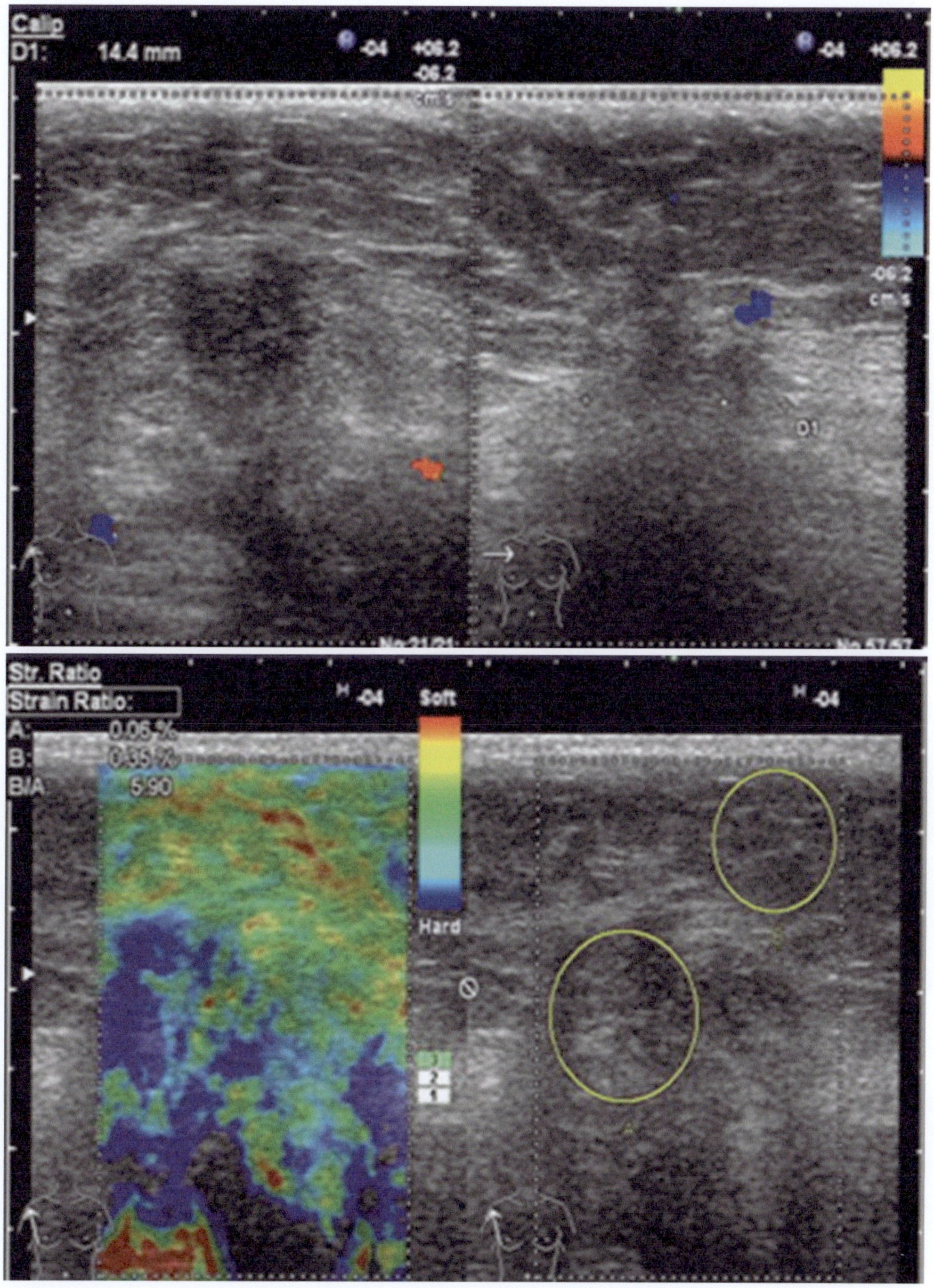

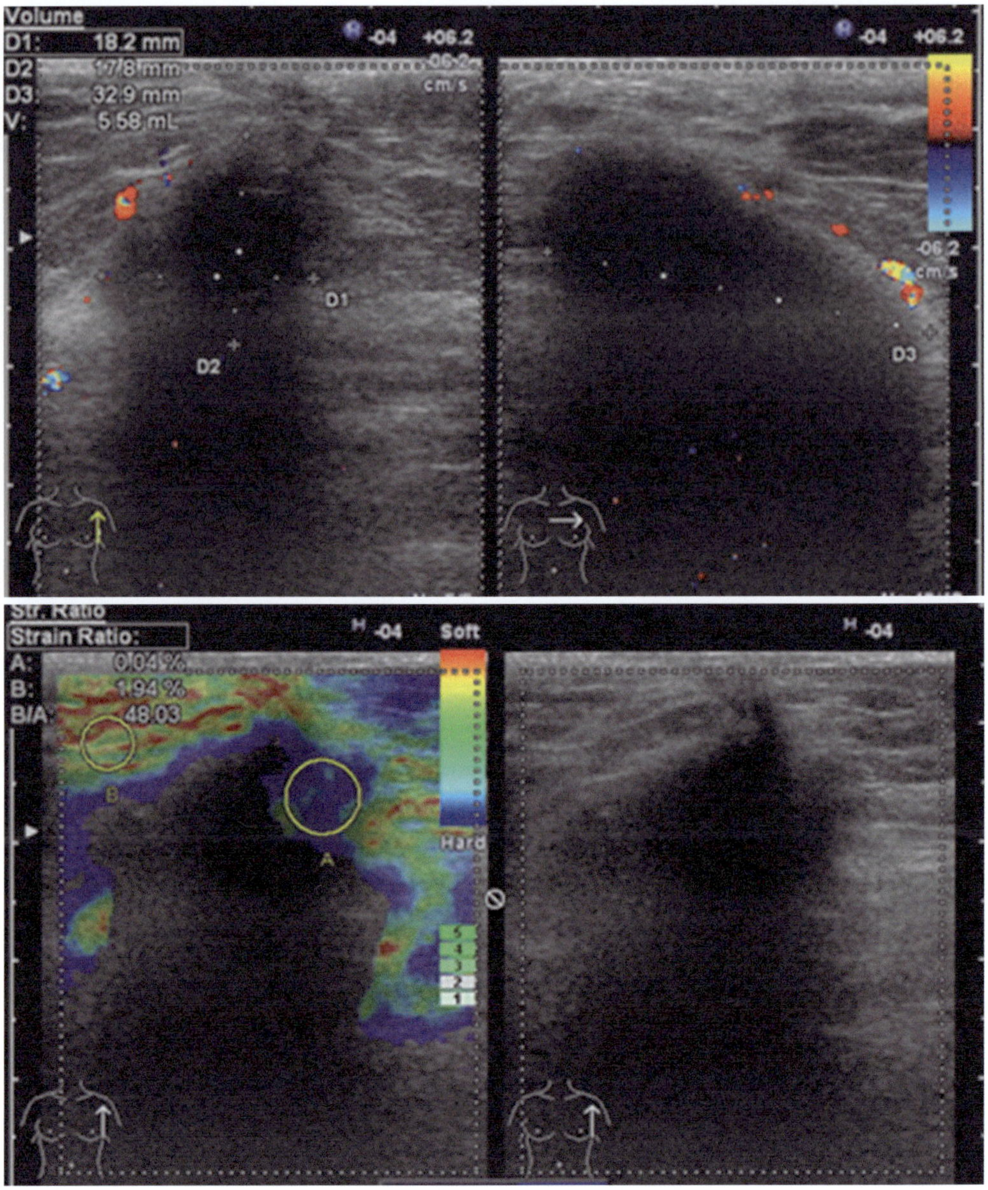

Fig. 9.35 A 62-year-old patient: pseudotumoral mass represented by chronic remnant fluid collection insufficiently drained after the surgical treatment, located under the axillary scar, presents a hard, fibrous contour, mimicking malignancy on US and RTSE, but without any internal Doppler signal; multiplanar reconstructions CT present even in the native acquisitions the hyperdense wall and the fluid density in the center of the left axillary lesion (*white arrow*)

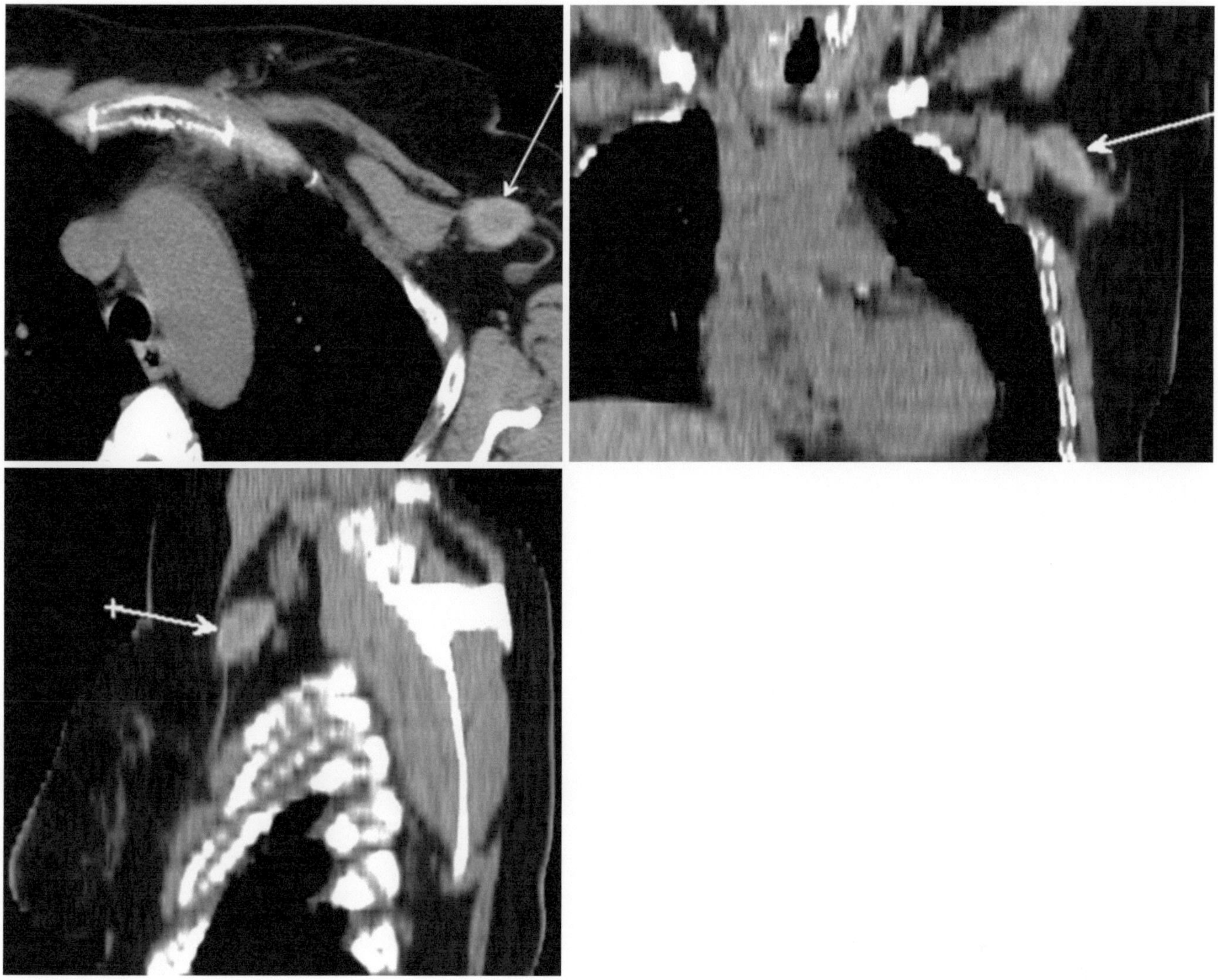

Fig. 9.35 (continued)

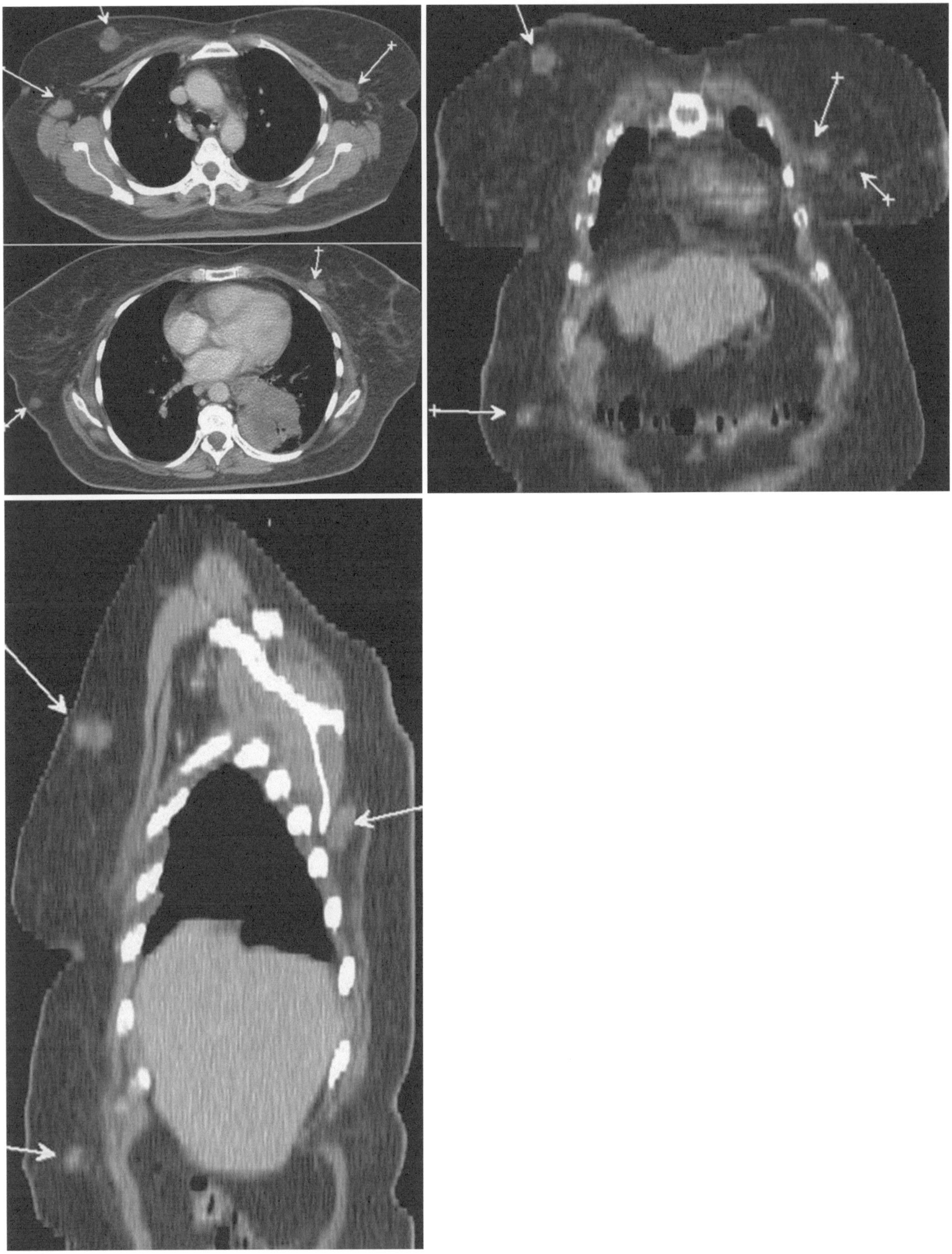

Fig. 9.36 Differential diagnosis: multiple subcutaneous metastases of breast cancer involving breast, thoracic, and abdominal regions are better demonstrated by multidetector CT with multiplanar reconstructions (*white arrows*); the axillae there are detected similar metastases not related to the lymph nodes

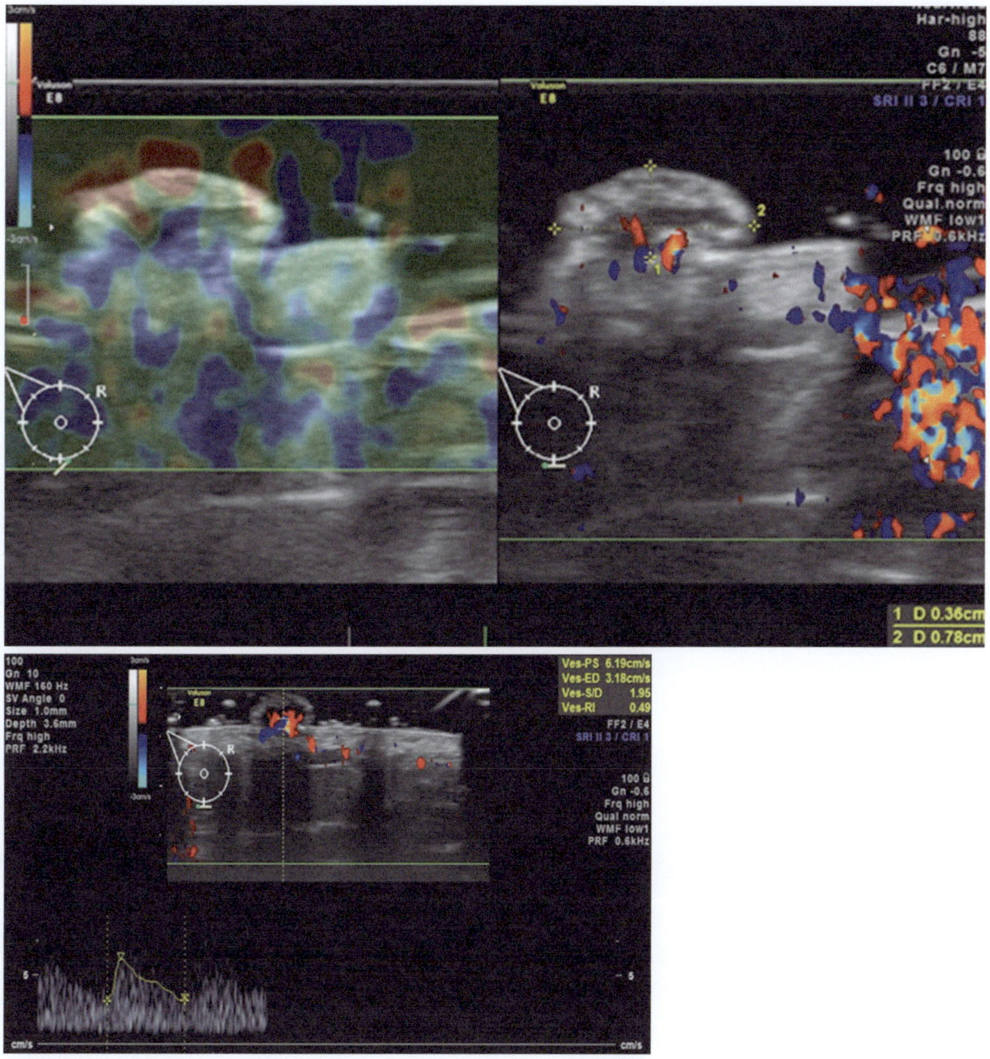

Fig. 9.37 Differential diagnosis: epithelioma in the submammary sulcus—the tumor is strictly located in the skin, without extension under the dermal basal membrane, and has a vascular axis and an intermediate strain (EPOSTM Vienna 2015, doi: 10.1594/ecr2015/C-0266 [1])

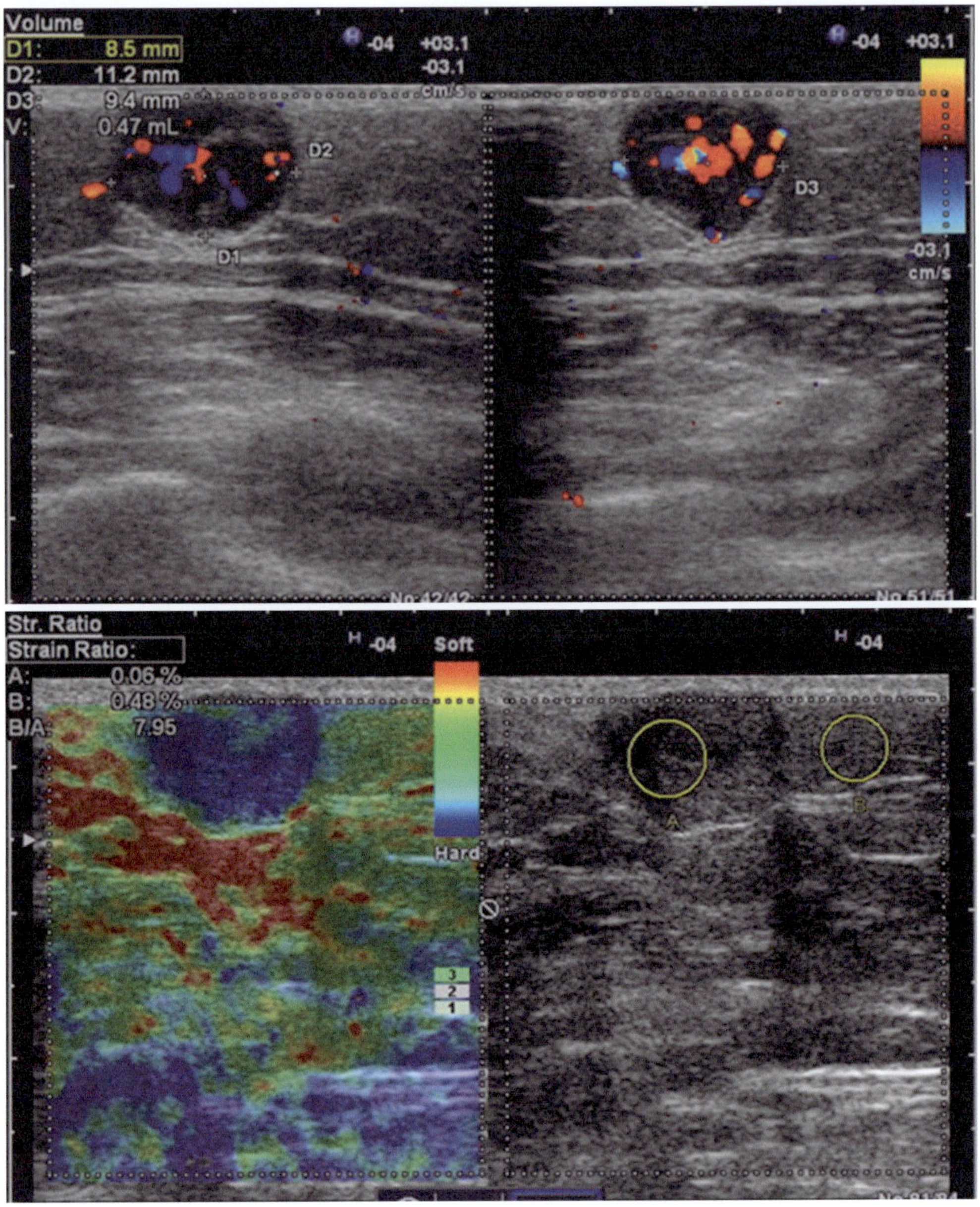

Fig. 9.38 Differential diagnosis: malignant melanoma—the lesion is located between the skin and the fascia superficialis, well delineated, hypoechoic, hypervascular, and with a score 4 Ueno; full US/FBU is useful in detecting small lesions, "buried" in the skin, clinical underestimated (EPOSTM Vienna 2015, doi: 10.1594/ecr2015/C-0266 [1])

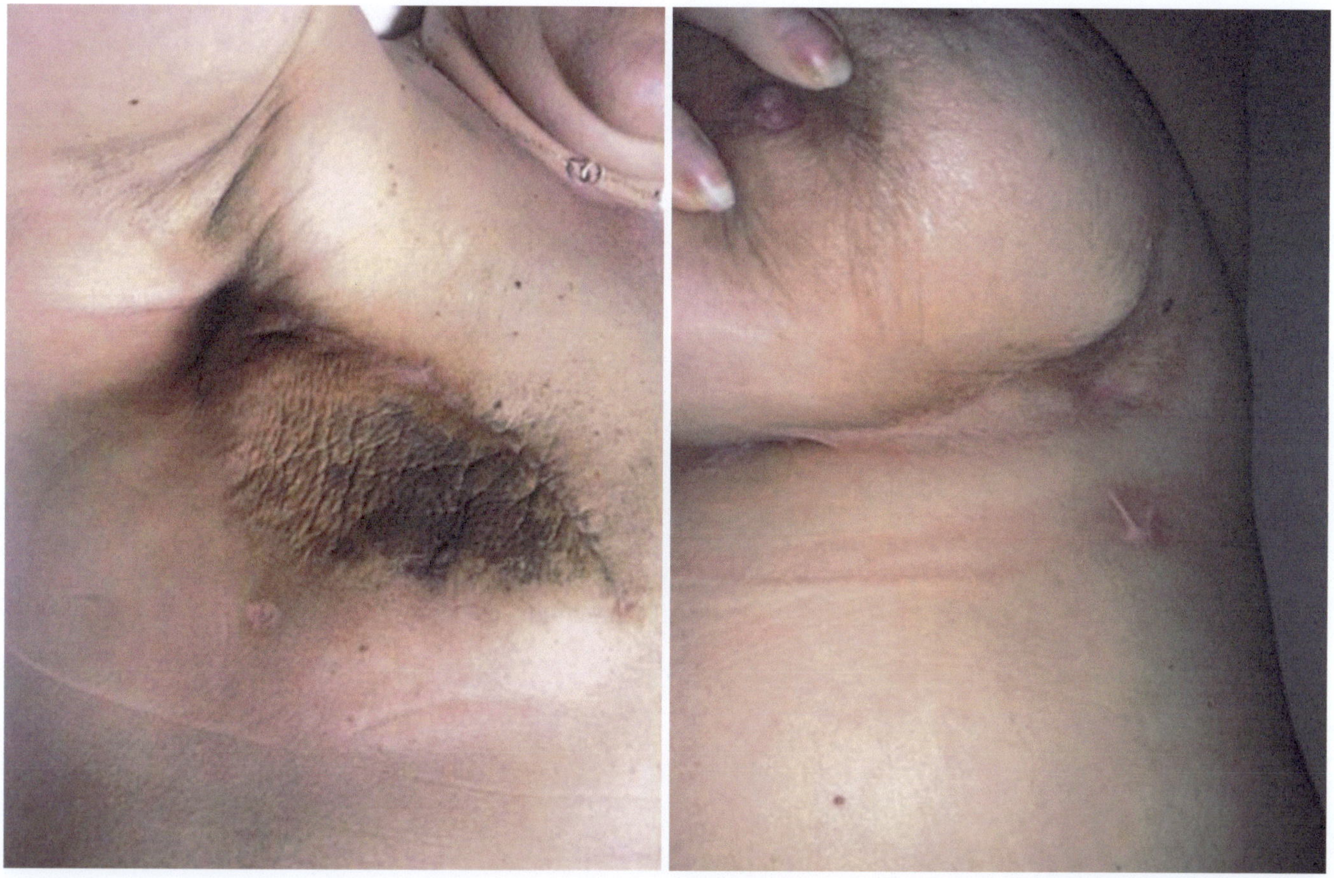

Fig. 9.39 *Left picture*: radical mammectomy followed by radiotherapy, with skin burns—pachydermatous thickening, itching, peeling, and brown pigmentation, partially reversible after several months. *Right picture*: conservative breast cancer surgery followed by radiotherapy presenting breast edema and erythema, skin depigmentation, and thickening with loss of elasticity

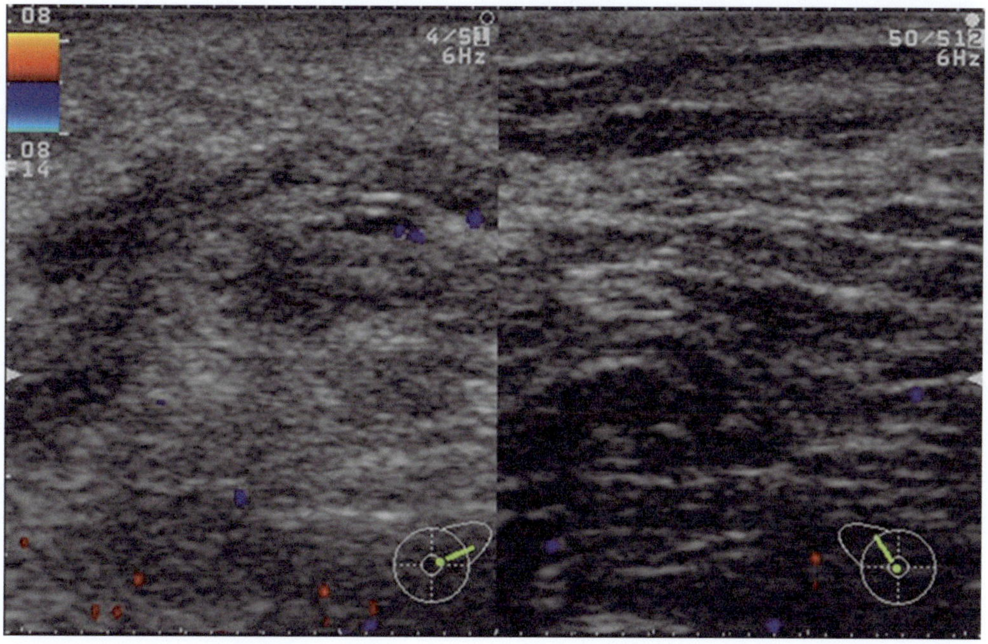

Fig. 9.40 Left breast loss of tissular differentiation and lymphedema with hyperechogenicity after conservative surgery with axillary lymphadenectomy and radiotherapy, compared with the right breast

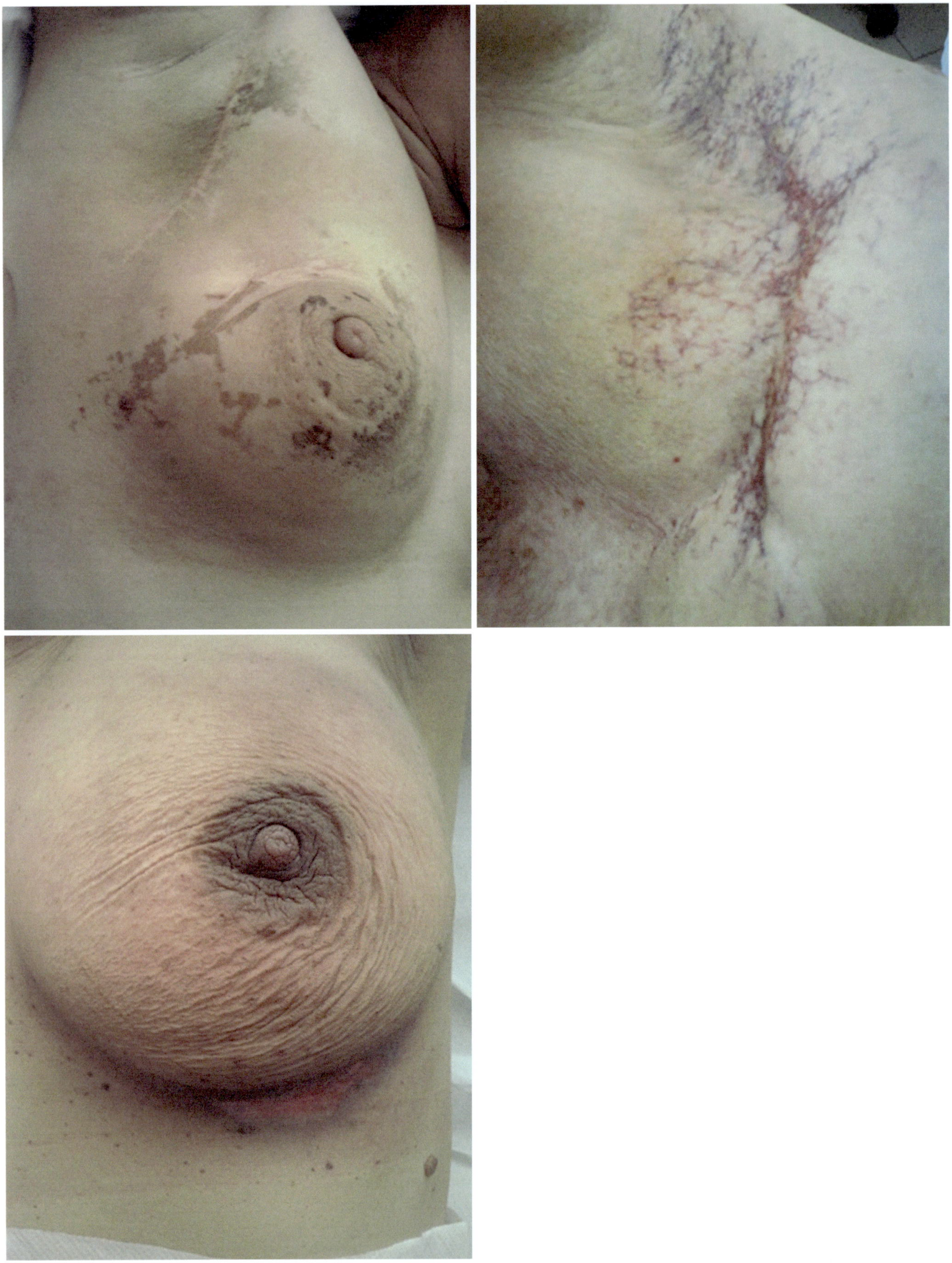

Fig. 9.41 Skin alterations after radiotherapy: inflammatory changes such as edema, erythema, and hyperthermia are usually reversible; pigmentation alterations such as brown geographic areas or depigmentation may be partially reversible. The ulcerations or necrosis are rare but dangerous, because of reduced tissular trophicity and delayed healing; skin vasculitis is a permanent sequel with only esthetical significance

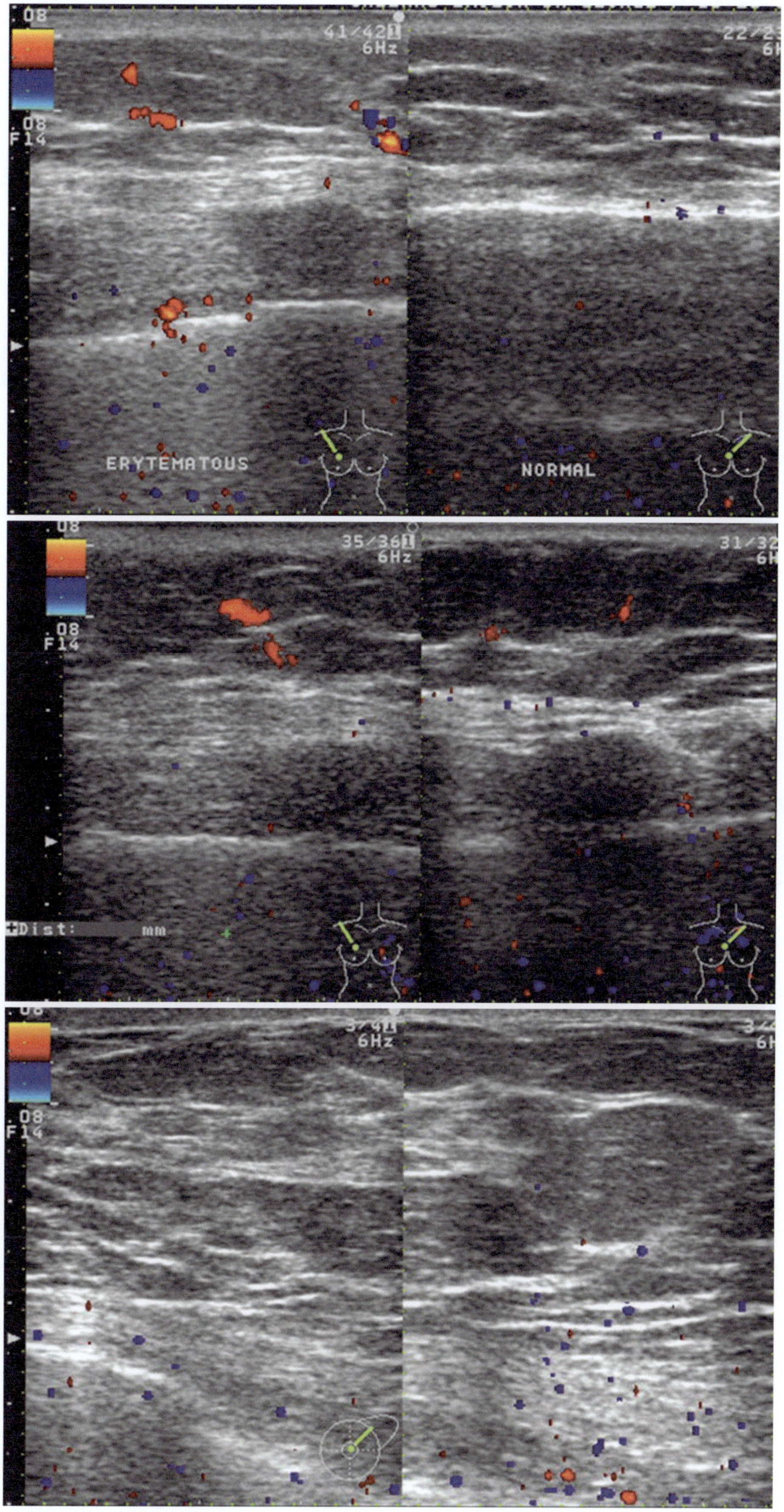

Fig. 9.42 A 76-year-old patient: right breast radiodermatitis strictly located at the irradiation field, clinically with polymorphous erythema; Doppler DE illustrates moderate diffuse hyper-vasculature associated with edema with thickening of all the breast structures: skin, subcutaneous and retromammary fat, breast lobar structures, and pectoral muscles. The limits of the irradiated with the normal nonirradiated tissues are well delimited clinically, and by US, the conserved regions are similar to those of the opposite left breast. US can be used as first intention method in the follow-up of local side effects after radiotherapy

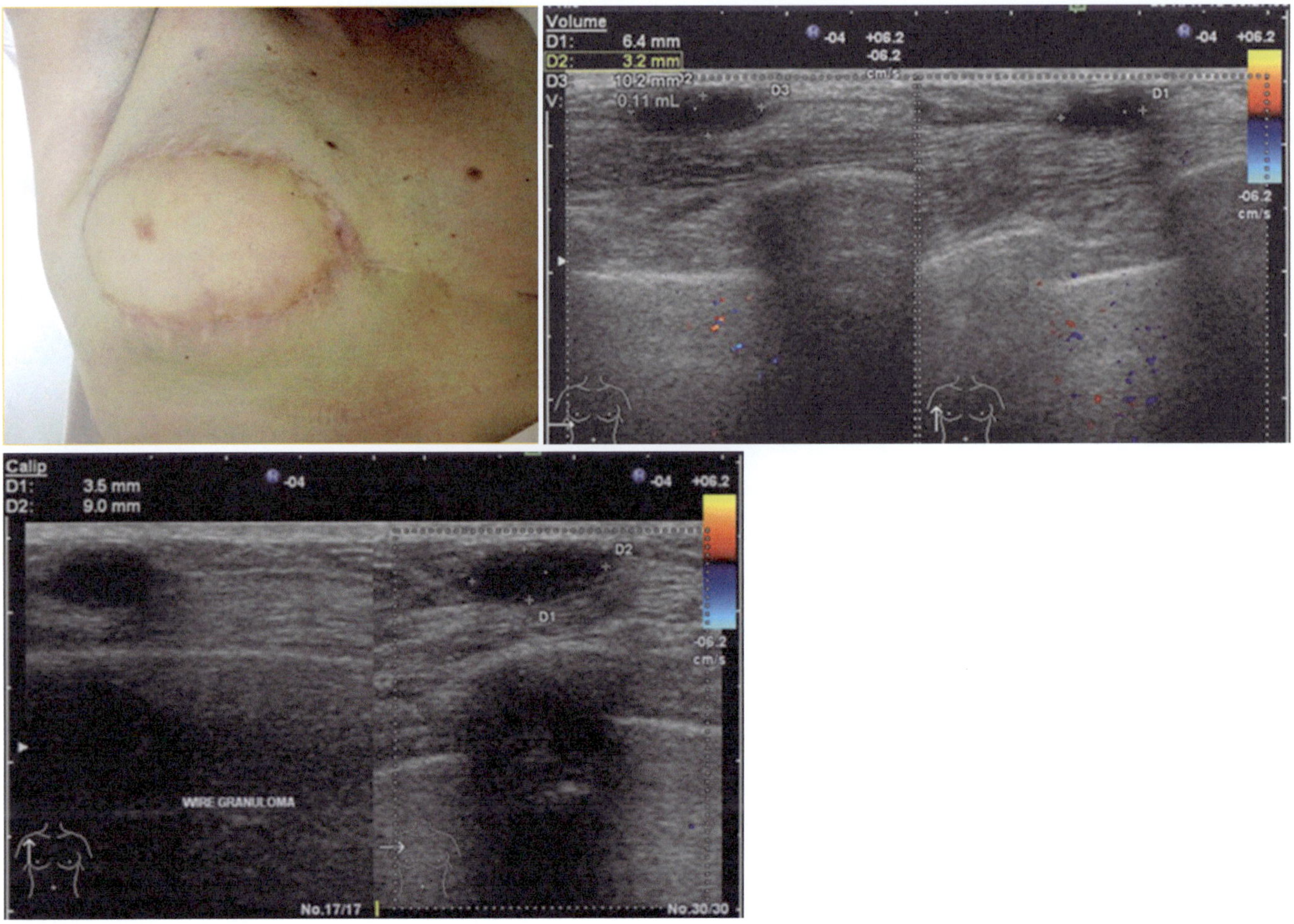

Fig. 9.43 Breast reconstruction with musculocutaneous flap; US survey is recommended for surgical evaluation and detection of the possible secondary malignancies. Suture granuloma with pseudocystic aspect, in the musculocutaneous layer, relatively unchanged after 2 years

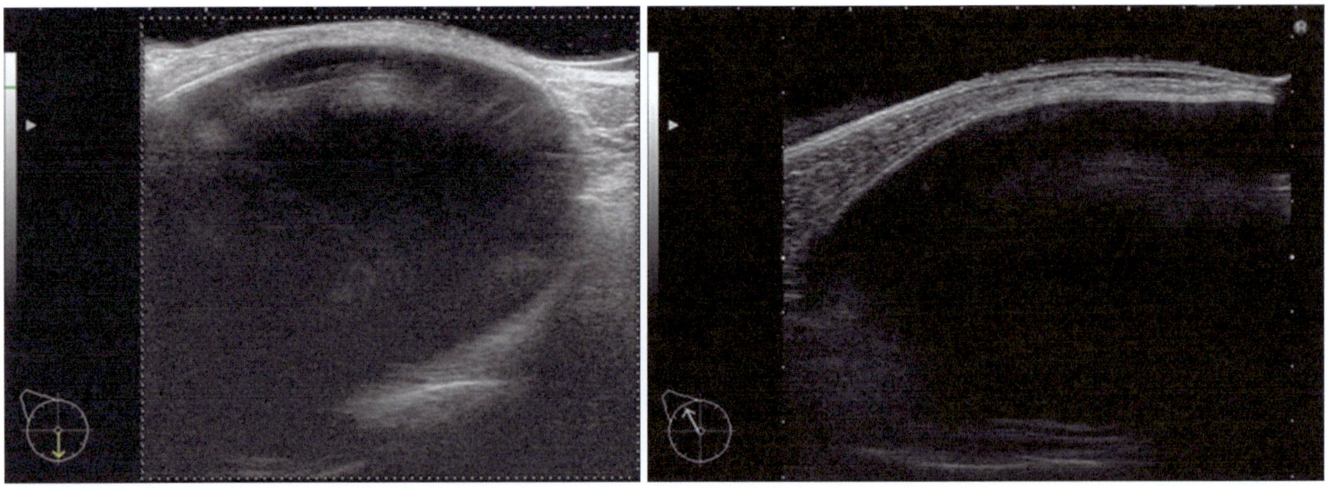

Fig. 9.44 A 35-year-old patient: second step in breast reconstruction with implant—the water bag adapted to the long linear transducer offers the accurate image of the capsule and contents of the prosthesis and the detailed information of the pectoral muscle and of the skin. This technique is painless and safer for the prosthesis as compared with mammography; the acquisitions are faster and cheaper than in the MRI technique

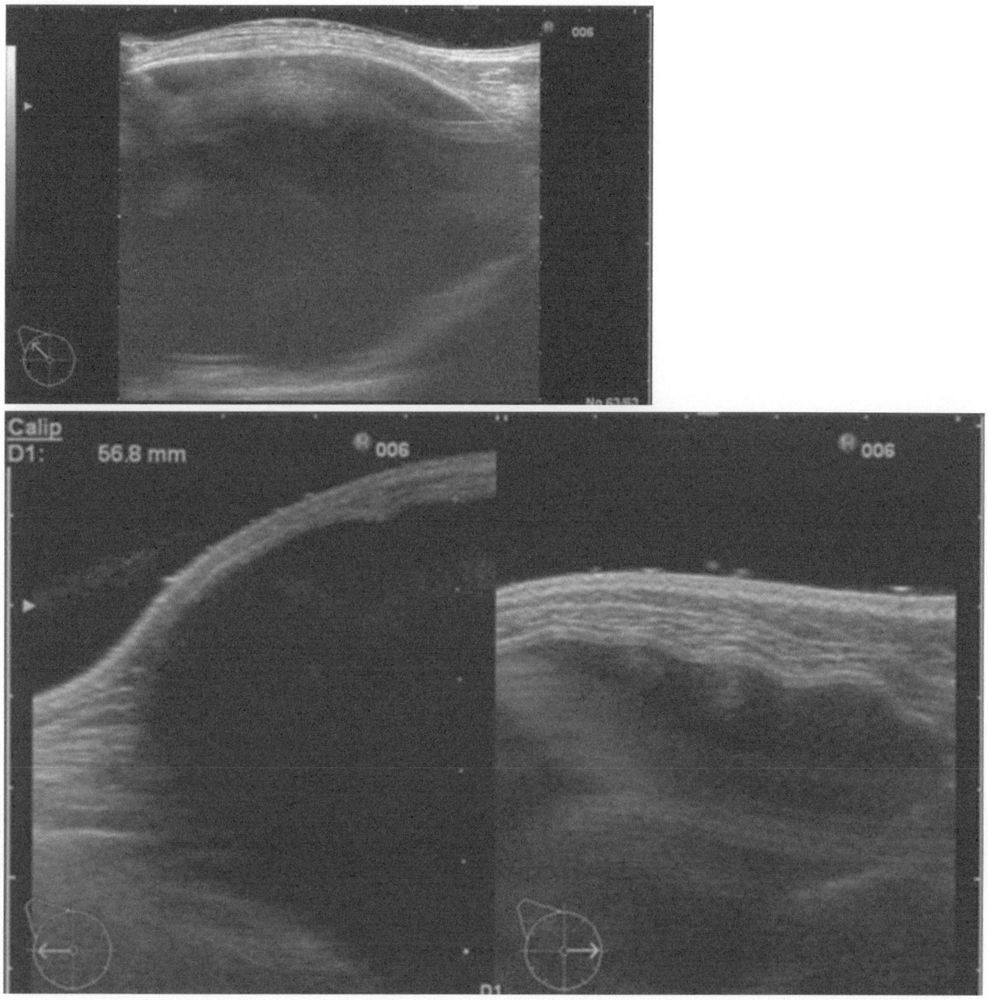

Fig. 9.45 The same case: follow-up examination after 12 months illustrates no malignant secondary lesions, but the prosthesis capsule has folds caused by pericapsular host tissular retraction; the changes are still small, and the surgical revision is not necessary

References

1. Georgescu AC, Andrei E (2015) Full breast ultrasonography as follow-up examination after a complex treatment of breast cancer. ECR Vienna, 2015; at EPOS™, Vienna. doi: 10.1594/ecr2015/C-0266
2. Michel T (2003) Practical ductal echography: guide to intelligent and intelligible Ultrasound imaging of the breast. Saned Editors, Madrid
3. Itoh A, Ueno E, Tohno E et al (2006) Breast Disease: Clinical Application of US Elastography for Diagnosis. Radiology 239:341–350
4. Amy D (2014) Chapter 4. Lobar ultrasonic breast anatomy. In: Francescatti DS, Silverstein MJ (eds) Breast cancer: a new era in management. Springer, New York. doi:10.1007/978-1-4614-8063-1_4
5. Georgescu A, Enachescu V, Bondari A, Bondari S, Manda A, Simionescu C (2011) A new concept: the full breast ultrasound in avoiding false negative and false positive sonographic errors. ECR, Vienna. doi:10.1594/ecr2011/C-0449
6. Aristida G (2012) Introduction in full breast ultrasonography – the unique integrated anatomical approach of breast imaging. SITECH, Craiova
7. Park S, Park HS, Kim SI, Koo JS, Park BW, Lee KS (2011) The Impact of a Focally Positive Resection Margin on the Local Control in Patients Treated with Breast-conserving Therapy. Jpn J Clin Oncol 41(5):600–608. doi:10.1093/jjco/hyr018
8. Han SY, Kim HH (2003) Parasternal sonography of the internal mammary lymphatics in breast cancer. In: 13th international congress on the ultrasonic examination of the breast. International breast ultrasound school. The 10th meeting of Japan Association of Breast and Thyroid Sonology
9. Fisher BJ, Perera FE, Cooke A et al (1997) Long-term follow-up of axillary node-positive breast cancer patients receiving adjuvant systemic therapy alone: patterns of recurrence. Int J Radiat Oncol Biol Phys 38(3):541–550
10. Arriagada R, Le MG, Rochard F (1996) Conservative treatment versus mastectomy in early breast cancer: patterns of failure with 15 years of follow-up data. Institut Gustave-Roussy Breast Cancer Group. J Clin Oncol 14(5):1558–1564
11. Obedian E, Fischer DB, Haffty BG (2000) Second Malignancies after Treatment of Early-Stage Breast Cancer: Lumpectomy and Radiation Therapy Versus Mastectomy. J Clin Oncol 18(12):2406–2412
12. Tot T (2007) The theory of the sick breast lobe and the possible consequences. Int J Surg Pathol 1:68–71
13. Vitung FA, Newman AL (2007) Complications in Breast Surgery. Surg Clin N Am 87:431–451
14. Berg WA, Gilbreath PL (2000) Multicentric and multifocal cancer: whole breast US in preoperative evaluation. Radiology 214:59–66
15. Cooper AP (1840) On the anatomy of the breast. Longman, Orme, Green, Brown, and Longmans, London (Special Collections, Scott Memorial Library, Thomas Jefferson University, http://jdc.jefferson.edu/cooper/)

10 Physiological and Pathological Aspects of Full Breast Ultrasonography in Men and Children

10.1 Male Breast Gynecomastia

Gynecomastia represents the development of the mammary bud in true mammary glandular structures in male, similar but usually incompletely developed as compared with female breast.

The normal male breast is represented by a small mammary bud, located retroareolarly, with hypoechoic aspect, usually with acoustic shadowing, surrounded by various amount of subcutaneous fatty tissue. No vascular signal could be detected by Doppler examination with usual transducers. Clinically, there is normal sensibility in the mammary area.

Gynecomastia may be suspected clinically by increasing of the mammary volume, simultaneously with the development of the nipple-areolar complex; the development may be continuous, but frequently it has alternate stages of calm and acute evolution. The active development is usually painful, and the patient addressability is increased, or the size of the breasts determines esthetical complaints.

Anatomically, gynecomastia is structured by the developed glandular parenchyma represented by branching ducts of the retroareolar bud; the breast ducts may have multiple branches, from the main ducts to ductules, but rarely the lobular structures can be identified, such as in severe hyperestrogenism. As in the female breast, the galactophorous ducts are surrounded by normal stroma containing new formation vasculature. The vasculature is proportional with the size of the breast and is more salient during the evolutive stage. These three elements in various proportions (mammary parenchyma, glandular stroma, and new formation vasculature) can be identified by Doppler DE and represent the essential findings for the positive diagnosis of gynecomastia [1].

The most frequent differential diagnosis is the *pseudogynecomastia*, which appears as an enlarged "breast tissue" represented by fatty tissue hypertrophy surrounding the small mammary bud. The other rare differential diagnosis is *mass-forming tumors*, and breast cancer in male is the most severe and usually the unique lesion treated. Breast tumors related to the mammary parenchyma are rare and develop almost always in preexistent changes of benign gynecomastia. Other tumors in the same area with no mammary origin are rare and are not correlated with the glandular mammary development.

Physiological gynecomastia has peak frequencies at three periods during the lifetime: in the neonatal period, in the adolescence, and in elderly men.

In the neonatal period, gynecomastia is due to influences from maternal estrogens across the placenta, and the spontaneous resolution occurs in 2–3 months.

During puberty, the peak frequency occurs at about the age of 13–14 years, and as many as 60 % of male adolescents are affected. Gynecomastia in a male adolescent typically resolves within months to 2 years. Logically, after 16 years, florid gynecomastia could be considered pathological.

In elderly men, physiological gynecomastia is not well defined, either concerning the limits of age or the evolution. In fact, it is generally difficult to differentiate the physiological from the pathological gynecomastia in elderly men, because the etiologic factors are combined. When present, the positive diagnosis of the physiological gynecomastia is made by exclusion of the main pathological etiologies.

Pathological gynecomastia is represented either by the "true" benign gynecomastia, which occurs in childhood, adulthood or elder male in other lifetime periods than the physiological changes, or by the malignant gynecomastia with associated malignant mass forming tumor; 65 % of breast masses are found in elderly man.

There are many conditions for the pathological breast development in boys and men, well known and with many classifications. Most authors admit that estrogen, acting through its receptor (ER), promotes ductal growth, while progesterone, also acting through its receptor (PR), supports alveolar development. It seems that low level of testosterone and the disequilibrium between estrogens and male hormones raise the risk of breast cancer in male, conditions found in undescended testes, orchiectomy, orchitis, testicular injury,

A. Colan-Georges, *Atlas of Full Breast Ultrasonography*, DOI 10.1007/978-3-319-31418-1_10

late puberty, and infertility [2]. Moreover, the association of the high blood cholesterol, rapid weight gain, benign breast conditions, and possibly obesity may be correlated with hormonal disequilibrium in some metabolic diseases including diabetes. Dyslipidemia combined with hyperestrogenemia is associated with men infertility [3]; similarly, in boys, adiposogenital syndrome associates the testosterone insufficiency with obesity. Any type of goiter is more frequently present in people with breast pathology of both sexes, but the mechanism is not very well explained [4, 5]. However, there are studies that demonstrate the correlation between hyperestrogenemia, goiter, and adrenal hyperplasia [6].

Rare cases present male hyperprolactinemia usually due to a pituitary microadenoma, with ductal ectasia containing milk secretion, but the nipple surges are usually absent due to hypoplastic pores [7].

Many patients without any internal endocrine pathology could present gynecomastia due to the food contamination with estrogens. Despite the negation of food producers, it seems that restriction to some contaminated aliments improves the patients' complaints and the clinical evolution is at least stopped. The ubiquitous environmental contaminants bisphenol A (BPA) and 4-nonylphenol (NPH) may promote adverse effects in humans triggering estrogenic signals in target tissues; thus, the results of the hormonal tests indicate that *the biological action of environmental estrogen such as BPA and NPH should be taken into account for the potential impact on human disease-like hormone-dependent breast cancer* [8]. The estrogenic effects of such industrial agents together with an increasing widespread human exposure should be taken into account for the potential influence also on hormone-dependent breast cancer disease [9].

Familial cases of gynecomastia could be assigned to some nutritional factors (food contaminants of estrogens), rather than to genetic factors; the differential diagnosis may be the clinical evolution after several months of dietary treatment.

The correct diagnosis of the pathological gynecomastia, either benign or malignant, includes the evaluation of its etiology; some cases may be considered as symptoms of a distant tumor that require for further examination. In some cases, gynecomastia is a sign of adrenal or testicular feminizing tumors with hyperestrogenism; in other cases, milk-secreting gynecomastia may reveal a pituitary prolactinoma [1].

The clinical appearance as a retroareolar painful lump has usually asymmetrical development, but rarely is found unilateral. Breast glands under estrogenic stimulation tend to grow, be sensitive, and be tender and may hurt. Usually, the diagnosis of gynecomastia is made by the physician by just simple observation and the presenting history. The visual inspection may identify as stages I–IV based on the Tanner grading system (Fig. 10.1). The breast is always palpated to ensure there are no hard masses present.

Mammography is sometimes used but without a significant role in the evaluation of breast mass in males, because a mammogram requires fairly decent sized breasts to be placed between the two mammographic plates and it is difficult to differentiate the eventual opacity as simple gynecomastia or tumoral lesion [10]. In addition, mammography could not be used in children.

The radiological findings of the breast male were classified according to the aspect of projections of the breast tissues on the plain-film or digital acquisitions [11, 12]:

- *Nodular glandular opacity (acute/florid phase)*
- *Dendritic opacity (chronic fibrotic phase)*
- *Diffuse glandular* (Fig. 10.2)

The Classical US The classical US is usually recommended for the identification of cysts, other fluids, or solid masses, but neglecting the glandular anatomy, it was not possible to analyze the types of benign gynecomastia, and being operator dependent, US was not considered as a reproducible, accurate method of diagnosis [13].

Usually, gynecomastia is presented on classical US scans performed directly over the palpable area in the breast as *hypoechoic tissue* in the subareolar region, considered as *breast tissue;* this appearance mimics the US findings of early breast development in female adolescents. US scan of the opposite breast may present a similar appearance, although the *hypoechoic tissue* may be less prominent, almost always coexisting bilateral more or less symmetrical gynecomastia.

The differential diagnosis of gynecomastia with other pathological masses is difficult to perform in the classical US, because the breast cancer usually is hypoechoic too, similar to the fatty tissue; the Doppler usefulness is not widely accepted, and most cases of breast cancer in males are usually misinterpreted. The lack of imaging diagnosis is compensated by breast biopsies, which are painful, with risk of hematoma up to 94 % 1 week after vacuum-assisted biopsy and 55 % after 3 weeks [14]; otherwise, because malignancies are rare in male breast, biopsies are usually unnecessary.

The FBU aspects of the three essential anatomical elements of gynecomastia are easily demonstrated; the technique of radial and antiradial scanning and the images' analysis are similar to the female breast [15]:

1. *The true mammary parenchyma* is represented by the retroareolar bud; it appears as a hypoechoic mass of pyramidal shape, the basis on the thoracic wall and the apex to the nipple; when gynecomastia is developing, the periphery of the bud is branching in ducts, more extended in the upper-outer quadrant; the initial branching is less specific, but the advanced stages present typical ducts with the hyperechoic central line representing the virtual lumen of

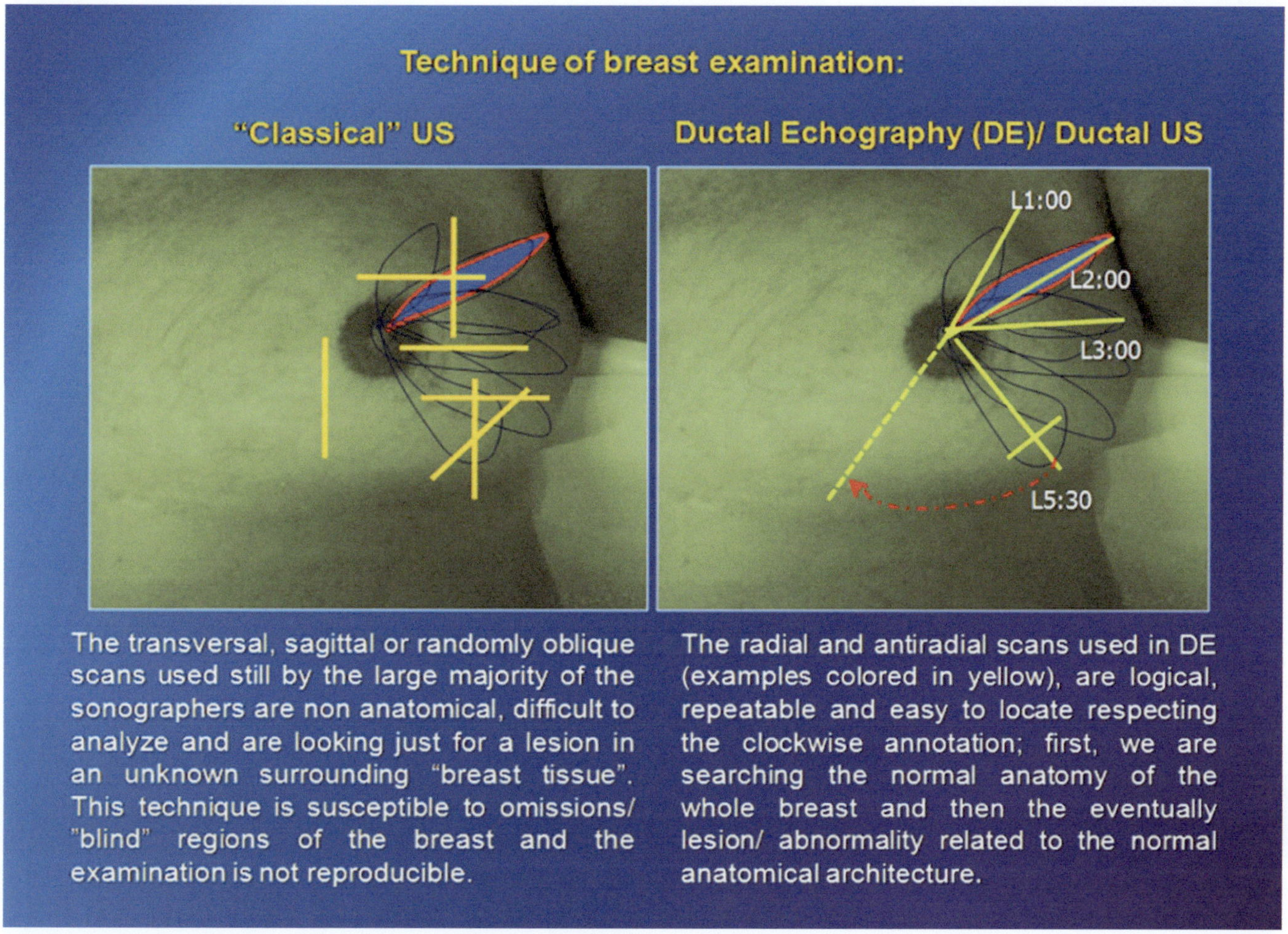

Fig. 10.1 Technique of examination of the male breast: "classical" US versus ductal echography (based on [16])

the "normal" ducts. The ducts may contain fluids, determining the ductal ectasia with the same appearance as in women: the secretions may appear transonic or more echoic, corresponding to serous up to milk secretions that are found in men with pituitary microprolactinoma. The lobules are usually not visualized, but they may appear in the advanced stages of gynecomastia or in relation with high hyperestrogenism. The salient lobules are associated with ductal thickening which is presumed as hyperplasia; in these cases, an adrenal or testicular feminizing tumor may be responsible for.

2. *The stromal component*, representing the connective, functionally supportive framework of the biological glandular cells (the mammary parenchyma); stroma represents in fact an amount of tissues containing connective cells, fibers, the arterial and venous vasculature, the lymphatic vessels, and the nerves, determining a general hyperechoic aspect. The presence of stroma in FBU appears as a hyperechoic structure surrounding the parenchymal bud and prolonged between its branches.

   Stromal development is simultaneous and proportional with the branching bud evolution, and its presence is essential to confirm a mammary glandular architecture, both in "true" gynecomastia and in premature thelarche; the specific glandular stroma is thick and with irregular borders, while the fatty tissue has only a thin hyperechoic conjunctive septae between large areas of hypoechoic fat.

3. *The new formation vasculature* is essential in the developing breast, such as gynecomastia or thelarche. Color and power Doppler are useful in confirming the diagnosis. The number and the size of the detected vessels are correlated with the size of the male breast and with the developing process intensity; the increasing vasculature becomes salient in the forming stages and the decreasing of the vascular network is significant for the stabilized, inactive stages. In gynecomastia, the spectral Doppler illustrates arterial velocimetry with low resistance and pulsatility flux indices, specific for the breast as "normal" anatomical organ, but this is unusual for the subcutaneous fatty tissue in pseudo-gynecomastia. The follow-up FBU

Fig. 10.2 The methods of diagnosis of gynecomastia (based on [16])

Clinical presentation	Age 60's, soft or hard, mobile or fixed, usually painless, subareolar usually eccentric, usually unilateral, recent evolution
Mammography	Limited applications due of breast size, does not visualise the ducts, rarely evidence of micro - calcifications, requires biopsy [10]: • Large mass: lobulated border • Small mass: spiculations
Breast MRI:	Less availability, does not visualise the ducts, use of paramagnetic contrast agents, requires biopsy
Classical US	The hypoechoic retroareolar eccentric mass similar to the "breast tissue" (incomplete characterisation), more or less regular contour, requires biopsy
Doppler Ductal US with RTSE = FBU	Pathological mass connected to ducts, new vasculature with tortuous shape, plunging artery with incidental angle and centripetal orientation; RTSE with score 4 or 5 Ueno/Tsukuba and high FLR over 5.00; biopsy ±

examination is useful in assessing the therapeutic response or the spontaneous resolution in newborn or teenager boy.

In a study of 2009, we presented an analysis of 47 cases of "true" benign gynecomastia examined by the FBU technique [1]; all the patients aged 8 months to 67 year old presented the elements of breast anatomy described, and particular cases were observed:

- Five cases of ductal ectasia correlated with hyperprolactinemia, from which one case had pituitary microprolactinoma.
- Seven cases of ductal-lobular hyperplasia, up to 3 mm, correlated with hyperestrogenism: one case presented an adrenal adenoma, three cases presented diffuse adrenal hyperplasia with hypercortisolemia and hyperestrogenemia, and three cases without internal hormonal disorders were considered as food hormonal contaminant changes and responded to dietary treatment (2 boys of 8 months and 4 years old, respectively, and a man of 38 years old).
- The rest of the 35 patients presented "simple" gynecomastia, with the three structural anatomical elements in various degrees of development; some cases were considered as "physiological," with spontaneous remission; others were included in various "pathological" degrees; some correlated with diabetes, obesity, goiter, liver insufficiency (increased conversion of androgens to estrogens in severe liver disease [17]), hormonal treatment of prostatic cancer, or dietary factors, especially particular animal fats (Figs. 10.3, 10.4, 10.5, 10.6, 10.7, 10.8, 10.9, 10.10, 10.11, 10.12, 10.13, 10.14, 10.15, 10.16, 10.17, 10.18, 10.19, 10.20, and 10.21).

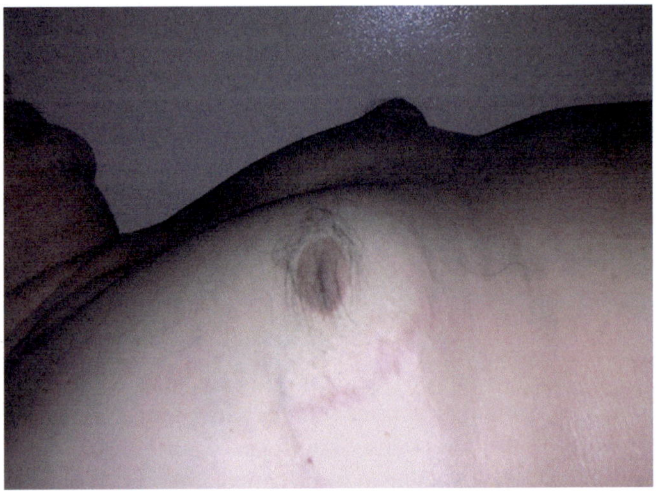

Fig. 10.3 Gynecomastia in adult with Tanner IV stage visible to the left breast; inverted right nipple following conservative surgery (unnecessary, because of the benign findings and bilateral evolution), with peripheral arcuate scar in the lowers quadrants

The treatment with spironolactone (Spironolactonum) determines a side effect as antiandrogenic activity, with about 5–30 % of male patients complaining of gynecomastia, impotence, or diminished libido [18]; the increased risk of male breast cancer was signaled about 40 years ago [19], but the incidence of cases is reduced because of the rare overall incidence of this disease.

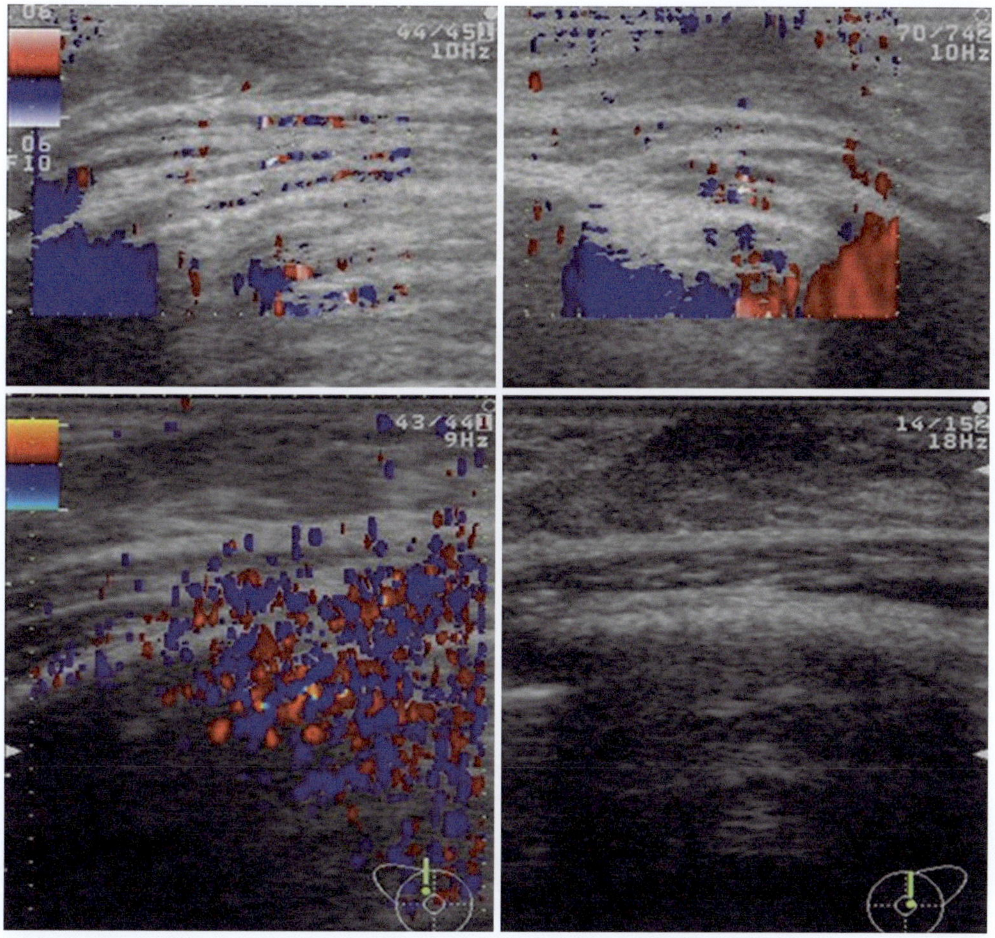

Fig. 10.4 Infantile gynecomastia: 1-year-old male with bilateral symmetrical mammary bud, probable of exogenous etiology (nutritional); motion Doppler artifacts are the inconveniences of the examination at this age, but the anatomy is well demonstrated (based on [16])

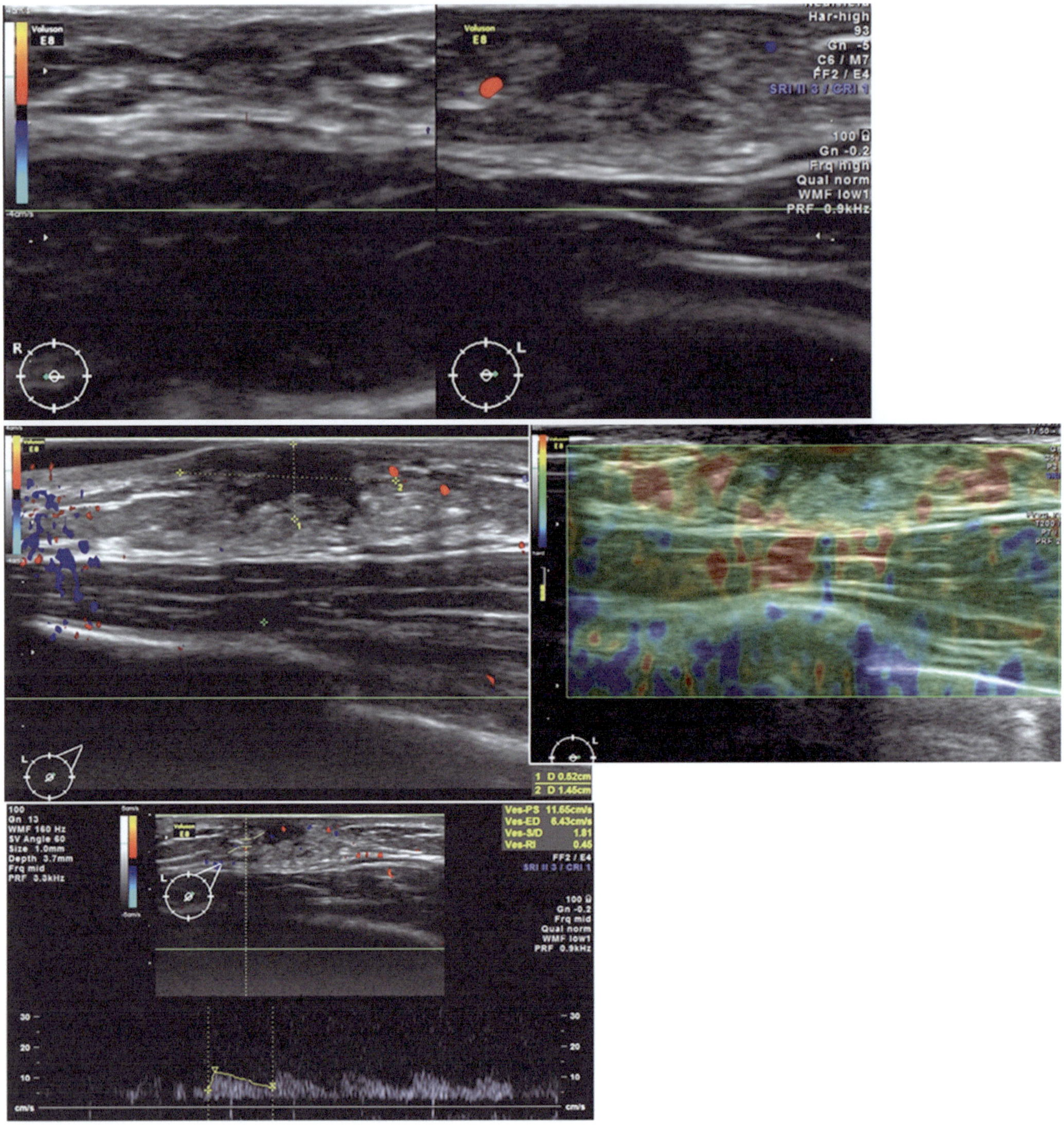

Fig. 10.5 Asymmetrical precocious pubertal gynecomastia in a 9-year-old boy: first development of the left breast, with the three anatomical elements (the branching bud, surrounding stroma, and new formation vasculature of low resistance velocity). Sonoelastography demonstrates the benign type of mammary strain

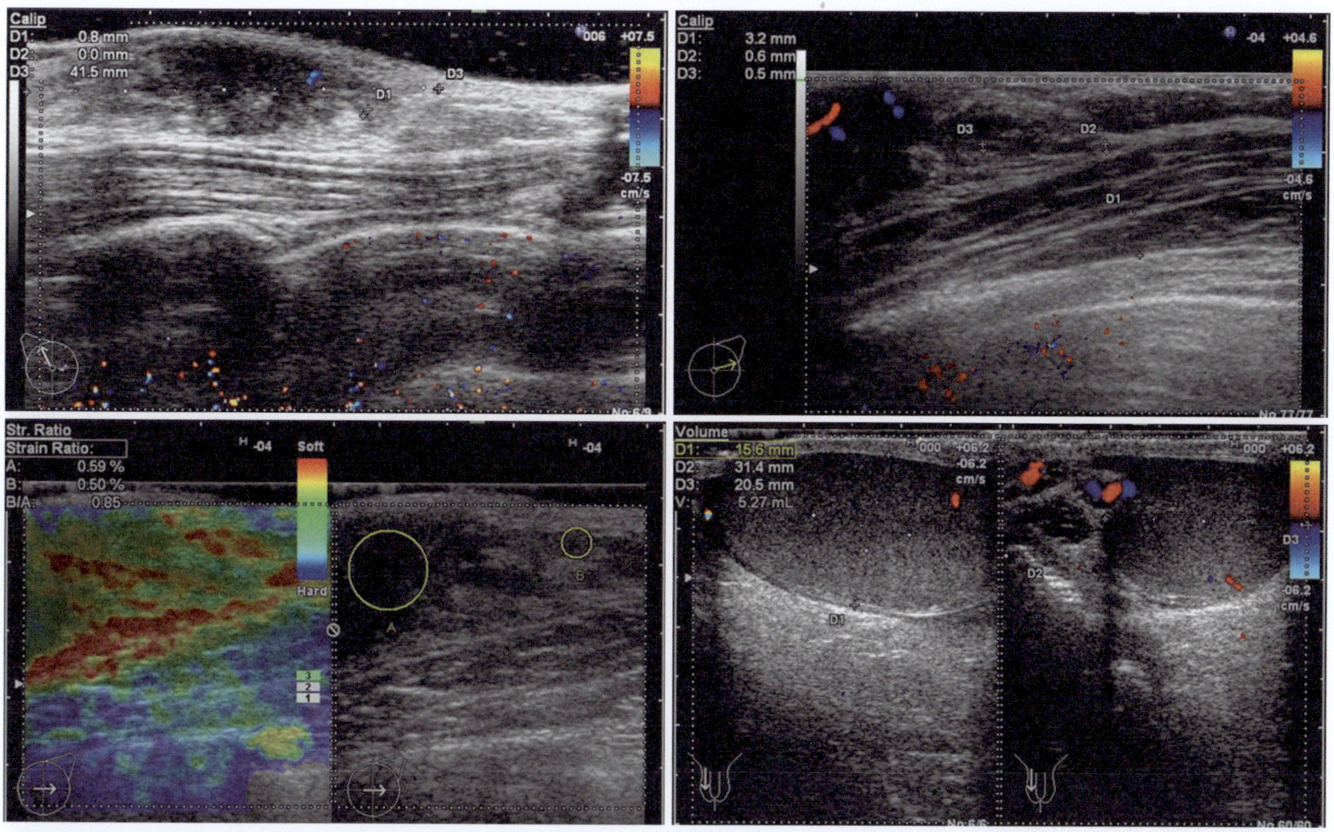

Fig. 10.6 Physiological pubertal gynecomastia in a 14-year-old boy: the testicular and epididymal size and vasculature are normal in puberty

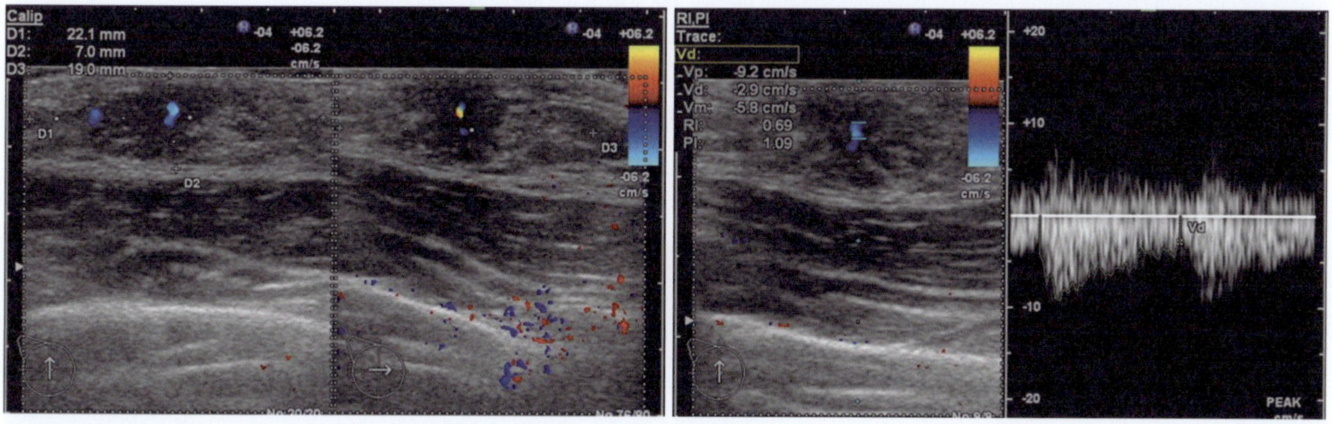

Fig. 10.7 Pubertal gynecomastia in a 13-year-old boy, with illustration of the three elements: parenchyma (branching of the mammary bud), glandular hyperechoic stroma, and new formation vasculature

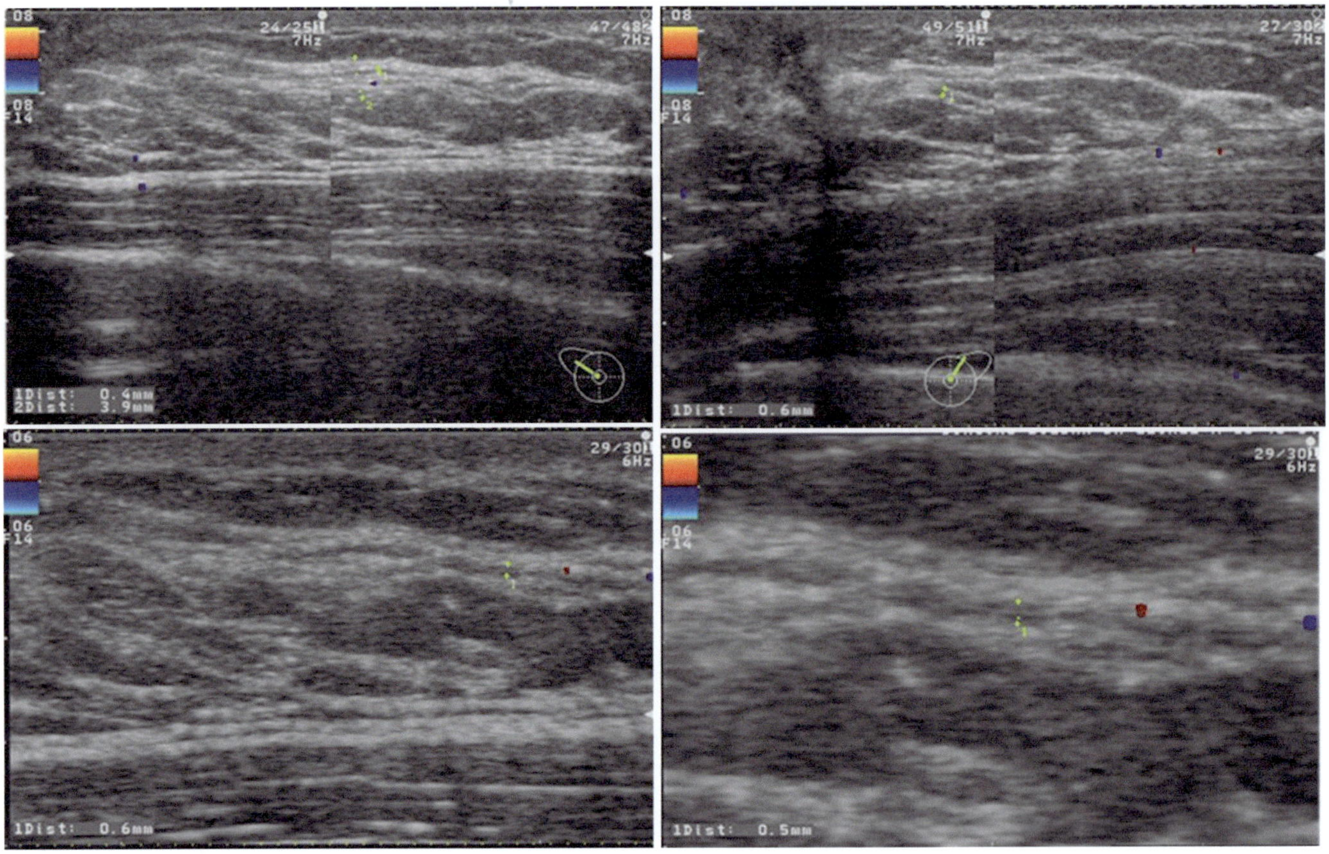

Fig. 10.8 Advanced pubertal gynecomastia in a 16-year-old boy: true mammary lobes with stroma and ducts containing the hyperechoic central line, a specific sign corresponding to the virtual lumen; despite the age, the size of the breasts is abnormal

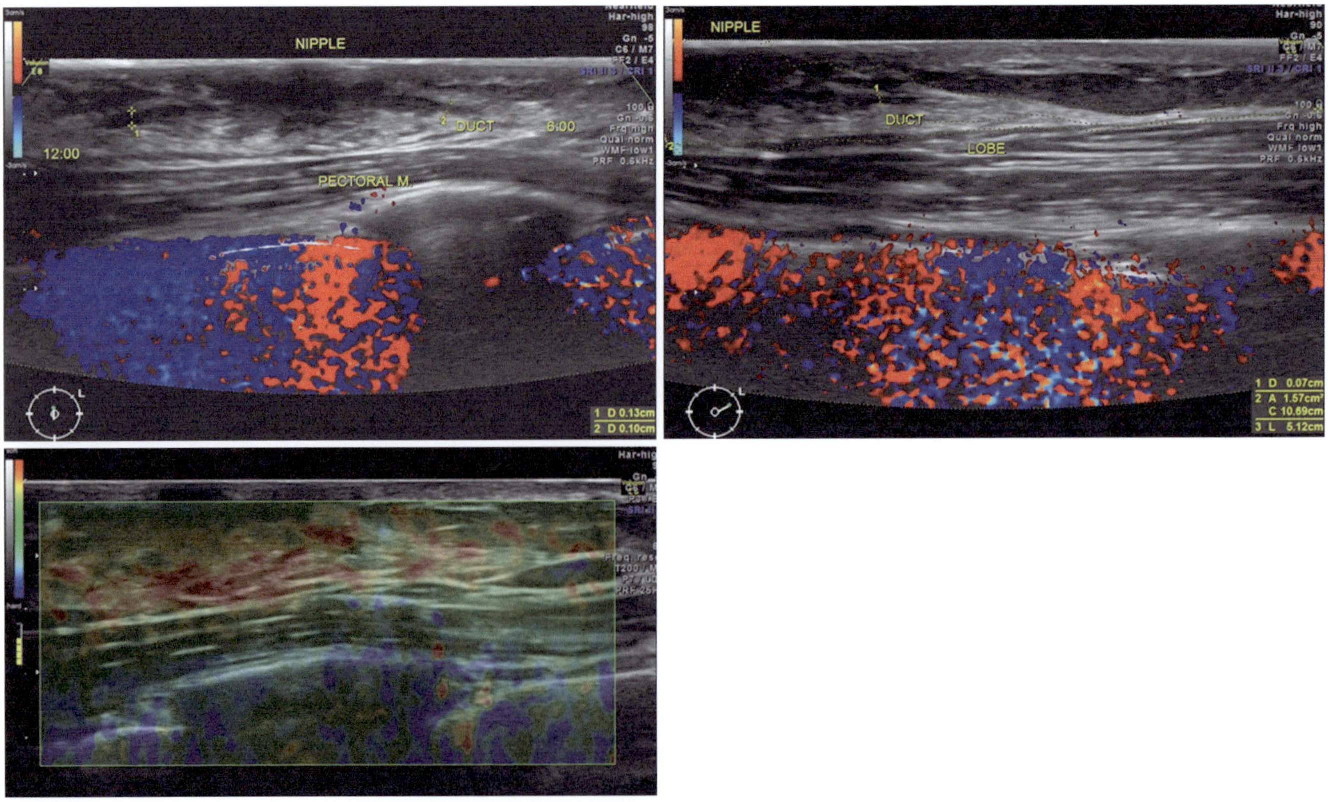

Fig. 10.9 A 65-year-old man with gynecomastia, without any pathologically proved etiology; the lobar anatomy is similar to the female pubertal breast, but the ductal diameters are usually thinner. Diagnosis: physiological gynecomastia in an older man

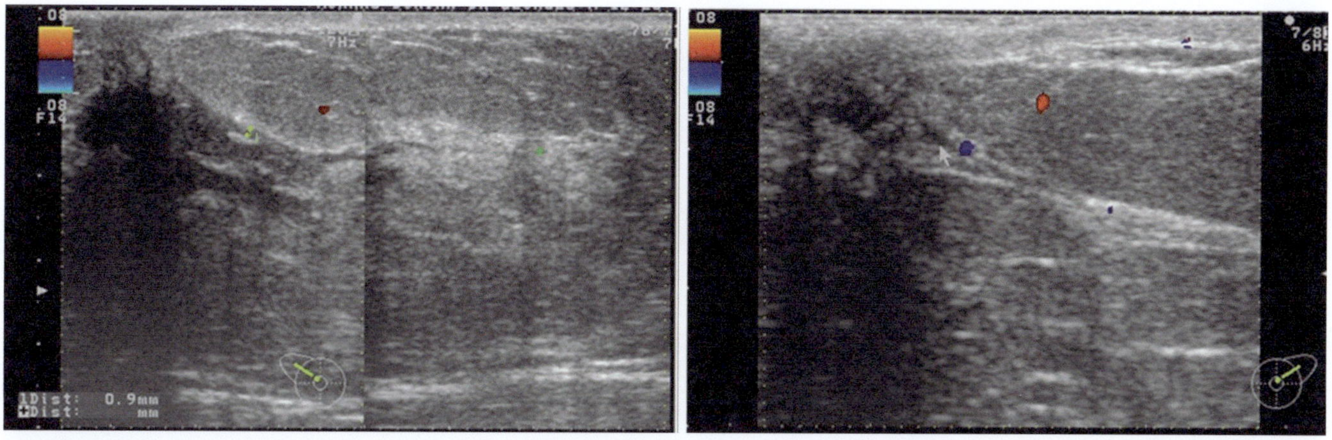

Fig. 10.10 Familial gynecomastia: 19-year-old son, presenting recent/florid gynecomastia with the three developing elements: branching ducts from the mammary bud, small amount of stroma, and visible new vasculature (based on [16])

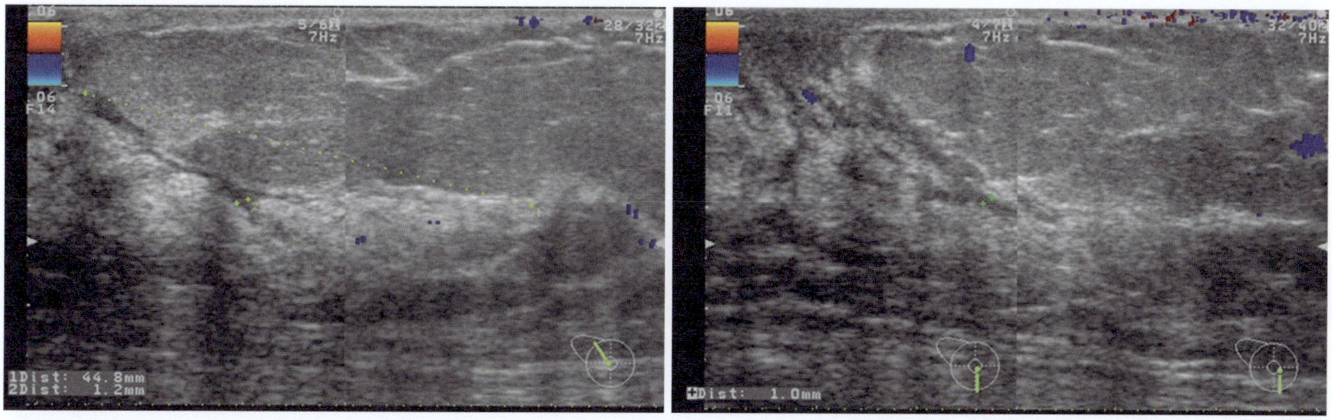

Fig. 10.11 Familial gynecomastia: 52-year-old father, with chronic gynecomastia for 4 years, presents mammary lobes with elongated ducts, irregular ductal thickening/hyperplasias; the hyperechoic stroma is larger, and there are thick premammary and retromammary fatty layers (type of heterogeneous breast in woman) (based on [16])

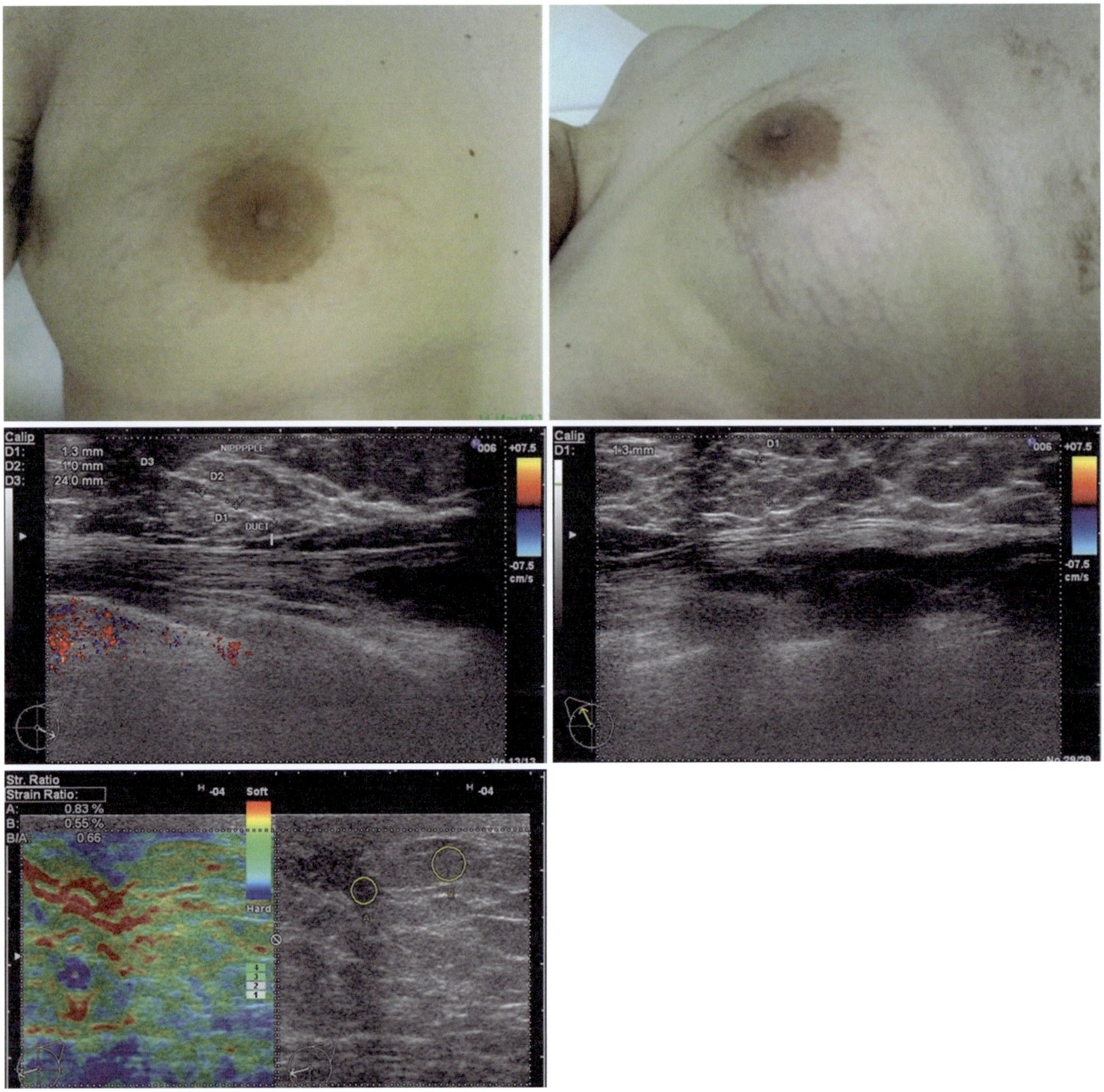

Fig. 10.12 "True" gynecomastia in a 54-year-old patient, with clinical signs of hypercortisolemia, the Cushing's syndrome: enlarged breasts with large areola demonstrate reddish stretch marks. FBU illustrates retroareolar branching bud: the ducts are typical, with the central hyperechoic line at DE, and sonoelastography delimits the breast parenchyma with score 1 Ueno and low FLR (based on [16])

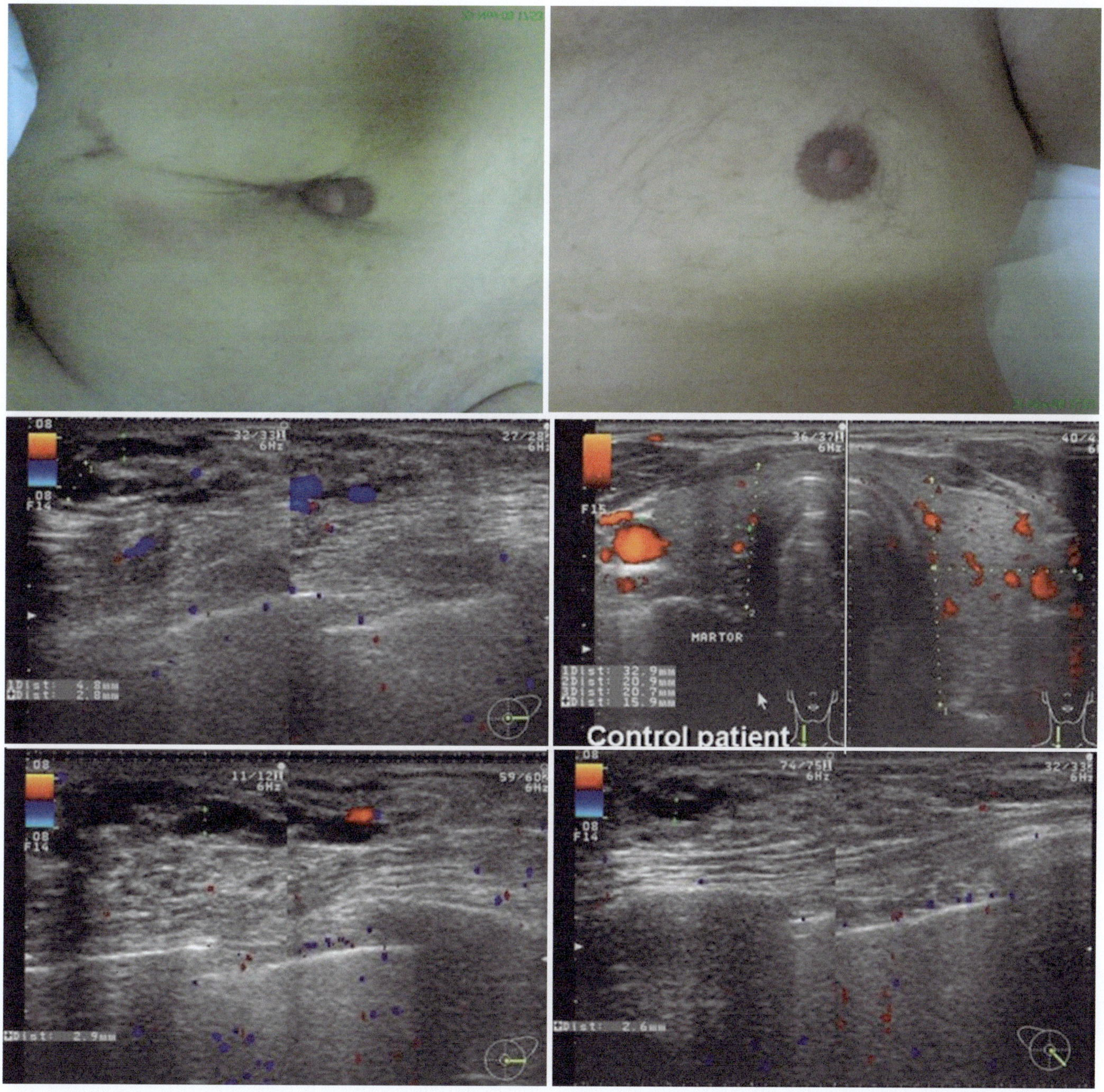

Fig. 10.13 Galactorrhea in man: 54-year-old male patient after right gynecomastia, misdiagnosed and partially removed (segmentectomy), with local evolution and finally contralateral development equally. The patient presented exophthalmia and Doppler US demonstrated diffuse goiter with moderate increasing of the Power Doppler signal compared to a control patient

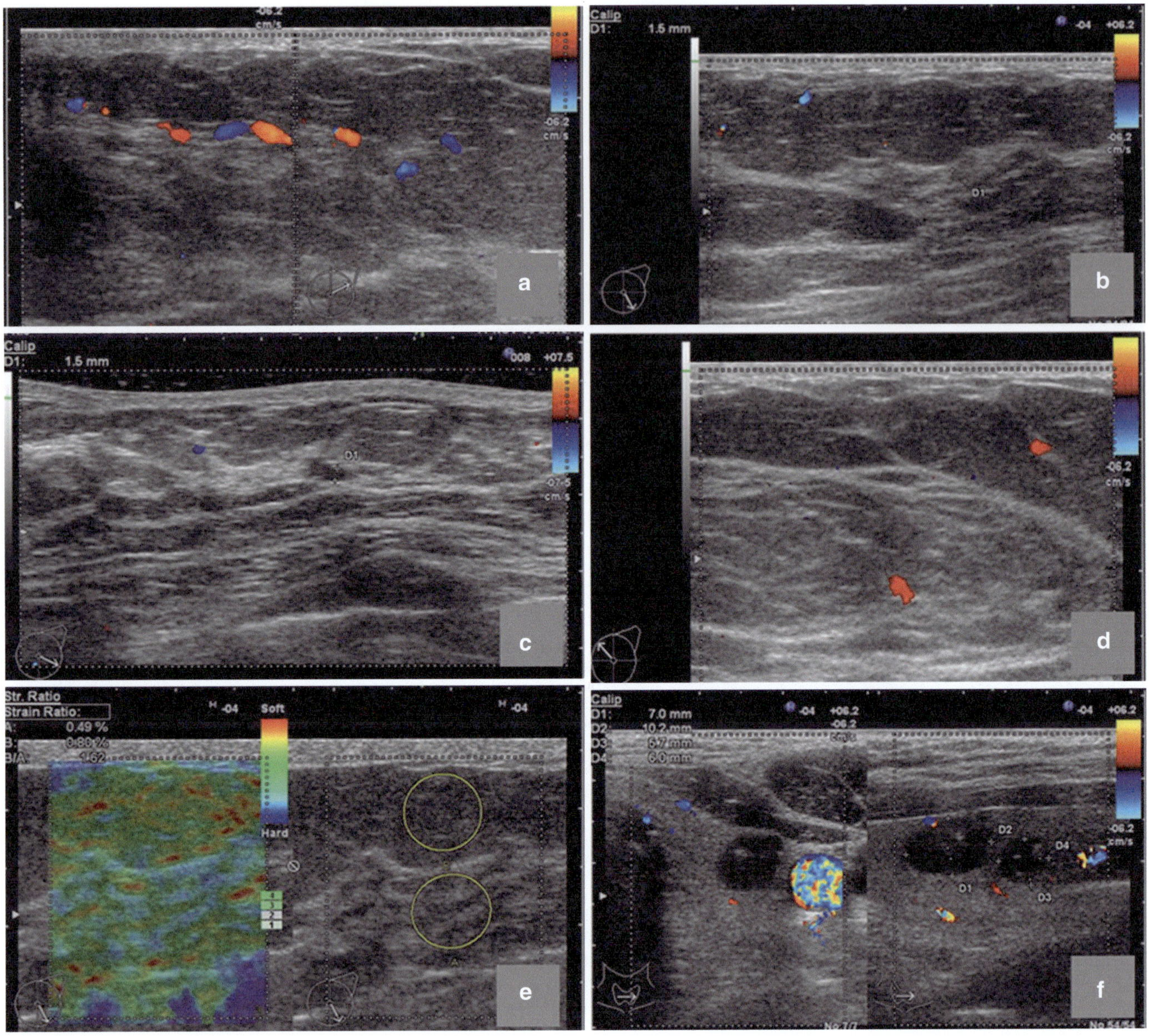

Fig. 10.14 FBU in a 43-year-old male: gynecomastia with stroma, ducts, and new vasculature (**a**); advanced stage presents terminal ductal-lobular specific units (**b**), small lobular hyperplasias (**c**), and Cooper ligaments with salient vasculature (**d**). Sonoelastography illustrates the normal parenchymal architecture in red-green and the mammary stroma in light blue, while the fatty tissue is more homogeneous (**e**). An associated colloid nodular goiter is present; a complex etiologic-pathogenic correlation has to be demonstrated (**f**) (based on [16])

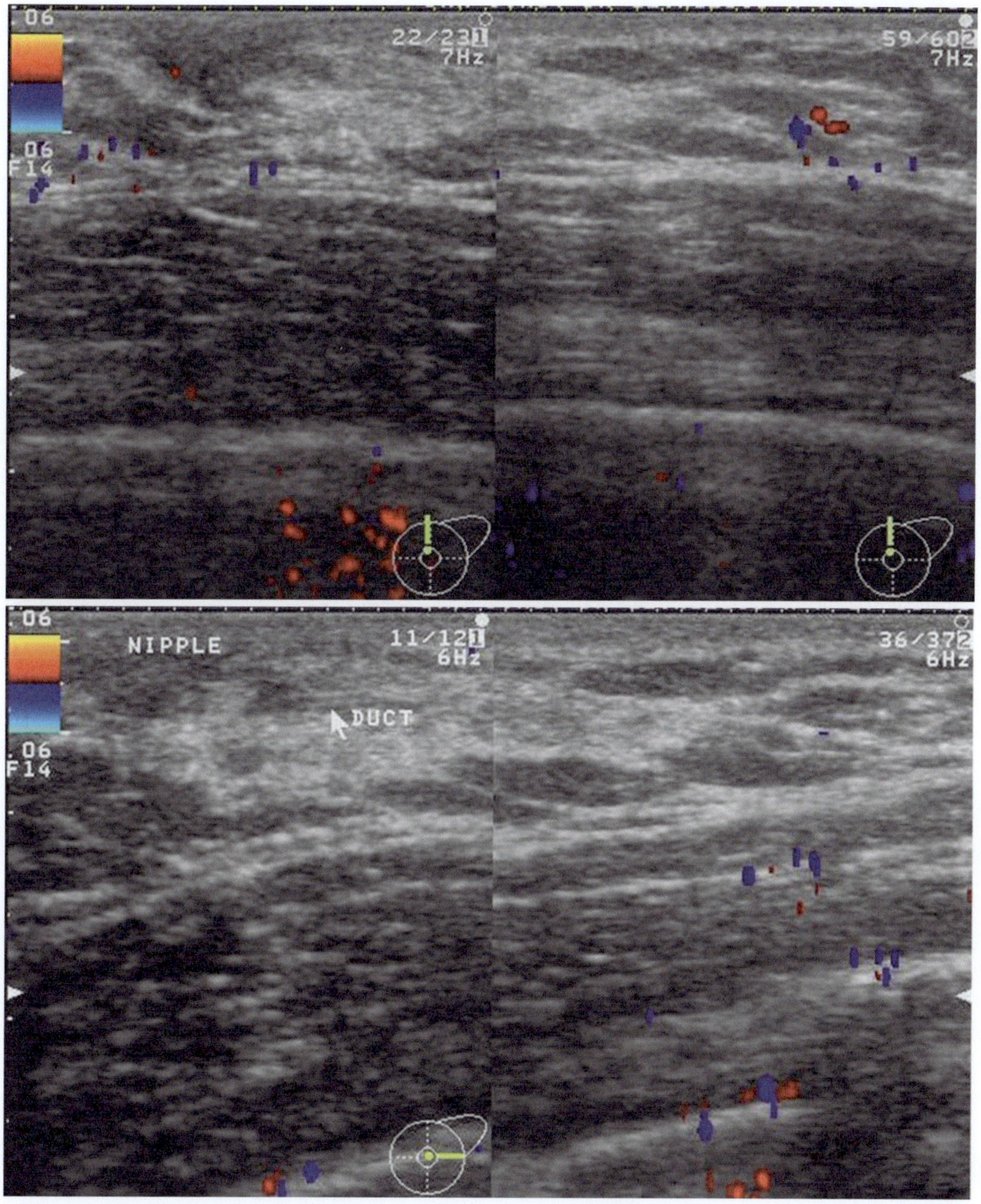

Fig. 10.15 Recent gynecomastia in a 33-year-old male patient with Cushing's syndrome: obesity, round-shaped face, cutaneous reddish stretch marks, folliculitis, and arterial hypertension; breast DE was performed in the general investigation for an associated infertility that could be correlated with these endocrine disorders [3]

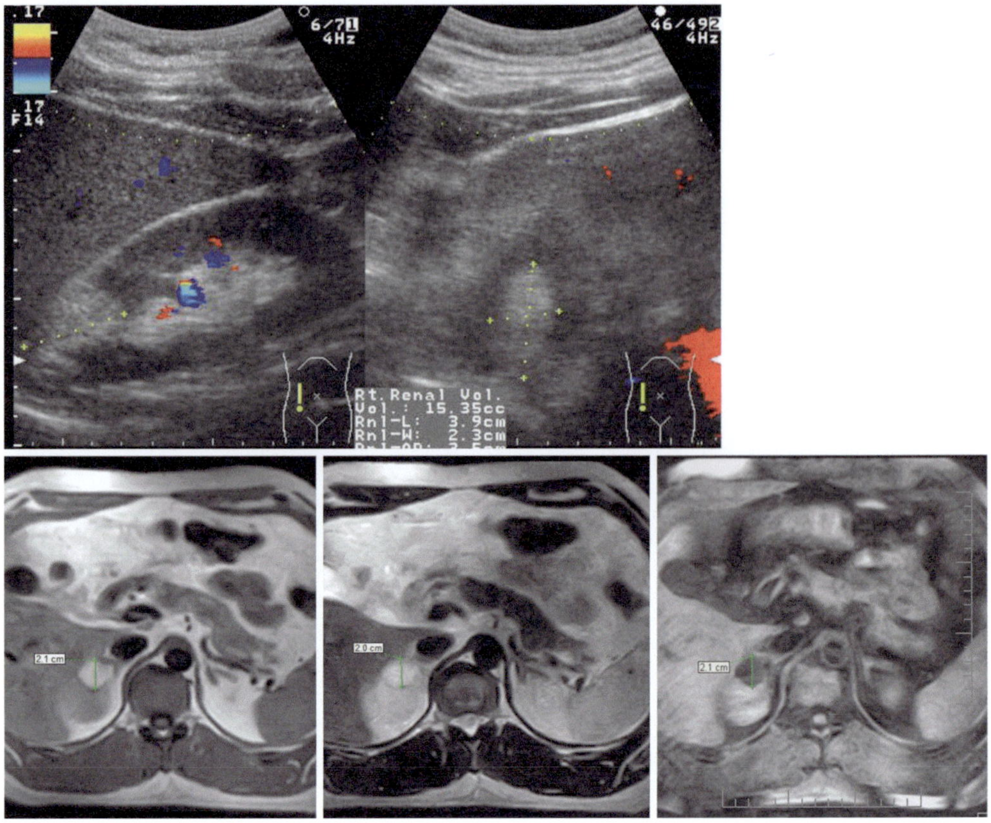

Fig. 10.16 Recent gynecomastia, the same case: increased values of E2 and plasmatic cortisone determined the research of the adrenals; first intention US demonstrated a right adrenal mass of 15.35 cc, with a lobulated contour, compression of the upper pole of the kidney parenchyma (pseudo-renal tumor), hyperechoic aspect, and no salient vasculature

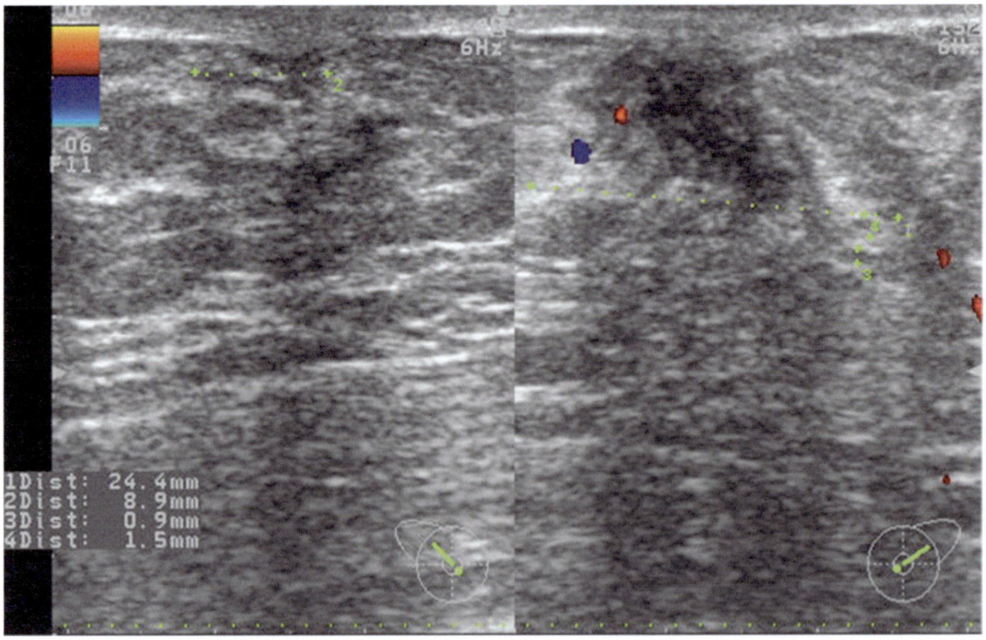

Fig. 10.17 Asymmetrical gynecomastia in a 58-year-old patient, with left breast branching mammary bud, new vasculature, and glandular stroma; the right mammary bud is typical "normal"

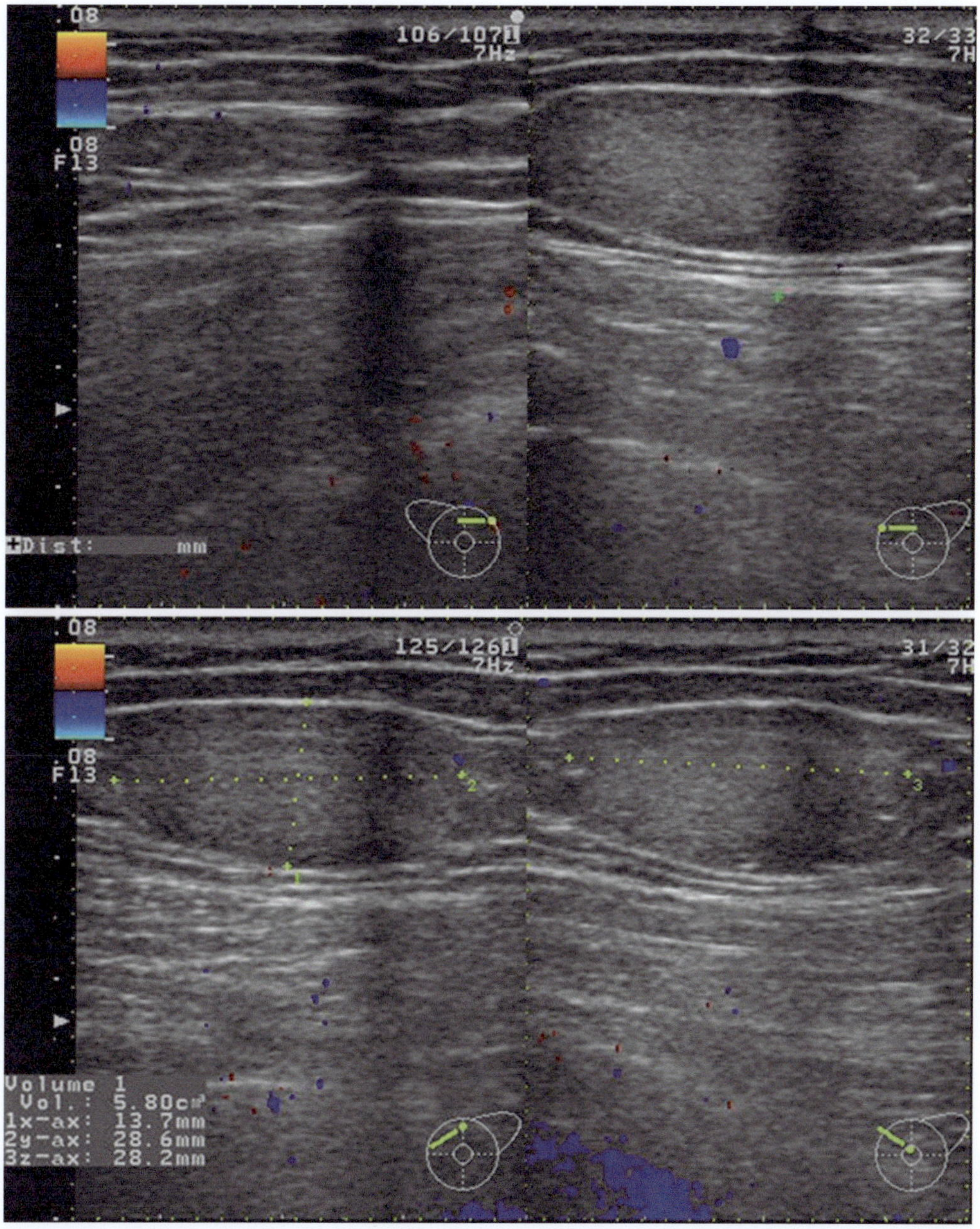

Fig. 10.18 Pseudo-gynecomastia: typical lipoma in the upper-inner left breast quadrant: homogeneous mass, izo-/hyperechoic, without salient vasculature

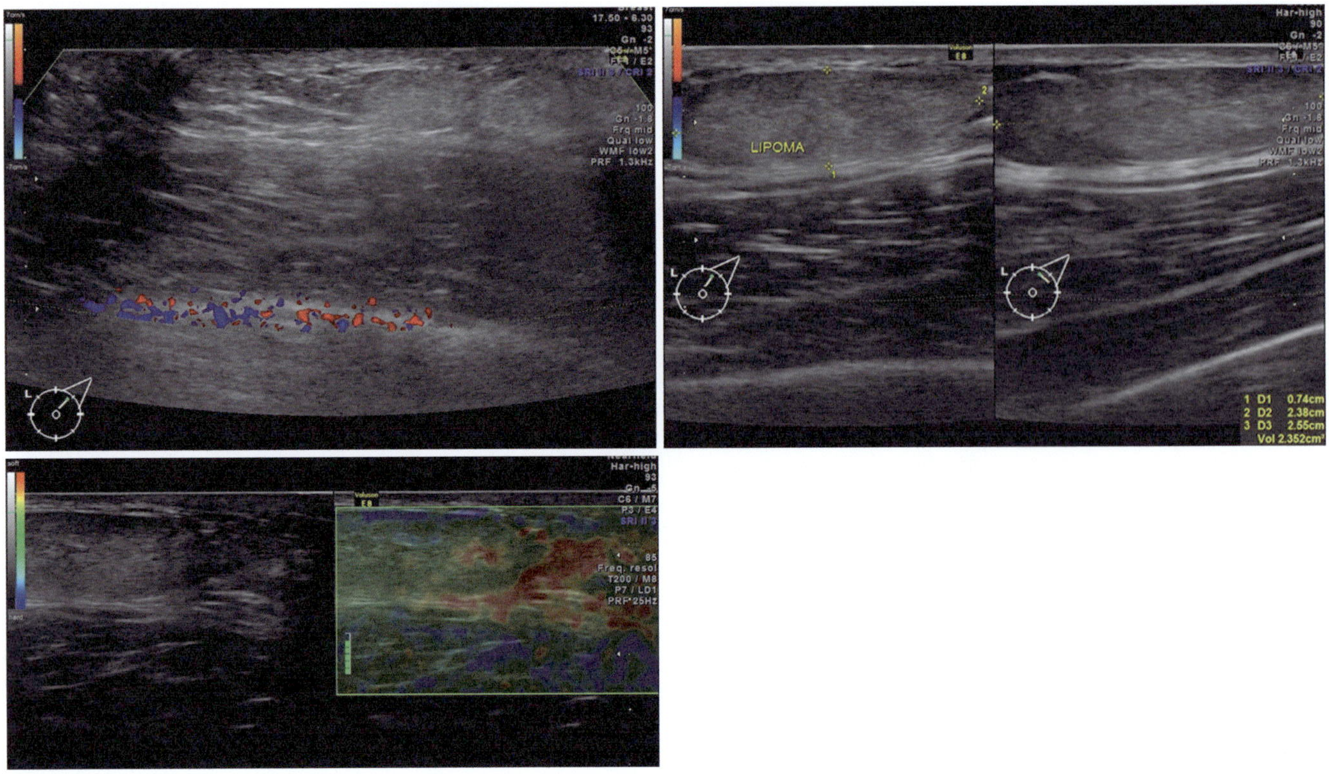

Fig. 10.19 FBU aspect of pseudo-gynecomastia in a 31-year-old man with a lipoma in the upper-outer left breast quadrant

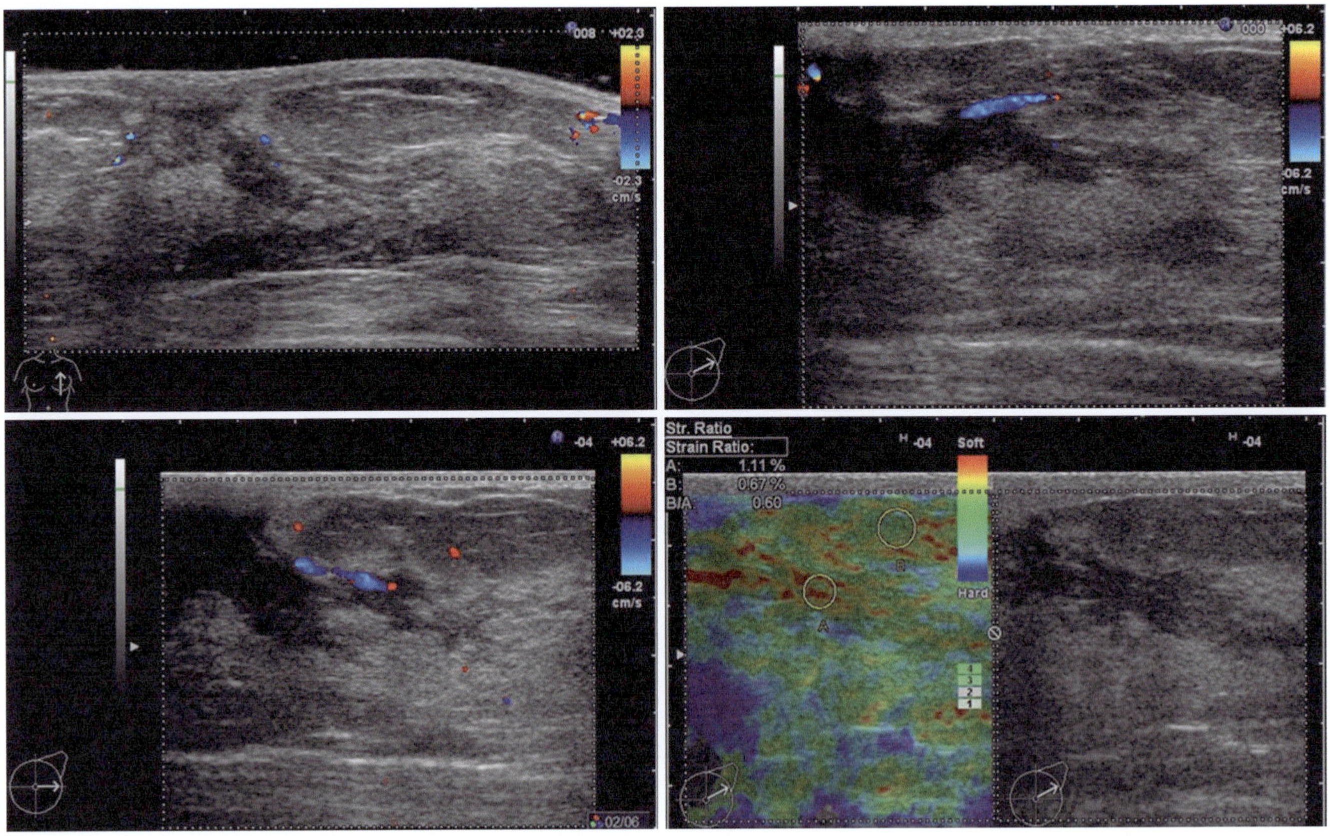

Fig. 10.20 FBU in a 63-year-old male: asymmetrical gynecomastia with advanced differentiation of the ducts and stroma on the right side, while the left mammary bud has a pseudotumoral hypoechoic aspect, with irregular margins, represented by the developing ducts, demonstrated by the RTSE with score 1 Ueno and very low FLR (0.60)

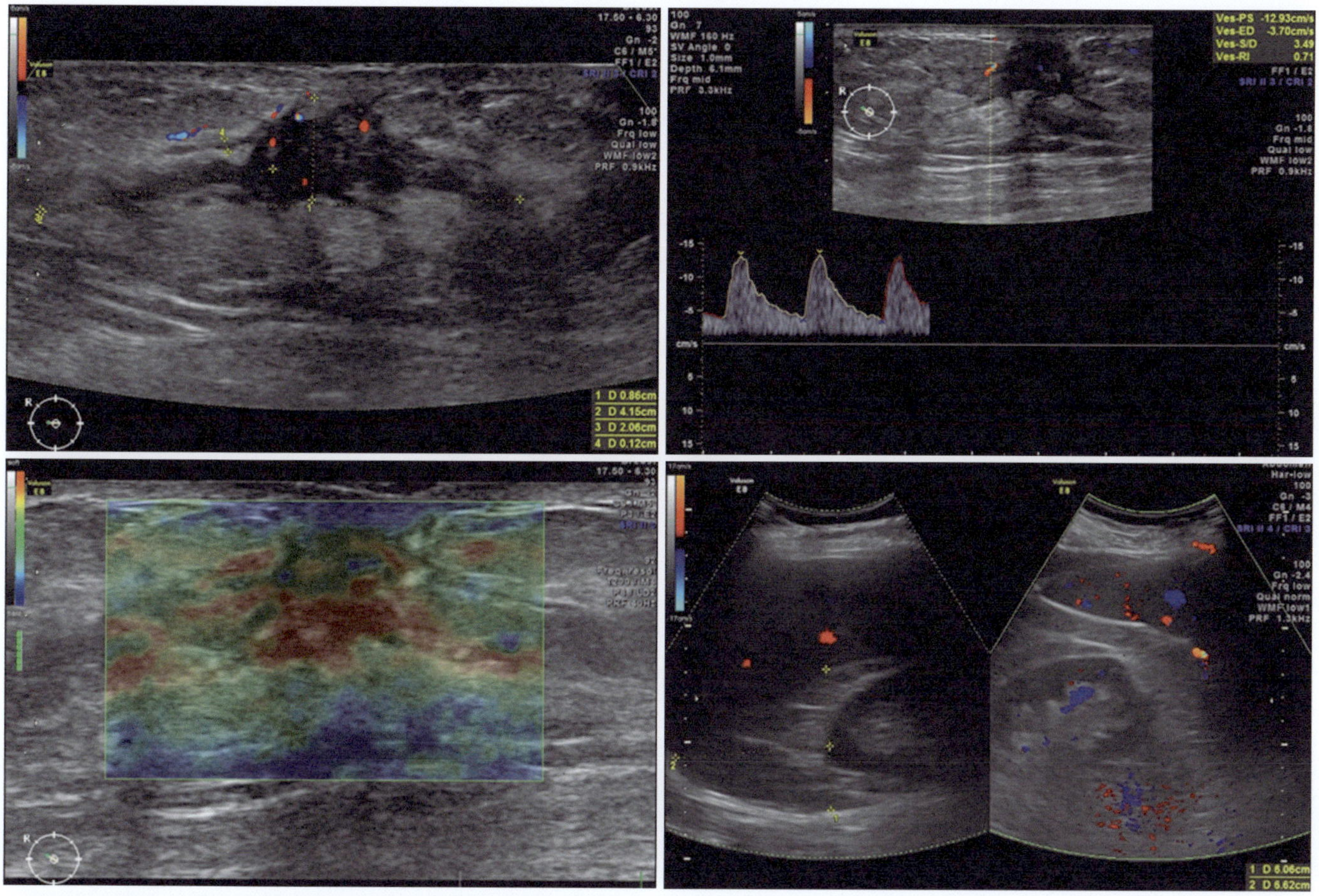

Fig. 10.21 FBU in a 64-year-old male, with pseudomalignant gynecomastia in 2D US; however, the new formation vasculature is peripheral, according to the periareolary vascular circle, and sonoelastography demonstrates a scoring type 1 Ueno for the branching bud, with normal increasing strain of the nipple-areolar complex

10.2 Breast Cancer in Man

The differential diagnosis of the "simple," benign gynecomastia with the male breast cancer or malignant gynecomastia is made using the same criteria as in women. Breast cancer in men is a rare disease, accounting for $\approx 1\,\%$ of all breast cancer cases [20], but it is severe because usually it is diagnosed in advanced stages or it is misinterpreted.

The risk factors for breast cancer in men may be grouped in genetic, metabolic, dishormonal, and environmental. Thus, the major genetic factors are acting similar to woman and include BRCA2 mutations, which are believed to account for the majority of inherited breast cancer in men; in some cases, Klinefelter syndrome and a positive family history may be present. There are suspected genetic factors such as AR gene mutations, CYP17 polymorphism, Cowden syndrome, and CHEK2 [20].

There are some general assumptions largely accepted in the literature:

- When it does occur, male breast cancer occurs in one breast and it is seen in elder males.
- In the majority of cases of gynecomastia, there is no cancer associated; however, any male over the age of 50 with a sudden increase in a single breast is suspected.
- Breast cancer in males presents just like in females: a mass is identified in a single breast, there is generally no pain or nipple discharge, but the mass may be hard to touch.
- The only way to tell if it is cancer is by a biopsy.

FBU aspect of breast cancer in men is similar to the cancer descriptors in woman; this technique is useful especially in demonstrating the connection between the abnormal mass/lesion with the ductal tree for certifying the breast etiology, and the radial scanning is helpful to precise the location upon the clockwise rotation; the aspect of the vasculature must be carefully analyzed to avoid overdiagnosis, and sonoelastography is recommended before any biopsy or surgical treatment. The ductal connection demonstration is essential in the diagnosis of male breast cancer, because similar to women, the majority of men's cancers are invasive ductal carcinomas [21, 22]. Papillary carcinomas are comparatively more common, and lobular carcinomas are rarer in men [23].

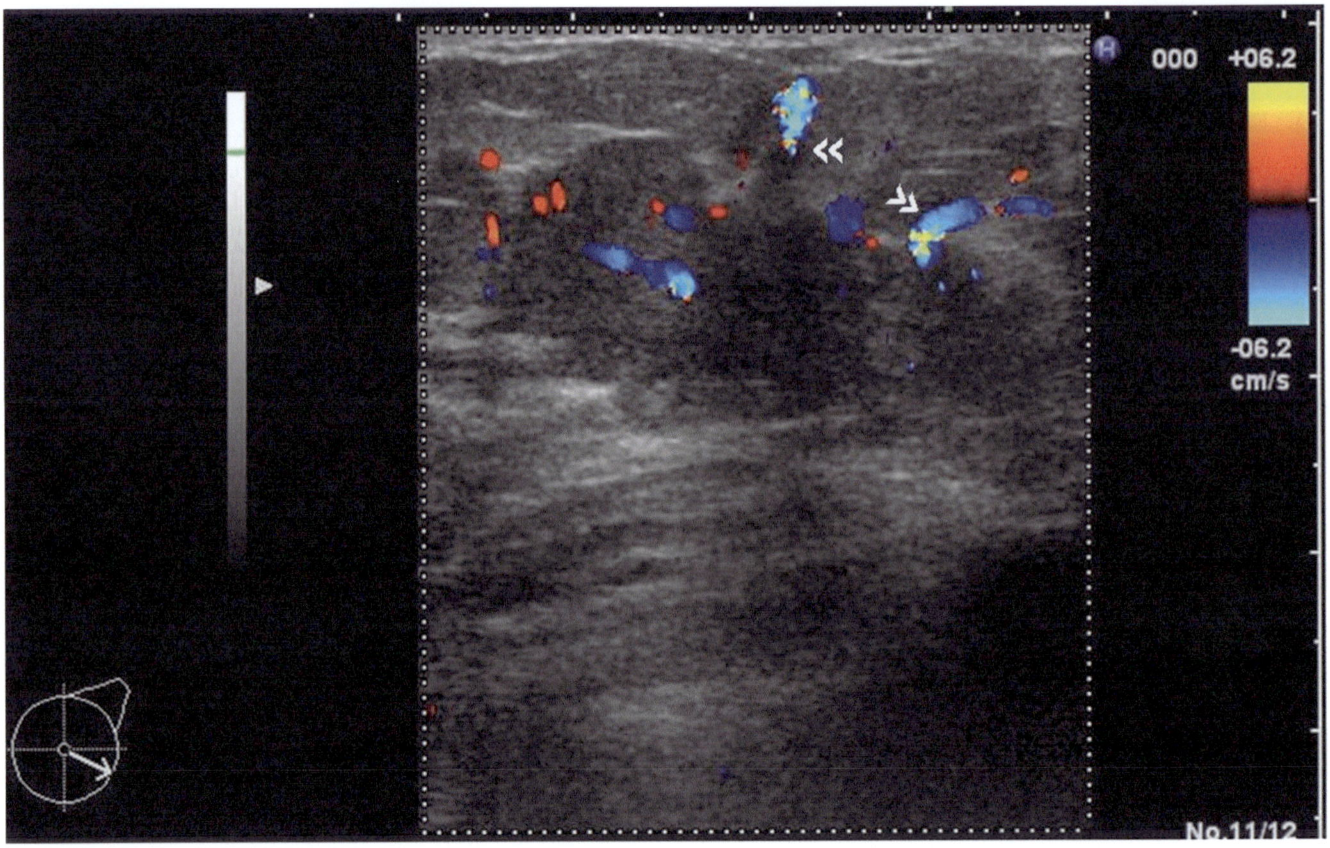

Fig. 10.22 Doppler US in a 52-year-old male demonstrates at L 4:00 a hypoechoic eccentric mass, with irregular spiculated borders represented by thickened connected ducts, the long axis parallel with the lobar radius and presenting malignant-type new vasculature: multiple vascular poles, with incident plunging angle, and tortuous course. The extension of the tumoral margins following the ducts and the vessels along the Cooper ligaments («) is highly predictive of malignancy. Sonoelastography would be concluding as an additional tool, avoiding unnecessary biopsies (based on [16])

In our experience, breast cancer in men is easier to detect than in women, because of the small breast volume usually without dense glandular structures surrounding the tumor; thus, the sensibility of the method is ≈100 %; the tumor stages of development at the patient presentation are earlier, due to the psychological factors; the associated axillary lymphadenopathy is detected in rare cases. We did not find multicentric or multifocal breast cancer in men, and the literature is poor relative to this aspect (Figs. 10.22, 10.23, and 10.24).

The vascular analysis by Doppler techniques is useful in the positive diagnosis of recent/florid gynecomastia and in the diagnosis of the pathological masses; some observations may be noted [16]:

- An overestimation of Doppler as a unique US finding should be avoided; however, the incident angle of the plunging artery may be considered as malignant sign [24], as well as enlarged tumoral vessels with aliasing flow.
- The value of Doppler or contrast-enhanced US (CEUS) is similar to contrast MRI of the breast, but Doppler is less expansive; however, the use of CEUS proved better results in the "classical" US and DE.
- Doppler characterization is useful in addition to the Stavros [25] and US BI-RADS criteria, because most pitfalls in breast US are due to neglecting the new formation vasculature (present in malignant lesions with benign Stavros criteria, absent in pseudomalignant lesions on classical US, or variant in indeterminate breast lesions).
- Doppler DE supplemented with sonoelastography represents the FBU, the only accomplished US examination of the breast and of the soft tissues, but there are some problems related to the not yet standardized technique: there are different machines with different software and scales of interpretation for the strain, and there are not yet enough trained sonographers in DE and sonoelastography.
- FBU is recommended before the biopsy and surgical treatment, especially in painful gynecomastia or pediatric patients, avoiding the inconvenient side effects such as pain, hematomas after biopsies [14], or scars.

It is assumed that men with gynecomastia may suffer from absolute or relative estrogen excess, and their risk for different associated malignancies may be increased.

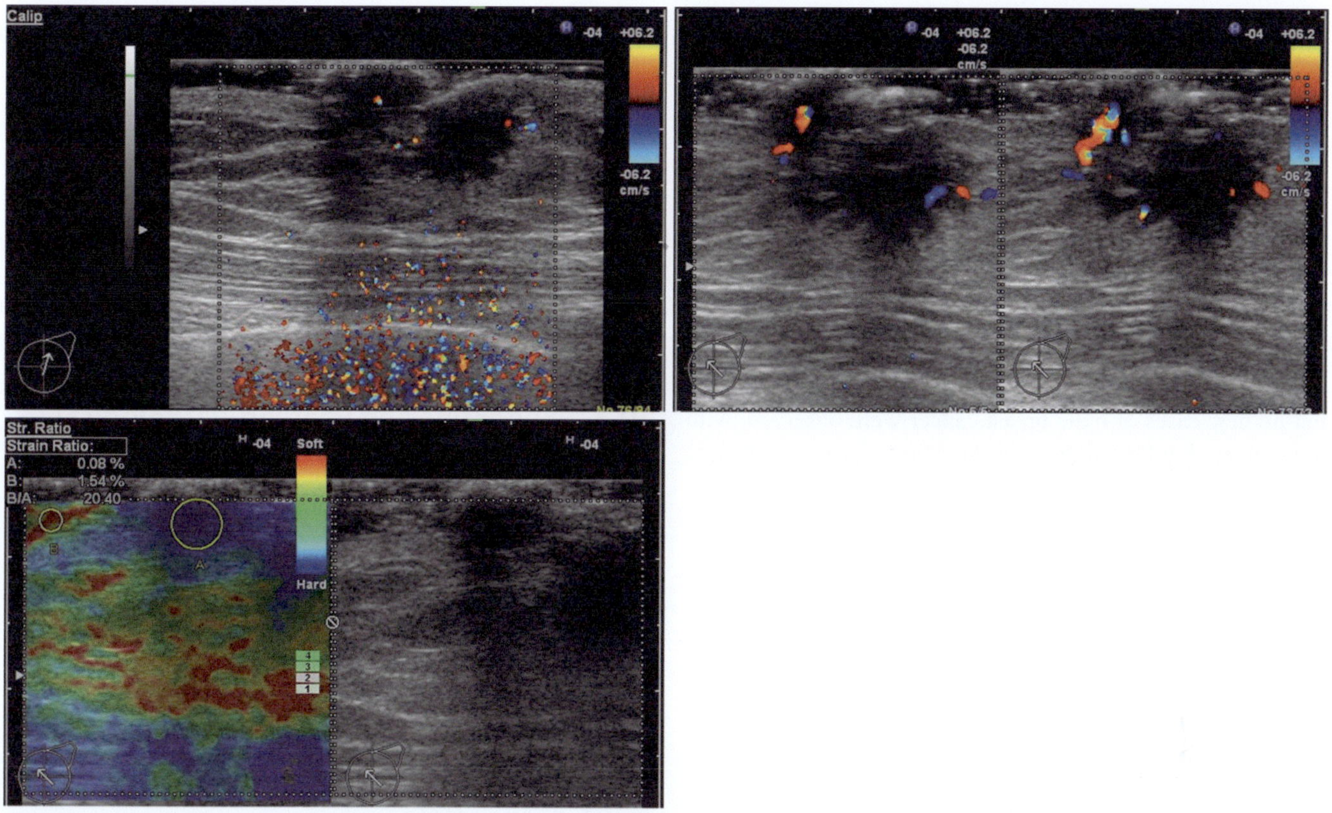

Fig. 10.23 L 5:00 central breast cancer in a 69-year-old male: FBU demonstrates the pathological mass with malignant features based on Stavros, connected to the nipple, with new formation vasculature and increased stiffness of the whole assembly tumor-connecting ducts-nipple

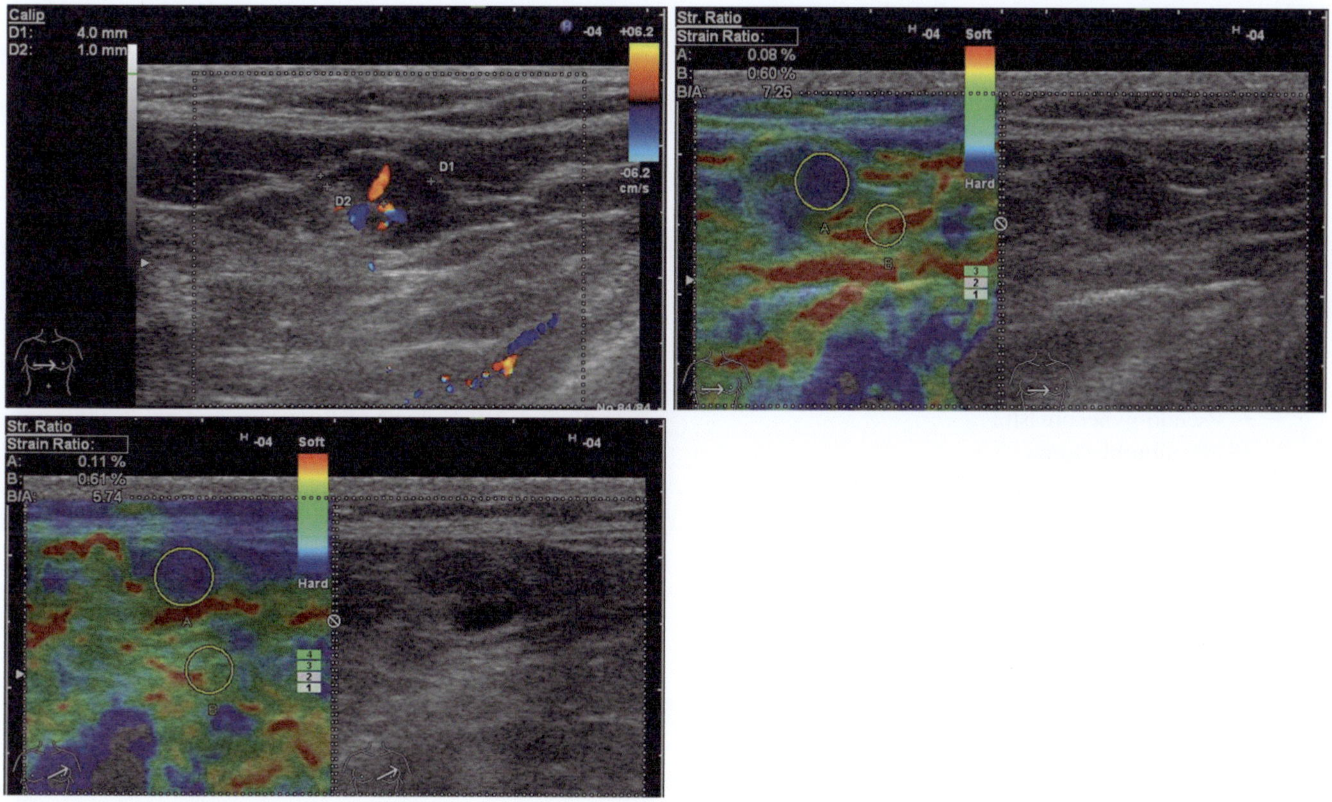

Fig. 10.24 The same case: suspected findings of intramammary lymph node in the lower-inner quadrant (*upper and middle images*) and left axillary lymph node (*bottom image*)

A study published in 2002 tested whether men with gynecomastia were at greater risk of developing cancer elsewhere [26]: a cohort of 446 men having a histopathologic diagnosis of gynecomastia following an operation for either unilateral or bilateral breast enlargement, between 1970 and 1979, was evaluated during a 20-year period, and at the end, the cohort constituted a significant value of 8375.2 person-years of follow-up time. The authors concluded there was a significant increased risk of testicular cancer and squamous cell carcinoma of the skin after more than 2-year interval in men which have been operated on for gynecomastia. In this cohort, there were 2 persons with initial breast carcinoma, but no new cases of male breast cancer were observed, with the explanation that diagnostic operations for gynecomastia may substantially have reduced this risk. We can observe the large proportion of unnecessary breast surgery (just 2 breast cancers from 446 cases, 0.44 %), which was justified as the main method of diagnosis in that period of time, as compared with the advanced developments in US available nowadays that offer a most accurate noninvasive diagnosis. The authors could not explain the risk of skin cancer, but they concluded that no improvement in prostatic cancer evolution was observed after estrogen therapy, which was responsible for gynecomastia.

For the differential diagnosis of male breast lesions, there are many classifications based on their risk of developing in male; a very useful classification based on the occurrence criterion was proposed by Olsson and col. [26]:

I. *Lesions that do occur in man* [26]
   A. Gynecomastia with parenchymal secondary lesions:
      - Ductal hyperplasia
      - Ductal ectasia (galactorrhea)
      - Papilloma
      - Adenoma
      - Fibrocystic changes
      - Diabetic mastopathy
      - Paget disease (more frequent as in women)
      - Breast cancer
   B. Non-gynecomastia
      - Pseudo-gynecomastia
      - Myofibroblastoma
      - Granular cell tumor (neural origin)
      - Epidermal inclusion cyst
      - Cystic lymphangioma
      - Varix
      - Leiomyoma
      - Lipoma
      - Pleomorphic hyalinizing angioectatic tumor of soft tissues

II. *Lesions that do not occur in man or are extremely rare* (rare cases with presence of the Lobules, as Precursory Lesions):
   - Fibroepithelial lesions:
     – *Fibroadenoma*
     – *Phyllodes tumor*
     – *Carcinosarcoma*
   - Lobular carcinomas

This classification does not include accidentally breast infections, from folliculitis to abscess, because the history and the clinical examination are usually concluding and the imaging diagnosis are not justified.

10.3 Endocrine and Imaging-Pathological Correlations in Gynecomastia

Because benign gynecomastia represents the most part of pathological male breast enlargement and the dishormonal etiology is the most frequent, DE is the method of choice before any interventional procedure, because the anatomical analysis offers the positive and differential diagnosis of gynecomastia and could characterize its subtypes (acute/florid, chronic, with or without additional masses), with recommendation for targeted hormonal tests and complementary imaging exams, reducing the time and the costs of the overall diagnosis [16].

The most important dishormonal changes implying gynecomastia were signaled:

- *Infertility:* A report of a positive correlation between E2 and FSH ($r=0.67$, $p<0.0001$) in a group of 106 infertile men [3] confirms the correlation of hyperestrogenism (gynecomastia) with infertility (hypogonadism). Based on that result, gynecomastia should be interpreted as a symptom, but also as a marker of treatment response in infertile man.
- *Goiter and pituitary pathology:* In daily practice, there are many cases with gynecomastia and goiter, with or without hormonal changes, and rarely may be associated hyperprolactinemia. Most cases are acquired diseases with expression predominantly in adulthood, with various etiologies, but a report of Benvenga and col. (2000) presented a 10-year-old boy with congenital adrenal hyperplasia and associated hyperplastic testicular adrenal rests, which had high serum concentrations of 17-OH progesterone (17-OHP), estradiol (E2), testosterone (T), and basal and TRH-stimulated TSH and PRL, but normal thyroid hormones (T3, T4, FT3, FT4) and thyroxin-binding globulin (TBG). This case suggests that E2 stimulates the secretion of basal and TRH-elicited TSH and PRL [6]. The importance of this study is the illustration of the pathogenic relation between E2 (gynecomastia) and TSH and PRL and also the possibility of the presence of a goiter with normal T3 and T4.

- *Hyperprolactinemia* in man has multiple etiologies [13], and the serum levels are generally correlated, in women and men, with the FBU aspect: the illustration of ductal ectasia with diffuse increased vasculature is correlated with high hormonal activity, while the low Doppler mapping is always correlated with normal prolactinemia, whether an associated chronic galactophoritis could be present [27]. Doppler DE could be a good follow-up examination for hyperprolactinemia, less expansive, and time-consuming than the serologic hormonal tests.
- *Hyperestrogenemia* may be related to the coronary thrombosis in man [28], similar to the menopausal hormonal substitution treatment. Inversely, if florid gynecomastia or ductal-lobular hyperplasia in men is demonstrated on DE, the serum concentration of E2 must be evaluated as a risk factor for thrombosis.
- Hyperestrogenemia in elderly should be firstly considered as pathological, and after exclusion of any associated etiology, it could be assumed as "physiological." Some cases could have complex etiology, with hyperestrogenemia masked by other symptoms and pathological markers. A report of a 71-year-old man with clinical signs of Kennedy disease, including dysarthria, dysphagia, palatal and oral mandibular fasciculations, lower-extremity weakness, gynecomastia, and testicular atrophy, proved the correlation with an increased estrogen level of 180–220 pg/mL [29]. This paper demonstrates the importance of gynecomastia as a symptom in elderly man.
- *Male breast cancer* coexists with gynecomastia, but there are confusions in the management of these diseases, while the classical methods of diagnosis could not demonstrate the benign mammary buds and ducts.

Gynecomastia in the general assumption is either a benign disease or a physiological breast development in male; however, 50 % of cases with gynecomastia are selected for mammography [10]. In elderly males, gynecomastia makes up 65 % of all breast lesions; 25 % is carcinoma and 10 % are other lesions. In fact, estrogen receptors are more commonly present in males with breast cancer than in women, occurring in 75–94 % of males with cancer [2].

Because the breast tissue in males responds to the hormonal stimulation, with growth of ducts and connective tissue resulting in gynecomastia, the overwhelming histological subtype of breast carcinoma in men is ductal or unclassified (93.7 %), followed by papillary (2.6 %). Infiltrating lobular carcinoma is rare in males, likely because of the rarity of terminal lobules in the male breast. The value of the FBU examination consists in the diagnosis of both gynecomastia and cancer, with visualization of nonpalpable infracentimetric tumors. In our experience, florid gynecomastia with salient new vasculature or the type with ductal hyperplasias are correlated with hyperestrogenemia at the time of the examination, while chronic gynecomastia with less vasculature may be associated with normal values of the steroid tests (Figs. 10.3, 10.4, 10.5, 10.6, 10.7, 10.8, 10.9, 10.10, 10.11, 10.12, and 10.13).

Doppler DE demonstrated large central ductal-ampullary ectasia up to 3–4 mm in diameter, peripheral thickened lobules connected to the ending ducts, and increased vascular Doppler signal with arterial and venous flow, similar to the lactating breast. Previous surgical treatment had proven milky ducts in the right breast (based on [1]) (Figs. 10.14, 10.15, and 10.16).

MRI examination demonstrated a right adrenal mass with heterogeneous hypersignal in axial T1WI and T2WI, with mark on the right kidney. WFT1 WI changes the character of the tumor in a heterogeneous hyposignal, demonstrating the lipid component of the tumor, almost pathognomonic for the benign adrenal adenoma (the "chemical shift sign") (based on [16]) (Figs. 10.17, 10.18, 10.19, 10.20, 10.21, 10.22, 10.23, and 10.24).

10.4 Pediatric Breast Disorders

The breast develops from the mammary bud that is formed in the first 6 weeks of life in utero. At birth, neonatal bud breast usually presents a small ductal branching with swelling, tenderness, and sometimes a minimal nipple surge, the so-called witch's milk, considered as physiological due to the maternal hormonal transplacental transfer. Further normal breast development does not occur until puberty, which usually occurs after 9 years old (Fig. 10.25).

Precocious breast development in girls represents precocious/premature thelarche and occurs before 8 years old. Developing breast bud mistaken for a mass could determine unsuitable surgical treatment finalized with amastia. The premature thelarche must be differentiated in the isolated form, considered as "benign," slowly progressive, from the premature puberty that refers to the appearance of physical and hormonal signs of puberty earlier than 8 years in girls and 9 years for boys. The precocious puberty is associated with pubarche (appearance of pubic hair in girls or boys younger than 7–8 years) and hormonal changes, as resulting risks of emotional distress, short stature because of rapid closure of the growing cartilages, presence of menses in girls, and increased libido in boys. In girls, US examinations may illustrate the development of the uterine body, with reversal of the index body/cervix >1 (in the prepubertal age, the index cervix/uterine body >2) and the development of multiple ovarian antral follicles (Figs. 10.25, 10.26, 10.27, 10.28, and 10.29).

Asymmetric development of breasts is usual, and it could be mistaken for a unilateral breast mass at clinical examination both in children and men and frequently is followed by biopsy and eventually surgical treatment. Breast biopsy in children must be carefully decided, because the secondary

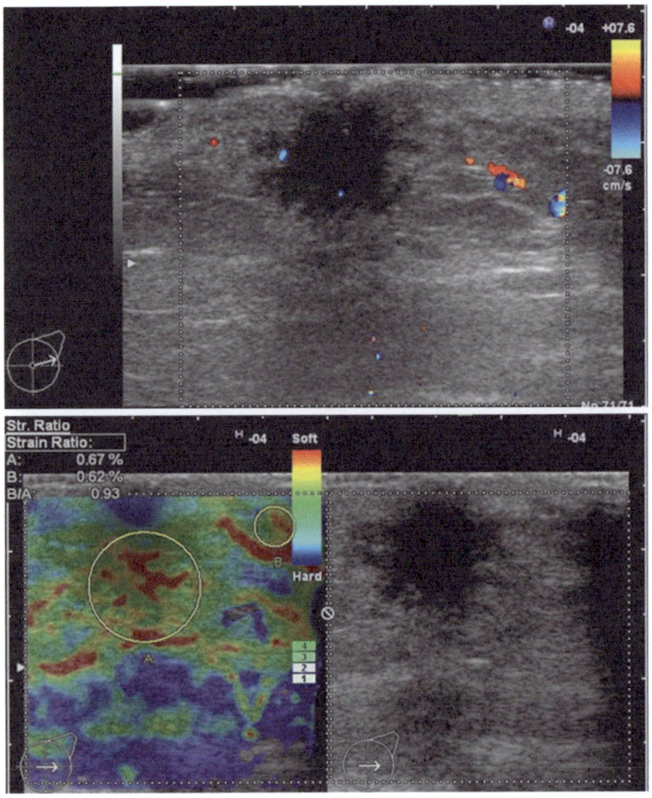

Fig. 10.25 FBU in a 10-year-old girl, normal thelarche: the mammary bud with peripheral branching ducts, surrounded by few amount of hyperechoic specific glandular stroma, containing many branches of new formation periareolary vasculature

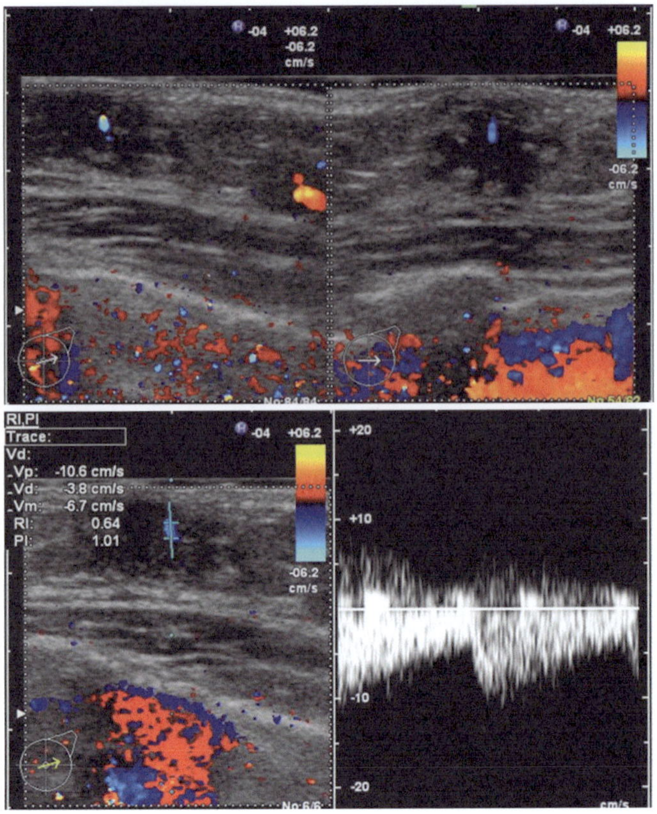

Fig. 10.26 Precocious thelarche in a 1-year-old girl, with similar Doppler US appearances with recent development

effects may be more important than in adults, due to the risk of hematomas [14] and to the effects of scar formation in a developing breast.

The premature thelarche has multiple etiologies, the most important being related to the precocious puberty that is determined by the secretion of high-amplitude pulses of gonadotropin-releasing hormone (GnRH) by hypothalamus.

Most cases of simple, isolated premature thelarche have no further complications, with most of these girls having normal puberty at a normal age.

The importance of the diagnosis of the true premature thelarche is the selection of the cases with risk of premature puberty, which must be further investigated for central nervous system abnormalities (tumors, inflammations, trauma, surgery, and congenital anomalies) [30]. Other causes seem to be familial inheritance, an increased body mass index, and an exposure to exogenous sex hormones (estrogens in poultry, phytoestrogens in soy products, environmental estrogen like agents such as pesticides and phthalates) [31]. To optimize visualization of the breast tissue, a linear-array high-MHz transducer should be used. For the evaluation of superficial lesions, using of a standoff pad or a generous mound of acoustic coupling gel to substitute for a standoff pad is helpful.

Normal US findings in children prior to thelarche were described in Chap. 3; there is the small hypoechoic mammary bud surrounded by the subcutaneous fatty tissue and with linear fibers of the pectoralis muscle located posteriorly. Subcutaneous fat demonstrates heterogeneous echotexture in a healthy infant. The ribs may also be seen as hypoechoic masses with associated shadowing, but they should not be mistaken for breast masses because they lie posterior to the pectoralis muscle; the cartilaginous parasternal rib segments may appear as hypoechoic well-shaped ovalar masses with posterior acoustic enhancement and marginal shadows (Kobayashi signs), mimicking benign lesions, but they are located posteriorly to the pectoral muscles, and no connection with the mammary bud can be demonstrated. When breast development starts, the breast bud appears as retroareolar pyramidal hypoechoic tissue that has small branches usually asymmetrically extended, mostly towards the upper-outer quadrant. The presence of the hyperechoic mammary stroma is always detected with new vasculature more or less salient, always beginning in the periareolary vascular circle, and with uniform distribution in the mammary quadrants (Figs. 10.28, 10.29, 10.30, 10.31, and 10.32).

In the pediatric and adolescent population, the literature and our results show that benign findings are the most

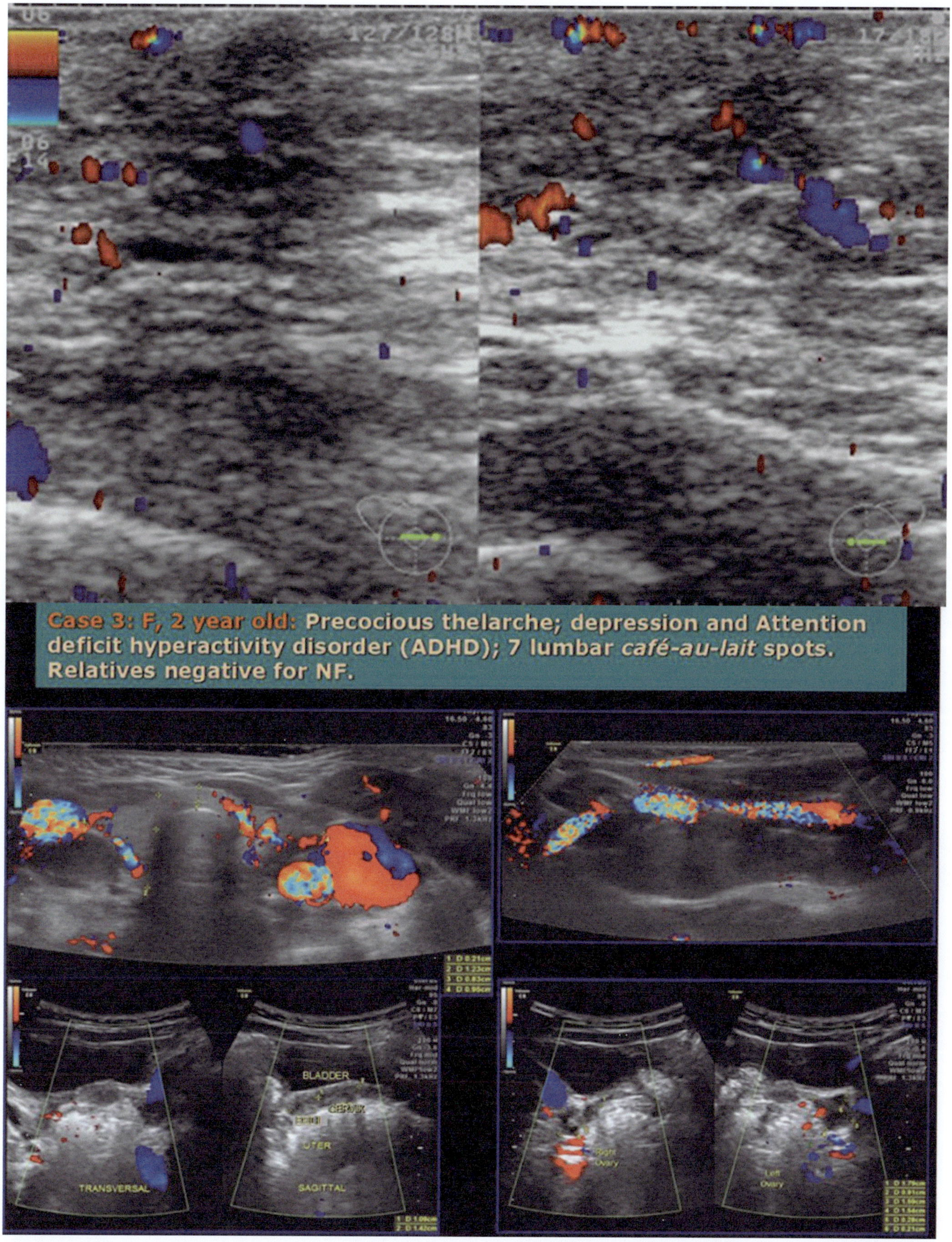

Fig. 10.27 Precocious puberty with precocious thelarche in a 2-year-old girl with neurofibromatosis 1 (the von Recklinghausen disease); the deep right cervical plexiform neurofibroma is displacing the right common carotid artery (based on [30])

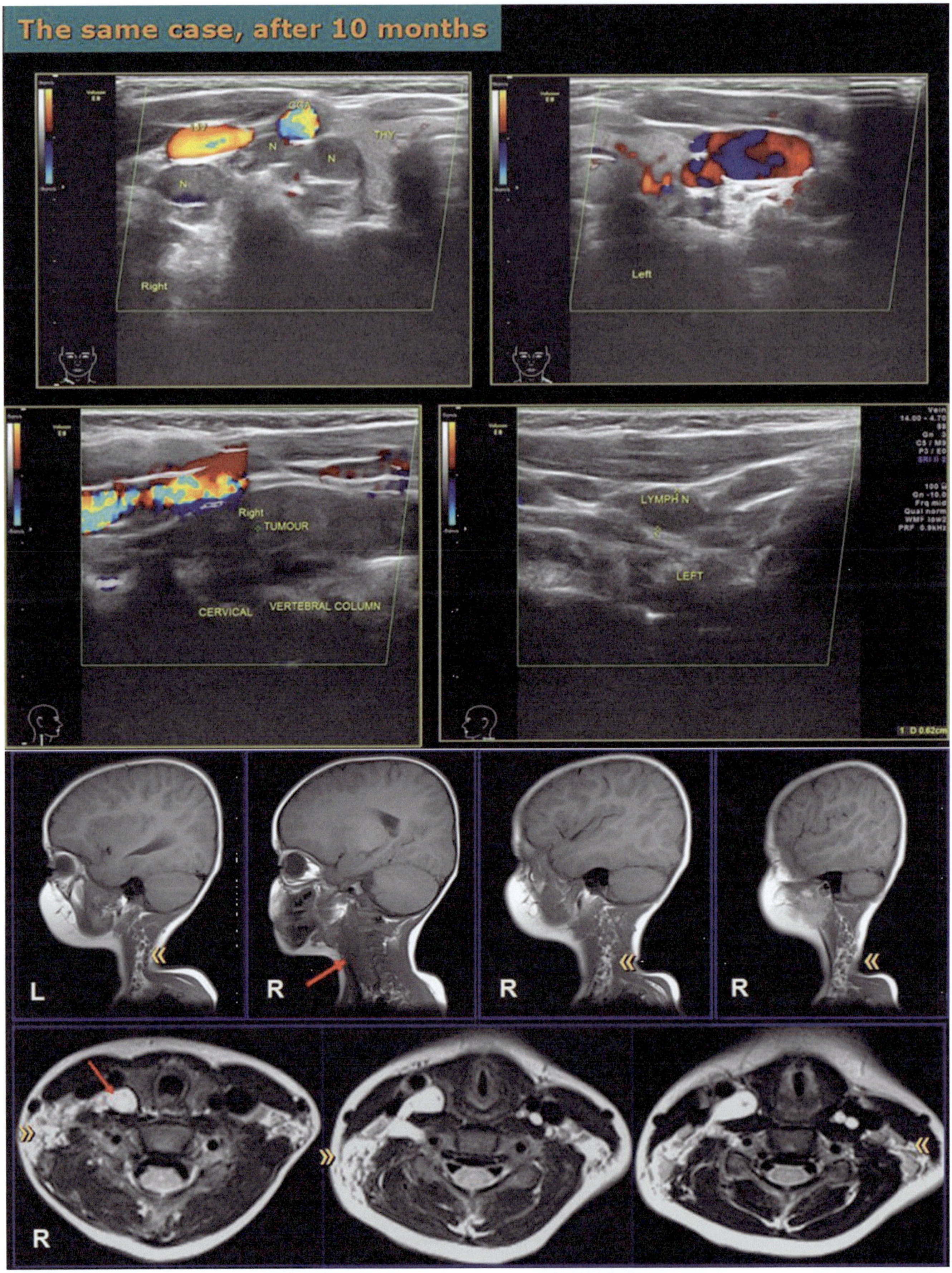

Fig. 10.28 Precocious puberty associated to neurofibromatosis 1, the same case: sagittal US scans illustrate the right plexiform neurofibroma and the left nodular tumors, similar to the sagittal T1WI and axial T2WI MRI scans; no evolution in the first 10 months (based on [30])

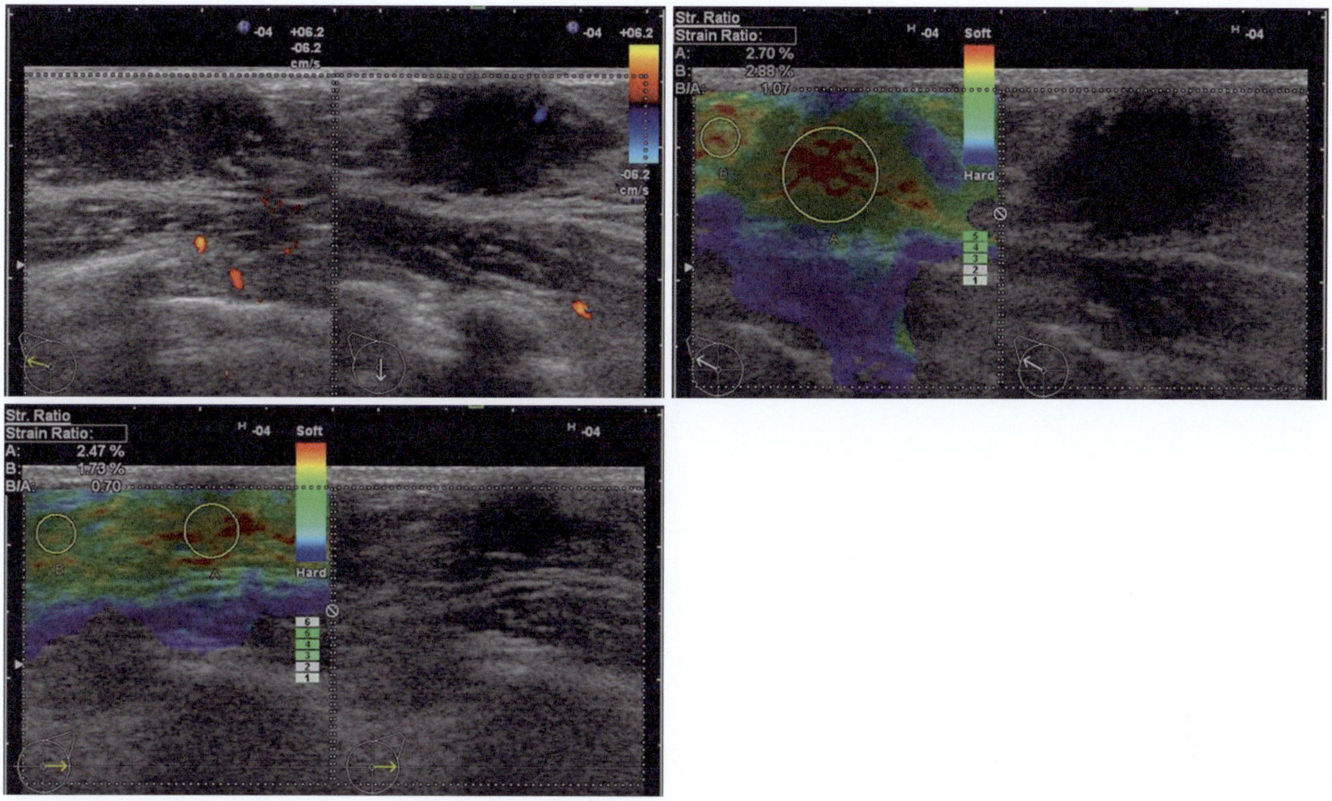

Fig. 10.29 Precocious thelarche in a 5-year-old girl, with asymmetrical development and pseudotumoral features; however, the peripheral ducts emerging from the hypoechoic mammary bud, which has benign posterior effects based on Kobayashi, are concordant with the benign score on sonoelastography

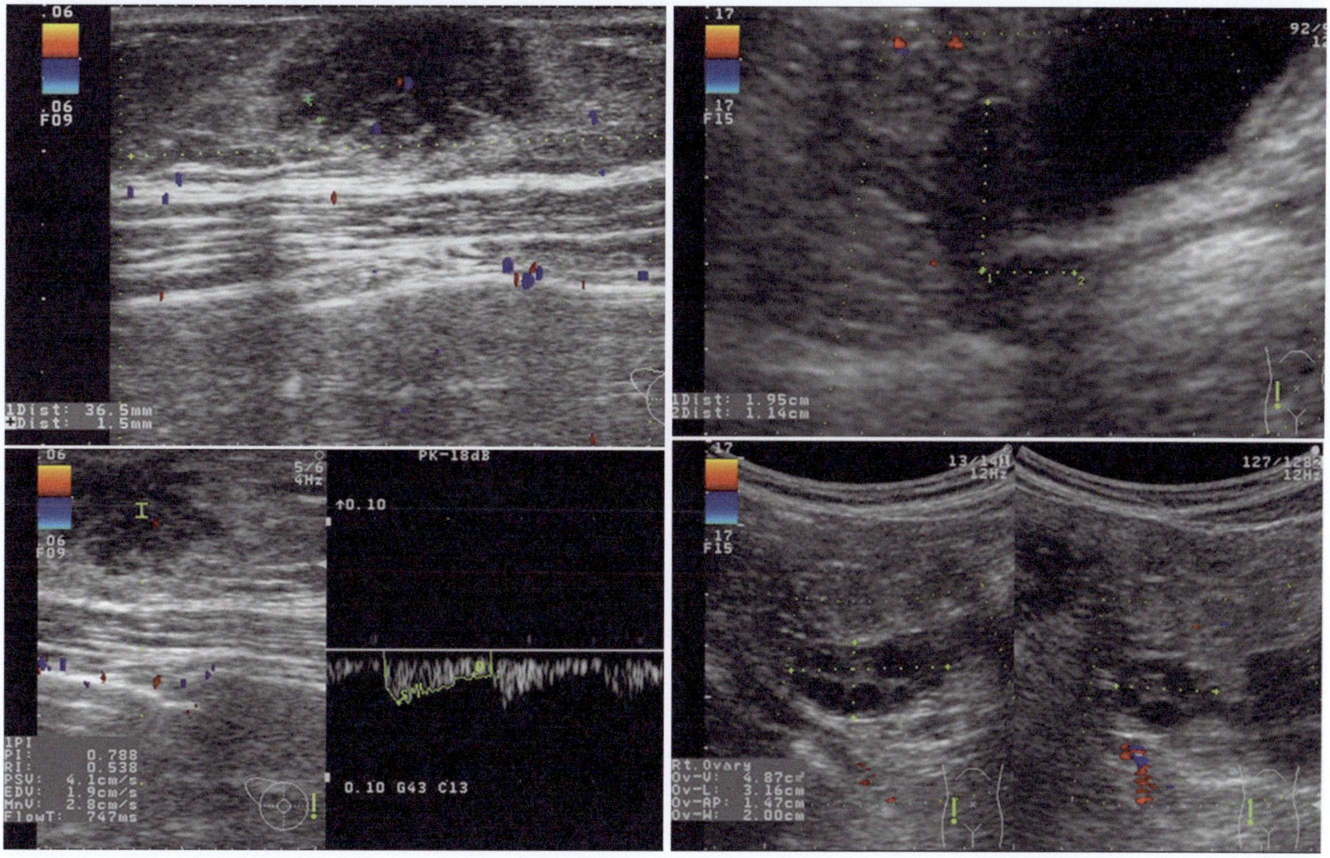

Fig. 10.30 Physiological thelarche in a 9-year-old girl, with uterine and ovarian simultaneous changes

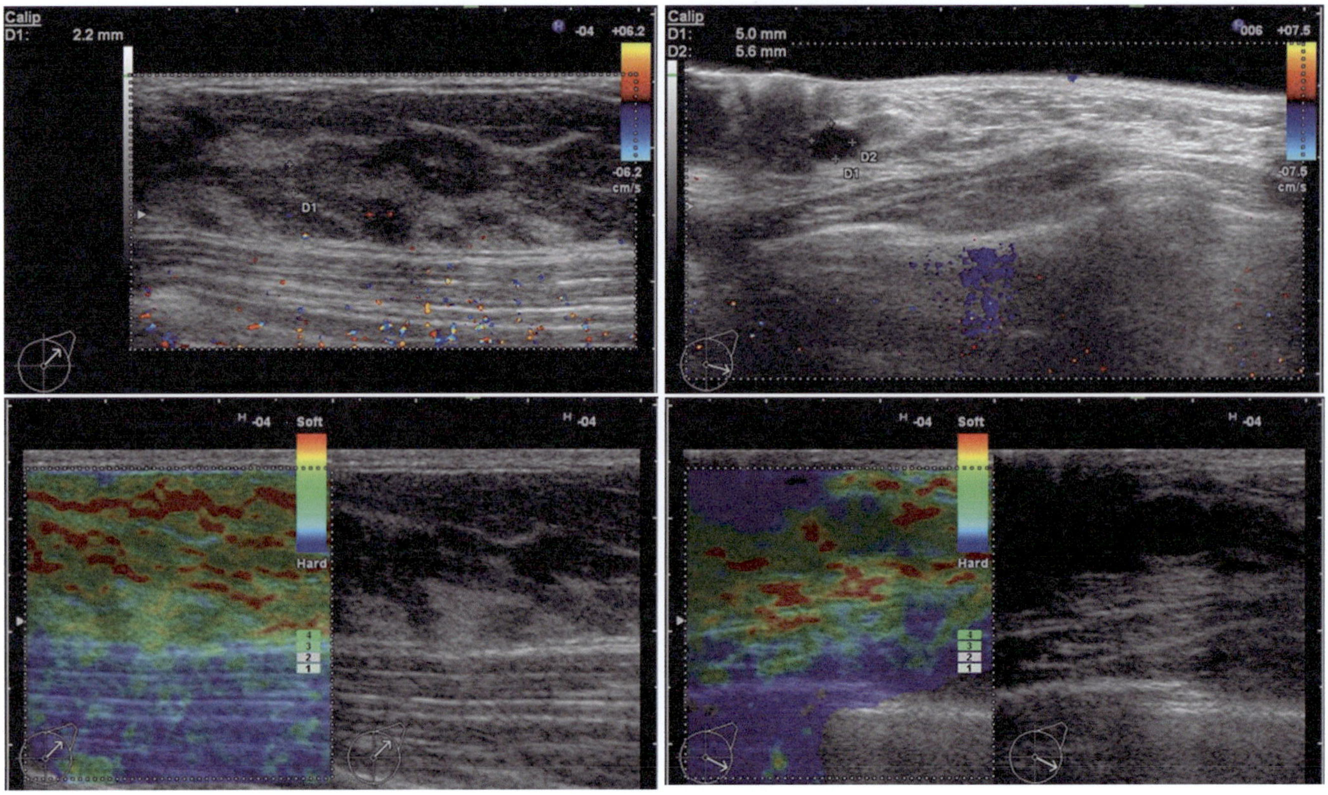

Fig. 10.31 Normal young pubertal breast in a 15-year-old: branching ducts and a remnant of the bud, with new vessels. RTSE shows high elasticity of the breast parenchyma

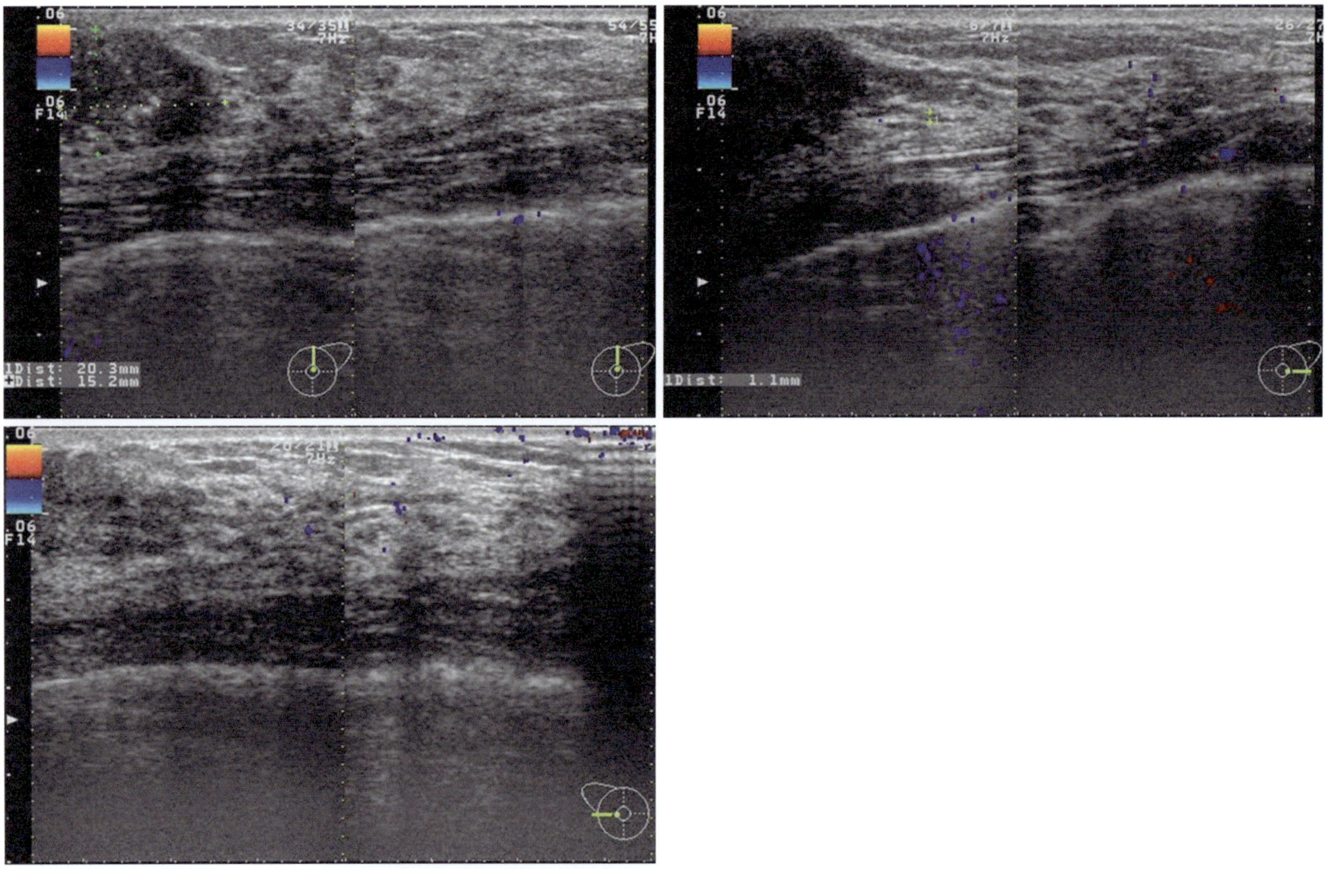

Fig. 10.32 Physiological thelarche: advanced stage of branching ducts in healthy 17-year-old patient; the remnant mammary bud has a pseudonodular aspect due to less developed mammary stroma in the retroareolar space, specific to the young breast type

common cause of symptomatic breast abnormalities. A careful physical examination with clinical follow-up and US helps in the evaluation of patient symptoms. Fibroadenomas are the most common solid breast masses excised in the pediatric and adolescent population, but the precise moment of the surgical treatment is unclear; we think that if the solid mass has no significant new vasculature and the size and growing evolution are not increased, then a conservative expectative treatment should be preferred in children and puberty, because of the possibility of spontaneous remission of the small lesions during breast development; moreover, fibroadenomas in young people are usually multicentric and multifocal, with asynchronous evolution, and each surgical treatment may increase the number of scars and may involve the breast growing process.

However, in the classical literature it is recommended in cases with US scans negative to base on the level of the clinical concern. Given the overwhelmingly benign causes, surgery should be the last resort and reserved only for lesions that are enlarged or have highly suspected features.

In the last years, given the development of the ultrasonographic machines, the knowledge of the sonographic appearance of physiological breast development and specific lesions in children and the young has acquired new acquisitions; as a consequence, breast sonography is nowadays most helpful in identifying and characterizing abnormalities and guiding further investigation.

A study of Aruna Vade and col. [32], concerning 20 adolescent girls between 13 and 19 years old who presented with palpable breast masses found to be solid at breast US, concluded that the classical US was not useful for predicting the histological diagnosis of all solid benign breast masses in adolescent patients. The Stavros sonographic criteria [33], however, were useful for predicting benignity in 65 % of the breast masses on which histopathologic examination was performed. We think not all benign findings in children must be surgically removed, especially when there are multiple nodular hyperplasias, because of inaesthetical risk of scars, risk of recurrence, and risk of damage relative to the finalizing of the developing breast. Moreover, this study is in accord with the specific literature and demonstrates the low specificity of the Stavros criteria in young breast when the glandular anatomy is neglected, the ductal connection is unknown, and the Doppler value is underestimated.

A detailed classification of the lesions found in 62 patients between 8 weeks and 20 years of age [34] after clinical and classical sonographic evaluation established four main groups of diagnoses: benign tumors (15), developmental disturbances (14), cystic changes (11), and inherent defects (7). In the remaining cases, the findings were no abnormality (9), nipple discharge without evidence of pathological or morphological correlates (3), abscesses (2), and epidermoid cyst (1). This study is significant because it demonstrates the absence of the malignancy, but it does not prove the accuracy of US in the differential diagnosis of benign findings; moreover, this study based on the classical US does not define the "developmental disturbances" or the "inherent defects" and cannot explain the nipple discharge, these limits being imposed by the nonanatomical sonographic examination.

Classical US is particularly helpful in characterizing cystic, inflammatory, and neoplastic lesions in children. Although most masses that occur in the pediatric breast are benign, *phyllodes tumor* may be benign or malignant. In adolescents, cystosarcoma phyllodes is rare, but it rests still as the most common malignant breast tumors. Phyllodes tumor is presented in the classical US as well-circumscribed, oval, or lobulated tumor with rapid grows; it develops from the periductal stroma, and it has a fibroepithelial structure, sometimes containing cystic areas.

After using US to evaluate breast masses in pediatric and adolescent patients, Weinstein and col. [34] reported the following findings: gynecomastia, cyst, fibroadenoma, lymph node, galactocele, ductal ectasia, and infection. They had no patients with malignancy, but citing Kronemer and col., they cautioned that, in rare cases, rhabdomyosarcoma, non-Hodgkin lymphoma, and leukemia may metastasize to the breast in children and adolescents [35].

Generally, most studies presented the occurrence especially of the solid masses and of no focal abnormality in symptomatic breasts for this group of age, while the cysts are more rare [34]; contrarily, as the women are aging, the incidence of simple cysts or fibrocystic dysplasia and of ductal ectasia is increasing. This aspect was not yet explained, but it is in contradiction with the occurrence of the cystic dysplasia based on *the sick lobe theory* that assumes the embryonic period [36].

The absence of the anatomical examination and interpretation of the breast in children determines the misdiagnosing of the classical US, which describes, for instance, in adolescents *glandular tissue, which is echogenic and surrounded by hypoechoic fat*, or *the glandular tissue is echogenic relative to the hypoechoic fat; this appearance mimics the breast tissue in an adult.* In fact, the specific *glandular tissue* in the breast is hypoechoic and represents the glandular parenchyma as in adulthood, which in children contains the mammary bud with branching galactophorous ducts, and lately completed at the end of the TDLUs with the glandular lobules. The glandular parenchyma is surrounded by the glandular stroma, which is itself well defined from the fatty tissue at the periphery and the glandular parenchyma in the central mammary area; the glandular stroma is hyperechoic due to the various components of the connective tissue and is similar in the developing breast with those of an adult breast. The glandular stroma is thicker than the stroma of the fatty tissue, represented by thin, linear hyperechoic *septa*, some with vascular signals on Doppler (Figs. 10.33, 10.34, 10.35, 10.36, 10.37, 10.38, 10.39, and 10.40).

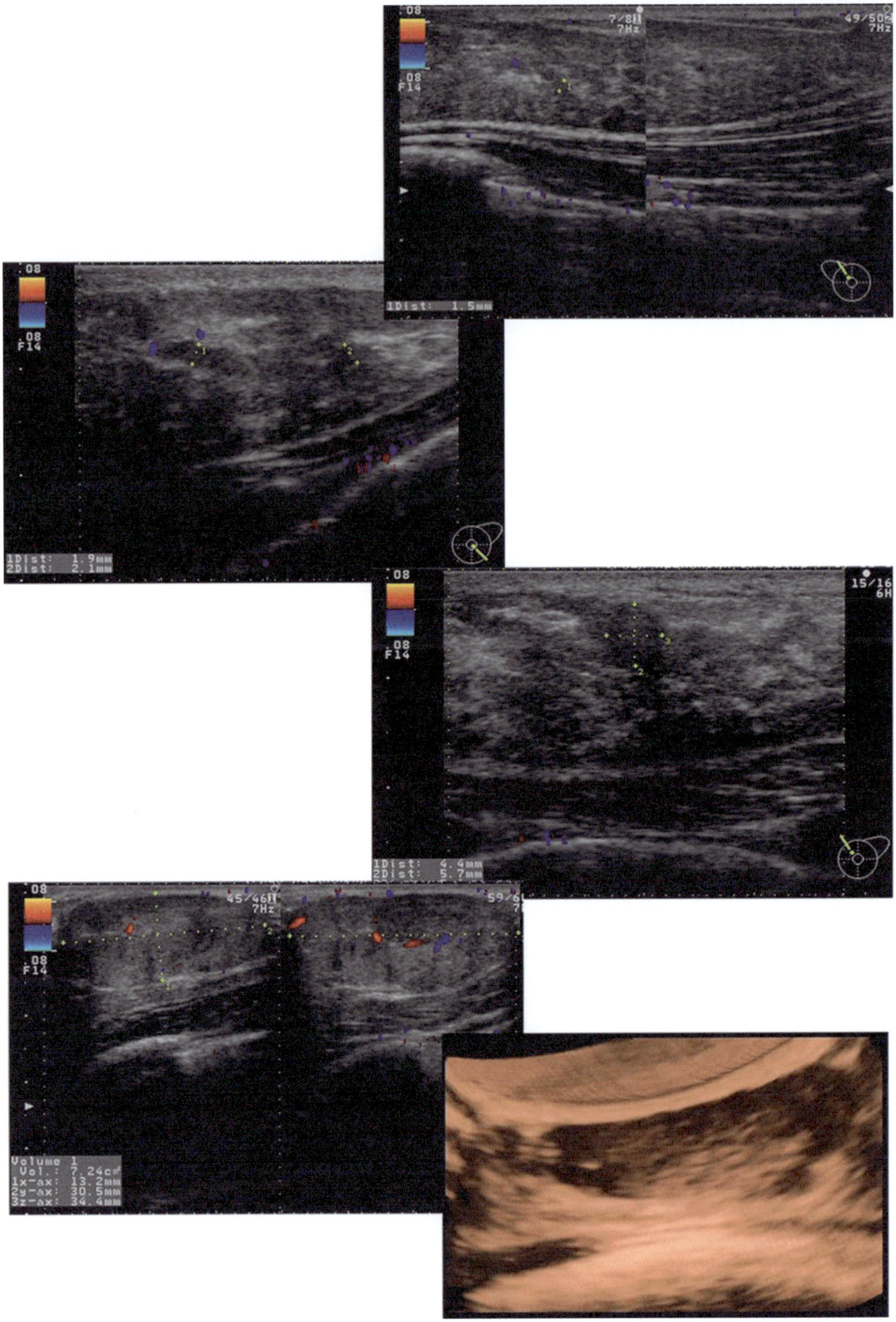

Fig. 10.33 A 15-year-old patient: dense young breast, with multiple fibroadenomas, on Doppler 2D US and 4D US

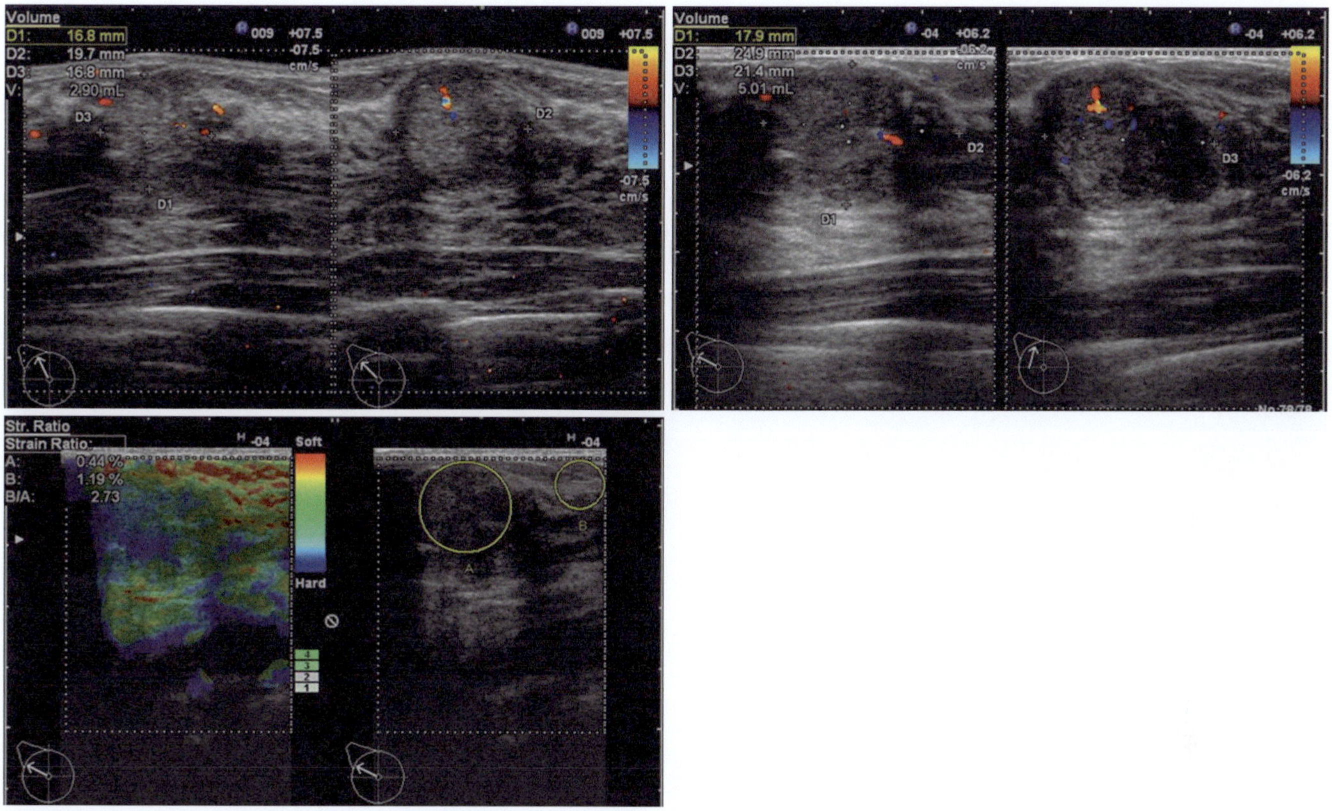

Fig. 10.34 A 15-year-old patient, the same case: R 11:00 normal developing breast, whereas at R 9:30, a solid nodule with 2D, color Doppler, and RTSE aspect of a benign lesion suggesting fibroadenoma

10.5 Malignancy of the Pediatric and Adolescent Breast

It is worldwide accepted that malignancies in the pediatric and adolescent populations are extremely rare. Potential malignancies in such patients may be either primary breast cancers or metastatic disease from other primary lesions. Primary breast cancer in patients younger than 20 years is exceedingly rare. Metastatic disease to the young breast occurs late in the course of a malignancy, because of the reduced vascularity in this period of life. Rhabdomyosarcoma, non-Hodgkin lymphoma, and leukemia are the most common primary tumors to metastasize to the breast in young patients [37]. When malignant breast mass occurs in this age group, it is more likely to be metastatic from a non-breast origin than a primary breast cancer [38].

The malignant findings of a mass have the same characters as in the adult population:

- *Irregular, angular, or microlobulated margins.*
- *Posterior acoustic shadowing.*
- *Exhibit vertical growth that is greater than horizontal growth.*
- *A rapidly enlarging mass should also be clinically suspected, although benign masses such as fibroadenomas may also grow over time.*

In a child or adolescent, especially those with a known history of a primary malignancy other than breast cancer, enlargement of even a circumscribed solid mass should be viewed with caution because it can be a metastasis to the breast; the differential diagnosis with precocious thelarche or gynecomastia may be clinical resolute by the absence of the breast pain. Chateil et al. [37] describe a variety of appearances for metastatic disease. In the classical US, some lesions are well circumscribed, but others exhibit more suspect features, such as posterior acoustic shadowing and vertical growth greater than horizontal growth. Among metastatic lesions, the most common US feature is heterogeneous echotexture.

None of the patients in our population had a malignant mass, but metastases from distant cancers are possible; moreover, axillary adenopathy may have extramammary

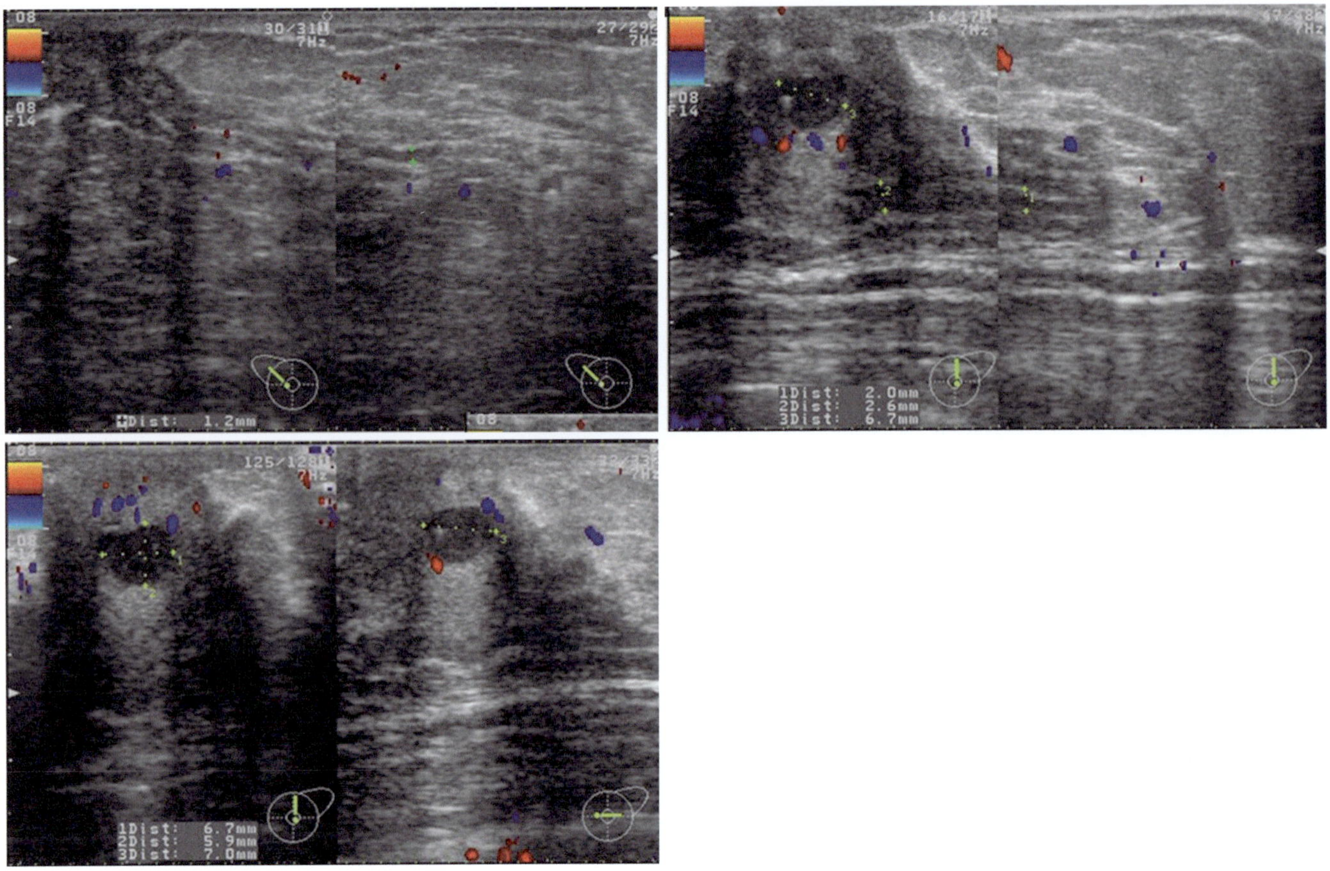

Fig. 10.35 Pathological thelarche in a 14-year-old girl: a 7 mm retroareolar fibroadenoma, located inside the mammary bud, hypoechoic with benign Kobayashi posterior effects, surrounded by new formation vessels. The ducts are distinct in the periphery, where the stroma is more developed than in the central region of the breast, typically for the thelarche

origins, and the breast involvement can be excluded after normal FBU. Despite the proved value in the assessment of the tissue strain in adults, sonoelastography is less applied in the pediatric investigation, mainly for the assessment of liver fibrosis, of the muscles in spastic neuropathy, of the thyroid, or of the peripheral lymph nodes. Further researchers will allow the use of sonoelastography in the diagnosis and therapeutic response monitoring of the soft tissue malignancies in pediatric breast included.

The connection with the ducts is proved by DE, and the developing process by accretion (new vessels) and concretion (fusion of the surrounding hypertrophic lobules) is obvious.

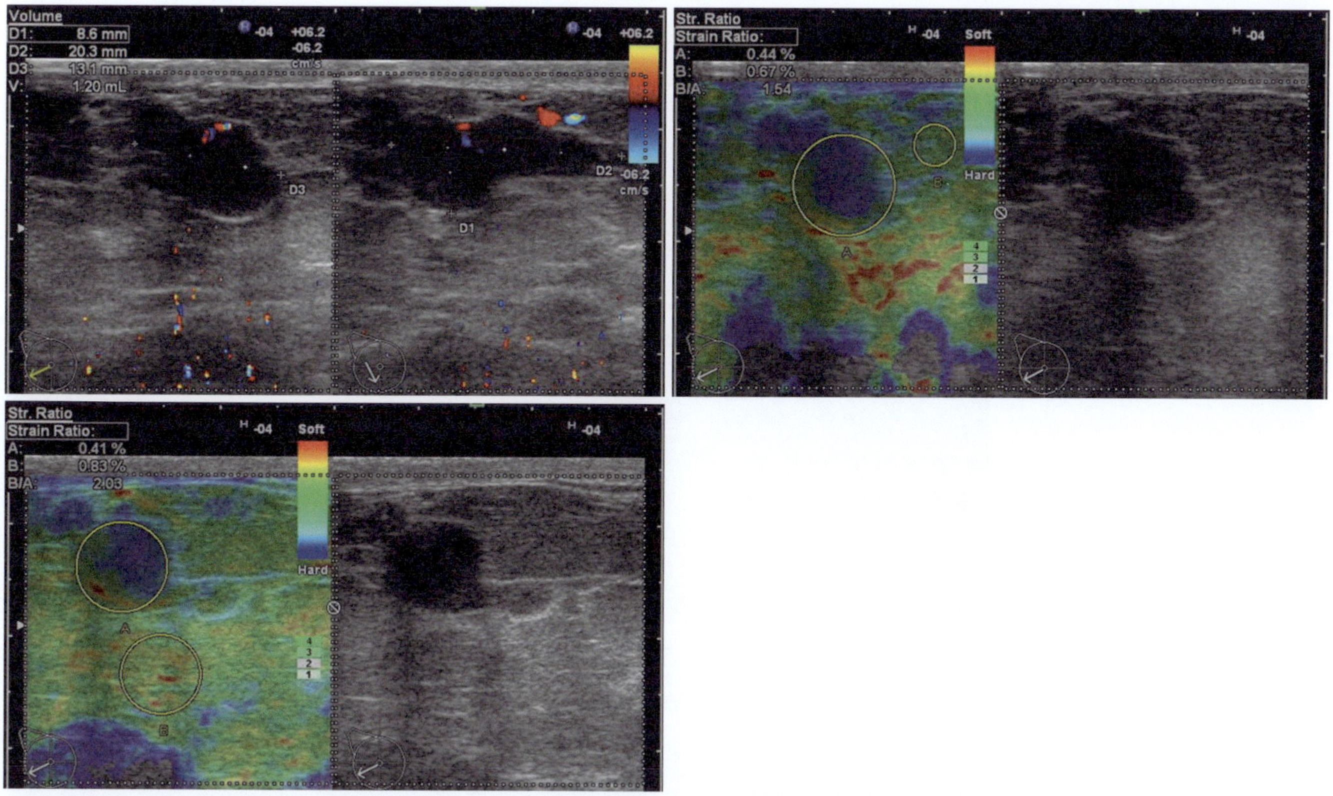

Fig. 10.36 Pathological thelarche in a 14-year-old girl: FBU illustrates at R 8:00 an enlargement of a ductal-ampullary segment, with ductal wall thickening with Doppler signal and fluid content; the BGR score based on Ueno and the low FLR are argued for benign findings with recommendation for a conservative treatment

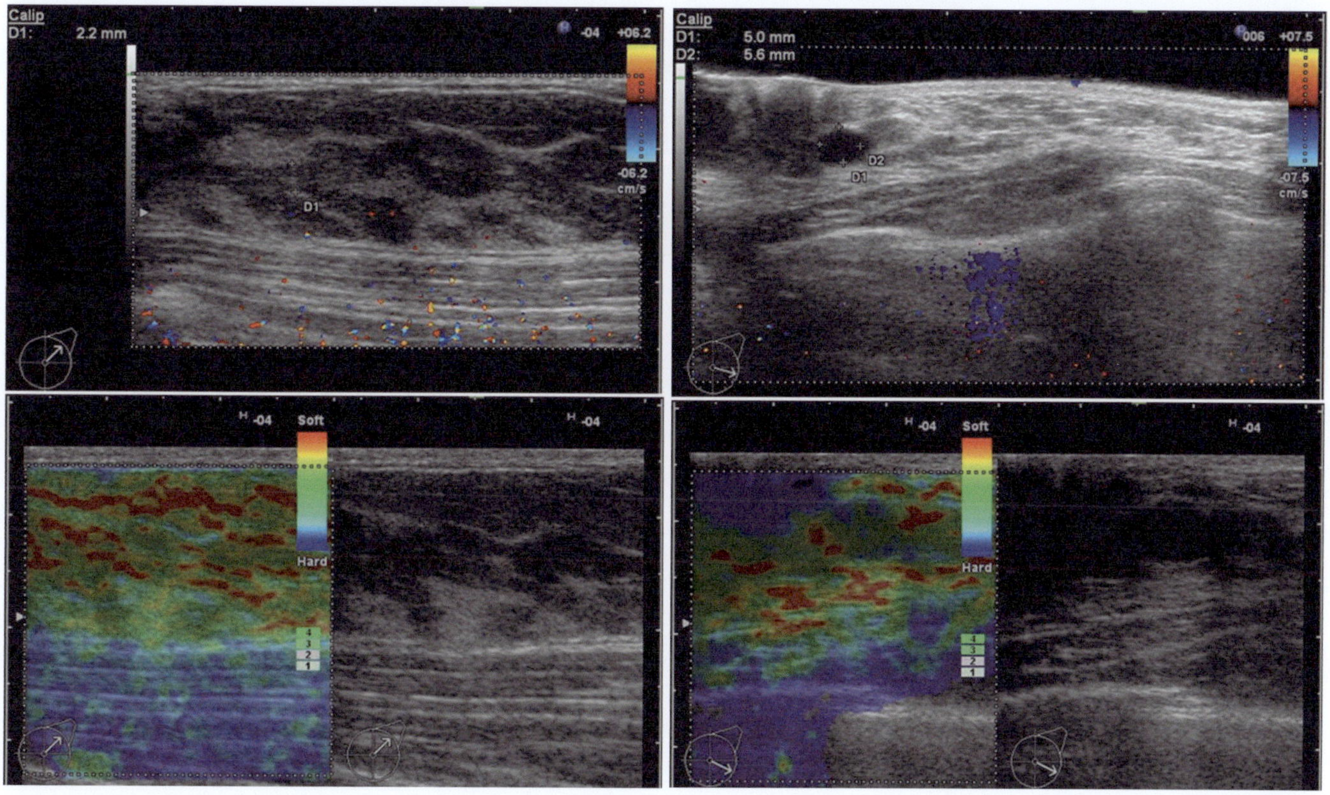

Fig. 10.37 Pathological thelarche in a 15-year-old girl: small cyst in the retroareolar region between the emerging ducts

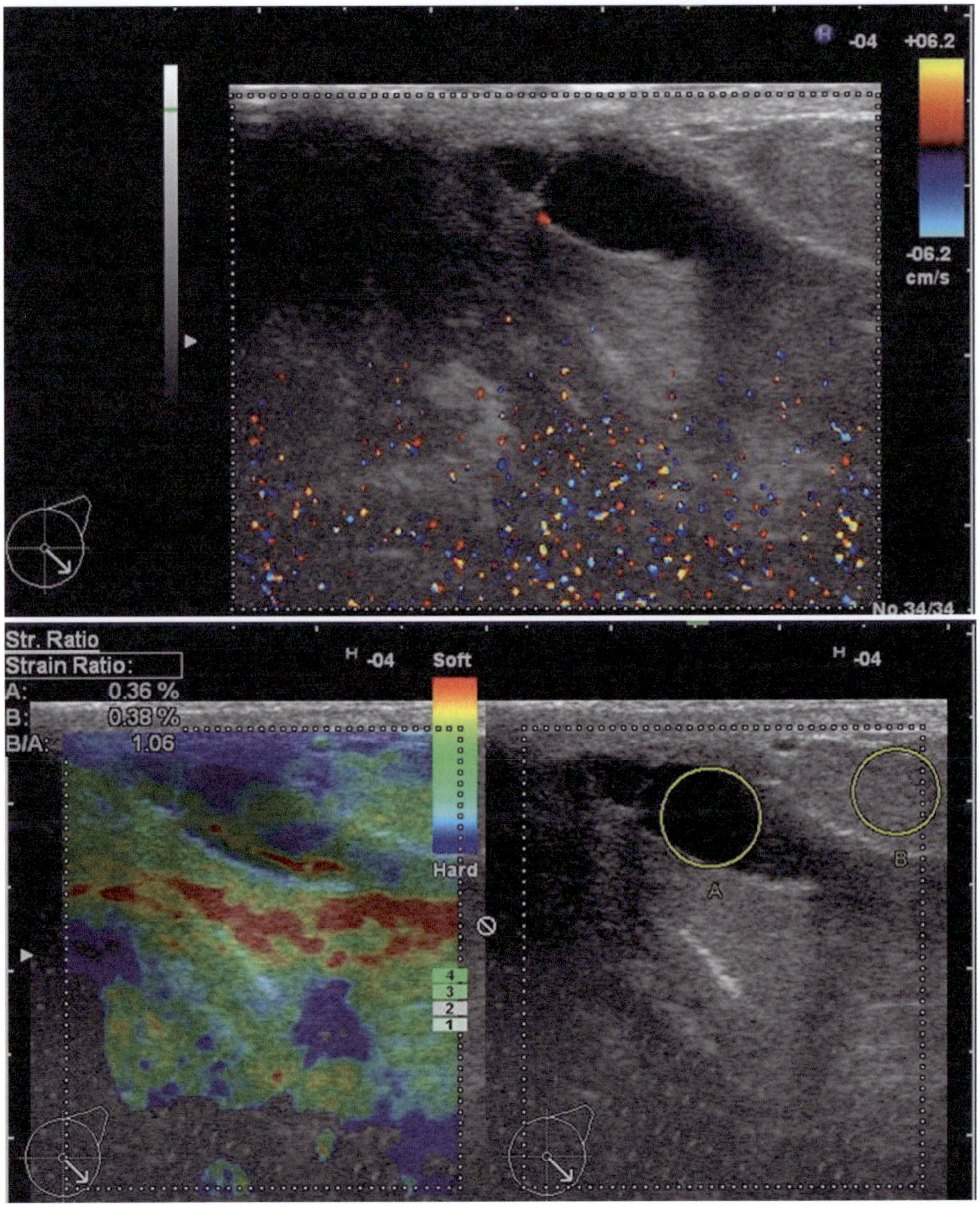

Fig. 10.38 Pathological thelarche in a 14-year-old patient: a couple of periareolary cysts with transonic content and thin walls in the L 5:00 radius, at the periphery of the mammary branching bud, with BGR score; the normal bud with intense hypoechogeneicity has high elasticity scored 1 Ueno

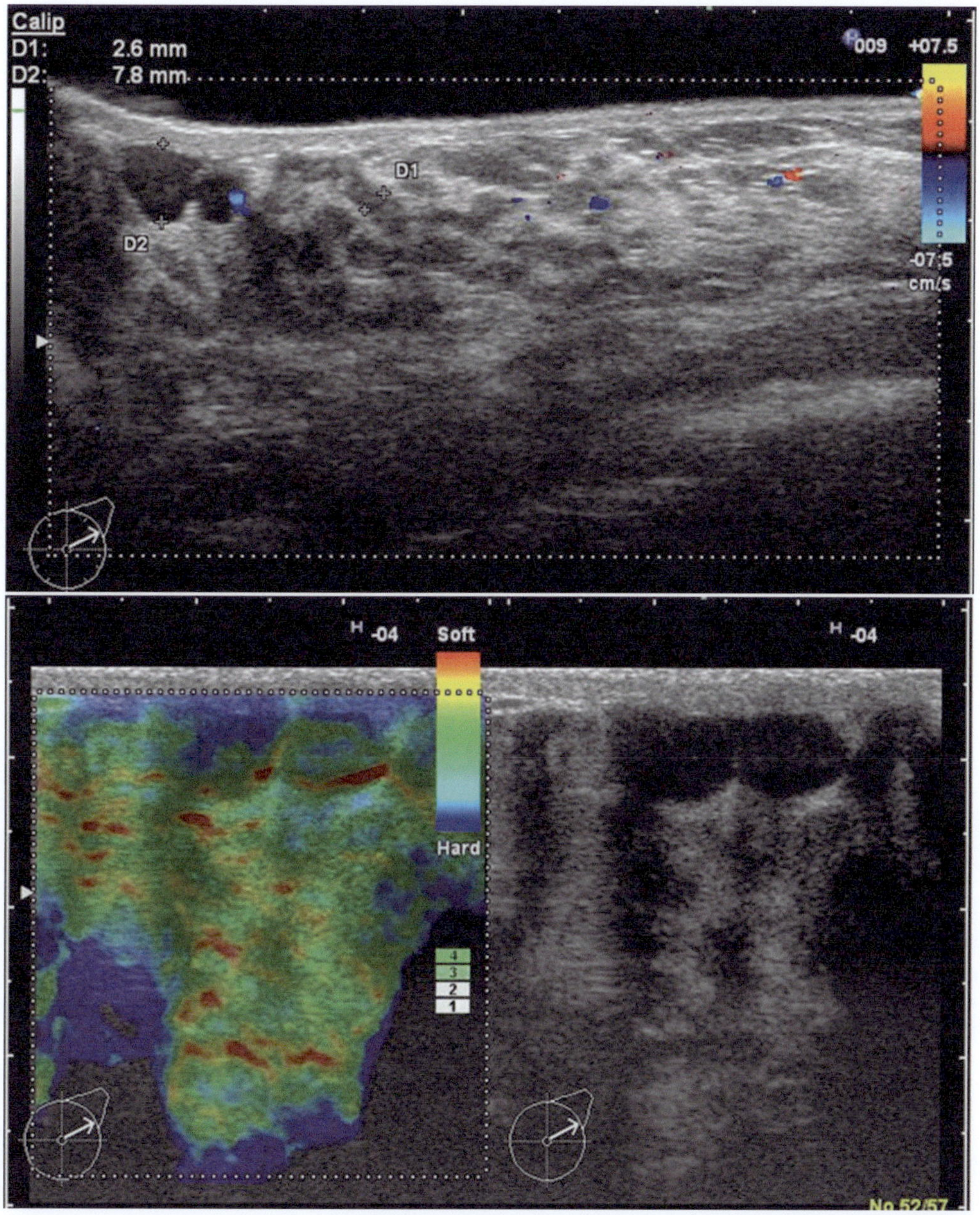

Fig. 10.39 Pathological thelarche in a 16-year-old girl: FBU illustrates at L 2:00 a young-dense type of mammary breast with thick ducts and large amount of glandular stroma and a periareolary couple of communicant cysts with fluid/debris level and BGR score

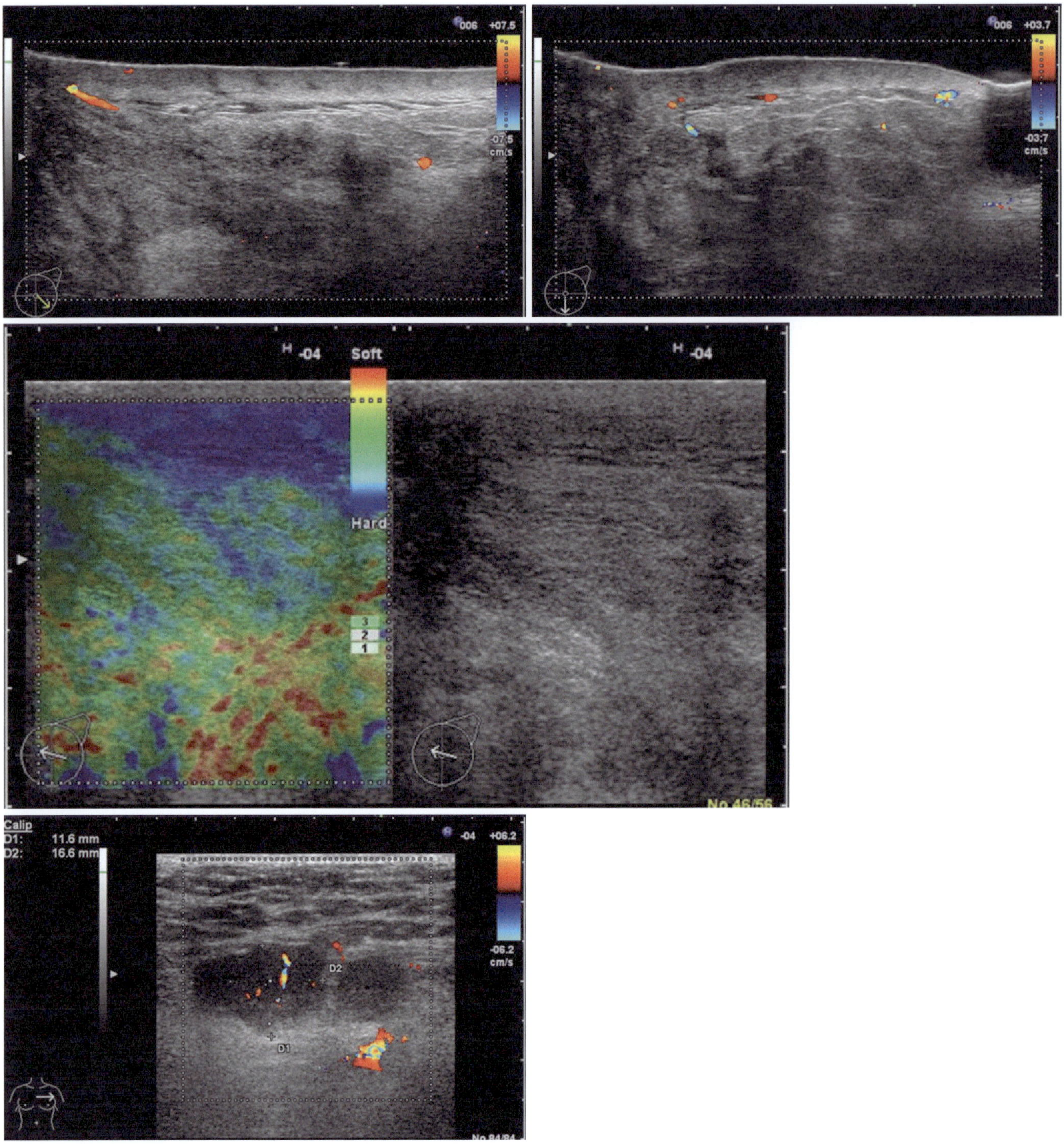

Fig. 10.40 Pathological thelarche in a 17-year-old patient with diffuse nonpuerperal mastitis: FBU illustrates the edema with thickening of the skin and lymphatic vessels in the premammary fatty tissue, an increase echogenicity of the glandular structures, salient diffuse vasculature, high stiffness of the superficial tissues (skin and fat), and a normal elasticity of the glandular region (ducts in *green*). The satellite axillary lymph nodes present reactive changes

References

1. Georgescu AC, Enachescu V (2009) The diagnosis of gynecomastia by Doppler Ductal Ultrasonography. Etiopathogenic, endocrine and imaging correlations – partial data. Med Ultrason 11(3):33–40
2. Thomas DB, Jimenez LM, McTiernan A et al (1992) Breast cancer in men: risk factors with hormonal implications. Am J Epidemiol 135:734–748. PubMed Abstract
3. Ramirez-Torres MA, Carrera A, Zambrana M (2000) High incidence of hyperestrogenemia and dyslipidemia in a group of infertile men. Ginecol Obstet Mex 68:224–229
4. Fujimoto Y, Hatama M, Tezuka K, Otani H et al (2005) Ultrasonic screening of the thyroid in the patients with breast complaints. In: Research and development in breast ultrasound. Springer, Tokyo, pp 167–169
5. Fujimoto Y, Kato Y, Maekawa H et al (1988) Ultrasonic screening of thyroid in the patients with breast complaints. J Ultrasound Med 7:39–S283
6. Benvenga S, Smedile G, Lo Giudice F et al (2000) Euthyroid hyperthyrotropinemia secondary to hyperestrogenemia in a male with congenital adrenal hyperplasia. Horm Metab Res 32(8):321–325, Page 50 of 50
7. De Rosa M, Zarrilli S, Di Sarno A et al (2003) Hyperprolactinemia in men. Clinical and biochemical features and response to treatment. Endocrine 20(1/2):75–82
8. Recchia AG, Vivacqua A, Gabriele S, Carpino A et al (2004) Xenoestrogens and the induction of proliferative effects in breast cancer cells via direct activation of oestrogen receptor alpha. Food Addit Contam 21(2):134–144
9. Vivacqua A, Recchia AG, Fasanella G, Gabriele S et al (2003) The food contaminants bisphenol A and 4-nonylphenol act as agonists for estrogen receptor alpha in MCF7 breast cancer cells. Endocrine 22(3):275–284
10. Evans GF, Anthony Y, Turnage RH et al (2001) The diagnostic accuracy of mammography in the evaluation of male breast disease. Am J Surg 181(2):96–100
11. Appelbaum AH, Evans GF, Levy KR et al (1999) Mammographic appearances of male breast disease. Radiographics 19(3):559–568
12. Cooper RA, Gunter BA, Ramamurthy L (1994) Mammography in men. Radiology 191(3):651–656
13. Berg WA (2006) Operator dependence of physician performed whole breast US: lesion detection and characterization. Radiology 214:355–365
14. Hertl K, Marolt-Musik M, Kocijancic I et al (2009) Haematomas after percutaneous vacuum assisted breast biopsy. Ultraschall in Med 30:33–36. doi:10.1055/s-2007-963724
15. Georgescu AC, Enachescu V, Bondari S (2010) The full breast Ultrasonography: an anatomical standardized imaging approach of the benign and malignant breast lesions. ECR, Vienna, EPOSTM. doi:10.1594/ecr2010/C-0434
16. Georgescu AC, Enachescu V (2010) The diagnosis of gynecomastia by Doppler ductal ultrasonography: etiopathogenic, endocrine and imaging correlations. ECR, Vienna, EPOSTM. doi:10.1594/ecr2010/C-0420
17. Renkes P, Gaucher P, Trechot P (1995) Spironolactone and hepatic toxicity. JAMA 273:376–377
18. Thompson D, Carter J (1993) Drug-induced gynecomastia. Pharmacotherapy 13:37–45
19. Loube SD, Quirk RA (1975) Letter: breast cancer associated with administration of spironolactone. Lancet 1:1428–1429
20. Weiss RJ, Moysich BK, Swede H (2005) Epidemiology of male breast cancer. Cancer Epidemiol Biomarkers Prev 14(1):20–26
21. Ruddy KJ, Winer EP (2013) Male breast cancer: risk factors, biology, diagnosis, treatment, and survivorship. Ann Oncol. doi:10.1093/annonc/mdt025
22. Burga AM, Fadare O, Lininger RA et al (2006) Invasive carcinomas of the male breast: a morphologic study of the distribution of histologic subtypes and metastatic patterns in 778 cases. Virchows Arch 449(5):507–512
23. Kornegoor R, Verschuur-Maes AH, Buerger H et al (2012) Molecular subtyping of male breast cancer by immunohistochemistry. Mod Pathol 25(3):398–404
24. Kujiraoka Y, Ueno E, Yohno E, Morishima I, Tsunoda-Shimizu H (2005) Incident angle of the plunging artery of breast tumors. In: Research and development in breast ultrasound. Springer, Tokyo, pp 72–75
25. Stavros AT, Thickman D, Rapp CL, Dennis MA, Parker SH, Sisney GA (1995) Solid breast nodules: use of sonography to distinguish between benign and malignant lesions. Radiology 196:123–134
26. Olsson H, Bladstrom A, Alm P (2002) Male gynecomastia and risk for malignant tumours – a cohort study. BMC Cancer 2:26. doi:10.1186/1471-2407-2-26
27. Georgescu AC, Andrei ME, Enachescu V, Bondari S (2013) New horizons in breast Doppler ductal echography: the positive and differential diagnosis of ductal ectasia, with etiopathological correlations. ECR, Viena, EPOSTM. doi:10.1594/ecr2013/C-0667
28. Phillips BG, Pinkernell HB, Jing T-Y (1996) The association of hyperestrogenemia with coronary thrombosis in men. Arterioscler Thromb Vasc Biol 16:1383–1387
29. Luo JJ (2007) Hyperestrogenemia simulating kennedy disease. J Clin Neuromusc Dis 9(2):291–296
30. Georgescu AC, Andrei ME, Manda A, Bondari S, Sendroiu I (2015) Contributions of imaging examinations in the diagnosis of the von Recklinghausen disease. ECR, Vienna, EPOSTM. doi:10.1594/ecr2015/C-1014
31. Kaplowitz PB, Kemp S, Windle LM, Levitsky LL et al (2014) Precocious puberty. Medscape, 14 Oct. http://emedicine.medscape.com/article/924002-clinical
32. Vade A, Lafita VS, Ward KA, Lim-Dunham JE, Bova D (2008) Role of breast sonography in imaging of adolescents with palpable solid breast masses. AJR Am J Roentgenol 191:659–663, © American Roentgen Ray Society
33. Bock K, Duda VF, Hadji P, Ramaswamy A, Schulz-Wendtland R, Klose K-J, Wagner U (2005) Pathologic breast conditions in childhood and adolescence evaluation by sonographic diagnosis. J Ultrasound Med 24:1347–1354, 0278–4297
34. Weinstein SP, Conant EF, Orel SG, Zuckerman JA, Bellah R (2000) Spectrum of US findings in pediatric and adolescent patients with palpable breast masses. Radiographics 20:1613–1621, © RSNA, 2000
35. Kronemer KA, Rhee K, Siegel MJ et al (2001) Gray scale sonography of breast masses in adolescent girls. J Ultrasound Med 20(5):491–496, quiz 498. [Medline]
36. Tot T (2007) The theory of the sick breast lobe and the possible consequences. Int J Surg Pathol 1:68–71
37. Chateil JF, Arboucalot F, Perel Y et al (1998) Breast metastasis in adolescent girls: US findings. Pediatr Radiol 28:832–835, CrossRef
38. Boothroyd A, Carty H (1994) Breast masses in childhood and adolescence: a presentation of 17 cases and a review of the literature. Pediatr Radiol 24:81–84, CrossRef

Index

A. Colan-Georges, *Atlas of Full Breast Ultrasonography*, DOI 10.1007/978-3-319-31418-1

MIX
Papier aus verantwortungsvollen Quellen
Paper from responsible sources
FSC® C105338

If you have any concerns about our products,
you can contact us on
ProductSafety@springernature.com

In case Publisher is established outside the EU,
the EU authorized representative is:
Springer Nature Customer Service Center GmbH
Europaplatz 3, 69115 Heidelberg, Germany

Printed by Libri Plureos GmbH
in Hamburg, Germany